Certified Clinical Medical Assistant (CCMA) Study Guide

EDITION 3.0

AUTHORS

Allison Threet, CHES

Lynnae Lockett, RN, RMA, CMRS, MSN

Jaime Nguyen, MD, MPH, MS

Danielle Scheetz, DC, CCMA

Christopher Touzeau, MS, FNP-C, NRP

Sharon Anton, PhD ABD, MSE, BSE, CPC

REVIEWERS

Beth Brand CMA, DOO, CNE

Lisa R. Davila, RN, MS

Mary Holliday, AAS CMA

Lynnae Lockett, RN, RMA, CMRS, MSN

Allison Threet, CHES

Sharon Anton, PhD ABD, MSE, BSE, CPC

Lauren Zappa, CMA

Jennifer Williams, MS, CMA (AAMA)

INTELLECTUAL PROPERTY NOTICE

National Healthcareer Association is a division of Assessment Technologies Institute, L.L.C. Copyright ©2023 Assessment Technologies Institute, L.L.C. All rights reserved. The reproduction of this work in any electronic, mechanical, or other means, now known or hereafter invented, is forbidden without the written permission of Assessment Technologies Institute, L.L.C. All of the content in this publication, including, for example, the cover, all of the page headers, images, illustrations, graphics, and text, are subject to trademark, service mark, trade dress, copyright, and/or other intellectual property rights or licenses held by Assessment Technologies Institute, L.L.C., one of its affiliates, or by third parties who have licensed their materials to Assessment Technologies Institute, L.L.C.

Current Procedural Terminology (CPT®) is a registered trademark of the American Medical Association.
CPT copyright © 2023 American Medical Association. All rights reserved.

PRODUCTION TEAM

Director of content: Kristen Lawler

Director of development: Derek Prater

Product strategy: Kathy Hunter

Project management: Meredith Derks

Content strategy: Kristiana Routh, Virginia Ferrari

Coordination of content review: Angie Kronlage, Jennifer Williams

Managers of editorial: Kelly Von Lunen, Tricia Lunt

Copy editing: Kya Rodgers, Rebecca Her, Bethany Robertson, Lindsey Casto

Illustrations: Randi Hardy, Six Red Marbles

Layout: Bethany Robertson

Media: Brant Stacy, Ron Hanson, Britney Frerking, Trevor Lund, Sarah Sutton

IMPORTANT NOTICE TO THE READER

The CCMA study guide provides the best insight on the type of content that will be included on the certification exam and can be an invaluable resource in your exam preparation. It is, however, a study guide. It should not be the only resource used in your studies, and it will not necessarily cover the specific construct of every question on the certification examination. Rather, it will provide the map to your success by presenting essential overviews of each topic included in the test plan.

Assessment Technologies Institute, L.L.C., is the publisher of this publication. The content of this publication is for informational and educational purposes only and may be modified or updated by the publisher at any time. This publication is not providing medical advice and is not intended to be a substitute for professional medical advice, diagnosis, or treatment. The publisher has designed this publication to provide accurate information regarding the subject matter covered; however, the publisher is not responsible for errors, omissions, or for any outcomes related to the use of the contents of this book and makes no guarantee and assumes no responsibility or liability for the use of the products and procedures described or the correctness, sufficiency, or completeness of stated information, opinions, or recommendations. The publisher does not recommend or endorse any specific tests, providers, products, procedures, processes, opinions, or other information that may be mentioned in this publication. Treatments and side effects described in this book may not be applicable to all people; likewise, some people may require a dose or experience a side effect that is not described herein. Drugs and medical devices are discussed that may have limited availability controlled by the Food and Drug Administration (FDA) for use only in a research study or clinical trial. Research, clinical practice, and government regulations often change the accepted standard in this field. When consideration is being given to use of any drug in the clinical setting, the health care provider or reader is responsible for determining FDA status of the drug, reading the package insert, and reviewing prescribing information for the most up-to-date recommendations on dose, precautions, and contraindications and determining the appropriate usage for the product. Any references in this book to procedures to be employed when rendering emergency care to the sick and injured are provided solely as a general guide. Other or additional safety measures may be required under particular circumstances. This book is not intended as a statement of the standards of care required in any particular situation, because circumstances and a patient's physical condition can vary widely from one emergency to another. Nor is it intended that this book shall in any way advise personnel concerning legal authority to perform the activities or procedures discussed. Such specific determination should be made only with the aid of legal counsel. Some images in this book feature models. These models do not necessarily endorse, represent, or participate in the activities represented in the images. THE PUBLISHER MAKES NO REPRESENTATIONS OR WARRANTIES OF ANY KIND, WHETHER EXPRESS OR IMPLIED, WITH RESPECT TO THE CONTENT HEREIN. THIS PUBLICATION IS PROVIDED AS-IS, AND THE PUBLISHER AND ITS AFFILIATES SHALL NOT BE LIABLE FOR ANY ACTUAL, INCIDENTAL, SPECIAL, CONSEQUENTIAL, PUNITIVE, OR EXEMPLARY DAMAGES RESULTING, IN WHOLE OR IN PART, FROM THE READER'S USE OF, OR RELIANCE UPON, SUCH CONTENT.

INTRODUCTION

More than $3 trillion is spent on health care in the U.S. each year. Health care is a big business. Qualified medical assistants, like you, will continue to be in demand. Medical assistants qualify for employment in a variety of settings, including hospitals, clinics, and private provider offices. Accepting the challenge to become a part of this growing field requires dedication and a willingness to continually update your skills. Having a medical assistant certification will help you support a successful career in this field. This study guide will help you prepare for the National Healthcareer Association (NHA) Medical Assistant (CCMA) Certification examination. To sit for the CCMA examination, you must have a high school diploma or a GED and complete a medical assisting training program (within the last five years). However, you may substitute 1 year of medical assistant experience in lieu of attending a formal training program. With this option, you must provide documentation that you worked as a medical assistant for at least 1 year. If you meet these criteria, you may register for the examination online at https://certportal.nhanow.com.

If your school is a registered NHA test site, you may be able to take a proctored exam via computer or in paper-pencil format. You also have the option to take the exam via computer at a PSI testing center. For more information about exam eligibility, see www.nhanow.com.

The key instructional content, or body of each chapter, follows the CCMA test plan. Following the key instructional content, there is a chapter summary that recaps the main points within the chapter. At the end of this handbook, a glossary defines the key words highlighted throughout, and drill questions assess your knowledge of the chapter subjects.

NHA MEDICAL ASSISTANT (CCMA) CERTIFICATION DETAILED TEST PLAN

This test plan is based on the 2021 Job Task Analysis Study. The tasks under each content domain are examples that are representative of the content. Items reflective of these stated tasks may or may not appear on the examination. Additionally, items that are reflective of tasks other than those included in the outline below may appear on the examination, as long as they represent information that is considered part of the major content domain by experts in the medical assistant profession. Refer to the full test plan at www.nhanow.com.

DOMAIN	% OF EXAM (# OF ITEMS)
1. Foundational Knowledge and Basic Science	10% (15 items)
2. Anatomy and Physiology	5% (8 items)
3. Clinical Patient Care	56% (84 items)
a. Patient Intake and Vitals (14 items)	
b. General Patient Care (28 items)	
c. Infection Control and Safety (15 items)	
d. Point-of-Care Testing and Laboratory Procedures (9 items)	
e. Phlebotomy (12 items)	
f. EKG and Cardiovascular Testing (6 items)	
4. Patient Care Coordination and Education	8% (12 items)
5. Administrative Assisting	8% (12 items)
6. Communication and Customer Service	8% (12 items)
7. Medical Law and Ethics	5% (7 items)
Total	150 items

Domain 1: Foundational Knowledge and Basic Science

HEALTH CARE SYSTEMS AND SETTINGS
- Roles, responsibilities, scope of practice, and titles of medical assistants
- Roles, responsibilities, scope of practice, titles, and credentials of medical providers and allied health personnel
- Licensing versus certification; maintenance of certification
- Types of health care organizations and delivery models (for example, outpatient/inpatient, patient centered medical home, collaborative care, accountable care organization, hospice, home health care, mobile health unit)
- Technology-based methods for providing health care and health information (for example, telehealth/virtual, patient portals)
- Health care payment models (for example, fee for service, value-based plans)
- General versus specialty health care and services
- Ancillary services and complementary therapies

MEDICAL TERMINOLOGY
- Common abbreviations, acronyms, and symbols
- The Joint Commission's (TJC) "Do Not Use" List
- Medical word building (roots, prefixes, suffixes, plurals)
- Lay terms and medical terms for common conditions, symptoms, and procedures
- Positional and directional terminology

BASIC PHARMACOLOGY
- Drug classifications (for example, diuretics, hypoglycemics, analgesics, over-the-counter), indications, commonly prescribed medications
- Drug classifications and schedules of controlled substances
- Differences between side effects and adverse effects; and between indications and contraindications
- Measurements (for both metric and standard systems) and dosage calculations, mathematical conversions/formulas
- Forms of medication (for example, tablets, patches, capsules)
- Look-alike/sound-alike medications
- Routes of medication administration
- Pharmacokinetics (absorption, distribution, metabolism, excretion)
- Rights of medication administration
- Principles of storage and disposal
- Sources of drug/medication information and FDA regulations

NUTRITION
- Dietary nutrients, suggested guidelines, and food labels
- Dietary needs related to diseases and conditions (for example, diabetes, kidney disease, celiac disease)
- Vitamins and supplements
- Eating disorders

PSYCHOLOGY
- Developmental stages
- Signs and symptoms of common mental health conditions (for example, anxiety, depression, PTSD, ADHD)
- Environmental and socioeconomic stressors
- Psychology of the physically disabled, developmentally delayed, and those who have diseases
- Defense mechanisms
- End of life and stages of grief

Domain 2: Anatomy and Physiology

BODY STRUCTURES AND ORGAN SYSTEMS
- Cell structure (for example, nucleus, cell membrane, cytoplasm, ribosomes, mitochondria, lysosomes)
- Anatomical structures, locations, and positions
- Structure and function of major body systems, including organs and their locations
- Interactions between organ systems, homeostasis

PATHOPHYSIOLOGY AND DISEASE PROCESSES
- Signs, symptoms, and etiology of common diseases, conditions, and injuries
- Diagnostic measures (for example, labs, imaging, biopsies) and treatment modalities (for example, infusion, chemotherapy, medication, surgery)
- Incidence, prevalence, risk factors, and comorbidities
- Epidemics and pandemics

Domain 3: Clinical Patient Care

PATIENT INTAKE AND VITALS

Tasks
- Ensure patient safety within the clinical setting.
- Identify patient.
- Complete a comprehensive clinical intake process, including the purpose of the visit.
- Measure and obtain vital signs.
- Convert measurements of vital signs.
- Obtain anthropometric measurements.
- Identify, document, and report abnormal signs and symptoms.

Knowledge of
- Patient identifiers (for example, name, date of birth [DOB], medical record number, last 4 digits of Social Security Number [SSN])
- Elements of a patient medical/surgical/family/social history
- Screenings and wellness assessments (for example, tobacco cessation, alcohol use, HIV screening)
- Mental health screenings (for example, mini mental state exam; anxiety and depression screening tools
- Blood pressure—methods for obtaining (manual, palpating, electronic), in-range and out-of-range values, common errors, and trouble-shooting methods
- Orthostatics—methods for obtaining, common errors
- Pulse—methods for obtaining in various locations, abnormal rhythms, in-range and out-of-range values
- Respiratory rate—methods for obtaining, in-range and out-of-range values, types of abnormal patterns (for example, apnea, hyperventilation, dyspnea)
- Pulse oximetry—in-range and out-of-range values, locations, and common errors
- Temperature—methods for obtaining in various locations, coordinating ranges, common errors
- Pain scale
- Menstrual status and last menstrual period
- Factors impacting vital signs (for example, age, medications)
- Conversion formulas for vital signs (for example, height, weight, temperature)
- Methods for measuring height, weight, BMI, and body and waist circumference; special considerations related to age, health, status, disability
- Pediatric measurements and growth chart

NHA MEDICAL ASSISTANT (CCMA) CERTIFICATION DETAILED TEST PLAN
Domain 3: Clinical Patient Care

GENERAL PATIENT CARE

Tasks

- Prepare examination/procedure room.
- Prepare and maintain a sterile field.
- Prepare patient for procedures, including providing education.
- Assist provider with general and specialty physical examination.
- Prepare and administer medications and/or injectables using nonparenteral routes.
- Prepare and administer medications and/or injectables using parenteral routes (excluding intravenous).
- Manage injection logs (for example, controlled substances, tuberculosis medications, immunizations).
- Perform staple and suture removal.
- Perform ear and eye irrigation.
- Administer first aid and basic wound care.
- Identify and respond to emergency/priority situations.
- Assist provider with patients presenting with minor and traumatic injury.
- Assist with surgical interventions (for example, sebaceous cyst removal, toenail removal, colposcopy, cryosurgery).
- Review provider's discharge instructions/plan of care with patients.
- Follow guidelines for sending orders for prescriptions and refills electronically, by telephone, fax, or email.
- Order and obtain durable medical equipment (DME) and supplies (for example, CPAP, wheelchair, hospital bed).
- Document relevant aspects of patient care in patient record.
- Operate basic functions of an electronic medical record/electronic health record (EMR/EHR) system.
- Implement updates in EMR/EHR (for example, quality measures, alerts, telemedicine, population health reporting).
- Enter orders using computerized physician order entry.
- Conduct telehealth or virtual screenings in the context of a telehealth/virtual visit.

Knowledge of

- Guidelines for establishing a sterile field
- Sterile techniques related to examinations, procedures, injections, and medication administration
- Positioning and draping requirements for general and specialty examinations, procedures, and treatments
- Equipment, supplies, and instruments required for general physical examinations
- Equipment, supplies, and instruments required for specialty examinations or procedures
- Patient instruction specific to procedures, including pre-and postprocedural instructions
- Modifications to patient care depending on patient needs (for example, assisting with ambulation and transfers for frail and disabled patients; using terms a child can understand for pediatric patients)
- Immunization schedules, requirements, and registries; adverse effects documentation and reporting
- Allergies (for example, medication, food, environmental); contraindications; type of reactions (mild, moderate, and severe); how to respond to allergic reactions or anaphylactic shock
- Dosage calculations related to injectables and oral medications
- Commonly used oral and parenteral medications, including forms, packaging, routes of administration, and rights of medication administration
- Methods of administration, techniques, procedures, and supplies related to eye and ear medications
- Storage, labeling, expiration dates, and medication logs
- Techniques (for example, needle angle, gauge, length) and injection site (for example, intramuscular, subcutaneous)
- Supplies and equipment related to injections
- Storage of injectables
- Techniques and instruments for suture and staple removal; types and sizes of sutures
- Instruments, supplies, and techniques related to eye and ear irrigation

- Commonly occurring types of injuries (for example, lacerations, abrasions, fractures, sprains, burns)
- Treatment for commonly occurring types of injuries (for example, bandaging, ice, elevation)
- Signs and symptoms of wound infection (for example, redness, pus, swelling, discharge) and wound stages
- Commonly occurring types of surgical interventions
- Signs and symptoms related to urgent and emergency situations (for example, diabetic shock, heat stroke, allergic reactions, choking, syncope, seizure)
- Emergency action plans (for example, crash cart, emergency injectables)
- Procedures to perform CPR, basic life support, and automated external defibrillator (AED)
- Legal requirements for content and transmission of prescriptions
- Electronic prescribing software, screening requirements for prescription refills
- Specialty pharmacies (for example, compounding and nuclear pharmacies; forms of medication available such as liquid, elixir, balm, ointment)
- Required components of medical records
- Prior authorizations for medication durable medical equipment (DME)
- Computerized Physician Order Entry (CPOE)
- Patient conditions appropriate for telehealth/virtual visit
- Modifications in care related to delivery of telehealth/virtual health care

INFECTION CONTROL AND SAFETY

Tasks
- Adhere to standard and universal precautions and guidelines related to infection control.
- Adhere to regulations and guidelines related to infectious diseases.
- Follow guidelines related to use of personal protective equipment (PPE), including donning and doffing.
- Adhere to guidelines regarding hand hygiene.
- Perform disinfection/sanitization.
- Perform sterilization of medical equipment.
- Perform appropriate aseptic techniques for various clinical situations.
- Dispose of biohazardous materials as dictated by Occupational Safety and Health Administration (OSHA) (for example, sharps containers, biohazard bags).
- Follow post-exposure guidelines (for example, needle safety guidelines, use of eyewash stations).

Knowledge of
- Common pathogens and nonpathogens
- Organisms and micro-organisms
- Infectious agents, chain of infection, modes of transmission, and conditions for growth
- Signs and symptoms of infectious diseases
- CDC guidelines for infectious disease (for example, prevention, reporting)
- Guidelines for exposure to bloodborne pathogens (for example, OSHA, American Hospital Association [AHA])
- Approaches for the control of infectious diseases, epidemics, and pandemics
- Universal precautions
- Standard precautions (for example, personal protective equipment)
- Handwashing techniques
- Alcohol-based rubs/sanitizer
- Sterilization techniques (autoclave, instrument cleaner, germicidal disinfectants, disposables) and principles for maintaining sterilization equipment
- Techniques for medical and surgical asepsis
- Order of cleaning and types of cleaning products
- Safety Data Sheets (SDS)
- Cautions related to chemicals
- Disposal methods
- Exposure control plan
- Logs (for example, maintenance, equipment servicing, temperature, quality control)

NHA MEDICAL ASSISTANT (CCMA) CERTIFICATION DETAILED TEST PLAN
Domain 3: Clinical Patient Care

POINT-OF-CARE TESTING AND LABORATORY PROCEDURES

Tasks
- Collect nonblood specimens (for example, urine, stool, cultures, sputum).
- Perform CLIA-waived testing.
- Recognize, document, and report in-range and out-of-range laboratory and test values.
- Match and label specimen to patient and completed requisition.
- Process, handle, and transport collected specimens.
- Perform vision and hearing tests.
- Perform allergy testing.
- Perform spirometry/pulmonary function tests (electronic or manual).
- Identify common testing errors leading to testing discrepancies or inaccurate results.

Knowledge of
- Point-of-care testing
- Information required on completed requisition and/or form per provider order (for example, type of test, date, time, diagnostic code)
- Specimen collection techniques and requirements
- CLIA-waived testing regulations
- Quality controls (internal and external)
- In-range and out-of-range laboratory and test values
- Preanalytical and postanalytical errors that affect testing results
- Elements related to vision and hearing tests
- Peak flow rates
- Scratch test and intradermal allergy test
- Requirements for transportation, diagnosis, storage, and disposal of specimens (for example, patient identifiers, site, test, chain of custody)

PHLEBOTOMY

Tasks
- Prepare patient for procedure.
- Verify order details.
- Select appropriate supplies for test(s) ordered (for example needle sizes, tubes).
- Determine venipuncture site accessibility based on patient age and condition.
- Prepare site for venipuncture.
- Determine order of draw.
- Perform venipuncture.
- Perform capillary puncture.
- Perform postprocedural care.
- Handle blood samples as required for diagnostic purposes.
- Process blood specimens for laboratory.
- Match and label specimen to patient and completed requisition.
- Recognize and respond appropriately to out-of-range test results.
- Prepare samples for transportation to a reference (outside) laboratory.
- Follow guidelines in distributing laboratory results to providers after matching patient to provider.

Knowledge of
- Blood components (for example, whole blood, plasma, serum platelets)
- Bloodborne pathogens
- Patient identifiers, content of requisition (for example, site or test, diagnostic code, dietary restrictions)
- Patient preparation (for example, fasting/nonfasting, medication use, basal state, positioning)
- Assessment of patient comfort/anxiety level with procedure
- Considerations related to special patient needs (for example, need for support person or witness, use of restraints, chain of custody)
- Medical conditions or history and medications affecting collection of blood
- Blood vacuum tubes required for chemistry, hematology, and microbiology testing
- Phlebotomy site preparation, including cleansing, wrapping, order of draw with microtubes

- Anatomy, skin integrity, venous sufficiency, contraindications
- Order of draw for venipuncture
- Insertion and removal techniques
- Evacuated tube, syringe, and butterfly methods
- Types of tubes, tube positions, number of tube inversions, and fill level/ratios
- Additives and preservatives
- Bandaging procedures, including allergies and skin types
- Preanalytical and postanalytical considerations pertaining to specimen quality and consistency
- Special collections (for example, timed specimens, medication levels, blood cultures, fasting)
- Centrifuge and aliquot
- Expected and unexpected test values; control values
- Equipment calibration
- Storage conditions related to sensitivity to light and temperature
- Requirements for transportation, diagnosis, storage, disposal
- Processing and labeling requirements
- External databases (for example, outside laboratories, reference sources)

EKG AND CARDIOVASCULAR TESTING

Tasks
- Prepare patient for EKG or ambulatory cardiac monitoring procedure.
- Identify types of leads and proper anatomical electrode placement.
- Perform EKG tests.
- Recognize abnormal or emergent EKG results (for example, dysrhythmia, arrhythmia, versus artifact).
- Assist provider with ambulatory cardiac monitoring (for example, stress test, Holter monitoring, event monitoring).
- Transmit results or report to patient's electronic medical record or paper chart and provider.
- Ensure proper functioning and storage of EKG equipment.

Knowledge of
- Techniques and methods for EKGs
- Procedures and instructions to minimize artifacts
- Artifacts, signal distortions, and electrical interference (for example, fuzz, wandering baseline)
- Preparation, positioning, and draping of patient
- Considerations related to patient characteristics (for example, anatomy, adult/pediatric, medical condition)
- Supplies needed (for example, paper, correct leads, razor, tape)
- Placement of limb and chest electrodes
- Signs of adverse reaction during testing (for example, signs of distress, elevated blood pressure, respiration)
- Abnormal rhythms or dysrhythmias associated with EKGs
- Waveforms, intervals, segment
- Calibration of equipment

Domain 4: Patient Care Coordination and Education

Tasks
- Review patient records prior to visit to ensure health care is comprehensively addressed.
- Ensure that documentation of preventive maintenance and screenings is included in patient record.
- Identify timelines and track recommendations for screenings and preventive maintenance (for example, mammogram, Papanicolaou (Pap) test, colonoscopy, immunizations).
- Assist provider with researching and supplying information on community resources for clinical and nonclinical services.
- Coordinate with health care providers and community-based organizations for continuity of care.
- Facilitate patient adherence (for example, continuity of care, follow up, medication adherence) to optimize health outcomes.

- Participate in team-based patient care (for example, patient-centered medical home [PCMH], accountable care organization [ACO]).
- Participate in transition of care for patients.
- Provide patient education via telehealth/virtual visit systems and processes.
- Provide education to patients on communicable disease prevention.

Knowledge of
- Preventive medicine, preventive screenings, and wellness
- Clinical quality measures
- Education delivery methods, instructional techniques, and learning styles for in-person and virtual visits
- Patient education related to nutrition and healthy eating, including restrictions, recommendations, and relation to medications
- Available resources for clinical services (for example, home health care)
- Resources and procedures to coordinate care and outpatient services
- Available community resources for non clinical services (for example, adult day care, transportation vouchers)
- Specialty resources for patient/family medical and cognitive needs
- Barriers to care (for example, socioeconomic, cultural differences, language, education)
- Roles and responsibilities of team members involved in patient-centered medical home (PCMH) and team-based care (TBC)
- Referral forms and processes
- Methods for the prevention of transmission communicable diseases

Domain 5: Administrative Assisting

Tasks
- Schedule and monitor patient appointments using electronic and paper-based systems.
- Determine the type of appointment needed.
- Prioritize appointment needs based on urgency.
- Monitor patient flow sheets, superbill, or encounter forms.
- Verify insurance coverage/financial eligibility.
- Identify and check patients in/out.
- Confirm appropriate diagnostic and procedural codes.
- Obtain and verify prior authorizations and precertifications (for example, for prescriptions, procedures, radiology).
- Prepare documentation and billing requests using current coding guidelines.
- Ensure that documentation complies with government and insurance requirements.
- Perform charge reconciliation (for example, enter charges, post payments, make adjustments, process accounts receivable).
- Bill patients, insurers, and third-party payers for services performed.
- Resolve billing issues with insurers and third-party payers, including appeals and denials.
- Manage electronic and paper-based medical records.
- Process office mail and faxes to appropriate staff member.
- Facilitate/generate referrals to other health care providers and allied health care professionals.
- Follow up patient calls and appointment confirmations.
- Enter information into databases or spreadsheets (for example, electronic medical record [EMR], electronic health record [EHR], Excel, billing modules, scheduling systems).
- Participate in safety evaluations and report safety concerns.
- Maintain inventory of clinical and administrative supplies.
- Activate and facilitate use of patient portals.
- Provide technical instruction on the use of telehealth/virtual visits and troubleshoot issues.

Knowledge of
- Types of office visits (for example, new patient, telehealth/virtual, annual wellness, specialty, sports/school physical), and requirements for each
- Screening methods to identify type of appointment needed
- Practice management systems and software (for example, EMR/EHR, scheduling software, paper-based filing systems, office storage for archived files)
- Requirements related to duration of visits (for example, purpose of visit, physician preferences)
- Sections of the medical record (for example, administrative, clinical, billing, procedural, notes, consents)
- Required documentation for patient review and signature
- Chart review
- Electronic referrals (for example, creation, requirements, administration)
- Financial eligibility, sliding scales, and indigent programs
- Government regulations (for example, promoting interoperability/meaningful use, Medicare Access and CHIP Reauthorization Act of 2015 [MACRA])
- CMS billing and documentation requirements
- Insurance fundamentals, including revenue cycle and incentive models
- Insurance terminology (for example, copayment, coinsurance, deductible, tier levels, explanation of benefits, medical necessity)
- Referral and insurance authorizations, pre-certification requirements (for example, surgical, diagnostics, labs)
- Diagnostic and procedural codes
- Third-party payer billing requirements
- Advanced beneficiary notice (ABN)
- Aging reports, collections due, adjustments, and write-offs
- Online banking for deposits and electronic transfers
- Auditing methods, processes, and sign-offs
- Data entry and data fields
- Equipment inspection logs, required schedules, and compliance requirements, including inspection by medical equipment servicers
- Telehealth/virtual visit technologies, barriers to access

Domain 6: Communication and Customer Service

Tasks
- Recognize the diversity of patient cultures and backgrounds when providing care.
- Recognize stereotypes and biases and interact appropriately with patients, colleagues, and others.
- Modify verbal and nonverbal communication for diverse audiences (for example, providers, coworkers, supervisors, patients and caregivers, external providers).
- Modify verbal and nonverbal communications with patients and caregivers based on special considerations (for example, pediatric, geriatric, hearing, vision, or cognitive impairment).
- Modify communications based on type of visit (for example, in-person, telehealth/virtual visits).
- Clarify and relay communications between patients and providers.
- Communicate on the telephone with patients and caregivers, providers, third-party payers using HIPAA guidelines.
- Prepare written/electronic communications/business correspondence.
- Handle challenging/difficult customer service occurrences.
- Utilize conflict management and complaint resolution to improve patient satisfaction.
- Engage in crucial conversations with patients and caregivers/health care surrogates, staff, and providers.
- Facilitate teamwork and team engagement.
- Demonstrate professionalism (for example, appropriate demeanor, clothing, language, tone).

Knowledge of
- Cultural, religious, psychosocial, and economic considerations impacting provision of care
- Gender identity and expression, pronoun use
- Patient characteristics affecting communication (for example, language barriers, age, developmental stage, cognitive, sensory, and physical impairments)
- Communication styles appropriate to oral, telephone, email, text communications
- Nonverbal cues for in-person and telehealth/virtual communication
- Communication cycle (clear, concise message relay)
- Therapeutic communication
- Interviewing and questioning techniques, including screening questions, open-ended, closed-ended, and probing questions
- Scope of permitted questions and boundaries for questions
- Active listening techniques
- Coaching and feedback, positive reinforcement of effective behavior
- Telephone etiquette
- Email etiquette
- Business letter formats
- Patient satisfaction surveys
- Techniques to deal with patients (for example, irate patients, custody issues between parents, chain of command)
- Conflict management and dispute resolution methods
- When to escalate problem situations
- Incident/event/unusual occurrence reports; documentation of event
- Cause and effect analysis (for example, risk management related to patient and employee safety)
- Professional presence (for example, appearance, demeanor, tone)

Domain 7: Medical Law and Ethics

Tasks
- Comply with legal and regulatory requirements.
- Obtain patient consent as needed. Adhere to professional codes of ethics.
- Obtain, review, and comply with medical directives (for example, advance directives, living will, health care proxy, medical order for life sustaining treatment).
- Protect patient privacy and confidentiality, including medical records.
- Adhere to legal requirements regarding reportable violations or incidents.
- Identify personal or religious beliefs and values and provide unbiased care.

Knowledge of
- Laws and regulations (for example, HIPAA, ACA, HERCA, Health Information Technology for Economic and Clinical Health [HITECH], 21st Century CARES Act, Controlled Substances Act)
- Patient's Bill of Rights
- Informed (verbal or written) and implied consent, including consideration for minors and those unable to give consent
- Advanced directives (for example, living will, do-not-resuscitate/do-not-intubate [DNR/DNI], Medical Orders for Life-Sustaining Treatment [MOLST] form)
- Power of attorney and legal guardianship
- Legal requirements related to maintenance, storage, and disposal of records
- Conditions for sharing information/release of information
- Criminal and civil acts; medical malpractice
- Mandatory reporting laws, sign and symptoms of abuse, triggers for reporting, and reporting agencies

Table of Contents

CHAPTER 1
Foundational Knowledge and Basic Science — 1

- OVERVIEW — 1
- HEALTH CARE SYSTEMS AND SETTINGS — 2
  - *Medical Assistant Roles, Responsibilities, Scope of Practice, and Titles* — 2
  - *Variables for the Scope of Practice* — 3
- PROVIDER AND ALLIED HEALTH ROLES, RESPONSIBILITIES, SCOPE OF PRACTICE, TITLES, AND CREDENTIALS — 4
  - *Physician Information* — 4
  - *Nurses* — 5
  - *Allied Health Professionals* — 5
- LICENSING VERSUS CERTIFICATION AND MAINTENANCE OF CERTIFICATION — 6
  - *Licensure vs. Certification* — 6
- TYPES OF HEALTH CARE ORGANIZATIONS AND DELIVERY MODELS — 7
  - *Inpatient and Outpatient* — 7
  - *Patient-Centered Medical Home* — 8
- TECHNOLOGY-BASED METHODS FOR PROVIDING HEALTH CARE AND INFORMATION — 9
  - *Telehealth and Virtual Visits* — 9
  - *Patient Portals* — 9
- HEALTH CARE PAYMENT MODELS — 10
  - *Fee for Service* — 10
  - *Value-Based Plans* — 10
- GENERAL VS. SPECIALTY HEALTH CARE AND SERVICES — 12
  - *General Health Care Services* — 12
  - *Specialty Health Care Services* — 12
- ANCILLARY SERVICES AND COMPLEMENTARY THERAPIES — 14
  - *Ancillary Services* — 14
  - *Complementary Therapies* — 14
- BASIC PHARMACOLOGY — 15
  - *Drug Classifications, Indications, and Commonly Prescribed Medications* — 15

TABLE OF CONTENTS

DRUG CLASSIFICATIONS AND SCHEDULES OF CONTROLLED SUBSTANCES — 17

SIDE EFFECTS, ADVERSE EFFECTS, INDICATIONS, AND CONTRAINDICATIONS — 18
- *Side Effects and Adverse Effects* — 19
- *Indications and Contraindications* — 19

METRIC AND STANDARD MEASUREMENTS, DOSAGE CALCULATIONS, AND MATHEMATICAL CONVERSIONS AND FORMULAS — 21
- *Metric System* — 21
- *Standard System* — 22
- *Dosage Calculations* — 22
- *Pediatric Dosage Calculations* — 23
- *Conversions and Formulas* — 24

FORMS OF MEDICATION — 26

LOOK-ALIKE AND SOUND-ALIKE MEDICATIONS — 27

ROUTES OF MEDICATION ADMINISTRATION — 28

PHARMACOKINETICS (ABSORPTION, DISTRIBUTION, METABOLISM, EXCRETION) — 29
- *Absorption* — 29
- *Distribution* — 29
- *Metabolism* — 30
- *Excretion* — 30

RIGHTS OF MEDICATION ADMINISTRATION — 30
- *Right Patient* — 30
- *Right Medication* — 31
- *Right Dose* — 31
- *Right Time* — 31
- *Right Route* — 31
- *Right Technique* — 32
- *Right Documentation* — 32

SOURCES OF MEDICATION INFORMATION AND FDA REGULATIONS — 32

NUTRITION — 33
- *Dietary Nutrients, Suggested Guidelines, and Food Labels* — 33
- *Dietary Nutrients and Suggested Guidelines* — 33
- *Food Labels* — 38

VITAMINS AND SUPPLEMENTS — 39

DIETARY NEEDS RELATED TO DISEASES AND CONDITIONS	42
Dietary Needs for Diabetes	42
Dietary Needs for Kidney Disease	43
Dietary Needs for Celiac Disease	45
EATING DISORDERS	46
Anorexia	46
Bulimia	47
Binge Eating	47
WRAP-UP	48

CHAPTER 2
Medical Terminology, Anatomy, and Physiology — 49

OVERVIEW	49
ANATOMY AND PHYSIOLOGY	50
Body Structure and Organ Systems	50
ANATOMICAL STRUCTURES, LOCATIONS, AND POSITIONS	52
Planes of the Body	52
Body Cavities	52
Body Quadrants and Regions	52
STRUCTURE AND FUNCTION OF MAJOR BODY SYSTEMS	53
Integumentary System	53
Skeletal System	54
Muscular System	57
Immune and Lymphatic Systems	57
Cardiovascular System	59
Urinary System	60
Gastrointestinal System	61
Respiratory System	63
Nervous System	63
Endocrine System	64
Reproductive Systems	65
INTERACTIONS BETWEEN ORGAN SYSTEMS AND HOMEOSTASIS	67
Homeostasis	67

TABLE OF CONTENTS

COMMON DISEASES, CONDITIONS, AND INJURIES	67
PATHOPHYSIOLOGY AND DISEASE PROCESSES	80
Diagnostic Measures and Treatment Modalities	80
EPIDEMICS AND PANDEMICS	81
MEDICAL TERMINOLOGY	81
Common Abbreviations, Acronyms, and Symbols	82
Abbreviations	83
Acronyms and Symbols	86
MEDICAL WORD BUILDING	86
Word Roots	87
Combining Root Words	90
Prefixes	90
Suffixes	91
COMMON TERMS	93
POSITIONAL AND DIRECTIONAL TERMINOLOGY	94
PSYCHOLOGY AND MENTAL HEALTH	95
Developmental stages	95
COMMON MENTAL HEALTH CONDITIONS	98
ENVIRONMENTAL AND SOCIOECONOMIC STRESSORS	99
Environmental Stressors	99
Socioeconomic Stressors	100
COMMUNICATION AND ACCOMMODATIONS	100
Physical Disability	100
Developmental Delay	101
Illness and Disease	102
DEFENSE MECHANISMS	102
END OF LIFE AND STAGES OF GRIEF	105
End-of-Life Struggles	105
Stages of Grief	105
WRAP-UP	107

CHAPTER 3
Patient Intake and Vitals — 109

- OVERVIEW — 109
- PATIENT SAFETY WITHIN THE CLINICAL SETTING — 110
  - *Identify Patient* — 110
- COMPREHENSIVE CLINICAL INTAKE PROCESS — 111
  - *Patient Medical, Surgical, Family, and Social History* — 111
- SCREENINGS AND WELLNESS ASSESSMENTS — 113
  - *Tobacco Cessation, Alcohol Use, HIV Screening* — 113
- MENTAL HEALTH SCREENINGS — 113
  - *Mini-Mental State Exam, Anxiety and Depression Screening Tools* — 113
- MEASURE VITAL SIGNS — 114
  - *Blood Pressure* — 114
  - *Pulse* — 118
  - *Respiratory Rate* — 120
  - *Pulse Oximetry* — 121
  - *Temperature* — 122
- PAIN SCALE — 124
- MENSTRUAL STATUS AND LAST MENSTRUAL PERIOD — 124
- PEDIATRIC MEASUREMENTS AND GROWTH CHARTS — 125
- OBTAIN ANTHROPOMETRIC MEASUREMENTS — 126
  - *Obtain Anthropometric Measurements* — 126
  - *Weight* — 126
  - *Height* — 127
  - *Body Mass Index* — 127
- IDENTIFY, DOCUMENT, AND REPORT ABNORMAL SIGNS AND SYMPTOMS — 128
- FACTORS AFFECTING VITAL SIGNS — 129
- WRAP-UP — 130

CHAPTER 4
General Patient Care: Part 1 — 131

- OVERVIEW — 131
- PREPARE EXAMINATION/PROCEDURE ROOM — 131
  - *General Physical Examinations* — 131
  - *Maintaining a Clean Examination Area* — 133
- SPECIALTY EXAMINATIONS OR PROCEDURES — 134
- PREPARE PATIENT FOR PROCEDURES — 136
  - *Patient Instruction* — 136
  - *Providing Patient Education* — 137
- ACCOMMODATION FOR PATIENT NEEDS — 138
  - *Older Adults* — 138
  - *Physical Disability* — 138
  - *Children* — 139
  - *Environmental Considerations* — 139
- ASSIST THE PROVIDER WITH EXAMINATIONS — 140
  - *Positioning and Draping* — 140
- PREPARE AND ADMINISTER NONPARENTERAL MEDICATIONS AND INJECTABLES — 143
  - *Dosage Calculations* — 143
- COMMONLY USED ORAL AND PARENTERAL MEDICATIONS — 146
  - *Medication Regulations and Best Practices* — 146
- EYE AND EAR MEDICATIONS — 148
  - *Eye Instillation* — 148
  - *Ear Instillation* — 149
- ALLERGIC REACTIONS — 149
  - *Types of Allergic Reactions* — 149
  - *Responding to Allergic Reactions* — 150
  - *Patient's Allergy Status* — 150

TABLE OF CONTENTS

PREPARE AND ADMINISTER MEDICATIONS – PARENTERAL ROUTES	**151**
Sterile Techniques	151
TECHNIQUES AND INJECTION SITE	**153**
Injection Sites	154
INJECTION SUPPLIES AND EQUIPMENT	**159**
Vials	159
Ampule	159
Syringes	160
STORAGE OF INJECTABLES	**161**
MANAGE INJECTION LOGS	**162**
Sample Medication Administration Record	162
STORAGE, LABELING, EXPIRATION DATES, AND MEDICATION LOGS	**163**
PERFORM EAR AND EYE IRRIGATION	**164**
Irrigation Instruments, Supplies, and Techniques	164
SEND ORDERS FOR PRESCRIPTIONS AND REFILLS	**165**
Legal Requirements for Content and Transmission of Prescriptions	165
ELECTRONIC PRESCRIBING SOFTWARE	**166**
SPECIALTY PHARMACIES	**167**
DOCUMENT CARE IN THE PATIENT RECORD	**169**
Required Components of Medical Records	169
OPERATE AN EMR/EHR SYSTEM	**170**
Implement Updates in an EMR/EHR	170
ENTER ORDERS USING COMPUTERIZED PHYSICIAN ORDER ENTRY	**171**
CONDUCT TELEHEALTH OR VIRTUAL SCREENINGS	**172**
Patient Conditions Appropriate for Telehealth/Virtual Visit	172
MODIFICATIONS FOR TELEHEALTH/VIRTUAL HEALTH CARE	**174**
WRAP-UP	**174**

TABLE OF CONTENTS

CHAPTER 5
General Patient Care: Part 2 — 175

- OVERVIEW — 175
- PREPARE AND MAINTAIN A STERILE FIELD — 175
- ASSIST WITH SURGICAL INTERVENTIONS — 178
- TECHNIQUES AND INSTRUMENTS FOR SUTURE AND STAPLE REMOVAL — 180
  - *Types and Sizes of Sutures* — 180
  - *Perform Suture and Staple Removal* — 181
- REVIEW PROVIDER'S DISCHARGE INSTRUCTIONS/PLAN OF CARE WITH PATIENTS — 183
- IDENTIFY AND RESPOND TO EMERGENCY/PRIORITY SITUATIONS — 184
  - *Commonly Occurring Types of Injuries and Treatment* — 186
  - *Administer First Aid and Basic Wound Care* — 188
  - *Wounds* — 189
  - *Wound Care* — 190
  - *Assist Provider with Patients Presenting with Minor and Traumatic Injury* — 193
- EMERGENCY ACTION PLANS — 194
  - *Procedures to Perform CPR, Basic Life Support, and Automated External Defibrillator (AED)* — 195
- ORDER AND OBTAIN DURABLE MEDICAL EQUIPMENT (DME) AND SUPPLIES — 197
  - *Prior Authorizations for Medication Durable Medical Equipment* — 197
- WRAP-UP — 198

CHAPTER 6
Infection Control and Safety — 199

- OVERVIEW — 199
- COMMUNICABLE DISEASES AND TRANSMISSION — 199
  - *Organisms and Micro-Organisms* — 200
  - *Common Pathogens and Nonpathogens* — 200
- INFECTION CONTROL GUIDELINES — 203
  - *Adhere to Standard and Universal Precautions and Guidelines Related to Infection Control* — 203
- FOLLOW GUIDELINES RELATED TO USE OF PPE — 206
  - *Donning Nonsterile Gloves* — 206
  - *Doffing Nonsterile, Contaminated Gloves* — 207

ASEPSIS — 207
- Aseptic Techniques for Various Clinical Situations — 207
- Techniques for Medical and Surgical Asepsis — 208

ADHERE TO GUIDELINES REGARDING HAND HYGIENE — 209
- CDC Hand Hygiene Recommendations — 209
- Handwashing Techniques — 210

PERFORM DISINFECTION/SANITIZATION — 211
- Order of Cleaning and Types of Cleaning Products — 212

PERFORM STERILIZATION OF MEDICAL EQUIPMENT — 214
- Sterilization Techniques and Maintaining Sterilization Equipment — 214

BIOHAZARD MATERIALS — 215
- Dispose of Biohazardous Materials — 215
- Personal Protective Equipment — 217

FOLLOW POST-EXPOSURE GUIDELINES (NEEDLE SAFETY GUIDELINES, USE OF EYEWASH STATIONS) — 218
- Exposure Control Plan — 218

WRAP-UP — 220

CHAPTER 7
Point-of-Care Testing and Laboratory Procedures — 221

OVERVIEW — 221

LABORATORY PROCEDURES — 221
- Laboratory Requisitions and Documenting Specimen Collection — 222
- Information Required on Completed Requisition — 222
- Departments in Clinical Laboratory — 222
- Demographic Information — 223

SPECIMEN COLLECTION — 223
- Point-of-Care Testing — 223
- CLIA-Waived Testing — 226
- Quality Controls — 227
- Collect Nonblood Specimens — 227

SPECIMEN PROCESSING AND TRANSPORTATION — 229
Requirements for Transportation, Diagnosis, Storage, and Disposal of Specimens — 229
Chain of Custody — 230

LABORATORY RESULTS — 231
Recognize, Document, and Report Laboratory and Test Values — 231
Common Testing Errors — 233
Preanalytical and Postanalytical Errors — 233

SPECIALTY TESTING — 234
Vision and Hearing Tests — 234
Allergy Testing — 236
Scratch Test and Intradermal Allergy Test — 236
Spirometry/Pulmonary Function Tests — 237
Peak Flow Rates — 238

WRAP-UP — 239

CHAPTER 8
Phlebotomy — 241

OVERVIEW — 241

PATIENT PREPARATION — 242

VERIFY ORDER DETAILS — 243
Patient Identifiers, Content of Requisition — 243

SELECT APPROPRIATE SUPPLIES FOR TEST(S) ORDERED — 244

BLOOD COMPONENTS — 246
Serum — 246
Plasma — 246
Clotted Blood — 246
Whole Blood — 246

DETERMINE ORDER OF DRAW — 247
Types of Tubes, Number of Tube Inversions, and Fill Level/Ratios — 247

TABLE OF CONTENTS

DETERMINE VENIPUNCTURE SITE ACCESSIBILITY — 248
- *Tourniquet Application* — 249
- *Site Restrictions* — 249
- *Skin Integrity and Venous Sufficiency* — 250

PREPARE SITE FOR VENIPUNCTURE — 250

PERFORM VENIPUNCTURE — 251

PERFORM CAPILLARY PUNCTURE — 251
- *Location of Capillary Punctures for Adults and Infants* — 252
- *Preparing the Site* — 252
- *Performing the Puncture* — 252
- *Order of Draw for Microcapillary Tubes* — 253

PERFORM POSTPROCEDURE CARE — 253
- *Bandaging Procedures* — 253

SPECIMEN INSTRUCTIONS — 254
- *Match and Label Specimen to Patient and Completed Requisition* — 254
- *Processing and Labeling Requirements* — 254

HANDLE BLOOD SAMPLES AS REQUIRED FOR DIAGNOSTIC PURPOSES — 255
- *Preanalytical and Postanalytical Considerations Pertaining to Specimen Quality and Consistency* — 255

PROCESS BLOOD SPECIMENS FOR LABORATORY — 256
- *Centrifuge and Aliquot* — 256

PREPARE SAMPLES FOR TRANSPORTATION TO A REFERENCE (OUTSIDE) LABORATORY — 257
- *Storage Conditions Related to Sensitivity to Light and Temperature* — 257
- *Requirements for Transportation* — 258

FOLLOW GUIDELINES IN DISTRIBUTING LABORATORY RESULTS — 258

RECOGNIZE AND RESPOND APPROPRIATELY TO OUT-OF-RANGE TEST RESULTS — 259

WRAP-UP — 259

CHAPTER 9
EKG and Cardiovascular Testing — 261

- OVERVIEW — 261
- ELECTROCARDIOGRAPH — 262
  - *Cardiology* — 262
  - *Waveforms, Intervals, and Segments* — 262
  - *Abnormal Rhythms* — 263
  - *Abnormal or Emergent EKG Results* — 264
  - *Artifacts, Signal Distortions, and Electrical Interference* — 265
- PATIENT PREPARATION — 266
  - *Prepare Patient for EKG or Ambulatory Cardiac Monitoring Procedure* — 266
  - *Preparation, Positioning, and Draping of Patient* — 266
  - *Supplies Needed* — 267
- PERFORM ELECTROCARDIOGRAPH — 269
  - *Lead Placement* — 269
  - *Types of Leads and Anatomical Electrode Placement* — 269
- PERFORM EKG TEST — 271
  - *Techniques and Methods for EKGs* — 272
  - *Signs of an Adverse Reaction During Testing* — 272
- TRANSMIT RESULTS OR REPORT — 273
  - *Transmit Results or Report to Patient's Electronic Medical Record or Paper Chart and Provider* — 273
- FUNCTIONING AND STORAGE OF EKG EQUIPMENT — 274
  - *Calibration of Equipment* — 274
- AMBULATORY CARDIAC MONITORING — 274
  - *Stress Testing* — 274
  - *Holter Monitoring/Event Monitoring* — 275
- WRAP-UP — 275

CHAPTER 10
Patient Care Coordination and Education — 277

- OVERVIEW — 277
- PATIENT CARE — 277
  - *Team-Based Patient Care* — 277
  - *Roles and Responsibilities* — 277
  - *Specific Roles of Team Members* — 279
  - *Support Staff* — 281
  - *Patients and Family Members* — 281
- PARTICIPATE IN THE TRANSITION OF CARE FOR PATIENTS — 282
  - *Resources and Procedures to Coordinate Care and Outpatient Services* — 282
- PREVENTIVE CARE — 282
  - *Preventive Medicine, Preventive Screenings, and Wellness Care* — 282
  - *Timelines and Recommendations for Screenings and Preventive Maintenance* — 283
- REVIEW PATIENT RECORDS PRIOR TO VISIT — 285
  - *Clinical Quality Measures* — 285
  - *Document Preventive Maintenance and Screenings* — 286
- EDUCATION AND COMMUNITY RESOURCES — 287
  - *Research and Supply Information on Community Resources* — 287
  - *Patient Education Related to Nutrition and Healthy Eating* — 287
  - *Resources for Clinical Services* — 288
- COORDINATE WITH PROVIDERS AND ORGANIZATIONS FOR CONTINUITY OF CARE — 288
  - *Available Community Resources for Non-Clinical Services* — 289
  - *Resources for Disabilities* — 289
- FACILITATE PATIENT ADHERENCE — 290
  - *Setting Up Appointments Following The Encounter* — 290
  - *Check in With the Patient or Family* — 290
  - *Barriers to Care* — 291
  - *Referral Forms and Processes* — 291

TABLE OF CONTENTS

PROVIDE EDUCATION TO PATIENTS ON COMMUNICABLE DISEASE PREVENTION	**292**
Prevention of Transmission of Communicable Diseases	292
TELEHEALTH TECHNOLOGIES	**293**
Patient Education via Telehealth or Virtual Visit Systems and Processes	293
Education Delivery Methods, Instructional Techniques, and Learning Styles	293
Learning Styles	293
Education Delivery Methods and Instructional Techniques	294
WRAP-UP	**294**

CHAPTER 11
Administrative Assisting — 295

OVERVIEW	**295**
PATIENT APPOINTMENTS	**295**
Practice Management Systems and Software	295
Schedule and Monitor Patient Appointments Using Electronic and Paper-Based Systems	297
IDENTIFY AND CHECK PATIENTS IN/OUT	**301**
Required Documentation for Patient Review and Signature	301
MANAGE ELECTRONIC AND PAPER-BASED MEDICAL RECORDS	**302**
Sections of the Medical Record	302
Monitor Patient Flow Sheets, Superbill, or Encounter Forms	302
Chart Review	303
OBTAIN AND VERIFY PRIOR AUTHORIZATIONS AND PRECERTIFICATION	**303**
Referral and Insurance Authorizations, Precertification Requirements	303
FACILITATE/GENERATE REFERRALS	**304**
Electronic Referrals	305

BILLING AND CODING — 305
Verify Insurance Coverage/Financial Eligibility — 305
Insurance Terminology — 306
Financial Eligibility, Sliding Scales, and Indigent Programs — 306

CONFIRM APPROPRIATE DIAGNOSTIC AND PROCEDURAL CODES — 307
Diagnostic and Procedural Codes — 307
Prepare Documentation and Billing Requests Using Current Coding Guidelines — 308

ENSURE DOCUMENTATION COMPLIES WITH REQUIREMENTS — 308
Government Regulations — 308
CMS Billing and Documentation Requirements — 309
Advanced Beneficiary Notice — 309

PERFORM CHARGE RECONCILIATION — 310
Insurance Fundamentals — 310

BILL PATIENTS, INSURERS, AND THIRD-PARTY PAYERS FOR SERVICES PERFORMED — 312
Third-Party Payer Billing Requirements — 312

RESOLVE BILLING ISSUES — 313

OTHER ADMINISTRATIVE DUTIES — 313
Follow-Up Patient Calls and Appointment Confirmations — 313
Process Office Mail and Faxes to Appropriate Staff Member — 314
Enter Information Into Databases or Spreadsheets — 315
Maintain Inventory of Clinical and Administrative Supplies — 315
Activate and Facilitate Use of Patient Portals — 317
Provide Technical Instruction on the Use of Telehealth/Virtual Visits and Troubleshoot Issues — 317
Participate in Safety Evaluations and Report Safety Concerns — 318

WRAP-UP — 318

TABLE OF CONTENTS

CHAPTER 12
Communication and Customer Service — 319

- OVERVIEW — 319
- COMMUNICATION — 320
  - Communication Cycle — 320
  - Therapeutic Communication — 320
  - Active Listening Techniques — 320
  - Oral, Telephone, Email, and Text Communications — 321
- COMMUNICATION BETWEEN PATIENTS AND PROVIDERS — 322
  - Interviewing and Questioning Techniques — 322
  - Scope and Boundaries — 322
  - Coaching and Feedback — 322
- CUSTOMER SERVICE — 323
  - Audience Considerations — 323
  - Nonverbal Communication — 323
  - Communication for Diverse Audiences — 324
  - Stereotypes and Biases — 324
  - Patient Cultures and Backgrounds — 325
- TYPE OF VISIT CONSIDERATIONS — 327
  - Nonverbal Cues in Telehealth — 327
  - Written and Electronic Communication — 327
- CRUCIAL CONVERSATIONS — 329
  - Incident/Event/Unusual Occurrence Reports — 330
  - Challenging Customer Service Occurrences — 330
  - When to De-Escalate Problem Situations — 330
  - Conflict Management and Complaint Resolution — 331
  - Cause-and-Effect Analysis — 332
- TEAMWORK — 332
  - Facilitate Teamwork and Team Engagement — 332
- PROFESSIONALISM — 333
  - Demonstrate Professionalism — 333
  - Professional Presence — 333
- WRAP-UP — 334

CHAPTER 13
Medical Law and Ethics — 335

- OVERVIEW — 335
- MEDICAL LAWS — 335
  - *Patient's Bill of Rights* — 335
- LAWS AND REGULATIONS — 337
- PROTECT PATIENT PRIVACY AND CONFIDENTIALITY — 340
  - *Legal Requirements for Maintenance, Storage, and Disposal of Records* — 340
- INFORMED AND IMPLIED CONSENT — 342
  - *Implied Consent* — 342
  - *Expressed Consent* — 342
  - *Informed Consent* — 342
- OBTAIN, REVIEW, AND COMPLY WITH MEDICAL DIRECTIVES — 343
  - *Advance Directives* — 343
  - *Living Will* — 344
- LEGAL REQUIREMENTS REGARDING REPORTABLE VIOLATIONS OR INCIDENTS — 346
  - *Criminal and Civil Acts* — 346
  - *Torts* — 347
  - *Mandated Reporting* — 348
  - *Abuse* — 348
- ETHICS AND VALUES — 350
- IDENTIFY BELIEFS AND VALUES AND PROVIDE UNBIASED CARE — 352
- WRAP-UP — 353

TABLE OF CONTENTS

IN PRACTICE
Patient Experience Coach ... 355
Case Studies ... 363
Quizzes ... 391

QUIZ 1: FOUNDATIONAL KNOWLEDGE AND BASIC SCIENCE	391
QUIZ 2: MEDICAL TERMINOLOGY, ANATOMY, AND PHYSIOLOGY	393
QUIZ 3: PATIENT INTAKE AND VITALS	396
QUIZ 4: GENERAL PATIENT CARE: PART 1	399
QUIZ 5: GENERAL PATIENT CARE: PART 2	402
QUIZ 6: INFECTION CONTROL AND SAFETY	405
QUIZ 7: POINT-OF-CARE TESTING AND LABORATORY PROCEDURES	407
QUIZ 8: PHLEBOTOMY	410
QUIZ 9: EKG AND CARDIOVASCULAR TESTING	412
QUIZ 10: PATIENT CARE COORDINATION AND EDUCATION	415
QUIZ 11: ADMINISTRATIVE ASSISTING	417
QUIZ 12: COMMUNICATION AND CUSTOMER SERVICE	420
QUIZ 13: MEDICAL LAW AND ETHICS	423
QUIZ ANSWERS	426

APPENDIX
Glossary ... 465
References ... 475
Index ... 477

CHAPTER 1
Foundational Knowledge and Basic Science

OVERVIEW

A medical assistant (MA) career can be exciting, rewarding, and successful. Career options and areas for development and growth are vast. To be set up for success, medical assistants must have a firm foundation of knowledge and understanding regarding numerous aspects of the medical field, the human body, and how to effectively work with others. Taking the time to learn foundational skills, including finding the most accurate and up-to-date information at any given time, will make a career as an MA much more impactful and effective.

This chapter will start by discussing health care systems and settings, focusing on the medical assistant's role. This includes understanding roles and responsibilities, discussion around certifications, and an overview of health care settings and delivery models that an MA may work within. Additionally, the chapter will give context to the greater health care team and options for care to guide understanding of the teammates and systems an MA is likely to encounter.

While medical assistants are not authorized to prescribe medications, supporting a patient's understanding of medications, managing clinic inventory, and, at times, administering medications are all important aspects of the medical assistant's role. This chapter will review fundamental pharmacology to begin building a working knowledge of common medications and how and why they are prescribed and to look at how medications work.

Nutrition and the major nutrients are the building blocks of life. Medical assistants must understand how nutrients impact overall health, how to discuss nutrition with patients, and where to seek resources for patient education. These topics will also be covered in this chapter.

Objectives

Upon completion of this chapter, you should be able to

- Identify the roles, responsibilities, scope of practice, and titles of medical assistants.
- Identify the roles, responsibilities, scope of practice, titles, and credentials of medical providers and allied health personnel.
- Differentiate licensing versus certification and identify maintenance of certification.
- Describe the types of health care organizations and delivery models (outpatient and inpatient, patient-centered medical home, collaborative care, accountable care organization, hospice, home health care, mobile health unit).
- Identify technology-based methods for providing health care and health information (telehealth, virtual patient portals).
- Differentiate health care payment models (fee-for-service, value-based plans).
- Differentiate general versus specialty health care and services.
- Describe ancillary services and complementary therapies.
- Identify medication classifications (diuretics, hypoglycemics, analgesics, over-the-counter), indications, and commonly prescribed medications.
- Describe medication classifications and schedules of controlled substances.
- Differentiate between side effects and adverse effects and indications and contraindications.
- Compute measurements (metric and standard systems), dosage calculations, mathematical conversions, and formulas.
- Identify forms of medication (tablets, patches, capsules).
- Identify look-alike and sound-alike medications.
- Identify routes of medication administration.
- Describe pharmacokinetics (absorption, distribution, metabolism, excretion).
- Summarize the rights of medication administration.
- Describe principles of storage and disposal.
- Identify sources of medication information and FDA regulations.
- Identify dietary nutrients, suggested guidelines, and food labels.
- Compare vitamins and supplements.
- Identify eating disorders.

HEALTH CARE SYSTEMS AND SETTINGS

The medical field can seem overwhelming. New terminology, legal concerns, direct or indirect patient care, unique processes, and high expectations can contribute to initial apprehension. However, this new role can be better understood through a holistic approach, looking at the health care system from all sides. In addition to understanding the role and *scope of practice*, it is crucial to understand the importance of the entire health care team. Knowing the skills and responsibilities of the various allied health and specialty providers strengthens the effectiveness and cohesiveness of the health care team. Each team member needs to respect and assist others in providing the best possible care for the patient.

Medical Assistant Roles, Responsibilities, Scope of Practice, and Titles

MA Roles

The role of an MA is primarily to work alongside a provider in an outpatient or ambulatory health care setting, such as a medical office. The MA can be cross-trained to perform both administrative and clinical duties. Administrative duties include greeting patients, scheduling, handling correspondence, and answering telephones. In addition, the MA is often responsible for obtaining medical histories from patients, providing patient education, performing laboratory tests, and preparing and administering immunizations. An MA achieves credentialing by passing a national *certification* exam.

MA Responsibilities

The responsibilities of an MA vary based on the setting in which they work. Duties can be primarily administrative, clinical, or a combination.

The medical assistant's role is constantly changing and evolving. In addition to traditional responsibilities, medical assistants are doing more patient navigation and care coordination work. In this role, medical assistants can guide patients as they journey through the health care system—helping them understand what is happening and what steps they need to take and helping them connect to the right specialists. To effectively support the patient in this way, the MA will often need to coordinate with other members of the patient care team, both within the clinic and externally with specialty care teams. The MA may ask questions on the patient's behalf to nurses and providers within the team to better understand the plan of care and provide the information to the patient in a clear, easily understood way. When coordinating with other teams, medical assistants can provide helpful context about the patient's social determinants of health and barriers to care, as well as support the patient in being scheduled appropriately and in a timely manner with specialists.

1.1 Administrative Duties

- Scheduling patient appointments
- Patient registration (demographics, payer information, compliance forms)
- Updating and working in patient records
- Sending claims to insurance
- Collecting patient responsibility amounts (copays, coinsurance, deductible)

1.2 Clinical Duties

- Collecting and processing lab specimens
- Performing diagnostic testing (EKG, spirometry)
- Preparing and cleaning examination rooms
- Preparing the patient for evaluation and procedure
- Measuring vital signs
- Preparing medications and administering immunizations

---

scope of practice. A specific set of standards that a medical professional may perform within the limits of the medical license, registration, and/or certification.

certification. Verification by an outside agency that an employer is following established guidelines and standards of care and providing the highest quality of care for their patients.

Scope of Practice

Scope of practice describes the duties delegated based on education, training, and experience. The scope of practice for the MA does not include the practice of medicine. Medical assistants should not perform duties they have not been trained or certified to do. Prior to practice, review the duties and restrictions related to medical assisting, which vary by state. Health care organizations may have stricter policies and procedures that they enforce, but they must comply with state regulations at minimum.

1.3 Take Note

The MA works under the supervision of a provider and performs tasks allowed by state and provider approval.

Variables for the Scope of Practice

Variables that affect the scope of practice for medical assistants include the regulations and policies issued by state medical boards. An MA with appropriate training may safely provide supportive services that are simple, routine medical tasks under the supervision of a licensed physician. In addition, the MA may only provide supportive services set forth by the medical office's organizational policies. These often include measuring height and weight, measuring vital signs, and performing various diagnostic and laboratory testing. Organizational policies must adhere to state and government guidelines to comply with current laws.

Titles

Over 50 years ago, medical providers began hiring assistants to support their medical practice. They recognized the need for administrative support. Over time, this turned into the MA role, combining administrative and clinical responsibilities. In 1956, a formal medical assistant association was formed and recognized by 15 states. The profession continued to evolve and was recognized by the U.S. Department of Education in 1978. At that time, training was completed on the job by the provider and other office staff. This eventually became time-consuming and expensive for providers, at which point formalized training and certification programs arose. Many clinical offices look to hire only those who have completed formal training and certification, ensuring they have the necessary skill set to work in patient care. Offices also follow specific guidelines requiring medical assistants to have current certification to input data regarding government insurance reimbursements into electronic health records.

Additional Certifications

Medical assistants can further their careers and extend their scope of work through continued education, leading to additional certifications, including the following.

- Certified medical administrative assistant (CMAA)
- Certified phlebotomy technician (CPT)
- Certified EKG technician (CET)
- Certified billing and coding specialist (CBCS)
- Certified electronic health records specialist (CEHRS)

CHALLENGE

1. Which of the following determines the scope of medical assistants?
   A. State medical boards
   B. Individual companies
   C. Physician the MA works under
   D. Credentialing organizations

   A is correct. While the provider the medical assistant works under and the organization who employs them may place stricter scope regulations on the medical assistant, all individual and company policies must comply with state regulations.

2. Why might a medical assistant pursue further certification?

   Obtaining additional certifications, such as CET and CBCS, will increase the scope of work for an MA and can lead to better job opportunities.

PROVIDER AND ALLIED HEALTH ROLES, RESPONSIBILITIES, SCOPE OF PRACTICE, TITLES, AND CREDENTIALS

Physician Information

When most people think of health care providers, they think of physicians, also known as doctors. All practicing doctors must be licensed in the state where they practice. To pursue a license, they must first complete eight years of school—four years of undergraduate college, followed by four years of medical or osteopathic school. Upon graduation, prospective physicians then move on to residency. Residency is a 2- to 7-year training period where they receive intensive on-the-job training with the direct oversight of a licensed physician. Finally, physicians must pass parts I, II, and III of the U.S. Medical Licensing Examination. There are two primary types of physicians: medical doctor (MD) and doctor of osteopathy (DO). Their scope of practice and responsibilities are nearly the same, though their training and expertise have slight variations.

- Medical doctors are allopathic providers and the most widely recognized type of doctor. They diagnose illnesses, provide treatments, perform procedures such as surgical interventions, and write prescriptions.

> **1.4 Physicians**
>
> *Role*
>
> *Doctor of Osteopathic Medicine (DO)*
> - Holistic approach to medicine
> - Training on osteopathic manipulative treatment
>
> *Doctor of Medicine (MD)*
> Scientific focus on diagnosis and treatment of medical conditions
>
> *Education*
> - 4-year undergraduate degree, generally science-based
> - 4 years of graduate school after passing the Medical College Acceptance Test (MCAT)
> - Graduate school consists of a 2-year medical education-based program and 2 years of clinical rotations
> - Residency program in a medical specialty (can last 3 to 7 years)

- Doctors of osteopathy complete requirements like those of MDs to graduate and practice medicine. In addition to modern medicine and surgical procedures, DOs use osteopathic manipulative therapy to treat patients.

In addition to physicians, there are two primary types of midlevel providers: physician assistants and nurse practitioners.

Physician Assistant

Physician assistants (PAs) must practice medicine under the direction and supervision of a licensed MD or DO, but they can make clinical decisions. In order to be licensed as a PA in the state of practice, individuals must first complete at least 4 years of college, followed by 2 years of PA school. Most PAs will focus on a specific specialty, such as cardiology or orthopedics.

Nurse Practitioner

Nurse practitioners (NP) provide basic patient care services, including diagnosing and prescribing medications for common illnesses. Nurse practitioners require advanced academic training beyond the registered nurse (RN) degree and have an extensive amount of clinical experience. In most states, NPs must work under the supervision of a physician, but in some states they can practice independently.

Nurses

Nurses are found in almost every health care setting.

A licensed practical nurse (LPN) must be licensed in their state. Typically, one year of schooling through an accredited program, along with passing a state board examination, is required to obtain an LPN license. LPNs are somewhat limited in their scope of practice, as the role is designed to be assistive. They can measure vital signs, administer some medications, and perform clinical care such as wound care. Often, the role of an LPN is to observe patients, recording and reporting on status changes. While they may work in many different settings, a primary use of LPNs recently is in long-term care settings due to the increasing number of older adults in the general population. In some states, and LPN may also be referred to as an LVN (licensed vocational nurse).

A registered nurse (RN) must complete more schooling in the form of an associate degree, diploma graduate, or baccalaureate degree. They, too, must pass a state board examination to be licensed. Due to the more intensive training, RNs have a much broader scope of practice than LPNs. RNs can work in clinical settings, public health agencies, administrative capacities, and educational settings.

Allied Health Professionals

Medical laboratory technicians perform diagnostic testing on blood, bodily fluids, and other specimens under the supervision of a medical technologist.

Medical receptionists check patients in and out, answer phones, schedule appointments, and perform other administrative tasks.

Occupational therapists assist patients who have conditions that disable them developmentally, emotionally, mentally, or physically.

Pharmacy technicians may perform routine medication dispensing functions that do not require the expertise or judgment of a licensed pharmacist. Pharmacy technicians must work under the direct supervision of a pharmacist.

Physical therapists assist patients in improving mobility, strength, and range of motion.

Radiology technicians use various imaging equipment to assist the provider in diagnosing and treating certain diseases.

CHALLENGE

1. Which of the following professions may have a scope that includes managing patient care independently? (Select all that apply.)
   A. Medical providers
   B. Physician assistants
   C. Nurse practitioners
   D. Osteopathic providers

   A and D are correct. Medical doctors (MDs) and osteopathic providers (DOs) are licensed physicians whose primary responsibility is to manage patient care. Nurse practitioners can also manage patient care independently in some states, though in most, they must work under the direction of a physician. Physician assistants have a similar scope of practice as NPs in most states but cannot manage patient care independently.

2. Match the allied health profession with the correct role description.

PROFESSION	DESCRIPTION
A. Medical laboratory technicians	1. Assist patients in regaining mobility.
B. Occupational therapists	2. Use imaging equipment.
C. Physical therapists	3. Assist patients who have disabilities.
D. Radiology technicians	4. Perform diagnostic testing on specimens.

   A: 4, B: 3, C: 1, D: 2
   Medical laboratory technicians perform diagnostic testing on blood, bodily fluids, and other specimens under the supervision of a medical technologist. Occupational therapists assist patients who have conditions that disable them developmentally, emotionally, mentally, or physically. Physical therapists assist patients in improving mobility, strength, and range of motion. Radiology technicians use various imaging equipment to assist the provider in diagnosing and treating certain diseases.

LICENSING VERSUS CERTIFICATION AND MAINTENANCE OF CERTIFICATION

Licensure vs. Certification

A medical school graduate must be licensed before beginning the practice of medicine. Being licensed by the state to practice medicine allows them to diagnose conditions and provide treatment. Licensing helps ensure that anyone providing medical care has the adequate knowledge and skill set to do so safely. It is important to understand the laws and regulations within each state to avoid violations of any kind.

Health Care Licensure

Licensure is regulated by state statutes through the medical practice acts. An MD, DO, or Doctor of Chiropractic degree is issued upon graduation from a medical or chiropractic institute.

Licensure for physicians is mandatory and controlled by a state board of medical examiners. Licensure may be accomplished by examination, *reciprocity*, or *endorsement*. Every state requires a written examination for MDs to practice. Some states grant the license to practice medicine by reciprocity, which automatically recognizes that the requirements were met by another state. Graduates of medical schools in the U.S. are licensed by the endorsement of the national board certification. Licensure by endorsement is granted on a case-by-case basis based on examinations. Graduates not licensed by endorsement must pass the state board exam.

As of 2022, no state requires medical assistants to be licensed. However, some states dictate that to complete specific services such as x-rays, individuals must have a license to perform that particular skill. For example, Florida does not require a medical assistant to have a license to collect prescribed routine laboratory specimens. However, in Washington, even nationally certified medical assistants must get licensing credentials through the Washington State Department of Health to perform phlebotomy or EKGs.

Certification

In addition, the government may require certification for the medical assistant to enter prescriptions into a computerized order-entry system. Advantages of certification include increased initial job placement, higher wages, and career advancement opportunities.

1.5 Take Note

Certification is generally optional, but some states require official education and training for a medical assistant to administer medication or perform phlebotomy procedures.

1.6 Take Note

Those certified through NHA have a valid certification for two years and must either retake the certification exam or complete 10 hours of continuing education to renew.

CHALLENGE

1. Which of the following describes the process for obtaining a medical license from one state based on requirements being met in another state?
   A. Reciprocity
   B. Examination
   C. Endorsement
   D. Graduation

   A is correct. Some states grant the license to practice medicine by reciprocity, which automatically recognizes that the requirements were met from another state.

2. What are the advantages of being certified as a medical assistant, even if it is not legally required in a state?

   Advantages of certification include increased initial job placement, higher wages, and career advancement opportunities. When employees hire a certified MA, they know they are already equipped with the foundational knowledge and experience to effectively manage their job responsibilities.

---

reciprocity. Agreement or arrangement that allows resident licensees of one reciprocal state to obtain a license in another reciprocal state.

endorsement. The process of a state/territory granting a license to an applicant who is licensed in good standing at the equivalent designation in another jurisdiction.

Maintaining a Certification

Once certification is obtained, it must be maintained to stay current. This ensures that medical assistants have the most up-to-date information about the medical field and provides validity to the overall profession. Each certification has different requirements for recertification, so medical assistants should understand and follow the recertification process of the organization sponsoring their certification.

TYPES OF HEALTH CARE ORGANIZATIONS AND DELIVERY MODELS

Inpatient and Outpatient

Inpatient care occurs while the patient is admitted to a hospital or facility. Ambulatory care refers to any care received in an outpatient facility. This includes many types of care settings.

Primary Care Clinics

Primary care clinics are outpatient care settings where patients are seen for routine type visits, including wellness checks, prevention counseling, chronic conditions, medication management, and minor acute needs. Primary care will be discussed in more detail later in the chapter.

Specialty Care Clinics

Specialty care clinics are outpatient facilities where patients who have complex or severe diseases and conditions are seen for routine visits by doctors who specialize in a specific disease or condition.

Home Health

Home health refers to specific types of care provided to those who cannot leave their home easily. Physical, occupational, and speech therapy are common types of home care. Skilled nursing is also common in the home health setting. It must be prescribed and overseen by a provider, typically a primary care provider (PCP). Home health is not used on an ongoing basis for a patient but is ordered for a set period based on an acute event, usually hospitalization. Home health orders include goals for the patient, such as managing their medications and ambulating safely. The service is complete when the goals are reached. Medical assistants working for the ordering provider are often responsible for submitting the order for home health, coordinating to ensure the patient is enrolled and scheduled, and assisting with the administrative aspects of the orders.

Mobile Health Units

Mobile health units bring health care to the communities that most need it and may otherwise lack access to the services provided. Teams working in a mobile health unit are equipped with means of transportation that allow for the setup and use of specialized medical equipment. There are mobile health units in the U.S. While this concept has been in use for services such as mobile stroke units, mobile urgent cares, and mobile mammogram buses, the COVID-19 pandemic brought this type of care to much of the country in the form of mobile testing and vaccination options.

Hospice

Hospice care is end-of-life care focused on comfort rather than curative efforts. Patients can qualify for hospice care if they have a terminal illness at the end stage. It can be delivered as outpatient or inpatient care. Typically, a patient will begin hospice outpatient but can transition to inpatient care as they need a higher level of care near the end of life.

Patient-Centered Medical Home

The *patient-centered medical home (PCMH)* is a care delivery model in which a PCP coordinates treatment to ensure patients receive the required care when and where they need it and in a way they can understand. This encompasses all aspects of care, from prevention and wellness education to acute illness and chronic disease management to end-of-life care. The PCMH is a team-based approach to health care in which a provider leads an interprofessional team to work collaboratively and effectively for their patients. Medical assistants are an integral piece of the PCMH team—assisting with direct patient care, care coordination, patient education, and administrative tasks essential to the model.

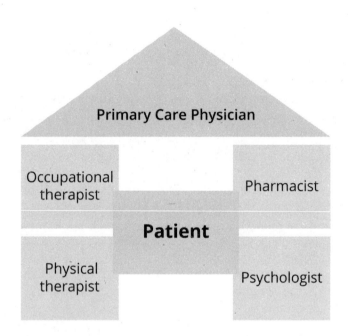

CHALLENGE

1. What are the primary benefits of mobile health units?

   > Mobile health units bring health care to the communities that most need it and may otherwise lack access to the services provided. They have been particularly helpful during the COVID-19 pandemic, as they can bring testing and vaccines to many communities and make these services as easy as possible to access and use.

2. Which of the following patients is receiving inpatient care?
   A. A patient completes diagnostic testing at a hospital and returns home following the test.
   B. A patient visits their primary care provider for a physical exam.
   C. A patient goes to a hospice facility for end-of-life care.
   D. A patient receives physical therapy in their home following hospitalization.

   > C is correct. Inpatient care occurs while the patient is admitted to a hospital or facility. Typically, a patient will begin hospice outpatient but can transition to inpatient care as they need a higher level of care near the end of life.

---

patient-centered medical home (PCMH). A partnership between a patient and their care team in which total health is the focus and not just a single condition. A health care team consists of a provider (physician, nurse practitioner, physician assistant), CMAA, CCMA, nurses, and pharmacist.

TECHNOLOGY-BASED METHODS FOR PROVIDING HEALTH CARE AND INFORMATION

Telehealth and Virtual Visits

Telehealth is health care delivered virtually, most commonly via video call. The increase in telehealth expanded to eliminate patients from coming in contact with communicable diseases, provide convenience, and allow patients in rural areas to obtain specialty care where it may not have been offered before. Telehealth can be an excellent option for patients and providers to review many aspects of care, but it does come with limitations.

Medical assistants may have multiple responsibilities when it comes to virtual visits. Scheduling virtual visits may require more time because the MA must gather or confirm the patient's email address, ensure the link has been sent, and review instructions. Some offices offer patients a test visit in which an administrator or MA will log into the link to ensure the patient can access it when it is time for their appointment. Medical assistants may also participate in the actual visit, just as they would with a standard office visit. This can include gathering a history, verifying medication and pharmacy information, setting an agenda, and following up with the patient on the next steps, such as referral or diagnostic testing coordination.

Patient Portals

Patient portals are a common feature in electronic health records. This feature allows patients to log into a patient-facing aspect of the EHR to view their personal health information, such as test results, visit notes, and patient education materials. Many patient portals include an option to securely message the health care team about concerns and plans of care. Some portals also allow patients to schedule appointments directly without needing to call the office. The benefits of patient portals include increased transparency about care, decreased wait times for patients to receive results, and reduced demand on the office staff due to direct access limiting the need for phone calls.

The MA may be responsible for uploading information to the portal, as well as assisting the patient with enrolling and getting set up with an account. Medical assistants should understand the portal's functionality and the clinic's policies and procedures around appropriate use.

1.7 Telehealth Appropriate

- Follow-up on medication adjustments
- Chronic condition review and discussion
- Patient education
- Evaluation of minor or common rashes and skin concerns
- Follow-up on new medical equipment, such as a CPAP machine
- Discussion of lab results

1.8 In-Person Evaluation Needed

- Diagnostic testing, such as imaging or lab work
- New pain symptoms
- Physical examination

CHALLENGE

1. Which of the following visits may be appropriate for telehealth? (Select all that apply.)
   A. Follow-up on medication adjustments
   B. Physical examination
   C. Patient education
   D. Review of lab results
   E. New pain symptoms

   A, C, and D are correct. Following up on medication adjustments to discuss how the patient is feeling, providing patient education, and discussing lab results may be completed over a video call, as the focus of these visits is primarily conversation. A physical exam and review of new pain symptoms, which often requires a physical exam, would be conducted in person for full efficiency.

2. Describe the medical assistant's role in patient portals.

   The MA is often responsible for assisting patients with enrolling in the portal. This includes having necessary paperwork completed, providing enrollment instructions, and reviewing how to use the portal to effectively interact with their health care team. The MA may also be responsible for uploading or updating data in the portal.

---

telehealth. The virtual delivery of health care services remotely.

HEALTH CARE PAYMENT MODELS

Fee for Service

The U.S. health care system is largely based on the *fee-for-service* model in which providers and medical facilities bill insurance and patients for the services provided. Every examination, medical service, test, and procedure has an associated procedural code and charge. These charges are managed through the provider's medical billing department and sent to the insurance (or directly to the patient) for payment. The insurance then charges the patient a predetermined amount for which they are responsible.

> **1.9 Take Note**
>
> The primary benefit of this model is that patients only pay for services they use. The risk of this model is that it can lead to unnecessary visits, tests, and procedures for the profit of those providing care.

Value-Based Plans

The health care system is increasingly moving toward *value-based plans* or care. The goals of value-based care are summarized in the Quadruple Aim.

- Improved patient outcomes
- Improved patient satisfaction
- Lower cost
- Health care professional well-being

Rather than costs being determined by each service, the cost is more holistic. This model prioritizes prevention and early intervention over complex intervention to prevent unnecessary downstream costs. Clinics and health care systems that adopt this model are rewarded financially for keeping patients healthy rather than making money based on visits, procedures, and interventions once the patient has become ill.

---

fee for service. System used by private insurance companies and not-for-profits in which insurance carriers determine the allowed charge either by a fee schedule or through service benefits that define covered services but not necessarily the exact payments.

value-based plan. Insurance coverage that changes the amount of reimbursement based on health outcomes of patients and the quality of the service they received.

1.10 Other Health Care Models

MODEL	DESCRIPTION
Managed care	An umbrella term for plans that provide health care in return for preset scheduled payments and coordinated care through a defined network of providers and hospitals.
Capitation (partial or full)	Patients are assigned a per-member, per-month payment based on age, race, sex, lifestyle, medical history, and benefit design. Payment rates are tied to expected usage regardless of how often the patient visits. Like bundled payment models, providers are incentivized to help patients avoid high-cost procedures and tests to maximize their compensation. Under partial- or blended-capitation models, only specific types or categories of services are paid based on capitation.
Health maintenance organization (HMO)	This plan contracts with a medical center or group of providers to provide preventive and acute care for the insured person. HMOs generally require referrals to specialists, as well as precertification and preauthorization for hospital admissions, outpatient procedures, and treatments.
Preferred provider organization (PPO)	These plans have more flexibility than HMO plans. An insured person does not need a PCP and can go directly to a specialist without referrals. Although patients can see providers in or out of their network, an in-network provider usually costs less.
Point-of-service (POS) plan	POS plans allow a great deal of flexibility for patients. They can self-refer to specialists and do not need an assigned PCP. Like PPO, the cost depends on whether the providers they see are within the plan's panel.

CHALLENGE

1. What is the primary difference between fee-for-service and value-based care?

   In fee-for-service models, the cost to the insurance and patient is determined by the cost of services provided. In value-based models, the cost is determined by the value to the patient and their long-term health.

2. Match the health care model with the correct description.

MODEL	DESCRIPTION
A. Managed care	1. Patients are assigned a per-member, per-month payment based on age, race, sex, lifestyle, medical history, and benefit design.
B. HMO	2. Plans that provide health care in return for preset scheduled payments and coordinated care through a defined network of providers and hospitals.
C. Capitation	3. An insured person does not need a PCP and can go directly to a specialist without referrals.
D. PPO	4. A plan that requires referrals to specialists, as well as precertification and preauthorization for hospital admissions, outpatient procedures, and treatments.

A: 2, B: 4, C: 1, D: 3
Managed care is an umbrella term for plans that provide health care in return for preset scheduled payments and coordinated care through a defined network of providers and hospitals. HMOs are health care plans that require referrals to specialists, as well as precertification and preauthorization for hospital admissions, outpatient procedures, and treatments. Capitation is a model in which patients are assigned a per-member, per-month payment based on their age, race, sex, lifestyle, medical history, and benefit design. Payment rates are tied to expected usage regardless of how often the patient visits. PPOs are health care plans in which an insured person does not need a PCP but can go directly to a specialist without referrals. Although patients can see providers in or out of their network, an in-network provider usually costs less.

managed care. System used by private and public insurance plans that controls health care cost and improves preventive care for its patients by having contracts with providers and medical organizations. The three types of managed care plans are health maintenance organization (HMO), preferred provider organization (PPO), and point of service (POS).

capitation. A managed care method of monthly payments to the provider based on the number of enrolled patients, regardless of how many encounters a patient may have during the month.

health maintenance organization (HMO). A medical insurance group that provides coverage of health care services for a period of time and a fixed annual fee.

preferred provider organization (PPO). A network of physicians, other health care practitioners, and hospitals that have joined together to contract with insurance companies, employers, or other organizations to provide health care to subscribers for a discounted fee.

point-of-service (POS). A type of managed care health insurance plan that is based on lower medical costs in exchange for more limited choice.

GENERAL VS. SPECIALTY HEALTH CARE AND SERVICES

General Health Care Services

General practitioners (GPs) are medical doctors who treat acute and chronic illnesses and provide patients with preventive care and health education. A GP may take a holistic approach to general practice that considers the biological, psychological, and social aspects relevant to the care of each patient's illness.

- Family practitioners offer care to the whole family, from newborns to older adults. They are familiar with a range of disorders and diseases. However, preventive care is their primary concern.

- Internists provide comprehensive care for adults, often diagnosing and treating chronic, long-term conditions. They also offer treatment for common illnesses and preventive care. Internists must have a broad understanding of the body and its ailments to diagnose conditions and provide treatment. Internists may focus on pediatric or adult medicine rather than provide care across the lifespan.

Specialty Health Care Services

Specialist care is used when a disease or diagnosis escalates beyond the area of expertise of a PCP. Specialists are providers focused on diagnosing and treating diseases and disorders of specific body systems.

1.11 Take Note

Medical assistants can interact with specialists by managing and coordinating referrals from primary care offices and directly supporting the specialist provider.

1.12 Specialist Care

SPECIALIST	FOCUS
Allergist	Evaluates disorders and diseases of the immune system, including **adverse reactions** to medications and food, anaphylaxis, problems related to autoimmune disease, and asthma
Anesthesiologist	Manages pain or administers sedation medications during surgical procedures
Cardiologist	Diagnoses and treats diseases or conditions of the heart and blood vessels
Dermatologist	Diagnoses and treats skin conditions
Endocrinologist	Diagnoses and treats hormonal and glandular conditions; often works with patients who have diabetes
Gastroenterologist	Manages diseases of the GI tract (stomach, intestines, esophagus, liver, pancreas, colon, and rectum)
Gynecologist	Diagnoses and treats internal reproductive system and fertility disorders
Hematologist	Diagnoses and treats blood and blood-producing organs, patients who have anemia, leukemia, and lymphoma
Hepatologist	Studies and treats diseases related to the liver, biliary tree, gallbladder, and pancreas

adverse reactions. Unwanted or undesired effects that are possibly related to taking a medication, usually secondary to the main effect of the medication.

1.12 Specialist Care *(continued)*

SPECIALIST	FOCUS
Neonatologist	Provides care of newborns, specifically those who are ill or premature
Nephrologist	Manages diseases and disorders of the kidney and its associated structures
Obstetrician	Provides care of patients during and after pregnancy
Oncologist	Treats and provides care for patients who have cancer
Ophthalmologist	Diagnoses and treats diseases and conditions of the eye
Orthopedist	Treats injuries and diseases of the bones, joints, muscles, tendons, and ligaments
Neurologist	Treats diseases and disorders of the brain and nervous system
Otolaryngologist	Treats diseases and conditions of the ear, nose, and throat
Pediatrician	Manages newborn to adolescent health
Psychiatrist	Diagnoses and treats mental disorders and conditions
Radiologist	Uses and interprets imaging to detect abnormalities in the body
Urologist	Manages disorders of the urinary tract

CHALLENGE

1. Which of the following specialists would a patient most likely see as a follow-up for a heart attack?
   A. Cardiologist
   B. Urologist
   C. Radiologist
   D. Hematologist

   A is correct. Cardiologists specialize in diagnosing and treating diseases and conditions of the heart and blood vessels, including heart attacks.

2. Match the specialist with the correct focus area.

SPECIALIST	FOCUS AREA
A. Dermatologist	1. Hormonal conditions
B. Endocrinologist	2. Mental health
C. Otolaryngologist	3. Skin
D. Psychiatrist	4. Ear, nose, and throat

   A: 3, B: 1, C: 4, D: 2
   Dermatologists specialize in conditions of the skin. Endocrinologists specialize in hormonal and glandular conditions. Otolaryngologists specialize in disorders and conditions related to the ear, nose, and throat. Psychiatrists diagnose and treat mental health conditions.

ANCILLARY SERVICES AND COMPLEMENTARY THERAPIES

Ancillary Services

Providing ancillary services in the provider's office adds convenience for patients and increases revenue for the organization. Ancillary services meet a specific medical need for a particular population.

- **Urgent care** provides an alternative to the emergency department. They cost less, have a shorter wait time, and are often conveniently located. Most have flexible hours and offer walk-in appointments. They are appropriate to use for non-life-threatening acute injuries and illnesses.
- **Laboratory services** perform diagnostic testing on blood, body fluids, and other specimens to conclude a diagnosis for the provider.
- **Diagnostic imaging** machines such as x-ray equipment, ultrasound machines, magnetic resonance imaging (MRI), and computerized tomography (CT) take images of body parts to further diagnose a condition.
- **Occupational therapy** assists patients who have conditions that disable them developmentally, emotionally, mentally, or physically. Occupational therapy helps the patient compensate for the loss of functions and rebuild to a functional level.
- **Physical therapy** assists patients in regaining mobility and improving strength and range of motion, often impaired by an accident, injury, or disease.

Complementary Therapies

Acupuncture involves pricking the skin or tissues with needles to relieve pain and treat various physical, mental, and emotional conditions.

Chiropractic medicine diagnoses and treats pain and overall body function through spinal manipulation and alignment.

Energy therapy is the calm method of clearing cellular memory through the human energy field, promoting health, balance, and relaxation. It centers on the connection between life's physical, emotional, and mental states found in various holistic healing techniques.

Dietary supplements contain one or more dietary ingredients, including vitamins, minerals, herbs, or other botanicals. A plant or part of a plant (flowers, leaves, bark, fruit, seeds, stems, roots, amino acids) is used for its flavor, scent, or potential therapeutic properties.

CHALLENGE

1. When and why may a patient benefit from going to urgent care rather than an emergency department?

   Urgent care costs less, has a shorter wait time, and is often conveniently located. Most have flexible hours and offer walk-in appointments. They are appropriate to use for non-life-threatening acute injuries and illnesses.

2. Which of the following ancillary services helps patients compensate for the loss of function due to injury, illness, or disease?
   A. Occupational therapy
   B. Physical therapy
   C. Urgent care
   D. Laboratory services

   A is correct. Occupational therapy assists patients who have conditions that disable them developmentally, emotionally, mentally, or physically. Occupational therapy helps the patient compensate for the loss of functions and rebuild to a functional level.

BASIC PHARMACOLOGY

Drug Classifications, Indications, and Commonly Prescribed Medications

The classification of medications is complex. Primarily, a medication's therapeutic action dictates the classification, but sometimes it is done by chemical formulations, body systems they act on, or symptoms the medication relieves. Some medications fall into more than one category. Gabapentin and pregabalin are good examples. Both medications are anticonvulsants; they treat seizures. However, they are also analgesics because they help relieve neuropathic (nerve) pain. Another example is hydrochlorothiazide, a diuretic—it helps eliminate excess fluid from the body. However, doing so can help lower blood pressure; thus, it is also an antihypertensive medication. Here are some of the most common classifications of medications medical assistants are likely to encounter.

1.13 Medication Classifications: Indications and Examples

MEDICATION CLASSIFICATION	INDICATION	EXAMPLES
Analgesics	Relieve pain	Acetaminophen, hydrocodone, codeine
Antacids/anti-ulcer	Gastroesophageal reflux disease (GERD)	Esomeprazole, calcium carbonate, famotidine
Antibiotics	Bacterial infections	Amoxicillin, ciprofloxacin, sulfamethoxazole
Anticholinergics	Smooth muscle spasms	Ipratropium, dicyclomine, hyoscyamine
Anticoagulants	Delay blood clotting	Warfarin, apixaban, heparin
Anticonvulsants	Prevent or control seizures	Clonazepam, phenytoin, gabapentin
Antidepressants	Relieve depression	Doxepin, fluoxetine, duloxetine, selegiline
Antidiarrheals	Reduce diarrhea	Bismuth subsalicylate, loperamide, dipehnoxylate/atropine
Antiemetics	Reduce nausea, vomiting	Metoclopramide, ondansetron
Antifungals	Fungal infections	Fluconazole, nystatin, miconazole
Antihistamines	Relieve allergies	Diphenhydramine, cetirizine, loratadine
Antihypertensives	Lower blood pressure	Metoprolol, lisinopril, valsartan, clonidine
Anti-inflammatories	Reduce inflammation	Ibuprofen, celecoxib, naproxen
Antilipemics	Lower cholesterol	Atorvastatin, fenofibrate, cholestyramine
Antimigraine agents	Relieve migraine headaches	Topiramate, sumatriptan, rizatriptan, zolmitriptan
Anti-osteoporosis agents	Improve bone density	Alendronate, raloxifene, calcitonin

1.13 Medication Classifications: Indications and Examples (continued)

MEDICATION CLASSIFICATION	INDICATION	EXAMPLES
Antipsychotics	Psychosis	Quetiapine, haloperidol, risperidone
Antipyretics	Reduce fever	Acetaminophen, ibuprofen, aspirin
Skeletal/muscle relaxants	Reduce or prevent muscle spasms	Cyclobenzaprine, methocarbamol, carisoprodol
Antitussives/expectorants	Control cough, promote the elimination of mucus	Dextromethorphan, codeine, guaifenesin
Antivirals	Viral infections	Acyclovir, interferon, oseltamivir
Anxiolytics (anti-anxiety)	Reduce anxiety	Clonazepam, diazepam, lorazepam
Bronchodilators	Relax airway muscles	Albuterol, isoproterenol, theophylline
Central nervous system stimulants	Reduce hyperactivity	Methylphenidate, dextroamphetamine, lisdexamfetamine
Contraceptives	Prevent pregnancy	Medroxyprogesterone acetate, ethinyl estradiol, drospirenone
Decongestants	Relieve nasal congestion	Pseudoephedrine, phenylephrine, oxymetazoline
Diuretics	Eliminate excess fluid	Furosemide, hydrochlorothiazide, bumetanide
Hormone replacements	Stabilize hormone deficiencies	Levothyroxine, insulin, desmopressin, estrogen
Laxatives, stool softeners	Promote bowel movements	Magnesium hydroxide, bisacodyl, docusate sodium
Oral hypoglycemics	Reduce blood glucose	Metformin, glyburide, pioglitazone
Sedative-hypnotics	Induce sleep/relaxation	Zolpidem, temazepam, eszopiclone

CHALLENGE

1. Which of the following medication classifications would be prescribed to treat high blood pressure in a patient?
   A. Bronchodilator
   B. Antihypertensive
   C. Contraceptive
   D. Antihistamine

   B is correct. Antihypertensives are medications used to treat high blood pressure, also known as hypertension.

2. Which of the following medication classifications is amoxicillin under?
   A. Antidepressant
   B. Antihypertensive
   C. Antidiarrheal
   D. Antibiotic

   D is correct. Amoxicillin is an antibiotic.

DRUG CLASSIFICATIONS AND SCHEDULES OF CONTROLLED SUBSTANCES

The federal *Controlled Substances Act (CSA)* created five schedules for controlled substances according to their potential for abuse and addiction. Only controlled substances are classified as scheduled. Medical assistants must understand these schedules, including the effect on how medications are prescribed and managed, to ensure they follow appropriate protocols and support the patient. Patients who need these medications may feel frustrated or shamed by the regulations in place if they need help understanding the reasons or believe the restrictions are personal. When a new controlled substance is prescribed, the MA can improve the patient experience by setting expectations and normalizing the experience.

Schedule I includes substances with a high potential for abuse and currently no approved medical use in the U.S. They are illegal, and providers may not prescribe them. These include heroin, mescaline, and lysergic acid diethylamide (LSD). Schedule I still includes cannabis (marijuana) even though it is legal for medical use with a prescription in many states. States can add substances to a schedule as a matter of state law, even if not included in federal scheduling. In the case of marijuana, the federal government does not federally prosecute those who use cannabis in states that allow it.

Schedule II includes substances that have a high potential for abuse, are considered dangerous, and can lead to psychological and physical dependence. Unlike schedule I drugs, schedule II drugs are approved for medical use. Schedule II drugs include morphine, methadone, oxycodone, hydromorphone, hydrocodone, fentanyl, and amphetamine. Schedule II prescriptions must be signed by hand, except as rules allow regarding distribution of electronic or printed prescriptions. Prescribers may electronically transmit prescriptions directly to the pharmacy in states where the prescription meets the requirement of state and federal regulations. Schedule II substances must be stored in a safe or steel cabinet of substantial construction. If the safe or cabinet is less than 750 pounds, it must be mounted or secured to something of substantial construction. The device should have an inner and outer door with locks for each door requiring different keys.

Schedule III includes substances with moderate to low potential for physical and psychological dependence. These include ketamine, anabolic steroids, acetaminophen with codeine, and buprenorphine.

Schedule IV includes substances that have a low potential for abuse and dependence. These include tramadol and benzodiazepines including diazepam, alprazolam, chlordiazepoxide, and clonazepam.

Schedule V includes substances that contain limited quantities of some narcotics, usually for antidiarrheal, antitussive, and analgesic purposes. These include diphenoxylate with atropine, guaifenesin with codeine, and pregabalin.

Schedule III, IV, and V controlled substances may not be filled or refilled more than 6 months after the date on which the prescription was issued and may not be refilled more than five times in 6 months.

For a current alphabetical list of all controlled substances and their CSA schedule number, go to the resources section of the Office of Diversion Control website.

Controlled Substances Act (CSA). Statute that identifies all regulated substances into one of five schedules depending on potential for abuse.

CHAPTER 1: FOUNDATIONAL KNOWLEDGE AND BASIC SCIENCE
Side Effects, Adverse Effects, Indications, and Contraindications

CHALLENGE

1. Match the schedules of drugs to the correct definition.

SCHEDULE	DEFINITION
A. Schedule I B. Schedule II C. Schedule III D. Schedule IV E. Schedule V	1. Substances that contain limited quantities of some narcotics, usually for antidiarrheal, antitussive, and analgesic purposes 2. Includes substances that have a moderate to low potential for physical and psychological dependence 3. Includes substances that have a low potential for abuse and dependence 4. Substances that have a high potential for abuse, are considered dangerous, and can lead to psychological and physical dependence 5. Includes substances that have a high potential for abuse and currently no approved medical use in the United States

A: 5, B: 4, C: 2, D: 3, E: 1
Schedule I drugs are the most strictly controlled, and schedule V are the least strictly controlled.

2. Which of the following schedules of medications can include refills on prescriptions? (Select all that apply.)
   A. Schedule I
   B. Schedule II
   C. Schedule III
   D. Schedule IV
   E. Schedule V

C, D, and E are correct. Schedule I drugs have no accepted medical use in the U.S. and therefore cannot be prescribed. Schedule II drugs have medical use and can be prescribed but cannot include refills. Schedules III to V can be prescribed with refills included on the original prescription.

SIDE EFFECTS, ADVERSE EFFECTS, INDICATIONS, AND CONTRAINDICATIONS

Medications can have good and bad effects.

- *Therapeutic effects* are the good effects—the ones for which providers prescribe them.

- *Side effects* are undesirable unintended actions on the body, such as nausea or dry mouth, and can limit the usefulness of the medication.

- Adverse effects are unintended, harmful actions of the medication, such as an allergic reaction, and prevent further use of the medication.

- Indications are the problems for which the provider prescribes a particular medication.

- Contraindications are symptoms or conditions that make a specific treatment or medication inadvisable or even dangerous.

- Precautions are problems that pose a lesser risk but require close observation and monitoring during medication therapy.

---

therapeutic effect. The helpful effect that the provider is hoping will help the patient to feel better.

side effect. A secondary reaction to the one intended.

Side Effects and Adverse Effects

Many people use side effects and adverse effects interchangeably, but there is a difference. Side effects develop predictably and are nearly unavoidable but not necessarily harmful. For example, a patient who takes diphenhydramine, an antihistamine, to relieve an itchy rash at bedtime sleeps better that night. Why? Because a side effect of diphenhydramine is sedation and sleepiness. So, advise caution when taking this medication prior to driving or operating machinery.

The expected therapeutic effect of lisinopril is a sustained reduction in blood pressure. Lisinopril can also cause many undesirable effects—some of them life-threatening. It is critical to review with a patient who is beginning medication therapy what side effects are the most common and which are serious enough to report to the provider immediately. With lisinopril, the patient might develop nausea, dizziness, or nasal congestion. These are common side effects and are likely to subside with time. However, immediate medical care is imperative if the patient develops swelling of the lips, face, and tongue. These could potentially indicate a fatal reaction to the medication.

With lisinopril, facial swelling is a rare effect due to the accumulation of a substance in the body that mimics anaphylaxis, a serious allergic reaction. Most medications have the potential to cause an allergic reaction.

- Mild allergic reactions usually manifest as itchy rashes.
- Serious allergic reactions involve spasms of the airways, swelling of the face and throat, and a serious decrease in blood pressure.

The patient's allergy history can explain the possibility of an allergic reaction. For example, if a patient has had a previous serious allergic reaction to eggs, they could have a serious allergic reaction to the flu vaccine because eggs have been used in some flu vaccines. For a serious or anaphylactic reaction, the patient needs epinephrine and medical attention. Medication allergies should be discussed, reviewed, and updated at every visit. Confirm allergies any time a prescription is written and prior to medication administration.

1.14 Take Note

Allergic reactions can be life-threatening, so advise all patients about seeking medical care immediately if they develop symptoms. An antihistamine, such as diphenhydramine, can help relieve a minor allergic reaction and is available over the counter.

Indications and Contraindications

The indication for a medication is the symptoms or reason a medication is prescribed, while contraindications are symptoms or conditions that make a particular treatment or medication inadvisable or even dangerous. The most common contraindication is hypersensitivity, a previous allergic reaction, to that medication. Other frequent contraindications include damage to or malfunction of a body system. For example, cirrhosis of the liver is a contraindication for taking acarbose, and hepatitis is a contraindication for taking duloxetine. Many other medications are toxic to the liver and require extreme caution with patients who have liver disease. These include acetaminophen, phenytoin, fluconazole, bupropion, penicillin, erythromycin, rifampin, ritonavir, lisinopril, and losartan.

Another important consideration is how a medication interacts with food or other medications. It is easy to confuse contraindications with interactions. For example, medications that are in the classification of a specific type of antidepressant, monoamine oxidase inhibitors (MAOIs), interact dangerously with foods that contain tyramine (avocados, smoked meats, wine, most cheeses).

CHAPTER 1: FOUNDATIONAL KNOWLEDGE AND BASIC SCIENCE
Side Effects, Adverse Effects, Indications, and Contraindications

MAOIs also interact adversely with other antidepressants, such as tricyclic antidepressants. Both interactions result in a hypertensive crisis. Examples of MAOIs are phenelzine, isocarboxazid, and tranylcypromine.

Grapefruit juice interacts with many medications, interfering with their metabolism, raising the levels of the medications, and producing toxicity. These medications include dextromethorphan, simvastatin, and sildenafil. Additionally, some herbal supplements interact with prescription medications. St. John's wort, an herbal supplement for mood and sleep disorders, reduces the effectiveness of warfarin and oral contraceptives.

Even more common are medications that interact with other medications. For example, if patients take propranolol with albuterol, both medications lose effectiveness. Aspirin and warfarin have anticoagulant effects, so taking both puts patients at risk of hemorrhage, or major bleeding. Many antibiotics—including ampicillin, sulfamethoxazole-trimethoprim, minocycline, and metronidazole—reduce the effectiveness of oral contraceptives.

For examples of medication indications, refer to the table of common medication classifications. Their actions apply to the common reasons for use, including pain, infection, muscle spasms, migraine headaches, anxiety, depression, or insomnia. Common potential adverse effects include gastrointestinal problems (nausea, vomiting, diarrhea, constipation). Some patients take medications with food to minimize these effects. Furthermore, if stomach irritation is a problem, taking a formulation with an enteric coating can help minimize the negative effects on the stomach. Also common are central nervous system effects (dizziness, headache, sedation, insomnia). Many medications cause changes in heart rate, blood pressure, vision, and hearing.

CHALLENGE

1. A patient has a prescription for medication to treat a bacterial infection. When taking this medication, the patient experiences nausea. Which of the following describes nausea caused by the antibiotic?

    A. Adverse reaction
    B. Side effect
    C. Allergic reaction
    D. Contraindication

    B is correct. Side effects are unintended responses to a medication, which are known, expected, and essentially harmless. The medication causes nausea in this case, but it is not dangerous to the patient, and despite the side effect, the medication is needed to treat the bacterial infection.

2. What are the differences between side effects and adverse reactions?

    A side effect is an unintended, undesirable action on the body caused by a medication, which is known and expected, as well as relatively harmless to the patient. Side effects may lead a patient to decline a medication but are not cause to avoid prescribing or recommending the medication. An adverse reaction is an unintended, harmful action of the medication, which may be unexpected and can cause death or long-term damage to the patient. Patients with known adverse reactions to medication should not be prescribed that medication.

METRIC AND STANDARD MEASUREMENTS, DOSAGE CALCULATIONS, AND MATHEMATICAL CONVERSIONS AND FORMULAS

Understanding systems of measurement and knowing how to calculate and verify medication dosages are essential skills for medical assistants. How often and what kinds of medications medical assistants will administer varies by practice setting, but these principles will help in discussions with patients about taking their medications at home. Patients might find measuring medications—especially liquid oral and injectable ones—challenging and need assistance.

Metric System

Most medication prescriptions and dosages will be in the metric system of weights and volume. However, some medication formulations in the apothecary and standard systems require conversions. Also, some prescriptions require dosage calculations based on a patient's weight in kilograms, especially for pediatric doses. So medical assistants need a working knowledge of conversions and calculations.

Prescriptions do not usually include length measurements, but there are exceptions. For example, the amount of nitroglycerin ointment to squeeze onto the application paper is a length measurement. Metric lengths are common in other clinical applications (measurements of wounds, distances to use in procedures).

The equivalency tables show the relationship various metric measurements have with each other.

1.15 Take Note

The metric system quantifies weight in kilograms (kg), grams (g), milligrams (mg), and micrograms (mcg). It measures volume in deciliters dL), liters (L), and milliliters (mL). Length is in kilometers (km), meters (m), centimeters (cm), and millimeters (mm). There are other metric values, but these are most used in practice.

1.17 Equivalency

UNIT	RELATIONSHIP TO BASE UNIT	DECIMAL VALUE/ WHOLE NUMBER
micro-	÷ 1,000,000	0.000001
milli-	÷ 1,000	0.0001
centi-	÷ 1,00	0.01
base unit	1	1
kilo-	× 1,000	1,000

1.16 Metric System Units

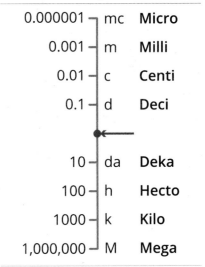

CHAPTER 1: FOUNDATIONAL KNOWLEDGE AND BASIC SCIENCE
Metric and Standard Measurements, Dosage Calculations, and Mathematical Conversions and Formulas

Standard System

Standard, or household, measurements of medications are still common, especially for liquid oral medications taken at home. Many liquid medications come with measuring cups with marked household and metric equivalents. Still, patients could misplace the cups and ask about using a teaspoon or tablespoon to measure the dosage. The table shows the most common equivalents for liquids and weight in this system.

1.18 Standard System

HOUSEHOLD VALUE	METRIC EQUIVALENT	HOUSEHOLD VALUE	METRIC EQUIVALENT
15 drops (gtt)	1 mL	1 pint	480 mL (about 500 mL)
1 teaspoon (tsp)	5 mL	1 quart	960 mL (about 1 L)
1 tablespoon (tbsp)	15 mL	1 gallon	3,830 mL
1 fluid ounce (oz), 2 tbsp	30 mL	2.2 pounds (lb)	1 kg
1 cup	240 mL		

Dosage Calculations

With all dosage calculations, always take time and recheck calculations. If there is any doubt, ask the provider or another medical assistant to check the calculations. The patient's well-being depends on accuracy in all calculations.

Ratio and Proportion

For calculating adult dosages, the proportion method works well.

For example, a provider prescribes diphenhydramine 50 mg for a patient who is having a mild allergic reaction. Available are 25 mg capsules. Here is how to determine how many capsules to give the patient.

If 25 mg equals 1 capsule (cap), then 50 mg equals how many (X) capsules?

$$\frac{25 \text{ mg}}{1 \text{ cap}} = \frac{50 \text{ mg}}{X \text{ cap}}$$

Cross-multiply and get the following.

$1 \times 50 = 25X$

$50 = 25X$

Then divide both sides of the equation by 25, and the result is 2 capsules.

Desired Over Have

Another common method for dosage calculation is the formula method, or desired over have. This involves thinking of the calculation as to what to give divided by what you have times the quantity you have. So, for that same prescription for diphenhydramine, the equation looks like this.

$$\frac{\text{Desired}}{\text{Have}} \times \text{Quantity} = X$$

$$\frac{50 \text{ mg}}{25 \text{ mg}} \times 1 \text{ cap} = X$$

$$\frac{50}{25} \times 1 = 2 \text{ capsules}$$

Pediatric Dosage Calculations

The most accurate method to determine medication dosage calculations for children is to use weight calculations.

Dosage by Weight

A provider prescribes diphenhydramine 5 mg/kg/day divided into four doses per day for a child who weighs 88 lb. Available is diphenhydramine oral liquid 12.5 mg in 5 mL. How much should the child receive per dose?

First, convert the child's weight to kg.

$$\frac{2.2 \text{ lb}}{1 \text{ kg}} = \frac{88 \text{ lb}}{X \text{ kg}}$$

Cross-multiply and get the following.

$$1 \times 88 = 2.2X$$

$$88 = 2.2X$$

Divide both sides of the equation by 2.2, and the equivalent is 40 kg. Multiply 5 mg by 40 kg to determine the daily dose.

$$5 \text{ mg} \times 40 \text{ kg} = 200 \text{ mg/day}$$

Divide the daily dose into four doses.

$$\frac{300 \text{ mg}}{4} = 50 \text{ mg/dose}$$

Then use either method to determine the amount of liquid medication to give the child. If 12.5 mg equals 5 mL, then 50 mg equals how many (X) mL?

$$\frac{12.5 \text{ mg}}{5 \text{ mL}} = \frac{50 \text{ mg}}{X \text{ mL}}$$

Cross-multiply and get the following.

$5 \times 50 = 12.5X$

$250 = 12.5X$

Divide both sides of the equation by 12.5, and the result is 20 mL.

Body Surface Area

Body surface area (BSA) is widely considered the most accurate way to calculate the dose based on weight for children up to age 12. The provider might calculate BSA using a nomogram and then use a formula to determine the pediatric dosage. Several formulas can be used to figure out the dose. The following is an example.

$$\frac{\text{BSA of child in m}^2}{1.7 \text{ m}^2} \times \text{adult dose} = \text{child's dose}$$

For example, using a BSA of 0.7 and an adult dose of 50 mg.

$$\frac{0.7 \text{ m}^2}{1.7 \text{ m}^2} \times 50 \text{ mg} = 20.5 \text{ mg}$$

20.5 mg is the child's dose. (Follow the rounding rules of the facility.)

Conversions and Formulas

There are several methods for converting one measurement to another within or between measurement systems. Within systems, simple arithmetic is usually sufficient. For example, if a provider prescribes 0.088 mg levothyroxine and the medication comes in micrograms (mcg), the conversion is simple. There is a three-decimal-point difference between milligrams and micrograms. Because the conversion is from a larger value (mg) to a smaller value, the decimal point moves three places to the right.

$0.088 \times 1,000 = 88$ mcg

The proportion method works well for other conversions between systems. This involves thinking of the conversion like this. If 2.2 lb equals 1 kg, then the number of pounds to convert, 66 lb, equals how many (X) kg? Another way to accomplish this calculation is to divide the weight in pounds by 2.2 (because 1 kg = 2.2 lb).

If a patient weighs 66 lb, how many (X) kilograms is this?

1 kg = 2.2 lb, therefore:

$$\frac{66 \text{ lb}}{1 \text{ kg}} = 30 \text{ kg}$$

Or:

$$\frac{2.2 \text{ lb}}{1 \text{ kg}} = \frac{66 \text{ lb}}{X \text{ kg}}$$

Cross-multiply and get the following.

$1 \times 66 = 2.2X$

$66 = 2.2X$

Then divide both sides of the equation by 2.2, and the result is 30 kg.

Here is another example.

The dosage of the medication is 15 mL, but the patient wants to measure it in teaspoons. If 5 mL equals 1 tsp, then 15 mL equals how many (X) tsp?

$$\frac{5 \text{ mL}}{1 \text{ tsp}} = \frac{16 \text{ mL}}{X \text{ tsp}}$$

Cross-multiply and get the following.

$1 \times 15 = 5X$

$15 = 5X$

Then divide both sides of the equation by 5, and the result is 3 tsp.

CHALLENGE

1. Which of the following measurement systems are most commonly used in prescription doses?
   A. Metric
   B. Apothecary
   C. Standard
   D. Household

   A is correct. Most medication prescriptions and dosages will be in the metric system of weights and volume.

2. Why is it important for medical assistants to understand how to convert metric measurements to standard measurements?

   Many at-home medications are prescribed or directed in metric doses. These medications typically come with measurement cups that indicate metric measurements, but patients may misplace these cups and call the clinic for advice on measuring the accurate dosage using standard measurements.

FORMS OF MEDICATION

Medications are available in a variety of formulations.

1.19 Common Medication Formulations

FORMULATIONS	ROUTE	FORMULATIONS	ROUTE
Aerosols	Inhalation	Mist	Inhalation, nasal
Caplets	Oral	Ointments	Topical, ophthalmic, otic, vaginal, rectal
Capsules	Oral	Patches	Topical
Creams	Topical, vaginal, rectal	Powders	Topical
Drops	Otic, ophthalmic, nasal	Powders for reconstitution	IV, IM, subcutaneous, ID
Dry powder for inhalation	Inhalation	Solid extracts, fluid extracts	Oral
Elixirs	Oral	Solutions	Oral, topical, vaginal, urethral, rectal
Emulsions	Oral	Sprays	Topical, nasal, inhalation, sublingual
Foams	Vaginal	Steam	Inhalation
Gels	Oral, topical, rectal	Suppositories	Vaginal, rectal
Injectable liquids	IV, IM, subcutaneous, ID	Suspensions	Oral
Liniments	Topical	Syrups	Oral
Lotions	Topical	Tablets	Oral, buccal, sublingual, vaginal
Lozenges	Oral	Tinctures	Oral, topical

CHALLENGE

1. Match the medication form to the correct route of administration.

FORM	ROUTE
A. Aerosol	1. Vaginal
B. Elixir	2. Nasal, otic, ophthalmic
C. Foam	3. IV
D. Injectable liquid	4. Oral
E. Drops	5. Inhalation
F. Patches	6. Topical

A: 5, B: 4, C: 1, D: 3, E: 2, F: 6
Aerosols are administered through inhalation. Elixirs are administered orally. Foams are administered vaginally. Injectable liquids are administered via IV or IM, subcutaneous, or ID. Drops are administered via nasal route, otic, or ophthalmic. Patches are administered topically.

LOOK-ALIKE AND SOUND-ALIKE MEDICATIONS

Be careful when handling and administering medications that have names or labels that look or sound alike. It is mandatory to check the medication label against the prescription to avoid making potentially serious medication errors.

Perform three checks before administering any medication.

- Check the medication against the prescription when the medication is selected.
- Check the medication and prescription when preparing the dose.
- Recheck the medication before restocking the bottle.

Make every effort to store these medications away from each other or add a labeling system to point out the extra caution staff should use when administering these medications. Often, a medication's brand name might be similar to another medication's generic name, such as clonidine and the brand name of clonazepam, Klonopin. Other pairs that can cause confusion are hydroxyzine and hydralazine or hydrocodone and hydromorphone.

For an extensive list of look-alike and sound-alike medications, see the tools section of the Institute for Safe Medication Practices website.

1.20 Strategies to Avoid Errors in Handling Look-Alike and Sound-Alike Medications

- Do not use abbreviations for medication names.
- Use "tall man" (mixed case) letters to emphasize parts of medication names that could cause confusion (cefoTEtan and cefOXitin).
- Change the appearance of look-alike medication names to alert staff to their differences.
- Create labels with indications or purposes for use, such as adding a "diuretic" label to hydrochlorothiazide packaging.
- Store look-alike or sound-alike medications in separate areas in medication cabinets or rooms.
- Alter computer selection screens to avoid having look-alike medication names appear consecutively.

CHALLENGE

1. Which of the following strategies are recommended for avoiding medication errors due to similar-sounding names? (Select all that apply.)
   A. Store all medications in alphabetical order.
   B. Use "tall man" letters.
   C. Use abbreviations for medication names.
   D. Create labels with indications for use.
   E. Alter computer selection screens to avoid look-alike medication names appearing consecutively.

   B, D, and E are correct. Using "tall man" letters, creating labels that indicate use, and altering computer selection screens are all recommended strategies for avoiding medication errors due to look-alike names. Health care workers should also not use abbreviations and should store look-alike medications in separate cabinets or rooms (rather than organizing them alphabetically) to reduce the risk of errors.

ROUTES OF MEDICATION ADMINISTRATION

Medical assistants use and discuss many different routes for using medications with patients. Providers must include the route of administration on every prescription to avoid undesirable effects that can occur with giving medication by the wrong route.

Medical assistants do not give medications by routes that require nurses or providers: intravenous, epidural, intrathecal, and others.

1.21 Take Note

The most common routes fall into two general categories: enteral (through the gastrointestinal tract) and parenteral (outside the gastrointestinal tract). Most commonly, parenteral refers to injections—intramuscular, intradermal, subcutaneous, and intravenous—but also includes routes like topical, vaginal, and inhalation.

1.22 Nonparenteral Routes

ROUTE	LOCATIONS	MEDICATION FORMULATION
Oral	Mouth, stomach, intestines	Mouth, stomach, intestines

1.24 Common Parenteral Routes for Medications—Injectable

ROUTE	LOCATIONS	MEDICATION FORMULATION
Intradermal	Skin of the upper chest, forearms, upper back	Injectable liquid
Intramuscular (IM)	Deltoid, vastus lateralis, ventrogluteal muscles	Injectable liquid
Subcutaneous (SQ or Sub-Q)	Upper arms, abdomen, buttocks, upper outer thighs	Injectable liquid

1.26 Common Parenteral Routes—Noninjectable

ROUTE	LOCATIONS	MEDICATION FORMULATION
Topical	On the skin	Gels, tinctures, solutions, ointments, lotions, creams, liniments, powders, patches, sprays
Vaginal/rectal	Vagina/vulva, rectum/anus	Suppositories, solutions, creams, ointments, gels, foams

1.23 Needle Insertions

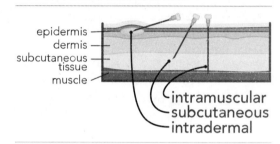

1.25 Areas of Subcutaneous Injections

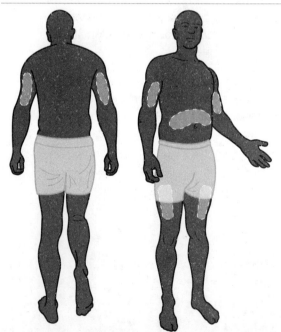

PHARMACOKINETICS (ABSORPTION, DISTRIBUTION, METABOLISM, EXCRETION)

Pharmacokinetics is the study of how medications move through the body. Understanding the four actions pharmacokinetics involves—absorption, distribution, metabolism, and excretion—helps with understanding a medication's onset of activity, the peak time of its effects, and how long its effects will last.

> **CHALLENGE**
>
> 1. Match the route with the correct location.
>
> | ROUTE | LOCATION |
> |---|---|
> | A. Intradermal | 1. Abdomen |
> | B. Intramuscular | 2. Forearm |
> | C. Subcutaneous | 3. Deltoid |
>
> A: 2, B: 3, C: 1
> Intradermal injections go into the skin of the upper chest, forearms, or upper back. Intramuscular injections go into muscles, such as the deltoid, vastus lateralis, and ventrogluteal muscles. Subcutaneous injections go under the skin.

Absorption

Through the process of absorption, the body converts the medication into a form the body can use and moves it into the bloodstream. For example, oral tablets or capsules move through the stomach or intestines to be absorbed. Oral liquids are absorbed the same way but have faster absorption because the fluids in the stomach do not have to break them down into an absorbable form.

The process of absorption also varies with the route. With IV administration, the medication goes directly to the bloodstream, so the onset of action is much quicker than other routes, which must first go through other systems, such as the skin or airways. At least some of every medication, even those for application on a skin rash or as eye drops, can end up in the bloodstream.

The speed of absorption depends on other factors as well, such as how easily the medication dissolves in fat. Medications that are highly fat-soluble pass more readily through cell membranes into the blood. Medications injected into muscle tissue are absorbed more quickly by the body due to blood circulation throughout the skeletal muscle. Another factor is the surface area available for absorption. The stomach has a smaller inner surface area than the intestines, so intestinal absorption is faster. Food slows the absorption of many medications and can inactivate some medications. Medications negatively affected by the gastrointestinal system require parenteral administration, such as by injection.

Distribution

Distribution is the transportation of the medication throughout the body. The bloodstream carries the medication to the body's tissues and organs. There are some barriers to medication distribution. The blood-brain barrier protects the brain from dangerous chemicals but can also make it difficult to get some therapeutic substances into brain tissues. On the other hand, some medications cross the placental barrier very easily, which is why many medications are risky for pregnant patients.

Metabolism

Metabolism changes active forms of the medication into harmless metabolites ready for excretion through urine or feces. The liver is the primary organ of metabolism, but the kidneys also metabolize some medications.

Many factors affect the ability to break down the chemicals in medications. These include the patient's age, how many medications they take, the health of various organs and tissues, and even genetic makeup.

Infants and older adults have the least efficient metabolism, so medication dosages must be modified to compensate for this variation.

Excretion

Excretion is the removal of a medication's metabolites from the body. The kidneys accomplish most of this through urine, but feces, saliva, bile, sweat glands, breast milk, and even exhaled air eliminate some medications. A medication's half-life is how long it takes for the processes of metabolism and excretion to eliminate half a dose of a medication. Some medications have very short half-lives, such as a few minutes, while others take days to leave the body. Knowledge of half-lives helps determine dosing intervals. If a patient does not receive the next dose before the half-life time, the therapeutic level of the medication will be too low (below the therapeutic range) to be effective.

CHALLENGE

1. Which of the four actions of pharmacokinetics affects the ability of a patient who is pregnant to take medications and why?

   Distribution is the transportation of the medication throughout the body. Because many medications can easily cross the placental barrier during distribution, the medications can reach the fetus, which may be dangerous.

2. Which of the following actions of pharmacokinetics changes active forms of the medication into harmless metabolites?
   A. Absorption
   B. Metabolism
   C. Distribution
   D. Excretion

   B is correct. Metabolism changes active forms of the medication into harmless metabolites ready for excretion through urine or feces.

RIGHTS OF MEDICATION ADMINISTRATION

The rights of medication administration are a collection of safety checks that everyone who administers medications to patients must perform to avoid medication errors.

Right Patient

Medical assistants should use two patient identifiers to verify that they are about to administer medication to the right patient. Then verify that data with the information on the medical or medication administration records. The most common verification method is asking patients to state their full name and date of birth. Other acceptable identifiers, such as a mobile phone number or a photo identification card, pertain only to that patient.

1.27 Take Note

It began as the five rights—the right patient, medication, dose, time, and route. Depending on the source, there are now up to twice that many. Most sources agree that the original five, plus the right technique and the right documentation, are the absolute essentials every time a person administers a medication to a patient.

Right Medication

Check the label three times to verify the medication name, strength, and dose—often referred to as the "three befores." This triple-check is essential every time someone gives a patient medication.

- The first time to check the medication label is when taking the medication container from the storage cabinet or drawer.
- The second is when taking the medication from its container to prepare to administer it.
- The third check is when putting the container back in storage or discarding it.

While checking the label, check the medication's expiration date to ensure it has not expired. Otherwise, the medication might be ineffective or even dangerous due to factors such as bacterial contamination. Never administer expired medication, and always dispose of expired medication according to facility guidelines and protocols.

Right Dose

Compare the dosage on the prescription in the patient's medical record on the provider's order with the dosage on the medication's label. If the dosage form available does not match what the provider prescribed, medical assistants must perform the mathematical calculations for administering the right dosage or find a medication container with a dosage form that matches the prescription. They must also double-check any calculations that seem questionable or that they are uncertain about and have another MA or the provider check them as well.

Right Time

In most office and clinic settings, medical assistants give medications right after the provider writes the prescription. Nevertheless, it is essential to confirm whether the medication has any timing specifications, such as the patient having an empty stomach or waiting several hours after taking another medication (such as an antacid) that might interact with the new medication. Make sure to prepare the patient for any immediate effects of the medication. For example, eye drops that dilate the pupils for an eye examination cause blurry vision and photophobia (sensitivity to light) after administration. The patient might not be able to drive until the effects wear off. If the patient does not have an escort or cannot wait in the facility long enough for the medication's effects to wear off, this is the wrong time to administer this medication.

Right Route

Medical assistants must compare the route on the prescription in the medical record with the administration route they are planning to use. Determine that the route is appropriate for the patient and that the medication formulation is right for that route. The correct route of administration can be confirmed with the medication's product insert from the manufacturer, the *Physicians' Desk Reference (PDR)*, or another reliable medication reference. As dictated by the medication's manufacturer, the route of administration must be adhered to.

Physicians' Desk Reference (PDR). Reference book that provides a guide to prescription medication information.

Right Technique

Medical assistants must know and understand the correct techniques for administering medications. For example:

- When administering an intramuscular injection, the correct angle of insertion of the needle is 90 degrees.
- The correct angle of insertion of an intradermal injection is 10 to 15 degrees.
- The correct angle for subcutaneous injections is 45 degrees.

Right Documentation

Always document administering medication after the patient receives it, not before. If the MA does not administer a medication as prescribed, the documentation must include this and why the patient did not receive it. Proper documentation includes date, time, quantity, medication, strength, method and location of administration, lot number, manufacturer, expiration date, and patient outcome, including any reaction or adverse effects a patient may have had to the medication, noting that the patient tolerated it well.

CHALLENGE

1. Which of the following are included in the original or fundamental rights of medication administration? (Select all that apply.)

   A. Right patient
   B. Right medication
   C. Right dose
   D. Right time
   E. Right route
   F. Right technique
   G. Right documentation
   H. Right assessment
   I. Right reason
   J. Right to know

   A, B, C, D, and E are correct. The right patient, right medication, right dose, right time, and right route were the original "five rights." Most sources also agree on the technique and documentation as important rights to include.

SOURCES OF MEDICATION INFORMATION AND FDA REGULATIONS

No health care professional can know everything about every medication. Because of this, medical assistants should have access to reliable, medically approved references they can refer to easily to find information regarding the medications they give. In addition to books and online resources, there are phone apps that have extensive information about thousands of medications. Medical assistants can also find extensive information in the package inserts that come with medications.

Physicians' Desk Reference

Each year, a new edition of the PDR is available. Publishers send free copies to providers' offices, and additional copies are available for purchase. It contains current, detailed information about thousands of medications. The PDR also has a product identification guide with color photographs of many medications. This is useful when patients bring medications to the office in secondary medication containers instead of pharmacy-issued packaging.

Online Medication References

Online sources (manufacturer's websites, government agencies, other online databases) are easy to access when medical assistants have questions about a medication or need more information to share with patients. Use only approved online resources to research medication information, especially when relating that information to patients. Consult providers regarding their preferred sites.

CHALLENGE

1. Where should a medical assistant look for reliable information on medications when needed?

   Medical assistants can find reliable, medically approved medication information through validated books and internet sources, approved phone apps, and package inserts.

NUTRITION

Dietary Nutrients, Suggested Guidelines, and Food Labels

Nutrients are essential food substances—the organic and inorganic materials the body needs for energy and cellular activities like growth, repair, disease resistance, fluid balance, and thermoregulation. Some nutrients, such as vitamins, minerals, and some amino acids, are essential, meaning the body cannot produce them. For example, some protein components must come from foods. Nonessential nutrients are those the body can make. Examples are vitamin D and cholesterol, which do not have to come from the diet.

The body has to break down all the nutrients in the diet into substances it can use. This process begins with digestion. Nutrients that contain calories are proteins, carbohydrates, and fats (lipids). Foods containing calories might contain other nutrients, but water, vitamins, minerals, and fiber do not contain calories. A balance of these nutrients in the diet is essential for everyone, especially for children, patients who are pregnant, and older adults.

Dietary Nutrients and Suggested Guidelines

There are six primary nutrients: water, carbohydrates, protein, fat, minerals, and vitamins. Below are details about each nutrient group. While previous dietary guidelines included daily intake recommendations, most resources have moved away from generalized recommendations. This is because it is now understood, better than ever, that there is no "one size fits all" recommendation regarding *nutrition*.

Guidelines have been released for the years 2020 to 2025. With this release, MyPlate removed all general recommendations for daily intake and replaced them with information about healthy eating based on life stage. To determine specific daily guidelines, individuals can go to myplate.gov and enter information to generate individualized guidelines. These personalized food plans take into account the following.

- Age
- Sex
- Height
- Weight
- Physical activity level

1.28 Take Note

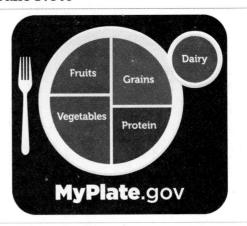

MyPlate (myplate.gov) is a resource developed and managed by the U.S. Department of Agriculture, which takes the most up-to-date Dietary Guidelines for Americans and creates patient-centered resources to distribute the information.

nutrition. The field of study focused on food and the substances in food that help people grow, recover from illnesses, and stay healthy.

Water

The human body is 50% to 80% water. People can survive longer without food than water. Although almost every food and beverage contains water, it is recommended that people still drink 2 to 3 L (64 to 96 oz) each day for optimal health.

Water has many functions, including transporting nutrients and oxygen throughout the body, helping remove waste, regulating body temperature through perspiration, and providing the basic component of blood and other bodily fluids. The body loses water throughout the day in urine, stool, sweat, and water vapor in breath—a total of 1,750 to 3,000 mL each day. Ideally, the body needs to balance intake and output, replenishing fluids the body eliminates with drinking water.

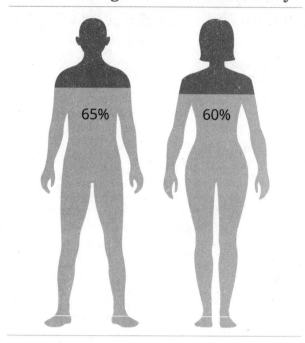

1.29 Percentage of Water in the Body

Protein

Proteins are large, complex molecules the body makes from amino acids, which are the natural compounds that plants and animal foods contain. There are three types of amino acids.

- Essential amino acids are ones the body cannot produce.
- Nonessential amino acids are ones the body can make from essential amino acids or as proteins break down.
- Conditional amino acids are not usually essential but might become essential when the body is undergoing stress or illness.

The body uses amino acids from proteins to repair and build tissues. They can also be used for energy if other sources (carbohydrates and fats) are unavailable. Using protein for energy is wasteful because, over time, the body will lose lean tissues, and muscle strength will diminish. Proteins also contribute to the body's structure, fluid balance, and creation of transport molecules. Each gram of protein provides four calories. Too little protein causes weight loss, malnutrition, fatigue, and increased susceptibility to infection. Too much protein will wind up as body fat or be converted to glucose. The body requires additional protein when recovering from burns, major infections, major trauma, and surgery. Additional protein is also important during pregnancy, breastfeeding, infancy, and adolescence.

Carbohydrates

Carbohydrates are organic compounds that combine carbon, oxygen, and hydrogen into sugar molecules and come primarily from plant sources. Carbohydrates comprise the majority of calories in most diets. Depending on their structure, they are either simple sugars (honey, candy, cane sugar) or complex carbohydrates (fruits, vegetables, cereal, pasta, rice, beans, whole-grain products).

The body uses carbohydrates primarily for energy for its cells and all their functions. Glucose is the simple sugar the body requires for energy needs, and the body burns it more completely and efficiently than it does protein or fat.

Through digestion, the body converts all other digestible carbohydrates into glucose. When the supply of glucose exceeds the demand, the body stores glucose in the liver as glycogen, a ready energy source when the body needs it. Each gram of carbohydrate provides four calories. Too little carbohydrate in the diet results in protein loss, weight loss, and fatigue. Too much can lead to weight gain and tooth decay.

Fats

Fats, or lipids, are a highly concentrated source of energy the body can use as a backup for available glucose. Fat molecules contain fatty acids.

Chemically, the distinctions between fatty acids and the types of fats they form are complex. For dietary purposes, the important difference is the degree of saturation.

- Unsaturated fatty acids are less dense and heavy. They are oils and have less potential for raising cholesterol levels (thus causing heart disease) than saturated fats. Unsaturated fats can be monounsaturated (olive, canola, and peanut oil) or polyunsaturated (corn, sunflower, and safflower oil).

- Trans fat is a fatty acid used to preserve processed food products. It is a byproduct of solidifying polyunsaturated oils (a process called hydrogenation) and raises LDL ("bad") cholesterol levels.

- Saturated fats are solid at room temperature. Primarily from meat products as well as palm and coconut oil, this type of fat also raises LDL. There is no cholesterol in other plant foods.

Fat is an important nutrient that is essential for the absorption of fat-soluble vitamins. Fats provide structure for cell membranes, promote growth in children, maintain healthy skin, assist with protein functions, and help form various hormone-like substances that have important roles, like preventing blood clots and controlling blood pressure. Stored fat has the protective function of insulating and protecting organs. Each gram of fat provides nine calories. Too little fat can cause vitamin deficiencies, fatigue, and dry skin. Too much fat can cause heart disease and obesity.

1.30 Simple vs. Complex Carbs

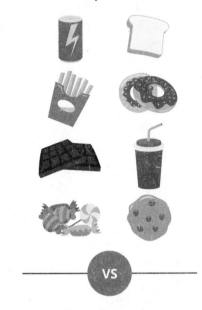

Simple carbs

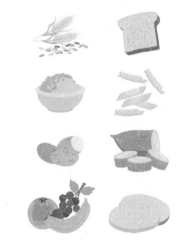

Complex carbs

Vitamins

Vitamins are organic substances the body needs for various cellular functions. Each vitamin has a specific role. Except for vitamins D, A, and B3, the body cannot make them or cannot make enough of them, so they have to be part of dietary intake to promote health and avoid deficiencies. Vitamins do not provide energy, but they are necessary for the body to metabolize energy.

The major classification of vitamins is according to their solubility. This means that their absorption, transportation, storage, and excretion depend on the availability of the substance in which they dissolve.

- Fat-soluble vitamins: A, D, E, K
- Water-soluble vitamins: B1, B2, B3, B6, folate, B12, pantothenic acid, biotin, C

Minerals

Minerals are inorganic substances the body needs in small quantities for building and maintaining body structures. They are essential for life because they contribute to many crucial life functions, like those of the musculoskeletal, neurological, and hematological systems. They provide the rigidity and strength of the bones and contribute to muscle contraction and relaxation. They also help regulate the body's acid-base balance and are essential for normal blood clotting and tissue repair. They are cofactors for enzymes, which means they assist those substances in performing their metabolic functions.

1.31 Food Sources of Vitamins

Vitamins	Food Sources
A	
B_1	
B_2	
B_5	
B_6	
B_9	
B_{12}	
C	
D	
E	
K	
PP	

1.32 Nutrient Food Sources

NUTRIENT	EXAMPLES OF FOOD SOURCES	NUTRIENT	EXAMPLES OF FOOD SOURCES
Water	Plain water; Vegetables; Fruit	Vitamin K	Green and leafy vegetables, dairy products, grain products, meat, eggs, fruits
Protein	Meat, poultry, and fish; Cooked beans; Eggs; Nuts, seeds, nut butters	Pantothenic acid	Meat, grains, legumes, fruits, vegetables
Carbohydrates	Whole grains; Vegetables; Fruits; Rice; Beans; Potatoes	Sodium	Beef, pork, sardines, cheese, green olives, sauerkraut
Fats	Fatty fish (tuna, salmon, sardines); Avocado; Olive oil	Potassium	Whole and skim milk, bananas, prunes, raisins
Vitamin A	Milk fat, meat, leafy vegetables, egg yolks, fish oil, orange and yellow fruits	Calcium	Milk and milk products, meat, eggs, cereals, beans, fruits, vegetables
Vitamin B (generalized)	Fish, meat, poultry, whole grains, seeds, nuts, yeast, avocados, bananas	Phosphorus	Milk, cheese, meat, poultry, cereals, nuts, legumes
Vitamin C	Berries, citrus fruits, green peppers, mangoes, broccoli, potatoes, cauliflower, tomatoes	Magnesium	Green leaves, nuts, cereal grains, seafood
Vitamin D	Sunlight, fortified milk, eggs, fish, liver	Iron	Soybean flour, beef, beans, clams, peaches
Vitamin E	Fortified cereal, nuts, vegetable oils, green and leafy vegetables	Iodine	Seafood, iodized salt, dairy products
Folate	Green and leafy vegetables, beans, asparagus, legumes	Zinc	Vegetables

Food Labels

To succeed in following strict guidelines for nutritional modifications (low sodium, adequate potassium), patients need to understand and use food labels. Reading food labels routinely can be a surprising realization of what is actually being consumed by the body.

The USDA requires food products to contain labels containing details about their contents. These nutritional facts must include specific elements.

- Serving size
- Calories per serving
- Grams of different types of fat
- Amounts of sodium, potassium, cholesterol, total carbohydrates, sugar, and protein
- Percentage of recommended daily values for some vitamins and minerals

Other information is voluntary, and requirements change from time to time.

When showing patients how to read food labels, emphasize that they should check the serving size and number of servings in the package. It is easy to mistake the list of calories and nutrients as the amount in the entire container when it might only be a small percentage of the container. Consider a bottle of a sports drink. After strenuous activity, thirst might dictate drinking the whole container, with the person thinking the amounts of sugar and sodium are reasonable. On closer inspection, those amounts are for one serving, and the bottle contains three servings.

1.33 Sample Food Label

Nutrition Facts		
8 servings per container		
Serving size		2/3 cup (55 g)
Amount per serving		
Calories		**230**
		% Daily Value
Total Fat	8 g	10%
Saturated Fat	1 g	5%
Trans Fat	0 g	
Cholesterol	0 mg	0%
Sodium	160 mg	7%
Total Carbohydrate	37 g	13%
Dietary Fiber	4 g	14%
Total Sugars	12 g	
Includes 10 g added sugar		20%
Protein	3 g	
Vitamin D	2 mcg	10%
Calcium	260 mg	20%
Iron	8 mg	45%
Potassium	235 mg	6%

Serving sizes often vary by manufacturer. These variations can be deceptive, so prepare patients to compare labels critically when choosing a food product. Also, check ingredient lists. The ingredients begin with the one the product contains the most of and then others in descending order.

Emphasize the components that are especially important for each patient's situation. Patients who are at risk for or have heart disease should be cautious about sodium and cholesterol. On the other hand, patients at risk for bone loss will want to check calcium amounts and opt for choices to increase their dietary calcium intake.

CHAPTER 1: FOUNDATIONAL KNOWLEDGE AND BASIC SCIENCE
Vitamins and Supplements

CHALLENGE

1. Match the nutrient with the correct description.

NUTRIENT	DESCRIPTION
A. Water	1. Large, complex molecules the body makes from amino acids
B. Protein	2. Inorganic substances the body needs in small quantities for building and maintaining body structures
C. Carbohydrates	3. Highly concentrated energy sources
D. Fats	4. Makes up 50% to 80% of the body
E. Vitamins	5. Organic compounds that combine carbon, oxygen, and hydrogen into sugar molecules
F. Minerals	6. Organic substances the body needs for various cellular functions

A: 4, B: 1, C: 5, D: 3, E: 6, F: 2
The human body is 50% to 80% water. Proteins are large, complex molecules the body makes from amino acids, which are the natural compounds that plants and animal foods contain. Carbohydrates are organic compounds that combine carbon, oxygen, and hydrogen into sugar molecules and come primarily from plant sources. Fats, or lipids, are a highly concentrated source of energy the body can use as a backup for available glucose. Vitamins are organic substances the body needs for various cellular functions. Minerals are inorganic substances the body needs in small quantities for building and maintaining body structures.

2. Which of the following aspects of food labels gives necessary context to all other information found on the label?
   A. Serving size
   B. Grams of fat
   C. Amount of sodium
   D. Percentage of the daily recommended value

A is correct. When teaching a patient about food labels, they must understand how to check the serving size. Serving sizes vary by manufacturer and can be misleading. Understanding the serving size will help the patient to know how much they are truly consuming in terms of all other categories listed on the food label.

VITAMINS AND SUPPLEMENTS

Vitamins and supplements are extremely common and are marketed to consumers as an easy way to improve health. The reality is that the best source of vitamins and nutrients needed for healthy living comes from whole foods, though many people take vitamin supplements in addition to their diet. The FDA monitors herbal and other supplements with much looser guidelines and monitoring than over-the-counter medications.

Patients should discuss any new vitamins or supplements with their provider before taking them. When reviewing medication lists during patient intake and the patient interview, ask about vitamin and supplement usage and document anything the patient takes. There can be dangers associated with taking them, such as interactions with prescription medications or negative impact on chronic conditions. A provider may recommend a supplemental vitamin, especially if the patient has a condition that reduces the ability to process that vitamin from natural food sources.

1.34 Common Vitamins and Supplements: Intended Benefits and Safety Considerations

VITAMIN/ SUPPLEMENT	FUNCTION/INTENDED BENEFIT	SAFETY CONSIDERATIONS
Vitamin A	Night vision, cell growth and maintenance, the health of the skin	Toxicity can occur if levels are too high, leading to headaches, peeling skin, and bone thickening.
Vitamin D	Calcium absorption, bone and tooth health, heart and nerve function	Toxicity can occur if levels are too high, leading to kidney failure, metastatic calcification, and anorexia.
Vitamin E	Protection of cells (including skin and brain), formation of blood cells	N/A
Vitamin K	Blood clotting, bone growth	Can counteract blood clotting medications, reducing their efficiency
Vitamin B1	Carbohydrate metabolism, heart, nerve, and muscle function	N/A
Vitamin B2	Fat and protein metabolism	N/A
Vitamin B3	Carbohydrate and fat metabolism	Toxicity can occur if levels are too high, leading to red, itching skin with tingling.
Vitamin B6	Enzyme assistance in the amino acid synthesis	Toxicity can occur if levels are too high, leading to peripheral neuropathy.
Vitamin B12	Protein and fat metabolism, nerve-cell maintenance, cell development	N/A
Vitamin C	Immunity, iron absorption, the structure of bones, muscle, and blood vessels	N/A
St. John's wort	Treatment for depression, anxiety, and sleep disorders	Some studies found it ineffective in its intended benefits (similar results to a placebo). No long-term safety studies have been conducted.

1.34 Common Vitamins and Supplements: Intended Benefits and Safety Considerations (continued)

VITAMIN/SUPPLEMENT	FUNCTION/INTENDED BENEFIT	SAFETY CONSIDERATIONS
Black cohosh	Relief of menopause symptoms, including hot flashes, night sweats, headaches, heart palpitations, and mood changes	Large doses can cause vomiting, dizziness, and headaches. Long-term studies have yet to be conducted (recommended to take for less than 6 months).
Melatonin	Melatonin is a naturally occurring hormone in the brain. Also can be taken as a supplement to potentially help with sleep regulation and combat aging (studies validate the support of sleep regulation but do not support anti-aging benefits).	Can result in drowsiness and headaches May interfere with conception
Willow bark	Pain relief (one of the main ingredients of aspirin comes from willow bark)	Do not exceed 240 mg/day Not safe for those who cannot tolerate aspirin
Glucosamine sulfate	Promote healthy cartilage formation to maintain or replace wear and tear on joints	No safety concerns Recent studies found glucosamine sulfate to be no more effective than a placebo in knee osteoarthritis.
Gingko biloba	Improve memory and mental function by increasing blood flow to the brain	Extremely high doses can lead to nausea, vomiting, and diarrhea.

CHALLENGE

1. Which of the following vitamins is known to improve night vision?
   A. Vitamin A
   B. Vitamin B12
   C. Vitamin C
   D. Vitamin D

   A is correct. Vitamin A has been shown to promote eye health, specifically concerning vision at night or in dark settings.

2. Match the supplement with the intended benefit.

SUPPLEMENT	INTENDED BENEFIT
A. St. John's wort	1. Improved memory
B. Black cohosh	2. Treatment for depression
C. Willow bark	3. Relief of menopause symptoms
D. Gingko biloba	4. Pain relief

   A: 2, B: 3, C: 4, D: 1
   St. John's wort treats depression, anxiety, and sleep disorders. Black cohosh relieves menopause symptoms, including hot flashes, night sweats, headaches, heart palpitations, and mood changes. Willow bark provides pain relief. Gingko biloba improves memory and mental function by increasing blood flow to the brain.

DIETARY NEEDS RELATED TO DISEASES AND CONDITIONS

In addition to factors such as age, sex, height, and weight, certain diseases also need to be considered when considering a healthy diet. When coaching a patient on nutrition, the patient's provider should approve recommendations to ensure they align with the patient's chronic conditions and treatment plans.

Dietary Needs for Diabetes

Type II diabetes is a chronic condition often connected to an individual's food intake. In the most general terms, diabetes is defined by the body's inability to turn food into energy properly. If caught and managed early, it is sometimes possible to entirely manage diabetes through diet. Over time, the need for medications increases, but careful blood sugar management through food intake can greatly reduce this need.

The goal of a healthy diet for a person who has diabetes is to control blood sugar levels, preventing blood sugar from going too high and too low. Careful planning and managing food intake can promote the stability and consistency of blood sugar.

General dietary guidelines for patients who have diabetes include the following.

- Eating several small, nutrient-dense meals consistently throughout the day.
- Avoiding or severely limiting foods high in added sugars. Properly balancing blood sugar is essential when high-sugar foods are consumed.
- Limiting foods high in carbohydrates, especially those with refined grains.
- Consuming more fiber. Fiber is an essential nutrient to help break down carbohydrates.

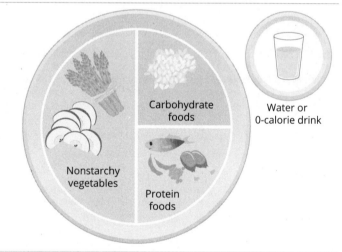

1.35 **MyPlate for Diabetes**

The CDC recommends following the plate method for easy diabetes management. The plate method centers around how to fill up a 9-inch dinner plate.

- ½ of the plate should be non-starchy vegetables, including green, leafy vegetables, cauliflower, or carrots.
- ¼ of the plate should be foods higher in carbs, ideally whole grains or other whole foods such as peas, potatoes, whole grain rice or pasta, beans, fruit, or yogurt.
- ¼ of the plate should be a lean protein such as chicken, turkey, beans, or tofu.
- Water is the best choice for a drink, but other zero-calorie (sugar-free) drinks can be substituted if strongly preferred.

Dietary Needs for Kidney Disease

Chronic kidney disease (CKD) is the gradual decrease in kidney function, and it impacts millions of Americans. It is most common in older adults as kidney function decreases. Many people may have early-stage (1 to 3) CKD without knowing it. As kidney function worsens and reaches stages 4 to 5, symptoms become more apparent, and the impact is greater. Annual blood work can help catch CKD early. Medications are typically not recommended in early stages, and diet is the primary intervention.

The U.S. Department of Health and Human Services recommends the following steps for altering a diet to prevent or mitigate further kidney damage (Note: Steps 1 to 3 should be implemented at any stage of CKD; steps 4 to 5 are most important for those in late-stage CKD.).

1.36 Dietary Modifications for Kidney Disease

STEP	ACTION/REASONS	OPTIMAL FOOD SELECTIONS
Step 1	Limit salt/sodium. • High blood pressure is a primary contributing factor to worsened kidney function. • Limiting sodium intake to less than 2,300 mg/day is optimal for those with CKD to prevent extra strain on the kidneys.	Swap prepared or packaged foods for fresh foods to avoid added sodium. Opt for salt/sodium-free spices to flavor food. Select foods with less than a 20% daily value of sodium. Rinse canned foods with fresh water before eating or cooking them.
Step 2	Be cautious with protein. • Protein is essential in any diet but also creates waste, which strains the kidneys. • Eat protein-rich foods with meals. • Discuss with your provider if animal-based or plant-based (or a combination) proteins are best.	Animal proteins • Chicken • Fish • Meat • Eggs • Dairy Plant proteins • Beans • Nuts • Grains
Step 3	Protect your heart. Eating heart-healthy foods will help prevent fat and cholesterol from building up in your heart, blood vessels, and kidneys.	Lean meats • Skinless poultry • Fish • Beans • Vegetables • Low-fat or fat-free milk products

1.36 Dietary Modifications for Kidney Disease *(continued)*

STEP	ACTION/REASONS	OPTIMAL FOOD SELECTIONS
Step 4	Minimize phosphorus intake. • As kidney function decreases, kidneys will no longer effectively filter out excess phosphorus levels. • Excess phosphorus in the blood can damage bones, leading to a higher risk of fractures, and can also damage blood vessels.	Low-phosphorus foods • Fresh fruits and vegetables • Bread, pasta, rice • Corn and rice cereals • Non-enriched rice milk Higher-phosphorus foods to limit • Meat, poultry, fish • Dairy • Bran cereals • Beans, lentils, and nuts
Step 5	Control potassium levels. • Severe kidney damage can lead to increased potassium in the bloodstream. • Potassium levels that are too high or too low can be very dangerous and damaging to the heart, muscles, and nerves. • Understanding potassium levels in food and discussing dietary changes related to potassium with a doctor are essential in late-stage CKD.	Lower-potassium foods • Apples • Peaches • White bread and pasta • White rice • Non-enriched rice milk Higher-potassium foods • Oranges • Bananas • Brown and wild rice • Bran cereals • Dairy • Whole-wheat bread and pasta • Beans and nuts

Source: https://www.niddk.nih.gov/health-information/kidney-disease/chronic-kidney-disease-ckd/prevention

Dietary Needs for Celiac Disease

Celiac disease is an autoimmune disorder in which individuals cannot safely consume gluten, a protein substance found naturally in wheat, barley, and rye. While many people may avoid gluten due to its potential to cause unpleasant bloating and digestion symptoms, those with celiac disease will incur damage to their small intestine if gluten is consumed. The primary treatment for celiac disease is eating a gluten-free diet.

Tips from the U.S. Department of Health and Human Services for those with celiac disease include the following.

- Look for foods labeled "gluten-free," "no gluten," "free of gluten," or "without gluten."
- Avoid foods made with ingredients that naturally contain gluten: wheat, barley, and rye. Be cautious of the following.
    - Baked goods
    - Baking mixes
    - Alcohols
    - Malt vinegar
    - Additives and flavorings
- Be cautious of cross-contact, especially when eating out at a restaurant.
- Prepare and store gluten-free foods separately from foods with gluten that other household members might be consuming.
- Opt for naturally gluten-free foods whenever possible, including the following.
    - Meat
    - Fish
    - Fruits and vegetables
    - Rice
    - Potatoes
    - Flour made from gluten-free foods, such as quinoa, buckwheat, soy, and nuts

CHALLENGE

1. The CDC's recommendations for food distribution for those with diabetes are based on a dinner plate of what size?
    A. 5 inches
    B. 7 inches
    C. 9 inches
    D. 12 inches

   C is correct. The plate method centers around how to fill up a 9-inch dinner plate.

2. Patients in which of the following stages of chronic kidney disease should monitor their phosphorus and potassium levels? (Select all that apply.)
    A. Stage 1
    B. Stage 2
    C. Stage 3
    D. Stage 4
    E. Stage 5

   D and E are correct. As kidney disease worsens, the kidneys are less able to filter out and maintain healthy levels of phosphorus and potassium in the blood. Patients in stages 4 and 5 of CKD must be cautious about this.

3. Which of the following foods would be the safest option for a person who has celiac disease?
    A. Whole-grain bread
    B. Malt vinegar
    C. Quinoa
    D. Beer

   C is correct. People living with celiac disease cannot safely consume gluten. Gluten is naturally found in wheat, barley, and rye. Bread, malt vinegar, and beer contain gluten unless specifically marked otherwise. Quinoa is a naturally gluten-free grain. Naturally gluten-free foods are always the safest option in the setting of celiac disease.

EATING DISORDERS

Medical assistants are likely to encounter patients who have eating disorders, which are food patterns that can impair health and well-being. The most common are anorexia nervosa, bulimia nervosa, and binge-eating disorder.

Anorexia

Anorexia nervosa affects people of all ages, genders, and races. Characteristically, patients are high achievers who exert severe control over their eating patterns. Often, there is a family history of anorexia and alcohol use disorder. Some patients have histories of childhood trauma, depression, major life changes, and high stress levels.

Warning signs and symptoms of anorexia nervosa include the following.

- Self-starvation
- Perfectionism
- Extreme sensitivity to criticism
- Excessive fear of weight gain
- Weight loss of at least 15%
- Amenorrhea (no menstrual periods)
- Denial of feelings of hunger
- Excessive exercising
- Ritualistic eating behavior
- Extreme control of behavior
- Unrealistic image of the self as obese

Medical assistants who observe or suspect any of these manifestations should alert the provider immediately, as this disorder can be life-threatening. Treatment involves hospitalization with parenteral nutrition or nasogastric feedings, plus psychotherapy. Educating the patient and family about nutrition is also essential.

Bulimia

Bulimia nervosa involves eating large amounts of food (binging) and then purging by self-induced vomiting, laxatives, or diuretics. It is controlling behavior, usually aimed at gaining control of weight. Sometimes it is caused by gaining some weight and dieting unsuccessfully to lose weight. People who have bulimia can feel guilty when they overeat or eat high-calorie foods and then attempt to alleviate the guilt by eliminating the food they eat. People who have this disorder often define their value as being thin and might previously have been thin. For a variety of reasons, they cannot control their eating habits. Those who seek treatment are most often in their 20s.

Warning signs and symptoms of bulimia nervosa include the following.

- Buying and consuming large amounts of food
- Purging after eating excessive amounts of food
- When dining with others, using the bathroom immediately after eating
- Using laxatives and diuretics
- Keeping weight constant while overeating fattening foods
- Mood swings
- Depression and guilt after binging and purging

Medical assistants who observe or suspect any of these manifestations should alert the provider immediately. Although this disorder is not life-threatening, it can cause lesions in the esophagus, erosion of tooth enamel, and electrolyte and hormone imbalances. Treatment involves psychotherapy, medication for anxiety and depression, dental work, nutrition counseling, and support groups.

Binge Eating

Binge eating disorder is similar to bulimia nervosa, without the purging behavior. With this disorder, people chronically overeat. The major manifestation is weight gain and obesity. Obesity increases the risk of heart disease, hypertension, type 2 diabetes mellitus, stroke, cancer, joint disorders, GERD, and sleep apnea. People who are obese often have heartburn, bloating, abdominal pain, diarrhea, and other gastrointestinal problems. With binge eating disorder, patients do not restrict their diet between binging episodes, often eat quickly until they are uncomfortably full, eat when not hungry, and eat alone due to feelings of shame and guilt about overeating. Food becomes an addiction or a coping mechanism, predisposing patients to alcohol and substance use disorders.

Medical assistants who suspect this disorder should alert the provider immediately. Treatment involves focusing on eating healthy food, self-acceptance, awareness of hunger and fullness, and engaging progressively in enjoyable physical activity. For some, keeping a food diary helps provide a realistic picture of how much food they consume. Discussion with a counselor about their feelings and emotions about eating can also help. Psychotherapy is effective in reducing the frequency and severity of binge episodes.

CHALLENGE

1. Match the eating disorder with the correct definition.

EATING DISORDER	DEFINITION
A. Anorexia nervosa	1. Binging and purging
B. Binge eating	2. Refusal to eat
C. Bulimia nervosa	3. Chronic overeating

A: 2, B: 3, C: 1
Anorexia nervosa is an eating disorder in which a patient refuses to eat over a period of time. Bulimia nervosa involves eating large amounts of food (binging) and then purging by self-induced vomiting, laxatives, or diuretics. Binge eating disorder is similar to bulimia nervosa, without purging behavior.

WRAP-UP

Success in the MA role is driven by a solid foundational knowledge of many different topics. The MA should understand their role and responsibility, including administrative and clinical responsibilities. They must also understand other roles of health professionals and their scope of work.

Understanding basic concepts of medication is also important for medical assistants. There are numerous medication classifications, typically categorized by the action of the medication. Medical assistants working with controlled substances must understand the five schedules, including the regulations around prescribing, storing, and disposing of each.

Due to similar-sounding names, many medications can be easily confused. Adhering to safety recommendations can help prevent medication errors. Follow the "three befores" and comply with the rights of medication administration when tasked with administering medication to a patient. If unsure of a medication, refer to reputable resources to obtain further information.

The MA must also know basic nutrition. Balanced nutrition plays a vital role in helping patients meet their greatest potential for health and wellness and managing many diseases and disorders. Every dietary nutrient—proteins, carbohydrates, fats, vitamins, minerals, and water—has an important function. With a proper understanding of nutrients, medical assistants can provide patients with approved information that may help them correct deficiencies, manage weight, and gain better control of acute and chronic health problems.

CHAPTER 2
Medical Terminology, Anatomy, and Physiology

OVERVIEW

A foundational understanding of the body components and systems is central to the MA role. In addition to understanding how the body should work, it is important to understand the many diseases, conditions, and deviations that can affect the body. Medical assistants do not diagnose or treat disease, but understanding common diseases, signs, symptoms, potential diagnostic measures, and treatments will equip medical assistants to better support providers and patients. This knowledge includes mental health conditions and basic psychology principles, because mental wellness is closely related to physical wellness. An ability to understand the big picture of what patients may experience and how to support them in these events is imperative to success.

Medical terminology is the language of the medical field and is an important aspect of understanding the body, disease states, and treatment options. Understanding how to form medical words will help explain the concepts of anatomy and physiology and allow understanding of new medical terminology encountered.

Objectives

Upon completion of this chapter, you should be able to

- Identify cell structure (nucleus, cell membrane, cytoplasm, ribosomes, mitochondria, lysosomes).
- Describe anatomical structures, locations, and positions.
- Compare structure and function of major body systems, including organs and their locations.
- Characterize interactions between organ systems and homeostasis.
- Identify signs, symptoms, and etiology of common diseases, conditions, and injuries.
- Recall diagnostic measures (labs, imaging, biopsies) and treatment modalities (infusion, chemotherapy, medication, surgery).
- Outline incidence, prevalence, risk factors, and comorbidities.
- Describe epidemics and pandemics.
- Define common abbreviations, acronyms, and symbols.
- Assemble medical word building (roots, prefixes, suffixes, plurals).
- Identify The Joint Commission's "Do Not Use" List.
- Define lay terms and medical terms for common conditions, symptoms, and procedures.
- Label positional and directional terminology.
- Differentiate developmental stages.
- Identify signs and symptoms of common mental health conditions (anxiety, depression, PTSD, ADHD).
- Describe environmental and socioeconomic stressors.
- Characterize psychology for those who have physical disabilities, developmental delays, and diseases.
- Describe defense mechanisms.
- Describe end of life and stages of grief.

ANATOMY AND PHYSIOLOGY

Body Structure and Organ Systems

Cell Structure

Cells are the building blocks of life. Every living thing starts as a single cell, which duplicates exponentially over time. Cells all have the same foundational components. Some cells have specific functions that require additional components.

2.1 Cell Structure

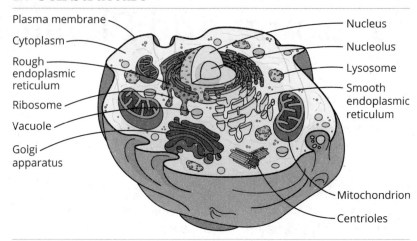

2.2 Primary Components of Human Cells

COMPONENT	DESCRIPTION	FUNCTION
Plasma membrane	Selectively permeable membrane (allows only certain substances through) made of phospholipids and proteins surrounding the entire cell	Separates the internal components of the cell from the surrounding environment Essential to the life of the cell
Cytoplasm	Gel-like fluid filling the inside of the cell that is comprised primarily of water, with electrolytes, metabolic waste products, and nutrients dissolved within it	Contains many suspended organelles, or cell structures Medium for chemical reactions
Nucleus	Large, spherical body near the center of the cell containing genetic material in the form of DNA	Control center of the cell Regulates cell activity Houses genetic material
Nuclear membrane	Double-layered, porous membrane surrounding the nucleus	Protects the nucleus, allowing in only specific materials
Nucleolus	Dark, dense body within the nucleus without an enclosing membrane; most cells contain one to four	Forms RNA and ribosomes
Mitochondria	Elongated, rod-shaped bodies filled with fluid, containing DNA Known as the "power plant" of the cell	Convert nutrients into energy for use by the cell/body; create adenosine triphosphate (ATP)
Ribosomes	Small granules of RNA found in the nucleolus or cytoplasm	Protein synthesis for both internal and external use
Cilia	Short, hair-like microtubules projecting from the cell membrane	Aid in the movement of substances along the surface of the cell
Flagella	Long, hair-like microtubules, projecting from the cell membrane	Move the cell itself, through a whip-like motion

2.2 Primary Components of Human Cells (continued)

COMPONENT	DESCRIPTION	FUNCTION
Endoplasmic reticulum	Complex connection of membranous fluid-filled, flat sacs and tubular channels	Transports materials throughout the cell
	Connects the cell membrane to the nucleus membrane, as well as some organelles	RER: Supports the synthesis and transport of proteins
	Comprised of the rough endoplasmic reticulum (RER) and smooth endoplasmic reticulum (SER)	SER: Supports the synthesis of some lipid molecules, including steroids
Golgi apparatus	Four to six flat membranous sacs, connected to the endoplasmic reticulum; typically found near the nucleus	"Packaging and shipping plant" of the cell
		Packages and releases materials secreted by the cell for external use
		Forms lysosomes for sure within the cell
Lysosomes	Sacs surrounded by membranes created by the Golgi apparatus	Digest waste materials including damaged materials found in the cell, old cell components, and materials entering the cell
Cytoskeleton	Comprised of protein microfilaments and microtubules	Maintains the shape and structure of the cell
		Keeps organelles in place and moves them throughout the cell as needed
Centrioles	Pair of rod-shaped bodies made of microtubules found near the nucleus	Participate in cell reproduction through the distribution of DNA to new cells

CHALLENGE

1. Match the cell component with its description.

CELL COMPONENT	DESCRIPTION
A. Plasma membrane B. Nucleus C. Mitochondria D. Golgi apparatus	1. Flattened membranous sacs connected to the endoplasmic reticulum 2. Elongated, rod-shaped bodies filled with fluid 3. Large, spherical body near the center of the cell 4. Made of phospholipids and proteins surrounding the cell

A: 4, B: 3, C: 2, D: 1
The plasma membrane is a selectively permeable membrane made of phospholipids and proteins surrounding the entire cell. The nucleus is a large, spherical body near the center of the cell containing genetic material in the form of DNA. Mitochondria are elongated, rod-shaped bodies filled with fluid, containing DNA. Golgi apparatus is four to six flattened membranous sacs, connected to the endoplasmic reticulum.

2. Which of the following cell organelles is responsible for transporting materials throughout the cell?

   A. Nucleolus
   B. Ribosomes
   C. Endoplasmic reticulum
   D. Mitochondria

   C is correct. The endoplasmic reticulum is a complex connection of membranous sacs and channels responsible for transporting materials throughout the cell.

ANATOMICAL STRUCTURES, LOCATIONS, AND POSITIONS

Familiarity with tissues, organs, and body systems aids in communicating with and providing optimal care for patients. Each of the divisions of the body has specific duties and locations. The human body can be studied according to each structure and how it functions.

Planes of the Body

Three main planes describe sections of the body and are also frequently used with various radiographic studies. These planes are used for discussing and documenting locations.

- *Sagittal plane:* Divides the body into left and right sides. Midsagittal refers to an equal division of left and right sides, running along the midline of the body.
- *Transverse plane:* Divides the body into upper and lower sections, not necessarily equally
- *Frontal plane:* Also called coronal plane, divides the body into anterior and posterior sections

2.3 Body Planes

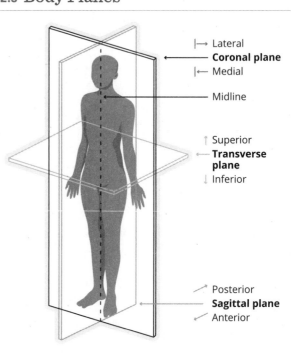

Body Cavities

The human body can be studied according to each division of five cavities and their internal organs.

- *Cranial cavity:* Within the skull; houses the meninges (brain)
- *Spinal cavity:* Traveling down the midline of the back and formed by the vertebrae, this contains the spinal cord
- *Thoracic cavity:* Within the chest; houses the lungs, heart, and major vessels
- *Abdominal cavity:* Within the abdomen; houses several major organs such as the stomach, liver, gallbladder, and intestines
- *Pelvic cavity:* Inferior to the abdominal cavity; houses the bladder and reproductive organs

Body Quadrants and Regions

The abdomen can be divided into four quadrants or nine regions, either of which is helpful as reference during physical examination of internal organs. Familiarity with each quadrant assists in correctly documenting a patient's chief complaint pertaining to issues related to the abdomen.

2.4 Body Quadrants

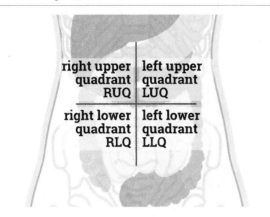

right upper quadrant RUQ	left upper quadrant LUQ
right lower quadrant RLQ	left lower quadrant LLQ

2.5 Body Regions

right hypo-chondriac region	epi-gastric region	left hypo-chondriac region
right lumbar region	umbilical region	left lumbar region
right iliac region	hypo-gastric region	left iliac region

STRUCTURE AND FUNCTION OF MAJOR BODY SYSTEMS

Body systems are groups of organs working together to perform complex tasks. When body systems perform efficiently, the body achieves *homeostasis*. When there is a disruption in the function of a body system, the result can be minor or significant, from a headache to organ failure. The following section reviews the components and functions of each body system.

> **CHALLENGE**
>
> 1. Match the body cavity with the body part it houses.
>
> | BODY CAVITY | BODY PART |
> | --- | --- |
> | A. Cranial cavity | 1. Liver |
> | B. Thoracic cavity | 2. Bladder |
> | C. Abdominal cavity | 3. Brain |
> | D. Pelvic cavity | 4. Lungs |
>
> A: 3, B: 4, C: 1, D: 2
> The cranial cavity is within the bony cranium and houses the meninges (brain). The thoracic cavity is within the chest and houses the lungs, heart, and major vessels. The abdominal cavity is within the abdomen and houses several major organs, such as stomach, liver, and gallbladder. The pelvic cavity is inferior to the abdominal cavity and houses the bladder.

Integumentary System

The following make up the integumentary system.

- **Skin:** Responsible for protection, temperature regulation, sensation, excretion, and vitamin D production

  ○ **Epidermis layer:** Outermost layer of epithelial tissue, covers the external surface of the body

  ○ **Dermis layer:** Thick layer beneath the dermis that contains arteries, veins, nerves

  ○ **Subcutaneous layer:** Loose, connective tissue composed of adipose tissue and lipocytes

- **Hair follicles:** Generate hair

- **Sebaceous (oil) glands:** Produce sebum to keep skin and hair soft and prevent bacteria from growing on the skin

- **Fingernails and toenails:** Protect the ends of fingers and toes

- **Sudoriferous (sweat) glands:** Produce sweat to aid in cooling the body

The largest organ of the body is the skin. Hair, nails, and glands are accessory organs of this system. The skin has several functions, which the accessory organs also aid in.

homeostasis. State in which the body's systems and biological processes maintain stability.

2.6 Layers of Skin

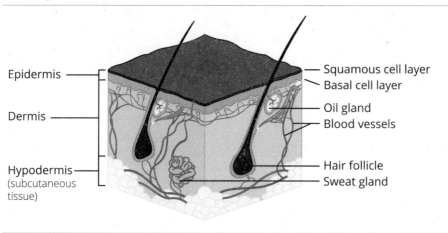

Skin Functions

- **Protection:** The skin is the body's first defense against illness and injury. It also protects the body's internal structures from dehydration and UV exposure.
- **Temperature regulation:** The skin plays a significant role in the body's ability to maintain and regulate its temperature. When a person is hot or cold, superficial blood vessels in the skin dilate or constrict to control the flow of blood to the surface of the skin, aiding in warming or cooling.
- **Excretion:** Perspiring aids in cooling the body but also results in the loss of water and minerals.
- **Sensation:** The skin is loaded with nerve receptors to detect sensations (heat, cold, pain).
- **Vitamin D production:** The body needs vitamin D to absorb calcium, which is needed for bone strength. Vitamin D comes from sun exposure to the skin.

Skeletal System

The skeletal system includes the following.

- **Axial skeleton:** The adult axial skeleton has 80 bones, including the skull, vertebrae, and ribs.
- **Appendicular skeleton:** The adult appendicular skeleton has 126 bones, including arms, legs, and pelvic girdle.
- **Ligament:** The ligaments attach bone to bone for joint stability.
- **Tendons:** The tendons join muscles to bones that help in moving extremities. Tendons in the muscular system help avoid muscle injury by absorbing some of the impact muscles take.
- **Connective tissue/cartilage:** This tissue maintains, protects, and gives form to other tissues and organs. Cartilage is a part of connective tissue found in the larynx and respiratory tract. It also covers and protects the end of long bones.

The skeletal system gives the body structure and posture, as well as protecting the soft internal organs from injury. The skeletal system also plays a key role by serving as attachment points for muscles in the body. This symbiotic relationship between bones and muscles often results in the systems being referenced as one (the musculoskeletal system). Bones of the skeletal system are classified by shape.

Bone Types

- **Long bones:** These bones have epiphysis, diaphysis, and medullary cavity containing yellow bone marrow. The ends of long bones are covered by articular cartilage to allow joint movement without causing friction. Examples: femur, humerus, tibia, fibula, ulna, radius

- **Short bones:** These are found in the wrists and ankles. Short bones are typically small and round. Examples: carpals, tarsals

- **Flat bones:** The majority of surface area of these bones are flat or slightly curved. Examples: skull, ribs

- **Irregular bones:** These include bones with an unusual shape that is typically related to its function. Examples: vertebrae, pelvis

- **Sesamoid bones:** These small, round bones are found in joints that are held in place by tendons. Example: patella

- **Red bone marrow:** Found within bones, marrow is responsible for producing new blood cells. This process is known as hematopoiesis. Bones also store calcium, which is essential for proper cell function.

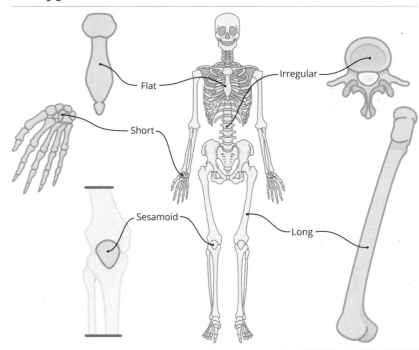

2.7 **Types of Bones**

Bones of the Appendicular Skeleton

- Upper extremities
  - Scapula
  - Clavicle
  - Humerus
  - Radius
  - Ulna
  - Carpals
  - Metacarpals
  - Phalanges
- Lower extremities
  - Pelvic girdle
  - Femur
  - Patella
  - Tibia
  - Fibula
  - Tarsals
  - Metatarsals
  - Phalanges

Bones of the Axial Skeleton

- Skull
- Cervical vertebrae
- Thoracic vertebrae
- Lumbar vertebrae
- Sacrum
- Coccyx
- Ribs

2.8 The Human Skeleton

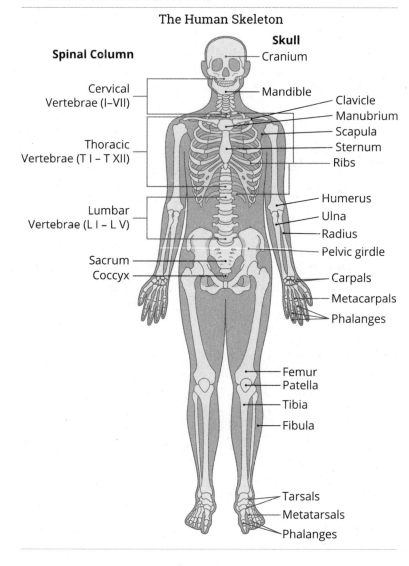

Muscular System

The muscular system is made up of the following.

- **Skeletal muscle:** Responsible for body movement; also called voluntary muscle or striated muscle
- **Smooth muscle:** Found within the walls of hollow organs and blood vessels and in the iris of the eye; also called involuntary muscle
- **Cardiac muscle:** Found only in the heart; cross-fibered to allow the heart to contract from the top and bottom to pump blood
- **Tendons:** Ends of skeletal muscles that attach the muscle to a bone

Muscles are responsible for movement, both voluntary (like walking) and involuntary (like digestion). The heart muscle is made of specialized fibers that allow it to function as a pump. The muscles and skeleton work together to provide posture, movement, and other essential body functions.

2.9 Types of Muscle

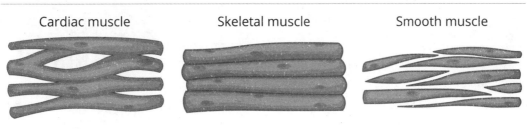

Immune and Lymphatic Systems

The lymphatic system includes the following.

- **Lymph nodes:** Small, glandular structures concentrated in the neck, axilla, and groin that produce and store lymphocytes. Lymph nodes are home to macrophages that filter lymph.
- **Lymph nodules:** Masses of lymphoid tissue comprised of macrophages and lymphocytes. Lymph nodules are not encapsulated like lymph nodes.
- **Thymus:** Located posterior to the sternum. The thymus is large in children and atrophies (shrinks) after adolescence. It is responsible for the production and maturation of T-cells.
- **Spleen:** Largest lymphoid organ, located in the upper-left quadrant of the abdomen. It is home to macrophages that filter the blood.
- **Interstitial fluid:** Tissue fluid found between cells. Once collected and filtered, it is called lymph.

2.10 Take Note

Creating immunity, or the ability to resist pathogens, is an essential function of the immune system. People are born with some immunity and develop more over time.

CHAPTER 2: MEDICAL TERMINOLOGY, ANATOMY, AND PHYSIOLOGY
Structure and Function of Major Body Systems

The immune system relies on the lymphatic system to prevent infections in the body. When a pathogen is detected, the lymphatic system begins activating the body's defenses. A major component of these defenses are B-cells and T-cells.

- *Antigen:* Foreign substance within the body
- *Antibody:* Protein the body creates in response to specific antigens
- **Immunoglobulins:** Antibodies
- **B-cells:** Type of lymphocyte that can recognize antigens and responds by turning into plasma cells; these plasma cells then create antibodies against specific antigens
- **T-cells:** Type of lymphocyte that can recognize antigens and attaches to them to attack the invading cells directly
- **Monocytes:** Engulf and destroy pathogens that have been coagulated with antibodies

Some immunity occurs from being exposed to pathogens, and other types of immunity are developed through immunizations. There are four primary types of immunity.

Types of Primary Immunity

- **Naturally acquired active immunity:** This occurs when a person has an infectious disease and then develops antibodies against the pathogen that caused the disease. The antibodies have a memory that prevents future infections by the same pathogen.
- **Artificially acquired active immunity:** This type of immunity is the result of administering a vaccination. The antibodies are activated by the vaccine and develop memory to recognize the pathogen in the future.
- **Naturally acquired passive immunity:** This is a short-lasting immunity transferred through the placenta and breast milk.
- **Artificially acquired passive immunity:** Also a short-lasting immunity, this is created by giving an exposed person antibodies containing blood products, as in an immune globulin.

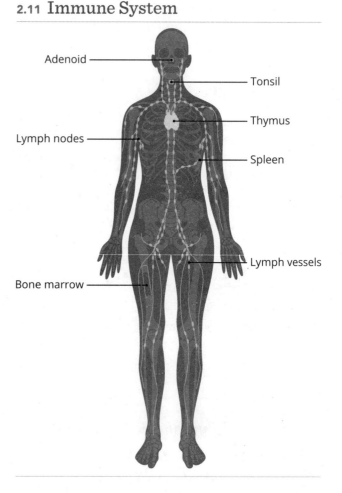

2.11 **Immune System**

antigen. Foreign substance within the body.

antibody. Protein the body creates in response to antigens.

Cardiovascular System

The cardiovascular system is made up of the following.

- **Heart:** Located within the central part of the chest (mediastinum) and functions as a pump to move blood throughout the body
- **Artery/Arteriole:** Thick-walled vessels that carry blood away from the heart. They propel blood with each contraction of the heart and are associated with various pulse points on the body. Smaller branches are arterioles.
- **Vein/Venule:** Vessels that carry blood toward the heart. They are thinner-walled than arteries and contain valves to prevent backflow. Smaller branches are venules.
- **Capillary:** The smallest blood vessels, which connect arterioles to venules. They aid in the exchange of oxygen and nutrients between blood and body cells.
- **Endocardium:** Innermost layer of cells that lines the atria, ventricles, and heart valves
- **Myocardium:** Muscular layer of the heart
- **Pericardium:** Outermost layer of the heart; a membrane that surrounds the heart and secretes pericardial fluid

2.12 Take Note

The average adult heart beats 60 to 80 times per minute while at rest.

2.13 Heart Anatomy

Labels: sa node, right atrium, pulmonary valve, av node, tricuspid valve, right ventricle, left atrium, bicuspid valve, aortic valve, bundle of His, left ventricle

The structures of the cardiovascular system work together to pump blood throughout the body. Blood carries essential oxygen and nutrients to cells and aids in eliminating cell waste. Blood travels to the heart to be pumped to the lungs for oxygen and then back to the heart to travel to the rest of the body.

The primary organ of the cardiovascular system is the heart. The heart is a muscle made up of three layers—the epicardium (outermost layer), myocardium (middle layer, thickest) and endocardium (inner layer, which is part of the electrical conduction system).

The heart contains four inner chambers. The right and left atria are the top chambers of the heart. The right atrium receives deoxygenated blood from the superior and inferior vena cava. The left atrium receives oxygenated blood from the pulmonary veins (the only veins in the body that carry oxygenated blood). The right and left ventricles are the bottom chambers of the heart. The right ventricle receives blood from the right atrium and sends deoxygenated blood through the pulmonary valve to the pulmonary artery and then to the lungs, where gas exchange occurs. The left ventricle receives blood from the left atrium and sends the oxygenated blood through the aortic valve to the aorta, which then branches off into smaller arteries that carry the blood to the body.

Between the right atrium and right ventricle is the tricuspid valve. Between the left atrium and left ventricle is the bicuspid (mitral) valve. The purpose of these valves is to prevent the backflow of blood into the atria when the ventricles contract.

Circulation of the blood occurs through two pathways—systemic and pulmonary circulation. Systemic circulation consists of arteries, arterioles, capillaries, venules, and veins in the body as a whole. Pulmonary circulation consists of arteries, arterioles, capillaries, venules, and veins going to, within, and coming from the lungs.

The heart contains its own electrical conduction system to keep the cardiac muscle contracting and blood flowing. This electricity can be mapped and analyzed to detect heart issues using an electrocardiogram (EKG).

The electrical impulse is generated by the sinoatrial (SA) node, also called the pacemaker of the heart.

From the SA node, the impulse travels to the atrioventricular node, also called the gatekeeper. From there, the impulse travels to the bundle of His and through the bundle branches located in the ventricular septum. Finally, the electrical impulse reaches the Purkinje fibers. These fibers cause the ventricles to contract and pump blood into the pulmonary artery and aorta. This entire process is the cardiac cycle.

Urinary System

The urinary system consists of the following.

- **Kidneys:** Located on either side of the vertebral column at the level of the top lumbar vertebrae, the kidneys are responsible for removing waste from the blood and producing urine.
- **Ureters:** These long tubes are responsible for carrying urine from the kidneys to the urinary bladder.
- **Urinary bladder:** This small muscular sac located within the pelvic cavity is responsible for storing urine.
- **Urethra:** This tube is responsible for carrying urine from the urinary bladder to the outside of the body and is longer in males due to pelvic shape and position of the prostate. The urinary meatus is located at the end of the urethra where urine exits the body.

2.14 Anatomy of the Urinary System

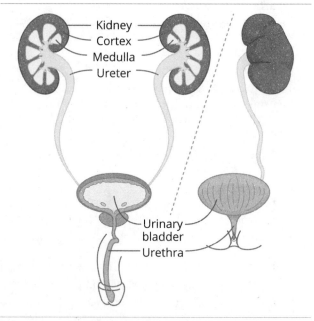

The urinary system is primarily responsible for filtering blood to remove waste products. This waste is then prepared for elimination by combining with water to form urine. Urine is produced in the kidneys and then stored in the urinary bladder to await elimination.

Gastrointestinal System

The gastrointestinal system is also known as the gastrointestinal tract. It begins with the mouth, or oral cavity. Digestion plays a vital role in the body's ability to maintain homeostasis. Water and nutrients are essential for proper function of body systems, as well as organ, tissue, and cellular function. The primary organs of the digestive system collectively make up the *alimentary canal*. There are also accessory organs of the digestive system that aid in various digestive functions.

2.15 Gastrointestinal System Anatomy

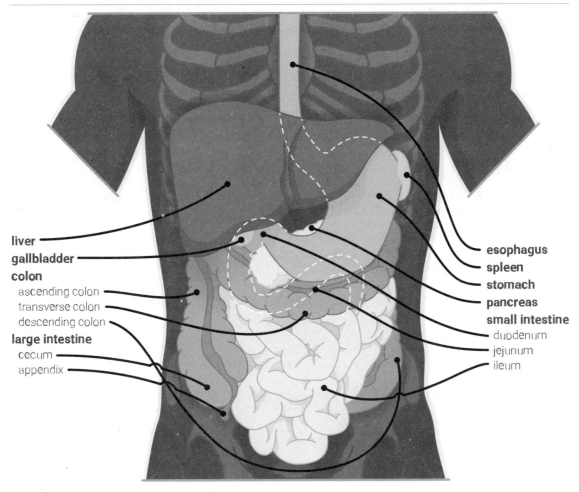

alimentary canal. The passage in which food passes through the body from the mouth to anus.

The following are part of the gastrointestinal system.

- **Mouth (oral cavity):** This is responsible for initiating digestion, both mechanical (chewing) and chemical (saliva).
- **Pharynx:** This includes the throat (the passageway for food between the oral cavity) and the esophagus (also part of the respiratory system).
- **Esophagus:** This muscular tube connects the mouth to the stomach. It uses wave-like contractions called peristalsis to propel food into the stomach.
- **Stomach:** Located below the diaphragm in the left upper quadrant (LUQ) of the abdominal cavity, the stomach receives food from the esophagus and continues breakdown using gastric juices. It then propels food to the small intestine. The stomach lining contains folds called rugae, allowing expansion.
- **Small intestine:** This organ takes up most of the space within the abdominal cavity and is primarily responsible for absorption of nutrients. It is divided into the following sections.
  - Duodenum
  - Jejunum
  - Ileum
- **Large intestine:** Also called the colon, the large intestine completes absorption and forms feces from solid waste products. It is divided into the following sections.
  - Cecum, which connects to the ileum, where the appendix is located
  - Ascending colon
  - Transverse colon
  - Descending colon
  - Sigmoid colon
- **Rectum:** This is the end of the colon that stores feces until defecation.
- **Anus:** This is the end of the rectum, which opens to the outside of the body to allow for elimination of feces.
- **Liver:** This large organ is located in the right upper quadrant (RUQ) of the abdomen. It produces bile needed to break down fats.
- **Gall bladder:** Located inferior to the liver, the gall bladder stores bile and connects to the duodenum.
- **Pancreas:** Posterior to the stomach and connected to duodenum, the pancreas produces enzymes that aid with digestion

Respiratory System

The following are part of the respiratory system.

- **Nose:** The nose is made of bones, cartilage, and skin. It contains small hairs called cilia to prevent large particles from entering.
- **Pharynx:** During respiration, air enters through the nose and mouth into the pharynx. The pharynx is also part of the digestive system.
- **Larynx:** Superior to the trachea, the larynx produces a person's voice.
- **Trachea:** Also called the windpipe, the trachea extends from the larynx and branches into bronchi. It is lined with cilia.
- **Lungs:** These two cone-shaped organs are located in the chest. The lungs contain bronchi, alveoli, and many blood vessels. The right lung is larger and divided into three lobes. The left lung has two lobes. Both lungs are surrounded by a membrane called pleura.

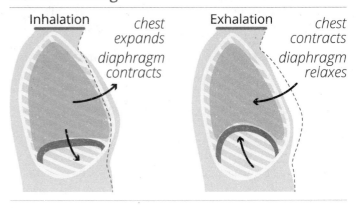

2.16 Breathing

The respiratory system functions by moving air into and out of the lungs, called respiration or breathing. The respiratory and cardiovascular systems work together to help deliver oxygen to the body via the blood and eliminate carbon dioxide. The exchange of oxygen and carbon dioxide within the lungs is external respiration, and the exchange within the hemoglobin of a red blood cell is internal respiration.

Nervous System

The nervous system contains the following

- **Brain:** The brain coordinates most body activities and is the control center for the body as well as thought, emotion, and judgment. It is divided into four lobes: frontal, parietal, occipital, and temporal.
- **Spinal cord:** The spinal cord provides a pathway for nerve impulses travelling to and from the brain and extends from the base of the brain to the lumbar vertebrae through the vertebral column.
- **Peripheral nerves:** The peripheral nerves include 12 pairs of cranial nerves and 31 pairs of spinal nerves branching off from the spinal cord. They carry nerve signals between the body and the brain.
- **Neuron:** The neuron is the functional unit of the nervous system.
- **Dendrites:** The dendrites have multiple branching structures.
- **Nucleus:** The nucleus directs cellular activities.
- **Cytoplasm:** The cytoplasm produces neurotransmitters and energy for the neuron.
- **Axon:** The axon stores neurotransmitters.

The nervous system controls all other body systems and is divided into two main sections—the central nervous system (CNS) and peripheral nervous system (PNS). The CNS includes the brain and spinal cord. The PNS is made of peripheral nerves found throughout the body.

The PNS is broken down further into two separate branches—the somatic nervous system and autonomic nervous system. The somatic nervous system controls the body's voluntary (skeletal) muscles. Afferent nerve cells, called neurons, carry information about the body's environment to the CNS. Efferent neurons carry responses from the CNS to the body to initiate action.

For example, if a person were to touch a hot stove, afferent neurons would carry the heat and pain sensations to the brain. The brain would process and respond using efferent neurons to signal the arm muscles to move the person's hand away from the source of the pain. The autonomic nervous system controls the body's automatic functions like breathing and digestion. The sympathetic branch controls the "fight or flight" response to stress. The parasympathetic branch returns the body to resting state after stress has been resolved and is responsible for maintaining homeostasis.

A neuron generates an electrical impulse when stimulated. The nervous system contains multiple neurotransmitters.

Endocrine System

The endocrine system is made of organs and glands that produce, store, and release *hormones*. Hormones are chemicals used by the body to increase or decrease activity of the hormone's specific target cells. This aids the body in maintaining homeostasis. There are two types of glands within the system: exocrine and endocrine. Exocrine glands release hormones into a duct for delivery to the target cells. Endocrine glands release hormones directly into the blood stream. There are many different organs that make up the endocrine system throughout the body.

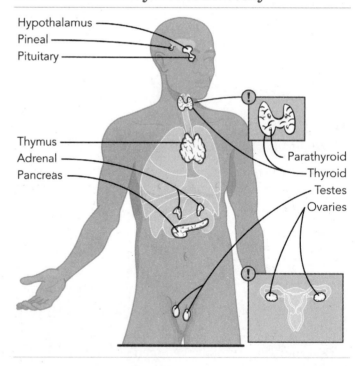

2.17 **Endocrine System Anatomy**

---

hormones. Chemicals used by the body to increase or decrease activity of the hormone's specific target cells.

Reproductive Systems

The male and female reproductive systems work together to achieve fertilization and produce offspring. Some intersex variations can occur in sex development in which there is a discrepancy between the external genitals and the internal genitals. The female and male reproductive system each contain structures and functions to aid in the reproductive process.

Male Reproductive Organs

The following organs are part of the male reproductive system.

- **Testes:** Produce sperm and testosterone; located below the pelvic cavity on the outside of the body, within the scrotum
- **Scrotum:** A pouch of skin that houses the testes
- **Penis:** External cylinder-shaped organ that moves urine and semen out of the body
- **Epididymis:** Coiled tube located superior to each testis; responsible for maturation of sperm cells
- **Vas deferens:** Connects the epididymis to the urethra
- **Seminal vesicles:** Sac-like organs that secrete seminal fluid that stimulate muscle contractions in the female reproductive organs to aid in propelling sperm forward
- **Prostate gland:** Surrounds the proximal urethra; contracts during ejaculation to aid in forward movement of sperm; secretes fluid that protects sperm within the vagina
- **Bulbourethral glands (Cowper's glands):** Inferior to the prostate gland; secrete fluid to lubricate the end of the penis to prepare for intercourse
- **Androgens:** Group of male sex hormones
- **Testosterone:** Most abundant and biologically active of male sex hormones

Female Reproductive Organs

The female reproductive system includes the following.

- **Ovaries:** Pair of oval-shaped organs located within the pelvic cavity; produce ova, estrogen, and progesterone
- **Fallopian tubes:** Muscular tubes with proximal opening near each ovary; connect distally to uterus; receive egg during ovulation
- **Uterus:** Hollow muscular organ, lies low in pelvic cavity; receives fertilized egg, which implants into uterine wall for fetal development. If no egg has implanted into the uterine wall, the uterine lining sloughs off, causing menstruation. The lower portion of the uterus is the cervix, which creates a barrier between the uterus and vagina and dilates during childbirth.
- **Vagina:** Muscular tube extending from the uterus to the outside of the body; expands during intercourse and childbirth

CHAPTER 2: MEDICAL TERMINOLOGY, ANATOMY, AND PHYSIOLOGY
Structure and Function of Major Body Systems

- **Labia majora:** Folds of skin and adipose tissue that protect other external genitalia
- **Labia minora:** Folds of skin within the labia majora, pinkish in color due to high blood circulation; form a hood over the clitoris
- **Clitoris:** Highly sensitive erectile tissue located anterior to the urethra
- **Perineum:** Area between the vagina and anus
- **Estrogen:** Group of sex hormones
- **Progesterone:** Hormone secreted by ovaries
- **Estradiol:** Most abundant and biologically active female hormone

The female reproductive cycle refers to a monthly fluctuation of hormones that aids in reproduction and prepares the uterus for carrying a child. When fertilization does not occur, menstruation takes place, and the process begins again.

CHALLENGE

1. Match the body system with its function.

BODY SYSTEM	FUNCTION
A. Skeletal	1. Control all other body systems
B. Integumentary	2. Move air in and out of lungs
C. Immune	3. Facilitate digestion
D. Cardiovascular	4. Remove waste products from blood
E. Urinary	5. Deliver blood to the body
F. Nervous	6. Protect the body from disease
G. Respiratory	7. Provide structure and posture
H. Gastrointestinal	8. Temperature regulation, sensation

   A: 7, B: 8, C: 6, D: 5, E: 4, F: 1, G: 2, H: 3
   The integumentary system has several functions, including protection, temperature regulation, and sensation. The skeletal system's purpose is to give the body structure and posture, as well as protect the soft internal organs from injury. The immune system activates when pathogens enter the body, to protect it from disease. The structures of the cardiovascular system work together to pump blood throughout the body. The urinary system is primarily responsible for filtering blood to remove waste products.

2. Which of the following classifications of bone describes the skull?
   A. Long
   B. Short
   C. Flat
   D. Irregular

   C is correct. Flat bones are bones in which most of the surface area is flat or slightly curved, such as the skull and ribs.

3. Order the steps of the cardiac cycle below into the correct sequence.
   A. Electrical impulse reaches the Purkinje fibers.
   B. Impulse travels to the AV node.
   C. Impulse travels into the ventricular septum.
   D. SA node generates an electrical impulse.
   E. Ventricles contract and pump blood into pulmonary artery and aorta.

   D, B, C, A, E
   The electrical impulse is generated by the sinoatrial (SA) node, also called the pacemaker of the heart. From the SA node, the impulse travels to the atrioventricular node, also called the gatekeeper. From there, the impulse travels to the bundle of His and through the bundle branches located in the ventricular septum. Finally, the electrical impulse reaches the Purkinje fibers. These fibers cause the ventricles to contract and pump blood into the pulmonary artery and aorta. This entire process is the cardiac cycle.

INTERACTIONS BETWEEN ORGAN SYSTEMS AND HOMEOSTASIS

When organs work together, they are referred to as systems. Body systems are responsible for all vital functions, including maintaining homeostasis.

Homeostasis

The nervous system and endocrine system are primarily responsible for achieving and maintaining homeostasis, but all body systems play a role.

Organ systems rely on each other in the achievement of homeostasis. When there is a disease or disorder within one body system, it will affect other systems and their ability to keep the body operating properly.

2.18 Take Note

Homeostasis is achieved when the body's systems and biological processes maintain stability. The body has built-in regulatory processes that react to external environmental changes to sustain balance.

CHALLENGE

1. Which of the following body systems are primarily responsible for achieving and maintaining homeostasis?
   A. Nervous and endocrine
   B. Immune and cardiovascular
   C. Integumentary and muscular
   D. Gastrointestinal and lymphatic

A is correct. The nervous and endocrine system are primarily responsible for achieving and maintaining homeostasis, but all body systems play a role.

COMMON DISEASES, CONDITIONS, AND INJURIES

A number of diseases, disorders, and abnormalities affect the various systems of the body. Medical assistants aren't expected to know and memorize all of them. Experience will bring familiarity with common diseases and disorders. These are a few of the most common diseases and disorders arranged by body system.

2.19 Conditions of the Integumentary System

DISEASE	SIGNS AND SYMPTOMS	ETIOLOGY	DIAGNOSIS	TREATMENT
Cellulitis	Skin of the affected area is swollen, red, and hot to the touch.	Bacteria (typically Streptococcus or Staphylococcus) enters the skin through cuts or abrasions and causes infection of connective tissue with severe inflammation of the skin.	Physical exam. Wound culture and blood tests can confirm bacterial etiology.	Resting the area, cutting away dead tissue if needed, antibiotics
Dermatitis	Red, itchy rash that may include blisters or oily scales	Allergic reaction to a specific allergen leading to inflammation of a region of the skin	Physical examination	Moisturizers. Steroid creams

2.19 Conditions of the Integumentary System (continued)

DISEASE	SIGNS AND SYMPTOMS	ETIOLOGY	DIAGNOSIS	TREATMENT
Eczema	Red, itchy skin Vesicular lesions (blisters) that may crust over	Believed to be caused by hereditary and environmental factors leading to inflammatory skin disease	Physical examination	Mild, fragrance-free soap and moisturizers, steroid creams, and antihistamines Goals of treatment are to heal the affected skin and mitigate recurrence.
Skin cancer: basal cell	Waxy bump or skin sore that does not heal within two months and continues to grow over time	Damage to DNA of basal cells caused by ultraviolet B (UVB) exposure from the sun and tanning beds	Physical examination and biopsy Early diagnosis is vital.	Surgical excision Liquid nitrogen freezing or curettage
Skin cancer: melanoma	A skin mole with specific characteristics Asymmetry: irregular shape Border: rough; irregular Color: nonuniform Diameter: More than ¼ inch	Excessive exposure to UVB rays	Physical examination and biopsy Early diagnosis is vital.	Surgery and radiation

2.20 Conditions of the Skeletal System

DISEASE	SIGNS AND SYMPTOMS	ETIOLOGY	DIAGNOSIS	TREATMENT
Sprain	Painful swelling or bruising of a joint area with decreased mobility	The joint being pushed outside of its normal range of motion, leading to joint and ligament damage	Physical exam with imaging	RICE • Rest • Ice • Compression • Elevation
Osteoporosis	Typically, there are no symptoms. Severe disease can lead to increased fractures and back pain.	Many factors including malnutrition, inadequate calcium intake/absorption, endocrine disorders, immobilization and lack of exercise, and aging can lead to bone loss, making bone weaker and more prone to fracture.	Measuring bone mineral density using a DEXA scan	Medications can slow bone loss and reduce the risk of fracture.
Osteoarthritis	Pain with movement in a specific joint Stiffness in joint following periods of inactivity Lack of flexibility	Degeneration (breakdown) of articular cartilage and changes in the synovial membrane	History, physical examination, and imaging	Physical therapy, exercise, and steroid injections can help relieve symptoms. Joint replacement may be needed if severe enough.
Rheumatoid arthritis	Systemic joint disorder typically starting with pain and decreased mobility in the smaller joints, such as fingers, before progressing to larger joints, such as knees and hips	Autoimmune disorder leading to changes in the connective tissues of the body, especially the joints *This may also be considered a disorder of the lymphatic/immune system.*	Physical examination, blood tests, and imaging	Physical therapy for mobility Medication to manage inflammation and pain
Gout	Red, hot, swollen joint Most common in the big toe	Excessive accumulation of uric acid in a joint, forming needle-like crystals in the joint	Aspiration of the joint to obtain and identify the crystals at a microscopic level	Anti-inflammatory medications and dietary adjustments

2.21 Diseases of the Muscular System

DISEASE	SIGNS AND SYMPTOMS	ETIOLOGY	DIAGNOSIS	TREATMENT
Muscular dystrophy	Chronic and progressive muscle weakness leading to eventual paralysis of muscle groups	Inherited or spontaneous genetic mutation in one of the genes involved with protecting muscle fibers from damage	Patient history, physical exam, muscle enzyme tests, electromyography, muscle biopsy, and genetic testing	Physical therapy, ambulatory devices, and medications to alleviate symptoms
Myopathy	Muscle weakness, cramps, stiffness, spasms, and tetany	Can result from many different disease processes	Based on symptoms. Focus is on understanding the underlying cause.	Treatment is dependent on the underlying cause. Physical therapy, medication therapy, support bracing, surgery, and massage all may help.
Myalgia	Muscle pain (broad term)	Several causes • Traumatic injury • Viral infection • Overuse or overstretching of muscle group • Medications and vaccines	Based on symptoms. Focus is on understanding the underlying cause.	Treatment is dependent on the underlying cause. Targeted symptomatic treatment includes massage, heat or cold therapy, and medication for pain and muscle relaxants.
Repetitive stress disorder (RSD)	Pain, tingling, numbness, swelling. Redness, loss of flexibility and muscle weakness	Repetitive tasks, forceful exertions, vibrations, mechanical compression and sustained uncomfortable positions can cause RSD.	Physical examination, patient history, and imaging	Early treatment: Anti-inflammatory medications, rest, splinting, and massage. Severe disease treatment: Surgery
Shin splint	Pain and swelling in the lower leg	Repeated stress of the tibia and connective tissues	Physical examination and patient history	RICE. Surgery if severe enough

2.22 Diseases of the Cardiovascular System

DISEASE	SIGNS AND SYMPTOMS	ETIOLOGY	DIAGNOSIS	TREATMENT
Anemia	Fatigue, dizziness, cold extremities, headache, irregular heartbeat	Most common cause is blood loss. Dysfunction in the creation of hemoglobin. Excessive destruction of red blood cells	Blood test	Depends on cause. Blood loss can be treated with a blood transfusion. Other causes may be treated through increase of iron or vitamin K.
Atherosclerosis	Chest pain, transient ischemic attacks (TIAs), peripheral artery disease, and kidney disfunction	Hardening of the arteries due to fatty deposits causing narrowing of vessels potentially due to high blood pressure, high cholesterol, smoking, diabetes, and other diseases	Physical examination, medical history, blood tests, Doppler ultrasound, EKG, stress test, angiogram, CT or MRI	Healthy diet, increased exercise, medications (cholesterol medication, beta blockers, ACE inhibitors, blood thinners, diuretics, calcium channel blockers), angioplasty, stents, endarterectomy, or bypass surgery
Congestive heart failure (CHF)	Fatigue, peripheral edema, shortness of breath	The heart's decreased ability to pump adequately due to coronary artery disease, high blood pressure, cardiomyopathy, valvular disease, or heart defects	Medical history, physical examination, blood tests, EKG, echocardiogram, and chest x-ray	Varies depending on the type and severity. Can include weight loss, controlling blood pressure, ACE inhibitors, and beta blockers
Hemophilia	Excessive bleeding, frequent bruising	An absence of clotting factors in the blood as the result of a genetic defect	Family history, physical examination, and blood tests	Replacement therapy to slowly infuse clotting factors into a vein
Hypertension	Higher than normal blood pressure, headaches, irregular heart rhythms, vision changes, or chest pain	Genetics, smoking, obesity, stress, too much salt intake	Consistently high blood pressure over two or three office visits over the course of one to four weeks	Medications, weight management, healthy diet, and stress reduction
Myocardial infarction (MI or heart attack)	Acute chest pain, nausea, vomiting, heartburn, and profuse sweating	Cardiac muscle becomes ischemic and dies, typically due to occlusion of the cardiac muscle because of atherosclerosis of the coronary artery.	EKG and blood tests	Fibrinolytic agents, diagnostic angiogram, stenting, and bypass surgery if severe enough

2.23 Diseases of the Urinary System

DISEASE	SIGNS AND SYMPTOMS	ETIOLOGY	DIAGNOSIS	TREATMENT
Acute renal failure	Decreased urine output, fluid retention, fatigue, shortness of breath, confusion, and nausea	Direct damage to the kidneys or other causes leading to a sudden change where the kidneys can no longer filter blood effectively, leading to dangerous levels of toxic waste in the body	Observation of urine output, blood tests, urinalysis, and other imaging	Correcting the underlying cause, medications, and hemodialysis in the setting of severe disease
Chronic renal failure	Early stages: No symptoms. Later stages: High blood pressure, feeling generally ill and fatigued	Chronic and progressive disease in which the kidneys cannot adequately filter blood due to many potential factors including diabetes, high blood pressure and glomerulonephritis	Blood test	Controlling blood pressure is the primary treatment to slow chronic renal failure. If it progresses far enough, hemodialysis will be needed.
Renal calculi (kidney stones)	Severe episodes of back and side pain, pain with urination. Dark or foul-smelling urine, nausea, frequent urination, fever, chills	Hard crystalline deposits forming in the urine due to abnormally high levels of certain substances in the body	Blood tests, urine tests, and imaging	Drinking water, pain relievers, and shock wave therapy in the form of lithotripsy to help break down and flush out the stones through urination
Urinary incontinence	Leakage of urine	Loss of bladder control leading to leakage of urine, sometimes triggered by coughing, lifting, or sneezing	Urinalysis, medical history, physical examination	Kegel exercises to strengthen muscles that control the bladder. Surgery (bladder sling)
Urinary tract infection (UTI)	Persistent urge to urinate, burning with urination, strong smelling cloudy urine, pelvic or flank pain	Infection in the urinary system most commonly caused by *Escherichia coli* (E. coli)	Urinalysis, urine cultures, and imaging	Antibiotics

2.24 Diseases of the Gastrointestinal System

DISEASE	SIGNS AND SYMPTOMS	ETIOLOGY	DIAGNOSIS	TREATMENT
Appendicitis	Pain in the lower, right abdomen, loss of appetite, nausea, vomiting, abdominal swelling, fever	Inflammation in the appendix due to blockage of the opening to the appendix, leading to rapidly multiplying bacteria in the appendix	Patient history, blood and urine tests, imaging	Surgical removal of the appendix
Celiac disease	Anemia, diarrhea, gas, bloating, weight loss, fatigue	Immune response triggered by gluten leading to damage of the small intestine and an inability to absorb nutrients	Physical examination, medical history, blood tests, antibody tests, and endoscopy with biopsy	Avoid gluten in any form
Colorectal cancer	Early stages: No symptoms. Later stages: Symptoms are nonspecific but can include fatigue, irregular bowel movements, blood in feces, cramps, bloating, and weight loss.	Cancer of the colon. Risk factors are a high-fat diet, family history, and inflammatory bowel disease.	Colonoscopy or barium enema	Early stages: Surgical removal of cancer cells. Advanced stages: Chemotherapy
Diverticulosis	Asymptomatic unless inflamed. When inflamed it is termed diverticulitis: pain in lower left abdomen, fever, chills, nausea, and vomiting.	Pouchlike herniations through the muscular wall of the colon caused by high pressure inside the colon pressing against weak areas of the colon wall	Typically discovered through colonoscopy	When inflamed, antibiotics are used for treatment.
Gastroesophageal reflux disease (GERD)	Heartburn, nausea after eating, difficulty swallowing	Lower esophageal sphincter muscle disfunction leading to stomach contents leaking back up the esophagus	Upper endoscopy, tests to measure amount of acid in the esophagus	Lifestyle/dietary changes, antacids. Surgery (severe cases)

2.25 Diseases of the Respiratory System

DISEASE	SIGNS AND SYMPTOMS	ETIOLOGY	DIAGNOSIS	TREATMENT
Acute respiratory distress (ARDS)	Shortness of breath, low blood pressure, and rapid breathing (following an injury)	Fluid buildup in the alveoli blocks oxygen from passing into the bloodstream following an acute injury, typically in those who are already critically ill or have had previous traumatic injuries.	Arterial blood gas analysis, chest x-ray	Oxygen therapy, mechanical ventilation, and antibiotics
Asthma	Wheezing, shortness of breath, chest tightness, and coughing	Airway inflammation causes lining of air passages to swell and tighten, leading to a reduction in the amount of air that can pass into and out of the lungs.	Pulmonary function tests	Medications, both inhaled and taken orally
Bronchitis	Shortness of breath, fever, chills, fatigue, coughing, and production of mucus	Acute: Caused by viral illnesses such as colds and flu Chronic: Caused by smoking	Physical examination in which the lungs are listened to via stethoscope, chest x-ray, pulmonary function tests	Acute: Typically resolves without intervention. Chronic: Respiratory therapy
Chronic obstructive pulmonary disease (COPD)	Chest tightness, productive cough, wheezing, shortness of breath with activity	Disease in which airflow into and out of the lungs is blocked, usually due to a combination of bronchitis and emphysema Primary cause is smoking.	Patient history, pulmonary function tests, chest x-ray, and CT scan	Smoking cessation, medication, and oxygen therapy
Rhinitis	Sneezing, coughing, runny nose, watering eyes, pressure in ears	Irritation and inflammation of the mucous membrane in the nose, along with excessive production of mucus Allergic rhinitis is triggered by allergens in the air.	Physical exam Allergists can help determine the cause of allergic rhinitis.	Antihistamines and corticosteroids

2.26 Diseases of the Nervous System

DISEASE	SIGNS AND SYMPTOMS	ETIOLOGY	DIAGNOSIS	TREATMENT
Alzheimer's disease	Memory loss, impaired judgement or language, inability to perform activities of daily living, inability to reason, paranoia, and agitation	Most common form of progressive dementia caused by progressive destruction on brain cells	No definitive diagnostic testing available. Diagnosis relies on medical history, physical exam, cognitive testing, brain scans, and lab tests.	No available treatment to cure the disease. Focus of care is on symptom management while ensuring the patient is comfortable, safe, and otherwise physically healthy.
Cerebral concussion	Distorted vision, headache, dizziness, nausea and vomiting, sensitivity to light or noise, inability to concentrate	Caused by traumatic injury to the brain	Physical and neurological exam	Observation and rest for seven to ten days.
Sciatica	Pain radiating from lumbar spine to the buttocks and down the back of the leg. Pain can be a dull ache or sharp, burning sensation.	Occurs from compression of the sciatic nerve, typically due to a herniated disc, bone spur, or tumor	Medical testing of muscle strength and reflexes. Imaging	Muscle relaxants, anti-inflammatory medications, physical therapy, corticosteroids
Cerebrovascular accident (CVA; stroke)	Symptoms vary depending on the area of the brain impact, but general symptoms are associated with the acronym FAST. Facial muscle weakness. Arm droop. Speech abnormalities. Time (occurs suddenly, treatment options limited by how quickly care can be initiated)	Caused by a decrease in blood supply to the brain or a rupture of a blood vessel in the brain	Neurologic examination, CT or MRI scan, Doppler ultrasound or arteriography	Immediate treatment involves restoring blood to the brain or reducing pressure on the brain (depending on the cause). Long-term treatment focuses on rehabilitation for quality of life.
Shingles	Blisters and pain on the skin in a bandlike pattern that follows the path of the affected nerves	Caused by the varicella zoster virus (also causes chicken pox). The virus can lie dormant for years following an infection of chicken pox, then reappear as shingles.	History, location of pain, and pattern of rash	Antiviral medications increase rate of healing. Pain relievers for symptom management

CHAPTER 2: MEDICAL TERMINOLOGY, ANATOMY, AND PHYSIOLOGY
Common Diseases, Conditions, and Injuries

2.27 Diseases of the Endocrine System

DISEASE	SIGNS AND SYMPTOMS	ETIOLOGY	DIAGNOSIS	TREATMENT
Cushing syndrome	Excessive fat deposits in the subscapular area and face	Most often caused by overuse of oral corticosteroid medications Can also be caused by hypersecretion of glucocorticoids from the adrenal cortex	Indications of high blood pressure, loss of muscle mass, glucose intolerance, and weight gain	Medications used to lower levels of glucocorticoids
Type 1 diabetes mellitus	Excessive thirst, frequent urination, extreme hunger, weight loss, fatigue, blurred vision, poorly healing wounds, numbness in hands and feet	Chronic condition caused by lack of insulin production This is a genetic, autoimmune condition that often develops in childhood and is commonly known as juvenile diabetes. *This may also be considered a disorder of the lymphatic/immune system.*	Blood tests to evaluate glucose metabolism	Monitoring blood sugar levels, insulin therapy, eating a healthy diet, and managing weight
Type 2 diabetes mellitus	Excessive thirst, frequent urination, extreme hunger, weight loss, fatigue, blurred vision, poorly healing wounds, numbness in hands and feet	Chronic condition caused by insulin resistance, due to a mix of genetics, obesity, and lifestyle choices Typically begins in adulthood but is being seen more often in adolescents	Blood tests to evaluate glucose metabolism	Monitoring blood sugar levels, eating a healthy diet, and managing weight Medications to lower blood sugar, such as metformin Insulin will be prescribed if the disease is uncontrolled or progresses.

2.27 Diseases of the Endocrine System *(continued)*

DISEASE	SIGNS AND SYMPTOMS	ETIOLOGY	DIAGNOSIS	TREATMENT
Hyperthyroidism	Sudden weight loss, rapid heartbeat, increased appetite, anxiety, tremor, sweating, frequent bowel movements, enlarged thyroid gland	Overproduction of the thyroid hormone by the thyroid gland	Physical examination, blood tests, radioactive iodine uptake test, and thyroid scans	Antithyroid medications, oral radioactive iodine
Hypothyroidism	Increasing tiredness, dry skin, constipation, and weight gain	Underproduction of the thyroid hormone by the thyroid gland	Blood test measuring thyroid stimulating hormone and thyroxine	Use of synthetic thyroid hormone levothyroxine
Graves' disease	Significant enlargement of the thyroid gland, increased heartbeat, muscle weakness, disturbed sleep, tremor, weight loss, anxiety, irritability, and bulging of the eyes	Caused by malfunction in the body's immune system that disrupts normal thyroid regulation, resulting in hyperthyroidism	Typically diagnosed by symptoms. Thyroid hormone tests may also be used.	Radioactive iodine therapy, antithyroid medications, beta blockers, and surgery

2.28 Diseases of the Reproductive System

DISEASE	SIGNS AND SYMPTOMS	ETIOLOGY	DIAGNOSIS	TREATMENT
Candidiasis	Vaginal itching, burning with urination, white vaginal discharge Often called a "yeast infection"	Overgrowth of the fungal microorganism *Candida albicans*	Testing of vaginal discharge	Over-the-counter or prescription medications
Ectopic pregnancy	Abdominal or pelvic pain with light bleeding Severe pain and bleeding are symptoms of emergent condition.	Zygote implantation in an area other than the uterine wall, most commonly in the uterine tubes	Physical examination, blood tests, and ultrasound	Termination of the pregnancy, as it is not viable and can rupture the uterine tube if allowed to develop far enough, which would require surgery
Endometriosis	Pelvic pain with menstruation, pain with intercourse, pain with bowel movements and urination, infertility	Occurs when pieces of endometrial tissue grow outside of the uterine lining, typically on the ovaries, intestines, or pelvic wall	Pelvic examination, ultrasound, and laparoscopy	Pain medication, hormone therapy, or laparoscopic surgery
Genital herpes	Pain, itching, and sores in the genital area Flu-like symptoms upon initial infection	Caused by the herpes simplex virus spread through sexual contact	Visual examination of sores, testing of sample from the sores	Incurable Medications, typically antivirals, can prevent or shorten outbreaks
Inguinal hernia	Bulging in the groin area accompanied by an aching sensation, pain with lifting, coughing, or movement, weakness, or pressure in the groin	A portion of the intestines protrudes thought a weak point of the abdominal wall.	Physical examination	If no symptoms, treatment is not indicated. Surgery to repair the hernia if symptoms present

2.28 Diseases of the Reproductive System (continued)

DISEASE	SIGNS AND SYMPTOMS	ETIOLOGY	DIAGNOSIS	TREATMENT
Cryptorchidism	Undescended testicles, when they fail to drop into the normal place of the scrotum	Some cases are unknown, others may be due to structural abnormalities, or there may be a mechanical problem.	Felt when conducting a physical examination	Only treatment choice is surgery and recommended after six months of age
Testicular torsion	When tissues surrounding the testicle are not well attached, causing the testes to twist around the spermatic chord cutting off blood flow to the testicle causing severe pain	Some causes are unknown. Some patients are born with no tissue holding the testes to the scrotum.	Found when conducting a physical examination	The spermatic cord needs to be untwisted to restore blood supply. Patients need to see a urologist, and surgery is necessary to correct.
Benign prostatic hyperplasia (BPH)	Enlargement of the prostate. Common later in life. Can cause uncomfortable urinary symptoms, urinary tract infections, or kidney problems	Causes are unknown but are believed to be linked to hormonal changes	Digital rectal examination, urine test, or prostate specific antigen test	Transurethral resection of the prostate

CHALLENGE

1. Which of the following diseases would be indicated if a patient presented with a waxy bump on the skin that has been growing for four months?
   A. Basal cell skin cancer
   B. Eczema
   C. Melanoma
   D. Cellulitis

   A is correct. The signs and symptoms of basal cell skin cancer are a waxy bump or skin sore that does not heal within two months and continues to grow over time.

2. What are the primary differences between diabetes mellitus types 1 and 2?

   Type 1 is a disorder in which the body lacks the ability to make insulin, whereas type 2 is a disorder in which the body is resistant to insulin. Type 1 diabetes, an autoimmune disorder, typically presents starting in childhood, whereas type 2 is not typically present until adulthood.

3. Which of the following conditions includes symptoms of excessive bleeding and frequent bruising?
   A. Hemophilia
   B. Myocardial infarction
   C. Congestive heart failure
   D. Atherosclerosis

   A is correct. Hemophilia is a disorder in which individuals lack clotting factors in the blood, leading to excessive bleeding and frequent bruising.

PATHOPHYSIOLOGY AND DISEASE PROCESSES

Diagnostic Measures and Treatment Modalities

To best assess and diagnose the pathophysiologic effects of a disease on the body, providers use a variety of diagnostic testing in conjunction with the patient's medical history and a thorough physical examination. Common tests include blood work, urinalysis, and diagnostic imaging (x-ray, ultrasound). When using an imaging modality that has radiation, there is some risk involved. However, it is generally considered minimal. It is the provider's responsibility to determine that the benefits of a radiologic procedure outweigh any risks involved. In addition, many diagnostic imaging procedures use alternate methods of image production that do not use radiation.

Diagnostic imaging studies that use radiation include x-rays, computed tomography (CT), angiography, mammography, and *nuclear medicine* studies. Diagnostic imaging that does not use radiation or radiologic waves includes magnetic resonance imaging (MRI), which uses an electromagnetic field to produce images, and ultrasound, which uses sound waves.

CHALLENGE

1. Which of the following diagnostic studies uses radiation? (Select all that apply.)
   A. X-ray
   B. Ultrasound
   C. CT scan
   D. Nuclear medicine
   E. MRI

   A, C, and D are correct. X-rays, CT scans, and nuclear medicine testing all use radiation. MRI uses magnetic waves. Ultrasound uses sound waves.

The use of contrast material is also common with diagnostic imaging. Many body structures appear dark on imaging studies (radiolucent) due to their lack of density. Contrast aids in making those structures more radiopaque (lighter/brighter), thereby making them easier for the radiologist to visualize on a radiograph. Contrast materials include air, barium, gadolinium, and iodine. These contrast substances can be administered orally, through injection, or intravenously.

Nuclear medicine is a type of diagnostic imaging that involves the administration of radioactive material called tracers (radiopharmaceuticals) to assess bodily functions. Examples of nuclear imaging include SPECT scan (used to assess brain damage following a stroke), PET scan (used to diagnose brain-related disorders and cancers), and MUGA scan (used to evaluate the condition of the heart muscle).

---

nuclear medicine. Type of diagnostic imaging that involves administration of radioactive isotopes that collect in areas of high metabolic activity.

EPIDEMICS AND PANDEMICS

Endemic disease is one that predominately spreads throughout a community at a normal rate. It may become an *epidemic* if the disease spreads rapidly to a large number of people. A pandemic is a worldwide outbreak of a disease, such as COVID-19.

Cough protocols, handwashing, and the use of hand sanitizer also aid in preventing the spread of disease and illness. Isolation precautions may also be implemented. Medical assistants are often involved in educating patients on these disease prevention measures. The *Centers for Disease Control and Prevention (CDC)* and *World Health Organization (WHO)* monitor disease outbreaks very closely to control the spread of illness before it reaches pandemic levels. WHO researches potential causative agents.

2.29 Take Note

An epidemic can turn into a pandemic if measures are not taken to keep the illness under control. However, vaccines can reduce the number of people that may become infected.

CHALLENGE

1. Which of the following organizations researches potential agents related to pandemics?
   A. World Health Organization
   B. Centers for Disease Control and Prevention
   C. Occupational Safety and Health Administration
   D. American Medical Association

   A is correct. The World Health Organization (WHO) researches potential causative agents related to pandemics.

2. What precautions can help prevent a pandemic?

   Vaccines reduce the number of people at risk. Cough protocols, handwashing, and the use of hand sanitizer also aid in preventing the spread of disease and illness.

MEDICAL TERMINOLOGY

Learning medical terminology might seem as daunting as learning another language. In a way, it is another language. When toddlers first start speaking actual words, they do not yet know what geography, philanthropy, or accountability mean. But with experience in listening and speaking, they learn to use and understand more words. They later notice connections among words—their prefixes, roots, and suffixes. As their vocabulary continues to expand, children usually master communication in their native language.

Medical assistants become fluent in medical terminology in much the same way, with one distinct advantage. They will first learn the basics in coursework and with learning activities such as this module. Here are the most common terms, abbreviations, acronyms, and symbols needed to begin to navigate communication in this new career. Learning how to dissect some terms into their prefixes, roots, and suffixes can also expand understanding of terminology much faster than learning each word individually, fast-tracking to mastery in medical terminology.

---

epidemic. Occurs when a disease spreads rapidly to a large number of people.

Centers for Disease Control and Prevention (CDC). National public health agency that protects the public's health.

World Health Organization (WHO). Agency that promotes health, and monitors and coordinates activities concerning health-related issues.

Common Abbreviations, Acronyms, and Symbols

Medical assistants see and use many abbreviations (a term that will refer here to symbols as well) in everyday practice. **The Joint Commission** and the Institute for Safe Medication Practices (ISMP) have put some abbreviations on their "Do Not Use" and "Error-Prone Abbreviations" lists. Avoiding these abbreviations is essential because of their potential for misunderstanding and medical errors. The following table includes examples of abbreviations that should not be used. (For the full lists, go to The Joint Commission and ISMP websites.)

2.30 Examples of Abbreviations to Avoid

DO NOT USE	USE INSTEAD
MS, MSO_4	Morphine
$MgSO_4$	Magnesium sulfate
Abbreviated medication name	Full medication name
Nitro	Nitroglycerin
u, U, IU	Units
x3d	For 3 days
cc	mL
Apothecary units	Metric units
od, O.D., OD	Daily or intended time of administration
q.d, qd, Q.D, QD, q1d, i/d	Daily
q.o.d., QOD	Every other day
Q6PM	6 p.m. daily
TIW, tiw	3 times weekly
HS	Half-strength, bedtime (hour of sleep)
SC, SQ, sub q	Subcutaneously
IN	Intranasal
IJ	Injection
OJ	Orange juice
@	At
&, +	And
/	Per
AD, AS, AU	Right ear, left ear, both ears
OD, OS, OU	Right eye, left eye, both eyes
D/C, dc, d/c	Discharge or discontinue

The Joint Commission. Accrediting body that focuses on quality improvement and patient safety, certifying health care organizations and programs in the U.S. including hospitals and health care organizations that provide ambulatory and office-based surgery, behavioral health, home health care, laboratory, and nursing care center services.

Abbreviations

Many other abbreviations are facility-specific but not universal. For example, one hospital might call its storage and processing area for medical products "central supply," while another might call it "materials management." So, "CS" has no meaning (or a different meaning) in Hospital B, and "MM" has no meaning (or a different meaning) in Hospital A. Likewise, Hospital A calls the surgery area the operating room (OR), while Hospital B calls it the surgical suite (SS). Yet another hospital uses "SS" to mean its department of social services.

Many acronyms go back to long-outdated usage. "Emergency room" became common parlance when there was literally one room—an emergency or accident room. Even though today's hospitals have an enormous emergency department (ED), "ER" is still in prevalent use today. Other terminology changes over time. What was once the recovery room (RR) is now the post-anesthesia care unit (PACU).

There are many common abbreviations that reflect current clinical practice and are primarily universal. Providers use many of these when writing orders, often on prescription pads, for diagnostic tests and procedures. Here is a list of many of those common abbreviations.

2.31 Common Abbreviations and Acronyms

ABBREVIATION/ACRONYM	MEANING	ABBREVIATION/ACRONYM	MEANING
Abd	Abdomen	C	Celsius
ABGs	Arterial blood gases	C&S	Culture and sensitivity
a.c.	Before meals	Ca	Calcium; cancer
ACLS	Advance cardiac life support	CABG	Coronary artery bypass graft
Ad lib	As desired	CAD	Coronary artery disease
ADHD	Attention deficit hyperactivity disorder	CBC	Complete blood count
AKA	Above-the-knee amputation	CC	Chief complaint
AMA	Against medical advice	CDC	Centers for Disease Control and Prevention
ASA	Aspirin	cm	Centimeter
ASAP	As soon as possible	CMS	Centers for Medicare and Medicaid Services
BE	Barium enema	CNS	Central nervous system
BKA	Below-the-knee amputation	CP	Chest pain
BM	Bowel movement	CPR	Cardiopulmonary resuscitation
BMI	Body mass index	c/o	Complains of
BP	Blood pressure	COPD	Chronic obstructive pulmonary disease
BPH	Benign prostatic hypertrophy	Csf	Cerebrospinal fluid
BPM	Beats per minute	CT	Computed tomography

2.31 Common Abbreviations and Acronyms (continued)

ABBREVIATION/ACRONYM	MEANING	ABBREVIATION/ACRONYM	MEANING
BRP	Bathroom privileges	Cv	Cardiovascular
BSA	Body surface area	CVA	Cerebrovascular accident (stroke)
BUN	Blood urea nitrogen	CXR	Chest x-ray
Bx	Biopsy	d	Day
c̄	With	D&C	Dilation and curettage
D/C, dc	Discharge, discontinue	HIV	Human immunodeficiency virus
DM	Diabetes mellitus	HPV	Human papillomavirus
DNR	Do not resuscitate	HTN	Hypertension
DOB	Date of birth	Hx	History
DTap	Diphtheria, tetanus, and acellular pertussis vaccine	I&D	Incision and drainage
Dx	Diagnosis	I&O	Intake and output
ECG, EKG	Electrocardiogram	ICU	Intensive care unit
ED	Emergency department	IUD	Intrauterine device
EEG	Electroencephalogram	K	Potassium
ENT	Ear, nose, and throat	KUB	Kidneys, ureters, bladder
F	Fahrenheit	L	Liter or left
FBS, FBG	Fasting blood sugar/glucose	lb	Pound
f/u	Follow up	LLE	Left lower extremity
FUO	Fever of unknown origin	LLL	Left lower lobe
Fx	Fracture	LLQ	Left lower quadrant
GI	Gastrointestinal	LMP	Last menstrual period
GTT	Glucose tolerance test	LUE	Left upper extremity
gtt	Drop	LUQ	Left upper quadrant
GU	Genitourinary	mg/dL	Milligrams per deciliter
GYN	Gynecology, gynecologist	MI	Myocardial infarction
H, hr	Hour	mL	Milliliters
Hct	Hematocrit	MM	Mucous membrane
HEENT	Head, ears, eyes, nose, throat	mm Hg	Millimeters of mercury
HF	Heart failure	MRI	Magnetic resonance imaging
Hgb	Hemoglobin	MS	Multiple sclerosis

2.31 Common Abbreviations and Acronyms (continued)

ABBREVIATION/ACRONYM	MEANING	ABBREVIATION/ACRONYM	MEANING
HIPAA	Health Insurance Portability and Accountability Act	N/V	Nausea/vomiting
NB	Newborn	RLL	Right lower lobe
NG	Nasogastric	RLQ	Right lower quadrant
NKA/NKDA	No known allergies/No known drug allergies	R/O	Rule out
NPO	Nothing by mouth (*nil per os*)	ROM	Range of motion
NS	Normal saline	RT	Respiratory therapy/therapist
NSAID	Nonsteroidal anti-inflammatory drug	RUE	Right upper extremity
OB	Obstetrics	RUQ	Right upper quadrant
OC	Oral contraceptive	Rx	Prescription
OOB	Out of bed	s̄	Without
OP	Outpatient	SOB	Shortness of breath
OT	Occupational therapy/therapist	Stat	Immediately
OTC	Over-the-counter	STI	Sexually transmitted infection
PA	Posteroanterior, physician assistant	Sx	Symptoms
p.c.	After meals (*post cibos*)	T&A	Tonsillectomy and adenoidectomy
PE	Physical examination, pulmonary embolism	TB	Tuberculosis
PID	Pelvic inflammatory disease	TIA	Transient ischemic attack
PMS	Premenstrual syndrome	Tx	Treatment
PO	By mouth	UA	Urinalysis
PRN	As needed	URI	Upper respiratory infection
PT	Physical therapy/therapist	UTI	Urinary tract infection
pt	Patient	VS	Vital signs
R	Right	WBC	White blood cell
RA	Rheumatoid arthritis	WNL	Within normal limits
RBC	Red blood cell	YO, y/o	Years old
RLE	Right lower extremity		

Acronyms and Symbols

Some medical symbols have fallen out of use because of their tendency toward misinterpretation, especially in handwriting. Some of those are on the "Do Not Use" and "Error-Prone Abbreviations" lists. Examples are the symbols for "greater than" and "less than" (> and <), as well as those for "greater than or equal to" and "less than or equal to" (≥ and ≤). Those lists also advise against using @ and &, as people can mistake them for the numeral 2. Likewise, the plus sign should not be used, because it can look like the numeral 4. When in doubt, spell it out. Here are a few symbols that medical assistants might still see in handwritten medical records. These can also be risky: ↑ could look like the numeral 7, ↓ could look like the numeral 1, and ° could look like the numeral 0.

2.32 Symbols

SYMBOL	MEANING
#	Pounds, number
↑	Increase
↓	Decrease
♂	Male
♀	Female
'	Feet
"	Inches
°	Degrees

CHALLENGE

1. Match each term with the common abbreviation.

TERM	COMMON ABBREVIATION
A. Hematocrit	1. lb
B. Treatment	2. K
C. Potassium	3. Hct
D. Pound	4. Tx

A: 3, B: 4, C: 2, D: 1

2. Match each term with the common abbreviation.

TERM	COMMON ABBREVIATION
A. Before meals	1. NPO
B. Nothing by mouth	2. PRN
C. As desired	3. a.c.
D. After meals	4. Ad Lib
E. By mouth	5. p.c.
F. As needed	6. PO

A: 3, B: 1, C: 4, D: 5, E: 6, F: 2

MEDICAL WORD BUILDING

As familiarity with medical terminology grows, it becomes easy to notice similarities among these terms. That is because many of them share common roots, prefixes, and suffixes. Putting together these components builds many medical terms. However, it doesn't work to just mix and match three components and find a word that is in universal use. For example, hemi- means half, narc means sleep, and -ism means condition. But a patient chronically getting half the amount of sleep they should get isn't heminarcism. There is no such word. Also, with some combinations, the result requires interpretation, because the literal meaning might vary a little from the actual meaning. An example is antibiotic, a combination of the prefix anti-, meaning against, and the *word root* bio, meaning life. Antibiotics are not incompatible with life. They kill a particular type of living organism: bacteria. Also, not all medical terms adhere to the *prefix*-root-*suffix* schema. However, looking at a word that has any one of those word components in it can offer a clue to what the term means.

word root. Core component of words that describe the basic meaning.

prefix. Word component that appears at the beginning of a word to change the meaning of the rest of the word.

suffixes. Word components that appear at the end of the word to change the meaning of the rest of the word.

Word Roots

Word roots are the core component of many words. Medical terms usually have one root but can have two or more.

For example, hem- means blood, and -rrhage means excessive flow. The "o" between the two creates the medical term hemorrhage, meaning excessive blood flow. Not all word roots relate to a body system or a body part, but the following tables lists some of the terms that do.

2.33 Take Note

Sometimes, when a root attaches to a prefix or suffix, it needs an extra vowel to combine the components. This vowel is known as a combining vowel.

Common Word Roots

2.34 Endocrine

WORD ROOT	MEANING
Aden	Gland
Pancreat	Pancreas
Thyr	Thyroid gland

2.35 Hematologic

WORD ROOT	MEANING
Hem, hemat	Blood
Phleb	Vein
Thromb	Clot

2.36 Integumentary

WORD ROOT	MEANING
Derm, dermat	Skin
Hidr	Sweat
Trich	Hair
Onych	Nail
Xer	Dry

2.37 Cardiovascular

WORD ROOT	MEANING
Angi	Blood vessel
Arteri, arter	Artery
Cardi	Heart
Vas	Vessel
Ven	Vein

2.38 Respiratory

WORD ROOT	MEANING
Bronch	Bronchial
Laryng	Larynx
Nas	Nose
Pleur	Pleura
Pneum, pneumon	Lungs, air
Pulmon	Lung
Rhin	Nose
Steth	Chest
Thorac	Thorax
Trache	Trachea

2.39 Neurologic

WORD ROOT	MEANING
Blephar	Eyelid
Cephal	Head
Cerebr	Cerebrum
Encephal	Brain
Esthesi	Sensation
Irid, ird	Iris
Mening, meningi	Membranes, meninges
Myel	Spinal cord, bone marrow
Myring	Eardrum
Neur	Nerve
Ocul, ophthalm	Eye
Ot	Ear

CHAPTER 2: MEDICAL TERMINOLOGY, ANATOMY, AND PHYSIOLOGY
Medical Word Building

2.40 Musculoskeletal

WORD ROOT	MEANING
Arthr	Joint
Brachi	Arm
Cervic	Neck
Chondr	Cartilage
Cost	Rib
Crani	Skull
Dactyl	Finger or toe
Fibr	Connective tissue
My	Muscle
Oste	Bone
Pod	Foot
Sacr	Sacrum
Spondyl, vertebr	Vertebra
Ten, tendin	Tendon

2.41 Gastrointestinal

WORD ROOT	MEANING
Abdomin	Abdomen
An	Anus
Appendic	Appendix
Bil, chol	Bile, gall
Col	Colon
Dent	Teeth
Enter	Intestines
Esophag	Esophagus
Gastr	Stomach
Gingiv	Gums
Gloss	Tongue
Hepat	Liver
Icter	Jaundice
Ile	Ileum
Lapar	Abdominal wall
Lingu	Tongue
Pancreat	Pancreas
Pepsia	Digestion
Phag	Eating, swallowing
Proct	Rectum
Splen	Spleen
Stomat	Mouth

2.42 Genitourinary/Reproductive

WORD ROOT	MEANING
Andr	Male
Colp	Vagina
Cyst	Bladder
Gravid	Pregnant
Gynec	Female
Hyster	Uterus
Mamm, mast	Breast
Metr	Uterus
Nephr	Kidney
Ov	Ovum
Oophor	Ovary
Orchid	Testicles
Prostat	Prostate gland
Pyel	Pelvis of the kidney
Ren	Renal/kidney
Salping	Fallopian tube
Ureter	Ureters
Ur	Urinary
Vesic	Bladder

2.43 Other

WORD ROOT	MEANING
Adip	Fat
Bio	Life
Carcin	Cancer
Cry	Cold
Dors	Back portion of the body
Gluc, glyc	Sugar
Hemi	Hernia
Hist	Tissue
Hydra	Water
Lact	Milk
Later	Side
Lip	Fat
Lith	Stone
Med, medi	Middle
Narc	Numbness, stupor, sleep
Necr	Death
Onc	Tumor
Path	Disease
Ped	Child; foot
Psych	Mind
Pyo	Pus
Pyr	Fever, heat
Septic	Infection
Therm	Heat

CHAPTER 2: MEDICAL TERMINOLOGY, ANATOMY, AND PHYSIOLOGY
Medical Word Building

Combining Root Words

A combining form is a word root with a combining vowel. Often, the combining vowel makes the medical term easier to pronounce. In most cases, the combining vowel is an "o," but it is sometimes "i" or "e." A combining form should be used when the last word root in a medical term connects with a suffix that begins with a consonant. When the word root connects with a suffix that starts with a vowel, just the word root should be used.

2.44 Combining Form Examples

WORD ROOT	COMBINING VOWEL	COMBINING FORM	SUFFIX	MEDICAL TERM
Col	O	Col/o	-stomy	Colostomy
Cephal	O	Cephal/o	-algia	Cephalagia
Col	O	Col/o	-ectomy	Colectomy
Cephal	O	Cephal/o	-dynia	Cephalodynia

When the suffix begins with a vowel, the word root is used. Examples include cephalalgia and colectomy. However, when the suffix begins with a consonant, the combining form is used, as in colostomy and cephalodynia. When connecting two word roots, always use the connecting vowel, even if the following word root begins with a vowel.

Prefixes

Prefixes are word components that appear at the beginning of a word to change the meaning of the rest of the word. They generally mean the same thing in each word they modify. Some medical terms have no prefix. An example is splenectomy, a combination of the word root splen, meaning spleen, and the suffix –ectomy, meaning removal. The following is a list of some of the common prefixes medical assistants will encounter.

2.45 Common Prefixes

PREFIX	MEANING	PREFIX	MEANING
A-, an-	Without	Ex-, extra-, exo-	Outside of
Ab-	Away, from	Hemi-	Half
Ad-	Toward	Hyper-	Above, excessive, increased
Ambi-	Both	Hypo-	Below, decreased, insufficient
Ante-	Before	Infra-	Beneath
Anti-	Against	Inter-	Between, among
Auto-	Self	Intra-	Within, during
Bi-	Two, twice, double	Levo-	To the left
Brady-	Slow	Macro-	Large
Circum-	Around	Mal-	Bad
Contra-	Against	Mega-	Exceptionally large

2.45 Common Prefixes (continued)

PREFIX	MEANING
De-	Down
Dys-	Painful, abnormal, difficult, bad
Endo-	Within, inside
Epi-	Above, on
Eu-	Normal, good
Multi-	Many
Neo-	New
Nulli-	None
Peri-	Around
Poly-	Many
Post-	After, behind
Pre-, pro-	Before, in front of
Presby-	Older age
Primi-	First
Pseudo-	False

PREFIX	MEANING
Meso-	Middle
Meta-	Over, beyond
Micro-	Small
Mono-	One
Quadri-	Four
Retro-	Behind, in back of
Sten-	Narrowed
Sub-	Under
Super-, supra-	Above, excess
Sym-, syn-	Together, with
Tachy-	Fast
Trans-	Across
Tri-	Three
Ultra-	Beyond, excess
Uni-	One

Suffixes

Suffixes are word components that appear at the end of the word to change the meaning of the rest of the word. Some medical terms have no suffix, such as appendix. Some medical terms combine a prefix and a suffix with no word root. An example is hemiplegia, a combination of the prefix hemi–, meaning half, and the suffix –plegia, meaning paralysis. The following tables list some of the common general suffixes medical assistants will encounter, as well as some that are more specific to clinical disorders and medical, surgical, and diagnostic procedures.

Common Suffixes

2.46 General

SUFFIX	MEANING
-age	Related to
-cidal, -cide	Pertaining to killing
-form	Shape
-fuge	Driving away
-iatry, -iatrist	Healing by a provider/healer
-ical	Pertaining to
-ion	Process

SUFFIX	MEANING
-logy, logist	Study of, one who studies
-ole	Little, small
-opia	Vision
-phylaxis	Protection, prevention
-pnea	Breathing
-therapy	Treatment
-uria	Urine

2.47 Surgery/Procedures

SUFFIX	MEANING
-centesis	Surgical puncture
-cise	Cut, remove
-clasis	Break down
-desis	Stabilization, binding
-ectomy	Removal, excision
-gram	Record
-graph	Instrument for recording
-graphy	Process of recording
-ion	Process
-lepsy	Seizure, convulsion
-lysis	Destruction, separation
-meter	Device for measuring
-metry	Process of measuring
-pexy	Fixation, to put in place
-plasty	Surgical repair, reformation
-scopy	Visual examination
-spasm	Involuntary twitch
-stasis	Stopping or controlling
-stomy	A new opening
-tomy	Incision
-tripsy	Crushing

2.48 Disorders/Conditions

SUFFIX	MEANING
-algia	Pain
-asthenia	Weakness
-cele	Swelling, herniation
-dynia	Pain
-ectasis	Dilation, expansion
-emesis	Vomiting
-emia	Blood condition
-gen	Producing
-ia, -ism	Condition of
-iasis	Presence of, formation of
-i	Inflammation
-malacia	Weakening or softening of
-mania	Obsessive preoccupation
-megaly	Enlargement
-oid	Seeming like
-ole	Small
-oma	Tumor
-osis	Condition, usually abnormal
-pathy	Disorder, disease
-penia	Deficiency, decrease
-phagia	Eating, swallowing
-phasia	Speech
-phobia	Fear
-plasia	Formation of
-plegia	Paralysis
-ptosis	Drooping, falling
-rrhage	Bursting forth
-rrhea	Flow, discharge
-rrhexis	Rupture
-sclerosis	Hardening condition
-trophy	Development

CHAPTER 2: MEDICAL TERMINOLOGY, ANATOMY, AND PHYSIOLOGY
Common Terms

CHALLENGE

1. Match the root with the correct meaning.

ROOT	MEANING
A. Aden	1. Bone
B. Chondr	2. Gland
C. Oste	3. Cartilage
D. Hepat	4. Liver

A: 2, B: 3, C: 1, D: 4

2. Match the root with the correct meaning.

ROOT	MEANING
A. Pepsia	1. Chest
B. Cyst	2. Bladder
C. Pyel	3. Digestion
D. Steth	4. Pelvis or kidney

A: 3, B: 2, C: 4, D: 1

3. Which of the following does the prefix presby- refer to?
   A. Older age
   B. Hospital
   C. Beneath
   D. Pain

   A is correct. The prefix presby- refers to older age.

4. Which of the following suffixes can be used to indicate a blood condition?
   A. -emesis
   B. -ectasis
   C. -emia
   D. -itis

   C is correct. The suffix -emia refers to a blood disorder (e.g., anemia).

COMMON TERMS

Usually, it is best to use lay terms instead of medical terminology when communicating with patients to ensure patients understand. Develop a knowledge base of lay terms associated with medical terms to effectively communicate with patients.

2.49 Medical Terms

MEDICAL TERM	LAY LANGUAGE
Hypertension	High blood pressure
Angina	Chest pain
Acute	New, urgent, sudden
Chronic	Ongoing
Alopecia	Hair loss
Cerebrovascular accident (CVA)	Stroke
Myocardial infarction	Heart attack
Edema	Swelling
CT scan	CAT scan
Cryotherapy	Freezing off
Abdomen	Stomach
Tachycardia	Fast heart rate, heart beating fast, heart racing

tachycardia. Heart rate greater than 100/min.

bradycardia. Heart rate less than 60/min.

2.49 Medical Terms (continued)

MEDICAL TERM	LAY LANGUAGE
Bradycardia	Low heart rate, heart beating slow
Hyperglycemia	High blood sugar
Hypoglycemia	Low blood sugar
GERD	Heartburn
Shortness of breath	Trouble breathing
Phalanges	Fingers and toes
Arrhythmia	Irregular heart rhythm
Erythrocytes	Red blood cells
Vertigo	Dizziness, room spinning, dizzy, lightheaded
Syncope	Fainting, temporary loss of consciousness
Deep vein thrombosis (DVT)	Blood clot
Osteoarthritis	Wear and tear
Amyotrophic lateral sclerosis (ALS)	Lou Gehrig's disease

> **CHALLENGE**
>
> 1. Which of the following is a patient likely referring to if they say they have "wear and tear" causing knee pain?
>   A. Osteoarthritis
>   B. Rheumatoid arthritis
>   C. Osteoporosis
>   D. Deep vein thrombosis
>
> *A is correct. Osteoarthritis is often referred to as "wear and tear" on joints by patients, as this was previously thought to be the cause of the condition.*

POSITIONAL AND DIRECTIONAL TERMINOLOGY

Knowledge of the medical terms that indicate directions and positions is essential for communicating in health care. For example, for various types of examinations and diagnostic procedures, not only must patients be positioned correctly or optimally, those positions and how the patient tolerated them must also be documented.

The following are lists of words medical assistants can use to help understand directional terms, as well as a list of terms that are essential for positioning.

2.50 Positional Terms

TERM	DEFINITION
Anatomical position	Standard frame of reference in which the body is standing up, face forward, arms at the sides, palms forward, and toes pointed forward
Supine	Lying face up
Prone	Lying face down
Dorsal recumbent	Lying facing upward with flexed knees, feet flat on floor
Fowler position	Sitting upright with back angled at 90 degrees
Semi-Fowler's position	Sitting with back angled at 45 degrees

anatomical position. Standard frame of reference in which the body is standing up, face forward, arms at the sides, palms forward, and toes pointed forward.

2.51 Directional Terms

TERM	DEFINITION
Anterior	Toward the front of the body, also known as ventral
Posterior	Toward the back of the body, also known as dorsal
Superior	Above; toward the head
Inferior	Below; toward the feet
Medial	Closer to the midline of the body
Lateral	Further from the midline of the body (toward the side)
Superficial	Closer to the surface of the body; more external
Deep	Farther from the body's surface; more internal
Proximal	Closer to the body's trunk
Distal	Further from the body's trunk
Dextrad	Toward the right
Sinistrad	Toward the left

CHALLENGE

1. Lying face-down could be described as which of the following positions?
   A. Prone
   B. Supine
   C. Anatomical
   D. Fowler position

   A is correct. The positional term prone refers to lying face-down.

2. What does anatomical position refer to?

   Anatomical position is the standard frame of reference in which the body is standing up, face forward, arms at the sides, palms forward, and toes pointed forward.

3. Match the direction term with the correct definition.

TERM	DEFINITION
A. Proximal	1. Toward the front of the body
A. Medial	2. Toward the left
B. Anterior	3. Pertaining to the belly side
C. Sinistrad	4. Closer to the body's trunk

A: 4, B: 3, C: 1, D: 2

PSYCHOLOGY AND MENTAL HEALTH

Developmental stages

One of the most generally accepted developmental theories is the work of *Erik Erikson*. His eight stages of development offer a guideline for identifying the psychosocial challenges patients face at different periods in their lives and the tasks they must master before successfully transitioning to the next stage of development. Erikson believed that society and culture affect how the personality of an individual develops and that successful completion of each stage supports the healthy development of the person's ego.

Trust vs. Mistrust

This is the psychosocial crisis for infants. Trust is the successful outcome of this stage. Mistrust is the unsuccessful outcome.

The developmental tasks for infants are to form an attachment with and develop trust in their primary caregiver and then generalize those bonds to others. They also begin to trust their own body as they learn gross and then fine motor skills. Achieving the tasks of this stage results in self-confidence and optimism that caregivers will meet the infant's basic needs. Nonachievement leads to suspiciousness and struggles with interpersonal relationships.

Erik Erikson. Psychologist who developed the concepts of stages of life based on a person's age.

Autonomy vs. Shame and Doubt

This is the psychosocial crisis for toddlers. Autonomy is the successful outcome of this stage. Shame and doubt are the unsuccessful outcome. During this stage, toddlers begin to develop a sense of independence, autonomy, and self-control. They also acquire language skills. Parents should be firm but tolerant with toddlers. Achieving the tasks of this stage results in self-control and voluntary delaying of gratification. Nonachievement leads to anger with self, a lack of self-confidence, and no sense of pride in the ability to perform tasks

Initiative vs. Guilt

This is the psychosocial crisis for preschoolers. Initiative is the successful outcome of this stage. Guilt is the unsuccessful outcome. During this stage, children look for new experiences but will hesitate when adults reprimand them or restrict them from trying new things.

Preschoolers have an active imagination and are curious about everything around them. Eventually they will start feeling guilt for some of their actions, which is part of the natural development of moral judgment.

Achieving the tasks of this stage results in assertiveness, dependability, creativity, and personal achievement. Nonachievement leads to feelings of inadequacy, defeat, and guilt and the belief that they deserve punishment.

Industry vs. Inferiority

This is the psychosocial crisis for school-age children. Industry is the successful outcome of this stage. Inferiority is the unsuccessful outcome. During this stage, children need to receive recognition for accomplishments to provide reinforcement and build self-confidence. If the achievements are met with a negative response, inferiority can be established. Children require acknowledgment of their successes. Achieving the tasks of this stage results in feelings of competence, self-satisfaction, and trustworthiness in addition to increased participation in activities and taking on more responsibilities at school, home, and the community. Nonachievement leads to feelings of inadequacy and the inability to compromise or cooperate with others.

Identity vs. Role Confusion

This is the psychosocial crisis for adolescents. Identity is the successful outcome of this stage. Role confusion is the unsuccessful outcome. During this stage, adolescents try to figure out where they fit in and what direction their life should take. If role confusion sets in, adolescents become followers, which can lead to poor decision-making. Achieving the tasks of this stage results in emotional stability, ability to form committed relationships, and sound decision-making. Nonachievement leads to a lack of personal goals and values, rebelliousness, self-consciousness, and a lack of self-confidence.

Intimacy vs. Isolation

This is the psychosocial crisis for young adults. Intimacy is the successful outcome of this stage. Isolation is the unsuccessful outcome. During this stage, young adults begin to think about partnership, marriage, family, and career. Lack of fulfillment in this key area of life can lead to isolation and withdrawal. Achieving the tasks of this stage results in the ability for mutual self-respect and love, intimacy, and commitment to others and to a career. Nonachievement leads to social isolation and withdrawal; multiple job changes or lack of productivity and fulfillment in one job; and an inability to form long-term, intimate, or close relationships.

Generativity vs. Stagnation

This is the psychosocial crisis for middle adults. Generativity is the successful outcome of this stage. Stagnation is the unsuccessful outcome. During this stage, adults continue raising children, and some become grandparents. They want to help mold future generations, so they often involve themselves in teaching, coaching, writing, and social activism. Achieving the tasks of this stage results in professional and personal achievements and active participation in serving the community and society. Nonachievement occurs when development ceases, which leads to self-preoccupation without the capacity to give and share with others.

Ego Integrity vs. Despair

This is the psychosocial crisis for older adults. Ego integrity is the successful outcome of this stage. Despair is the unsuccessful outcome. During this stage, most adults retire; their children, if they have any, no longer live at home. Many will volunteer to retain a feeling of usefulness. Their bodies experience age-related changes, and health becomes a major concern, especially as friends and loved ones die. Achieving the tasks of this stage results in wisdom, self-acceptance, and a sense of self-worth as life draws to a close. Nonachievement leads to dissatisfaction with one's life, feelings of worthlessness, helplessness to change, depression, anger, and the inability to accept that death will occur.

CHALLENGE

1. Match the successful outcome to the unsuccessful outcome within the same development stage.

SUCCESSFUL	UNSUCCESSFUL
A. Trust	1. Inferiority
B. Autonomy	2. Stagnation
C. Initiative	3. Shame and doubt
D. Industry	4. Mistrust
E. Identity	5. Guilt
F. Intimacy	6. Despair
G. Generativity	7. Isolation
H. Ego integrity	8. Role confusion

   *A: 4, B: 3, C: 5, D: 1, E: 8, F: 7, G: 2, H: 6
   The correct sequence is trust vs. mistrust, autonomy vs. shame and doubt, initiative vs. guilt, industry vs. inferiority, identity vs. role confusion, intimacy vs. isolation, generativity vs. stagnation, and ego integrity vs. despair.*

2. In which of the following Erikson's stages of development is poor decision-making most likely to be experienced?

   A. Trust vs. mistrust
   B. Autonomy vs. shame and doubt
   C. Industry vs. inferiority
   D. Identity vs. role confusion

   D is correct. During identify vs. role confusion, adolescents try to figure out where they fit in and what direction their life should take. If role confusion sets in, adolescents become followers, which can lead to poor decision-making.

COMMON MENTAL HEALTH CONDITIONS

Mental health is as important as physical health when it comes to overall wellness. Mental health refers to a person's cognitive abilities, behaviors, and emotions. Mental health conditions and illnesses can be caused by biological issues (such as genetics), environmental issues (such as learned behaviors, poor coping mechanisms, traumatic experiences), or a combination of both. There are over 300 recognized mental illnesses, many with overlapping symptoms. Understanding how to interact empathetically and effectively with a patient suffering from a mental illness is key for medical assistants (and all health care professionals). This involves being patient and professional in all interactions, building trust with the patient, and working together with the patient and provider to understand appropriate and helpful language and actions to communicate with each individual patient effectively. Treatment includes medications and behavior therapies.

2.52 Common Mental Health Conditions

CONDITION	DESCRIPTION	SIGNS AND SYMPTOMS	TREATMENT
Depression	Mood disorder that can be caused by a chemical imbalance in the brain	Extreme sadness, fatigue, lethargy, hopelessness, pain, digestive issues, extreme lack of motivation (even with activities and hobbies that previously were enjoyable), thoughts of suicide	Typically managed best with a combination of therapy, healthy lifestyle, and medication
Attention-deficit/hyperactivity disorder (ADHD)	Chronic condition that typically begins in childhood but can impact individuals throughout their life	Inattention in which the individual struggles to regulate attention and focus, making it difficult to follow directions and stay organized. Hyperactivity and impulsivity can present as constant fidgeting, excessive talking, and struggling with quiet activities. More commonly diagnosed in boys	Medications and behavior therapies
Anxiety	Disorders that lead to extreme feelings of worry and fear, to the point that the person's ability to function and respond to typical situations is inhibited	Uncontrolled levels of stress, fast heart rate, sweating, and being consumed by worry	Therapy, healthy lifestyle, and medication
Post-traumatic stress disorder (PTSD)	A condition resulting from a traumatic or terrifying event. Not everyone who experiences a traumatic event will develop PTSD. War veterans; people who have experienced physical, emotional, or sexual abuse; people who have lived through an attack or natural disaster; and those who have lost a loved one might experience PTSD.	Intrusive memories (such as flashbacks to the event), negative changes (negative thoughts and hopelessness), changes in reactions (new and potentially aggressive behaviors), trouble with concentration and sleep, self-destructive behaviors, and avoidance (avoiding places, people, or experiences associated with the negative event; avoiding loved ones; avoidance of discussing the event)	Psychotherapy, exposure therapy, and medication

CHALLENGE

1. Which of the following mental health conditions involves difficulty focusing and struggling with quiet activities?
   A. Anxiety
   B. Depression
   C. Post-traumatic stress disorder (PTSD)
   D. Attention-deficit/hyperactivity disorder (ADHD)

   D is correct. The most common signs of ADHD are inattention, hyperactivity, and impulsivity.

2. How many mental health conditions are currently recognized?
   A. 50 to 100
   B. Over 300
   C. About 500
   D. Over 1,000

   B is correct. There are over 300 recognized mental illnesses.

ENVIRONMENTAL AND SOCIOECONOMIC STRESSORS

A stressor is anything that causes anxiety or stress. Many things in the environment cause stress, as do psychological factors (grief, depression, loss, guilt). Even things that are positive (taking a vacation, having an intimate experience, graduating from college) can be stressors. Coming to a health care facility can create a great deal of stress for a patient. This can be reflected by an increase in blood pressure in the office that is not reflected in the patient's readings from home, commonly called white-coat syndrome. This is an objective indication of the patient's anxiety.

Environmental Stressors

Environmental stressors, or physical stressors, include situations that cause enough stress to become obstacles to achieving goals or having positive experiences. Things in the environment (air pollution, ultraviolet rays from excessive sun exposure, overcrowding, language and cultural barriers, discrimination) cause the body physical stress.

Events in the environment (death of a loved one, theft, vandalism, motor-vehicle crashes, physical assault, job, school problems) can also cause stress. Major disasters (fires, floods, tornadoes, earthquakes, hurricanes, war) can result in PTSD, which causes anxiety, insomnia, anger, loss of interest in daily activities, and flashbacks to the traumatizing event.

Even though a stressor might originate from the environment, the mind interprets the severity of the situation and helps the person cope with it in a positive way. From there, people deal with the stressor based on their perception, experience, and resources they have available to them. When they cannot cope with the situation or do not have adequate support systems, they can develop any number of negative outcomes.

environmental stressor. Situation that causes enough stress to become an obstacle to achieve goals or have positive experiences.

CHAPTER 2: MEDICAL TERMINOLOGY, ANATOMY, AND PHYSIOLOGY
Communication and Accommodations

Socioeconomic Stressors

Many people undergo a great deal of stress over financial situations. Life is expensive; sometimes it seems like an endless cycle of working and struggling to meet expenses and pay debts. Just when it seems that getting ahead financially is within reach, a sudden unexpected expense (medical bills, vehicle repair) or a job loss eliminates the possibility of economic balance, and the expenses and debt may pile up. Even people who have not had a great deal of socioeconomic stress in their lives can suddenly find themselves in a stressful situation due to retirement, changes in the economy that lead to a loss of investments, identity theft, lack of job security, involuntary job loss (getting fired), or the loss of a home or vehicle. Medical assistants encounter patients who have minimal health insurance and find the out-of-pocket costs of many diagnostic procedures, treatments, and medications beyond what they can afford.

CHALLENGE

1. Which of the following is an example of a socioeconomic stressor?
   A. Loss of a vehicle
   B. Death of a loved one
   C. Fear of doctor's offices
   D. Air pollution

   A is correct. Socioeconomic stressors are those related to financial situations. Loss of a vehicle can be very expensive and make it difficult to manage daily tasks and responsibilities if a new one cannot be afforded easily.

2. Why do similar stressors affect people differently?

   The mind interprets the severity of the situation and helps the person cope with it in a positive way. People deal with the stressor based on their perception, experience, and resources they have available to them.

COMMUNICATION AND ACCOMMODATIONS

A general understanding of the principles of therapeutic communication is helpful when working with all patients. For example, medical assistants can encourage patients to express their feelings by reflecting patients' statements back to them in a way that promotes further communication. It is also helpful to make observations and offer recognition of positive changes. These techniques promote positive communication. Patients can also have specific types of problems that require special consideration and techniques. The medical assistant helps build and nurture the relationship with all health care staff.

Physical Disability

Medical offices and facilities are legally required, according to the Americans with Disabilities Act, to have appropriate access for patients who use wheelchairs or other assistive devices. These include marked parking spaces, ramps, and accessible bathrooms with large stalls and handrails. Medical assistants can ensure these patients are comfortable and able to function well in their surroundings by organizing common areas. The patients will feel more at ease, and it will be easier to build therapeutic relationships with them. They will see the office staff has anticipated their needs and facilitated their navigation throughout the office.

Many patients who have disabilities experience instances of people making tactless remarks or asking inappropriate questions. Only ask questions regarding their disability as part of a medical evaluation or history gathering. Instead of asking "How did that happen to you?" ask "What can I do to assist during your visit?" Being over-solicitous can come across as insincere. Be prepared to provide any necessary accommodations, but do not make assumptions. Ask the patient what they require and respect their answer.

Office Organization Strategies

- Create enough gaps between the chairs in the waiting areas and along walls for safe wheelchair access, maneuvering, and parking.

- Do not place any area rugs or throw rugs where patients walking with assistive devices or navigating with wheelchairs will encounter them.

- Eliminate metal or wooden sills in doorways. Replace them with graduated rubber coverings that provide a smoother surface for wheels to transition over.

- Remove any objects that would interfere with complete swiveling of wheelchairs.

- Position reading materials at a height where patients in wheelchairs can reach them easily.

- Provide sturdy bars or rails along walls for patients who have difficulty walking or have balance issues.

- For patients who have vision loss, provide Braille signs and reading materials along with large-print materials. Use descriptive language when speaking with these patients and avoid touching without verbally alerting the patient first.

- For patients who have hearing loss, offer services such as online appointment scheduling. Patients might be able to communicate well in person but have considerable difficulty hearing and understanding speech on the telephone, making scheduling difficult. Stand directly in line with the patient's face when speaking, not from the side or behind them. Pronounce words clearly to allow the individual to see lip movements as well as hear what is said. Do not shout. Clarity of speech is much more important in facilitating understanding. If a sign-language interpreter is requested, by federal law, the office must provide an interpreter.

- For patients who have service animals, remember that these animals are not pets. If others attempt to speak to, touch, or interact with these animals, intervene as necessary and educate that service animals are on duty and things that distract them from their duties are inappropriate.

- Have accommodations ready for any patient who requests them. Ask the patient what type of accommodation they prefer before providing assistance.

Developmental Delay

The first step when working with patients who have mental or emotional disabilities is to determine how they communicate and what level of communication they understand. Family members and caregivers can assist with this, but do not assume the patient is incapable of communicating. Always address the patient first. Remain calm, avoid showing impatience, and speak at a consistent volume. Any time you cannot understand something the patient says, ask for clarification. Advocate for patients and always treat them with respect and empathy. Provide accommodations to meet patients' needs and ask how to assist during their visit.

Illness and Disease

Individuals who have chronic or terminal illness are under an extreme amount of stress. Casual, routine opening lines like an excessively cheerful "How are you doing today?" can provoke defensive responses like, "How do you think I'm doing? I'm dying." Even if the patient doesn't say that, they might think it. Instead, welcome these patients warmly and respect their dignity. Treat them with kindness and care at all times.

Offer support and empathy, and allow the patient to set the tone of the conversation. Never say you know how the patient feels. All feelings are unique to the individual, so to express this belittles the person and shows a lack of respect for their individuality. Listen carefully to the patient, maintain eye contact, and always ask how to help. Prior to beginning medical data collection, use a broad opening like, "What would you like to talk about today?" How the patient answers will help set the tone for the remainder of the interaction.

Make sure the patient has all the services they need, such as hospice referrals, meal-delivery services, and home health assistance. Support groups and community services can also help; these services can provide social experiences and an outlet for dying patients and their families.

CHALLENGE

1. What accommodations can support a patient who has hearing loss?

   Services such as online appointment scheduling can be very helpful. Patients might communicate well in person but have considerable difficulty on the telephone, making scheduling difficult. Position directly in line with the patient's face when speaking, not from the side or behind them. Pronounce words clearly to allow the individual to see lip movements as well as hear what is said. Do not shout. Provide a sign-language interpreter if requested.

2. Which of the following would be an appropriate action for the medical assistant to take when working with a patient who has a developmental disability?

   A. Stay calm.
   B. Speak louder.
   C. Speak to the family member instead.
   D. Change the subject.

   A is correct. When communication begins and a patient becomes agitated or confused, remain calm. Avoid showing impatience or speaking louder, which can increase the patient's agitation. Any time the MA cannot understand something the patient says, ask for clarification. Family members can help, but the patient should never be ignored.

DEFENSE MECHANISMS

Defense mechanisms are coping strategies people use to protect themselves from negative emotions such as guilt, anxiety, fear, and shame. Individuals are generally unaware that they are using these responses to stress. Developing the ability to recognize these defense mechanisms and the emotions behind them can help medical assistants tremendously in understanding patients and helping to meet their needs.

2.53 Take Note

Defense mechanisms can be adaptive and help the individual change or adjust as they come to terms with the stressor. Maladaptive defense mechanisms hinder change and adjustment.

---

defense mechanisms. Coping strategies individuals use to protect themselves from negative emotions such as guilt, anxiety, fear, and shame.

2.54 Common Defense Mechanisms

DEFENSE MECHANISM	MEANING	EXAMPLE
Apathy	Indifference; lack of interest, feeling, concern, or emotion	"I don't care what she puts in my evaluation, it won't change anything."
Compensation	Balancing a failure or inadequacy with an accomplishment	"I ate a lot of candy yesterday, but I also ate a big green salad."
Conversion	Transformation of an anxiety into a physical symptom that has no cause	"I get a severe headache every time I see my ex with his new wife."
Denial	Avoidance of unpleasant or anxiety-provoking situations or ideas by rejecting them or ignoring their existence	"I am healthy and fit. There is no way I have cancer, so I don't need all those tests."
Displacement	Redirection of emotions away from the original subject or object onto another, less-threatening subject or object	"I had enough trouble handling that last patient. I don't need to deal with this malfunctioning copier right now."
Dissociation	Disconnection of emotional importance from ideas or events and compartmentalizing those emotions in different parts of awareness	"I'm always getting into fights with my neighbors, which is odd because I teach an online course in conflict resolution."
Identification	Attribution of characteristics of someone else to oneself or the imitation of another	"I could pass that certification test just like she did, and I haven't even studied the material."
Intellectualization	Analysis of a situation with facts and not emotions	"He didn't break up with me because he didn't love me. He just had too much on his plate at work at the time."
Introjection	Adoption of the thoughts or feelings of others	"My dad says I should stand up for myself, so I am going to be more assertive."
Physical avoidance	Keeping away from any person, place, or object that evokes memories of something unpleasant	"I can't go to that hospital because that's where my father died."
Projection	Transference of a person's unpleasant ideas and emotions onto someone or something else	"She leaves more charts incomplete than I do, so why am I getting this warning?"
Rationalization	Explanation that makes something negative or unacceptable seem justifiable or acceptable	"My partner drinks every night to make himself less anxious about work."
Reaction formation	Belief in and expression of the opposite of one's true feelings	"I really hate being in the military, but I always sign some people up at recruitment events."
Regression	Reversion to an earlier, more childlike, developmental behavior	"I can't do all that paperwork, and you can't make me."

CHAPTER 2: MEDICAL TERMINOLOGY, ANATOMY, AND PHYSIOLOGY
Defense Mechanisms

2.54 Common Defense Mechanisms (continued)

DEFENSE MECHANISM	MEANING	EXAMPLE
Repression	Elimination of unpleasant emotions, desires, or problems from the conscious mind	"They tell me I was hurt in that robbery, but I can't remember anything about it."
Sarcasm	Use of words that have the opposite meaning, especially to be funny, insulting, or irritating	"You have a nice office if you like working in caves."
Sublimation	Rechanneling unacceptable urges or drives into something constructive or acceptable	"When I was a kid, I used to like to pull wings and legs off insects I'd catch. Now I am a biology teacher."
Suppression	Voluntary blocking of an unpleasant experience from one's awareness	"The doctor said I need more tests, but I'm going to take my vacation first."
Undoing	Cancelling out an unacceptable behavior with a symbolic gesture	"I had a big fight with my wife last night, but I'm going to buy her some flowers on my way home today."
Verbal aggression	Verbal attack on a person without addressing the original intent of the conversation	"Why would you ask me that when you can't even control your children?"

CHALLENGE

1. Which of the following defense mechanisms is shown in the statement "I haven't picked up my insulin because my blood sugar is always high and nothing will help"?
    A. Apathy
    B. Projection
    C. Sarcasm
    D. Verbal aggression

   A is correct. Apathy is defined as indifference, or a lack of interest, feeling, concern, or emotion. In this example, the patient understands they have diabetes but does not feel any interest in concern or interest in managing it, because nothing has seemed to work before.

2. Match the defense mechanism with the correct definition.

DEFENSE MECHANISM	DEFINITION
A. Compensation B. Identification C. Rationalization D. Regression	1. Attribution of characteristics of someone else to oneself or the imitation of another 2. Explanation that makes something negative or unacceptable seem justifiable or acceptable 3. Reversion to an earlier, more childlike, developmental behavior 4. Balancing a failure or inadequacy with an accomplishment

A: 4, B: 1, C: 2, D: 3
Compensation is a method of balancing a failure or inadequacy with an accomplishment. Identification is the attribution of characteristics of someone else to oneself or the imitation of another. Rationalization is an explanation that makes something negative or unacceptable seem justifiable or acceptable. Regression is the reversion to an earlier, more childlike, developmental behavior.

END OF LIFE AND STAGES OF GRIEF

As people age and their physiologic abilities and reserves dwindle, they tend to seek more health care services.

After age 60, many people start to think about their own mortality. They realize that so much of their life is behind them, and they begin to wonder how many "good years" they have left. For many, their adult children live long distances away and have families and careers of their own. It gradually becomes more difficult for older adults to continue to work, maintain their home, and—depending on what health conditions they have—participate in activities they enjoy as well as activities of daily living. They worry that minor issues, like forgetting to buy an item they need at the grocery store or misplacing their keys, mean they are developing dementia. Those whose capacity for independent living has diminished can become victims of elder abuse, which can involve neglect or physical abuse, often perpetrated by caregivers or family members who are overwhelmed with the burden of caring for the aging individual.

Many older adults deal with constant grief as friends, neighbors, and family members die. They may also grieve for themselves—for their younger, healthier days and for the abilities they are losing or have lost. They hear many clichés, such as "Just take one day at a time," "Don't worry about what hasn't happened yet," and "You're only as old as you feel." However, these platitudes offer little comfort to older adults grappling with the grim realities of aging.

All patients need support when they encounter the health care system, and older adults are a unique population because they face so many challenges toward the end of life. The physical challenges are real, and the feelings of grief can be overwhelming. This leads to a major health concern for older adults: depression.

End-of-Life Struggles

Many older patients have chronic or terminal illnesses that influence them to prepare for the end of life. Patients should arrange for end-of-life care, funeral, burial, and cremation services. If the person has a dependent, such as a partner, the dying person will need to make financial or caregiving arrangements. The person also needs to have advance directives in place, as well as a will and a durable power of attorney for health care document available. These preparations bring the reality of the end of life into sharp focus and generally put the patient and loved ones into a state of anticipatory grief. This means that they are feeling the emotions and reactions that grief causes before the loss occurs.

Stages of Grief

Just like with developmental stages, several theorists have defined the various stages of grief. The most well-known theory is the five stages of grief Elisabeth Kübler-Ross defined as a result of her extensive experience in working with dying patients. Awareness of these stages can help medical assistants understand what grieving patients are experiencing, whether the loss is the death of a loved one, body part or function, finances, home, or any number of other losses that have a strong and lasting effect on the person.

Not everyone grieves in the same way. While one person might navigate through the stages of grief one by one and in sequence, others can be in more than one stage simultaneously. Some might skip one or more stages. The duration of the process is also highly variable. There is no right way to grieve. The stages of grief that Kübler-Ross defined are as follows.

Denial
During this stage, the grieving person cannot or will not believe that the loss is happening or has happened. They might deny the existence of the illness and refuse to discuss therapeutic interventions. Thought processes reflect the idea of "No, not me." Support the patient without reinforcing the denial. It might help to give the patient written information about the disease and treatment options with the approval of the provider.

Anger
During this stage, the grieving person might aim feelings of hostility at others, including health care staff (because they cannot fix or cure the disease). Thought processes reflect the idea of "Why me?" Do not take the patient's anger personally. Instead, help them understand that becoming angry is an expected response to grief.

Bargaining
During this stage, the grieving person attempts to avoid the loss by making a deal, such as wanting to live long enough to attend a particular family occasion. The patient might also be searching for alternative solutions. They are still hoping for their previous life, or life itself, or at least a postponement of death. Thought processes reflect the idea of "Yes, me, but..." Listen with attention and encourage the patient to continue expressing their feelings.

Depression
During this stage, the reality of the situation takes hold, and the grieving person feels sad, lonely, and helpless. For example, they might have feelings of regret and self-blame for not taking better care of themselves. They might talk openly about it or might withdraw and say nothing about it. Thought processes reflect the idea of "Yes, it's me." Sit with the patient and do not put any pressure on them to share their feelings. Convey support and understanding. Referrals to a support group or for counseling can be helpful.

Acceptance
During this stage, the grieving person comes to terms with the loss and starts making plans for moving on with life despite the loss or impending loss. They are willing to try to make the best of it and formulate new goals and enjoy new relationships. If death is imminent, they will start making funeral and burial arrangements and might reach out to friends and family who have not been a part of their recent years of life. There might still be some depression, but there might also be humor and friendly interaction. Thought processes reflect the idea of "Yes, me, and I'm ready." Offer encouragement, support, and additional education to the patient and their family and friends during this time.

CHAPTER 2: MEDICAL TERMINOLOGY, ANATOMY, AND PHYSIOLOGY
Wrap-Up

CHALLENGE

1. During which of the following stages of grief might it be most helpful to give the patient written materials?
   A. Denial
   B. Anger
   C. Bargaining
   D. Depression
   E. Acceptance

   A is correct. During denial, the patient might deny the existence of the illness and refuse to discuss therapeutic interventions. Support the patient without reinforcing the denial. It might help to give the patient written information about the disease and treatment options.

2. Which of the following stages of grief involves feeling sad or hopeless?
   A. Denial
   B. Anger
   C. Bargaining
   D. Depression
   E. Acceptance

   D is correct. During the depression stage, the reality of the situation takes hold, and the grieving person feels sad, lonely, and helpless.

3. Which of the following stages of grief involves asking the question "why me?"?
   A. Denial
   B. Anger
   C. Bargaining
   D. Depression
   E. Acceptance

   B is correct. During the anger stage, thought processes reflect the idea of "Why me?"

WRAP-UP

A strong knowledge of body systems and physiological processes is an important aspect of working as a medical assistant. Medical terminology serves as a building block to this foundational knowledge. Understanding common root words, prefixes, and suffixes will allow an MA to be more immersed in the field of medicine and equipped with a necessary skill set to understand future topics, trainings, and encounters.

Disease, illness, and injury are threats faced by people every day in every community. The accurate diagnosis of conditions, effective treatment, management, and disease prevention are the cornerstones for quality medicine and health care. All health care workers commit to the safe and reliable treatment of sick and injured patients. A strong foundational knowledge of disease, risk factors, and disease prevention will aid an MA throughout their career and make them an invaluable part of any health care team.

CHAPTER 3
Patient Intake and Vitals

OVERVIEW

Medical assistants in ambulatory care provide quality patient care, interact effectively with patients, ensure safety, and assist the provider as necessary. This module focuses on highlighting areas that are considered critical knowledge to know and apply in the health care setting.

A medical assistant who works in the clinical area of the office must complete several activities prior to the provider examining the patient. Although patient encounters are individualized, the medical assistant follows a consistent intake procedure to ensure patient safety and preparedness for the encounter.

Vital signs are taken during each intake process and serve as key indicators of homeostasis. Alterations in values could indicate a precursor of illness or disease. Factors such as stress, food or liquid intake, medical conditions, age, and physical activity can affect vital signs. It is extremely important to be accurate in obtaining vital signs as well as have knowledge of normal and abnormal values to effectively communicate with the provider and deliver education to patients. Accurate documentation serves as a key communication tool among health care professionals.

Objectives

Upon completion of this chapter, you should be able to

- Outline patient identifiers (name, date of birth, medical record number, last four digits of social security number).
- Characterize elements of a patient's medical, surgical, family, and social history.
- Identify screenings and wellness assessments (tobacco cessation, alcohol use, HIV screening).
- Identify mental health screenings (Mini-Mental State Exam) and anxiety and depression screening tools.
- Describe methods for measuring (manual, palpating, electronic), expected reference ranges, common errors, and troubleshooting methods.
- Describe orthostatic methods for obtaining common errors.
- Describe pulse methods for measuring in various locations, abnormal rhythms, and expected reference ranges.
- Describe respiratory rate methods for measuring, expected reference ranges, and types of abnormal patterns (apnea, hyperventilation, dyspnea).
- Describe pulse oximetry expected reference ranges, locations, and common errors.
- Describe temperature methods for measuring in various locations, coordinating ranges, and common errors.
- Describe the pain scale.
- Identify menstrual status and last menstrual period.
- Indicate factors impacting vital signs (age, medications).
- Calculate conversion formulas for vital signs (height, weight, temperature).
- Describe methods for measuring height, weight, body mass index, and body and waist circumference, with considerations related to age, health, status, and disability.
- Calculate pediatric measurements and growth chart.

---

vital signs. Metrics (temperature, pulse, respiration, blood pressure) used to evaluate a patient's overall health status.

PATIENT SAFETY WITHIN THE CLINICAL SETTING

The importance of safety in the ambulatory care setting cannot be underestimated. Make every effort to maximize the safety of patients and staff to prevent injury and avoid litigation. Planning for environmental emergencies, such as fires and natural disasters, is essential to protect human life. This involves identifying emergency policies and evacuation plans and having emergency equipment easily accessible.

In an emergency, pay particular attention to the safety of children, older adults, and patients requiring accommodations. Children are prone to falls and injuries involving sharp objects, choking on small items, or touching electrical outlets. When preparing the patient prior to being seen by the provider, take precautions to avoid a child falling from the examination table. Maintain visual and physical contact with patients until they return to their parent or guardian.

Patients may need assistance walking or getting onto an examination table. Some patients might also need supervision while waiting to be seen. Restrooms should be equipped with handrails and emergency alert buttons; if they are not available and there is a safety concern, someone should be with or near the patient.

For all patients, be alert for potential hazards and take measures to maximize patient safety.

Identify Patient

A patient's medical record contains demographics that require verification at each visit. Demographic information includes name, address, telephone number, insurance information, and emergency contact. Each established patient has a medical record. Some electronic medical record systems identify patients by an assigned medical record number, making each patient unique within the health care system.

The first step in ensuring safety is proper patient identification. The Joint Commission stresses the need to use two methods of identification to validate that care and treatment are delivered to the correct patient. The most common method is to have patients state their full name and date of birth. Avoid saying the patient's name and then asking them to confirm it. A patient could respond to the wrong name, especially in a time of crisis, stress, or illness.

When dealing with financial issues, such as billing, a common form of identification is to ask for the patient's full name and verify the last four digits of their Social Security number. Rarely does anyone ask for the full Social Security number due to issues related to confidentiality. Name and birth date are the two most common identifiers used when face-to-face and receiving care.

CHALLENGE

1. Which of the following are the two most common identifiers used to confirm patient identity?

   A. Name and Social Security number
   B. Name and birth date
   C. Name and address
   D. Social Security number and birth date

   B is correct. The two identifiers that should be used to identify patients are name and birth date.

2. A patient enters the medical office. The medical assistant greets them and verifies the patient's name, address, telephone number, insurance information, and emergency contact. This specific information describes which of the following?

   A. Personal information
   B. Medical record
   C. Demographics
   D. Patient identifiers

   C is correct. This information is the patient's demographic information within the electronic health record that will be verified each visit for any changes.

COMPREHENSIVE CLINICAL INTAKE PROCESS

Patient Medical, Surgical, Family, and Social History

The patient screening process can also be referred to as rooming patients. It is the process of gathering initial information from the patient. Depending on the type of visit, the amount of information collected during the screening process varies, but all patients should have a minimum screening, including the *chief complaint* and medication review, at each visit.

A chief complaint, also referred to as chief concern, is *subjective* information documented in the medical record in the patient's own words. This is likely the first piece of information the medical assistant records that identifies the reason for the visit. "Please tell me why you are coming in today" and "What brings you to the office today?" are open-ended questions that elicit the chief complaint. The patient's response of "My stomach hurts" would be subjective information. When recording a patient's chief complaint, use quotation marks when indicating anything directly stated by the patient.

Routinely ask patients to bring all medications or a current list of medications to the office for appointments. This helps the MA compare medications being taken to those in the medical record and ensures patients follow the correct instructions.

Medication reconciliation is a formal process necessary at every office visit. Comparing the patient's list of medications to the medical record is a safety measure that reduces the risk of improperly prescribing an incorrect or contraindicated prescription, including medication interactions and adverse reactions.

3.1 Take Note

Subjective information is usually described and experienced by the patient and is not measurable.

3.2 Health Record Information Section

The sections of the health record include the following.

Administrative section
- Patient information/demographics
- Financial and insurance information
- Correspondence

Clinical section
- Past medical history/family history/social history/occupational employment
  - Medical history: past illnesses, surgeries
  - Family history: illnesses or diseases relevant to the immediate family
  - Social history: diet, exercise, caffeine intake, smoking, use of alcohol or recreational drugs
  - Occupational history: any occupational employment hazard or exposures
- Orders/referrals
- Clinical data
- Progress notes
- Diagnostic imagining information
- Laboratory information
- Medication list/allergies

---

chief complaint. Primary reason for the office visit.

subjective. Information gathered from what a patient communicates.

medication reconciliation. Comparing the patient's list of medications to the medical record as a safety measure to reduce the risk of improperly prescribing an incorrect or contraindicated prescription, including medication interactions and adverse reactions.

CHAPTER 3: PATIENT INTAKE AND VITALS
Comprehensive Clinical Intake Process

Patients can develop an allergy at any time. Educate the patient on identifying any unusual reactions when starting a new medication. Ask what allergies the patient has and what type of reaction occurred. For example, gastrointestinal upset, previous anaphylactic reactions, or hives, as this will help the provider determine if an allergic reaction is likely to occur in the future. Document the allergy status in the medical record. Avoid exposing a patient to a substance that can lead to an allergic reaction or life-threatening anaphylaxis. Most electronic formats offer safety measures of alerting the provider if a prescribed prescription could cause a reaction. In a paper chart, flag the patient's allergy in several areas. It is often noted in red ink or using red allergy stickers.

A personal and family history is completed at or prior to the first office visit. This document contains information reported by the patient as a starting point for the provider collecting the patient's *objective* information. Objective information is observed or can be measured. A patient's past medical history is objective information because it is documented and measured within their health record. When a patient completes a health history form, the MA will ensure that it is complete and answer any patient questions. This documentation identifies any predispositions to diseases and conditions and forms an overall picture of the patient's health based on past events. Although this extensive history is usually only completed once, routinely review it when a patient attends appointments and determine whether changes or updates need to be included. Many clinics request that patients update their medical history forms annually.

CHALLENGE

1. A patient states they smoke two packs of cigarettes per day. This finding should be recorded in which of the following sections?
   A. Social history
   B. Past medical history
   C. Chief complaint
   D. Family history

   A is correct. Nicotine usage is an assessment related to the patient's social history.

2. Which of the following is objective information? (Select all that apply.)
   A. Stomach pain
   B. Blood pressure 128/74 mm Hg
   C. Nausea
   D. Heart rate 88/min
   E. Weight 175 lb

   B, D, and E are correct. Blood pressure, heart rate, and weight are information that can be measured and documented, which makes them objective data. Stomach pain and nausea are subjective because that is what the patient reports.

3. Which of the following is an example of what the medical assistant may be responsible for documenting? (Select all that apply.)
   A. Review of systems
   B. Medical history
   C. Family history
   D. Social history
   E. Chief complaint

   B, C, D, and E are correct. The medical assistant is responsible for documenting the medical, social, and family history and chief complaint. The provider will review the systems.

objective. Information that can be observed or measured.

SCREENINGS AND WELLNESS ASSESSMENTS
Tobacco Cessation, Alcohol Use, HIV Screening

When screening a patient, ask specific questions about their lifestyle. The patient's responses can trigger the need for a wellness screening or assessment. Screenings have increased throughout the years. Increased data collection requirements focus on prevention and quality patient care. Patients will be interviewed regarding their use of alcohol, tobacco, caffeine, recreational drugs or other chemical substances, and sexual practices. Also, question the patient about their occupational history to identify any hazards to which they may have been exposed during their employment, such as asbestos. Various types of machinery could pose a potential risk of injury and impact their health status. In addition, ask the patient about diet and exercise to provide greater detail regarding their health status. Be aware that the patient may not be comfortable answering these questions or even refuse to answer some of these questions. Attempt to ask the questions again or document "patient declined to answer" in the patient's medical record.

CHALLENGE

1. While reviewing a patient's health history form, the medical assistant noticed they did not complete the social and occupational history part of the form. Why might a patient not complete this portion of the form, and what should the medical assistant do?

   The patient may have missed that part of the health history form or be uncomfortable answering some questions. Explain the importance of getting all the information and ask the patient if they need help answering the questions. The patient has the right to refuse to answer the questions.

MENTAL HEALTH SCREENINGS
Mini-Mental State Exam, Anxiety and Depression Screening Tools

Mental health screenings assess the patient's safety and mental status. Depression screening asks questions about the patient's moods, thoughts, and feelings. The Patient Health Questionnaire-2 (PHQ-2) focuses on the patient's frequency of depressed mood over two weeks. If the patient's answers reflect a positive response to depression, the medical assistant can proceed to the Patient Health Questionnaire-9 (PHQ-9). This screening asks additional questions to assess if the patient meets the criteria for a depressive disorder diagnosis. Older adult patients could require a mini-mental examination to evaluate for dementia or other degenerative disorders.

Depression can be difficult to recognize. Therefore, one must know the common symptoms.

Anxiety is a common emotional response for many people. Anxiety can be a response to fear or an unfamiliar situation. For example, some patients have "white coat syndrome," which is anxiety related to seeing a health care provider for an evaluation. Anxiety can vary from mild to severe symptoms. The GAD-7 questionnaire is for general anxiety and used to screen patients for anxiety.

3.3 Common Depression Symptoms

- Difficulty going to sleep, staying asleep, or getting up in the morning
- Profound sadness and fatigue
- Change in appetite
- Loss of energy

3.4 Common Anxiety Symptoms

- Heightened ability to observe or make connections
- Difficulty focusing on details
- A sense of panic
- Irritability
- Feeling cold, sweaty
- Heart palpitations
- Shortness of breath

CHAPTER 3: PATIENT INTAKE AND VITALS
Measure Vital Signs

CHALLENGE

1. Which of the following is a common sign of depression?
   A. Feeling anxious or nervous
   B. Binge eating
   C. Profound sadness and fatigue
   D. Illogical thought patterns

   C is correct. The most common sign of depression is sadness and fatigue. The other symptoms listed are signs of depression that are less common.

2. A 16-year-old patient has come to the office reporting lower abdominal pain. As the MA interviews the patient, they notice the patient seems to have difficulty concentrating on the conversation. The patient constantly looks toward the closed door of the exam room and asks the medical assistant several times whether the provider is nice. Which of the following is a likely reason for the patient's behavior?
   A. Depression
   B. Physical abuse
   C. Anxiety
   D. Substance abuse

   C is correct. The patient is expressing signs of anxiety. This patient may be experiencing white coat syndrome.

MEASURE VITAL SIGNS

Blood Pressure

Blood pressure measures the force of the blood circulating through the arteries. Blood pressure readings can impact decisions related to the patient's treatment or the need for additional diagnostic tests. Equipment used to determine blood pressure manually includes a sphygmomanometer (a blood pressure cuff) and stethoscope. Electronic equipment can interpret blood pressure without the use of *auscultation*.

Systolic and *diastolic* pressure readings are phase I (the first sound heard, systolic) and V (the final sound heard, diastolic) of the Korotkoff sounds. Korotkoff sounds are distinct sounds that are heard throughout the cardiac cycle. In phase II, there is a swishing sound as more blood flows through the artery. In Korotkoff phase III, sharp tapping sounds are noted as more blood surges. In phase IV, the sound changes to a soft tapping sound, which begins to muffle.

Blood pressure is usually taken with the patient in a sitting position. Different contributing factors can potentially cause errors or influence blood pressure readings. Using the wrong cuff size can impact the systolic and diastolic pressure up to 6.9 mm Hg. If a patient has their legs crossed while taking their blood pressure, the systolic blood pressure may be raised by 2 to 8 mm Hg. The position of the arm can influence the blood pressure reading. If the arm is above the heart level, the reading is lowered. If the arm is lower than the right atrium (dangling at their side), the reading will be artificially elevated. If the patient holds their arm up, the muscular tension will raise the pressure. The arm should be resting on the table or chair next to them at the same level as the heart to avoid these errors.

3.5 Take Note

Measured in millimeters of mercury (mm Hg), the systolic pressure is recorded when the first sharp tapping sound is heard, when the blood begins to surge into the artery that has been occluded by the inflation of the blood pressure cuff. The diastolic pressure is noted when the last sound disappears completely and the blood flows freely.

---

auscultation. Listening with a stethoscope.

systolic. Measurement of force while the heart is contracting; top number on a blood pressure reading.

diastolic. Measurement of force while the heart is relaxing; bottom number on a blood pressure reading.

The palpatory method can be used in emergent situations when the blood pressure cannot be auscultated (heard). The systolic pressure may be checked by feeling (palpating) the radial pulse rather than hearing it (auscultating) with a stethoscope. The blood pressure cuff is placed in the usual position (one inch above the bend in the elbow, or antecubital space) and palpates the radial pulse, noting the rate and rhythm. Inflate the cuff until the pulse disappears, then add 30 mm Hg more inflation to get above the systolic pressure. Do not remove the fingers from the pulse or change the pressure of the fingers. Carefully watch the gauge while slowly releasing the pressure in the cuff and wait until the first pulse beat is felt. Note the reading on the gauge and document the first pulse felt as the systolic pressure. For example, if the MA first felt the pulse return at 104 mm Hg, the palpated blood pressure would be 104/P, with P indicating that the systolic reading was palpated. Accurately determine blood pressure both manually and electronically with the understanding that the palpatory method is usually only used in emergent situations.

Blood pressure readings vary based on age, internal conditions, and external influences. Genetics also play a role in a predisposition to developing hypertension. Blood pressure tends to rise with aging.

3.8 Portable Aneroid Sphygmomanometer

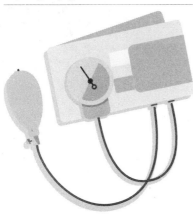

3.6 Factors That Can Influence Blood Pressure and Cause Hypertension

- An increase in blood volume can increase a person's blood pressure, while a decrease in blood volume can decrease a person's blood pressure.
- Peripheral resistance can increase blood pressure. The lumen of the blood vessels becomes smaller, making it more difficult for blood to pump through the blood vessels, causing an increase in blood pressure.
- The overall condition of the heart muscle impacts blood pressure. When the heart muscle gets overworked and becomes weakened, it is unable to contract and provide the force it needs to pump the blood effectively, and the pressure in the vessels tends to increase to maintain an adequate level of circulating blood and oxygen to meet the supply and demand of nutrients the body needs.

3.7 Common Causes of Errors and Troubleshooting Blood Pressure Readings

- The limb used for measurement is positioned above the heart rather than at the heart level.
- The bladder in the cuff is not completely deflated before a reading is started or retaken.
- The pressure in the cuff is released too rapidly.
- The patient is nervous or anxious.
- The patient drank coffee or smoked a cigarette within 30 minutes of the blood pressure measurement.
- The cuff is applied improperly.
- The cuff is too large, too small, too loose, or too tight.
- The bladder is not centered over the artery, or the bladder bulges out from the cover.
- There was a failure to wait for 1 to 2 minutes between measurements.
- The instrument is defective.
  - Air leaks in the valve
  - Air leaks in the bladder
  - Aneroid needle not calibrated to zero

Contraindications for limb selection
- One-sided mastectomy: Use the arm on the side not impacted by the mastectomy.
- Bilateral mastectomy: Use leg.
- Lymphedema: Use leg.
- Dialysis fistula: Use arm that is not affected.

3.9 Blood Pressure Expected Reference Range by Age

AGE CATEGORY	SYSTOLIC (MM HG)	DIASTOLIC (MM HG)
Birth	67 to 84	35 to 53
Infant (1 to 2 months)	72 to 104	37 to 56
Toddler (1 to 2 years)	86 to 106	42 to 63
Preschooler (3 to 5 years)	89 to 112	46 to 72
School-age (6 to 9 years)	97 to 115	57 to 76
Preadolescent (9 to 11 years)	102 to 120	61 to 80
Adolescent (11 to 15 years)	110 to 131	64 to 83
Adult (15+ years)	Less than 120	Less than 80

3.10 Stages of Hypertension

BLOOD PRESSURE CATEGORY	BLOOD PRESSURE (MM HG)
Normal	**Systolic (upper number):** Less than 120 AND **Diastolic (lower number):** Less than 80
Prehypertension	**Systolic:** 120 to 139 OR **Diastolic:** 80 to 89
High Blood Pressure (Hypertension) Stage 1	**Systolic:** 140 to 159 OR **Diastolic:** 90 to 99
High Blood Pressure (Hypertension) Stage 2	**Systolic:** 160 or higher OR **Diastolic:** 100 or higher
Hypertension Crisis (Emergency care needed)	**Systolic:** Higher than 180 OR **Diastolic:** Higher than 110

3.11 Aneroid Sphygmomanometer

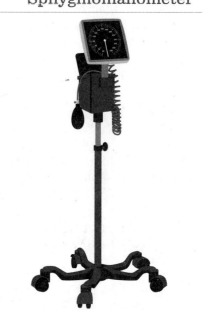

3.12 Blood Pressure Cuff Sizes

UPPER ARM CIRCUMFERENCE	BP CUFF SIZE
8.7 to 10.2 inch	Small Adult
10.6 to 13.4 inch	Adult
13.8 to 17.3 inch	Large Adult
17.7 to 20.5 inch	X-Large Adult

CHALLENGE

1. Which of the following Korotkoff phases is indicative of the diastolic recording?
   A. Phase I
   B. Phase II
   C. Phase III
   D. Phase IV
   E. Phase V

   E is correct. All sounds disappear in phase V. Note the gauge reading when the last sound occurs and record it as diastolic.

2. Which of the following can occur if the wrong size blood pressure cuff is used?
   A. The systolic and diastolic can be impacted by up to 6.9 mm Hg.
   B. The blood pressure can be elevated by up to 9.5 mm Hg.
   C. The systolic will be elevated by up to 6 mm Hg, and the diastolic will remain the same.
   D. The diastolic will be lowered by 9 mm Hg, and the systolic will remain the same.

   A is correct. Using the wrong cuff size can impact the systolic and diastolic pressure up to 6.9 mm Hg

Orthostatic Hypotension

Methods for Obtaining Common Errors

Orthostatic hypotension, also known as postural hypotension, is a significant drop in blood pressure during positional changes, particularly when the patient is moving from lying down to sitting or from sitting to standing. In addition to a decrease in blood pressure, there is an increase in pulse rate. It can lead to the patient falling or even passing out if severe enough. Dehydration, heart disease, diabetes, some medications, and nervous system disorders are all causes of orthostatic hypotension.

If the provider is concerned about orthostatic hypotension, they may ask the MA to measure orthostatic vital signs. To do so, check the patient's blood pressure and pulse rate while lying down, sitting upright, and standing. Wait for 2 to 5 minutes before checking each position to allow the vital signs to regulate and adjust to the change in position. An increased pulse rate of at least 10 beats per minute (bpm) and a decreased blood pressure of at least 20 points between positions indicate orthostatic hypotension.

When checking orthostatic vital signs, the medical assistant should keep the patient's arm on a bed or table, as having the patient hang their arm down can lead to a false high blood pressure reading. Additionally, watch the patient closely and monitor for signs of dizziness and any other indications that the patient is close to falling or passing out. If this occurs, help the patient back to a safe position—either sitting or lying down—and talk to the provider. Do not continue with the test if it is unsafe for the patient.

CHALLENGE

1. A 56-year-old patient came in reporting dizziness. The physician ordered orthostatic vital signs only in the lying and standing positions. In the lying position, the patient's vitals were heart rate 90/min and blood pressure 130/80 mm Hg. In the standing position, the patient's vitals were heart rate 115/min and blood pressure 108/68 mm Hg. Did the patient have a positive test for orthostatic hypotension? Explain why.

   Yes, the patient had a positive test for orthostatic hypotension. The patient had a greater than 10/min increase in heart rate and greater than 20 mm Hg drop in blood pressure, which indicates a positive test.

orthostatic hypotension. A significant drop in blood pressure during positional changes, particularly when the patient is moving from lying down to sitting or from sitting to standing; also known as postural hypotension.

Pulse

Heart rate, also known as the pulse rate, is the number of times the heart beats per minute. The second and third fingers of the dominant hand should be used to palpate the pulse. The number of beats is counted for one full minute to obtain the patient's pulse rate.

There are nine various pulse points throughout the body. The three most common sites to palpate a pulse include the following.

- The radial pulse, located on the thumb side of the wrist, is the most common site for taking an adult pulse.
- The brachial pulse, inside the upper arm, is the most common for measuring pulse in children and using to measure blood pressure.
- The carotid, located in the neck just below the jawbone, is most common for use in emergency procedures.

Other locations to palpate a pulse include the following.

- Temporal artery located on the side of the forehead
- Femoral artery located on the inner groin area
- Popliteal artery located behind the knee
- Posterior tibial artery located behind the ankle
- Dorsalis pedis artery located on top of the foot

In addition to palpation, the pulse can be determined through auscultation. The apical pulse is measured by listening with a stethoscope to the heartbeat at the apex of the heart. The apical pulse is commonly measured in children, infants, and adults with irregular heartbeats. The apical pulse is measured for 1 full minute.

Pulse rates depend on the patient's condition and age. Time of day, activity level, and medications can also affect heart rate. As identified in the chart, average heart rates tend to slow with age.

3.13 Take Note

Pulse is evaluated on rate, rhythm or regularity, and volume or strength. A pulse can be described as 70/min (rate), regular (rhythm), and thready (strength). Thready reflects a pulse as difficult to detect or faint. Bounding describes a pulse as being very strong.

3.14 Locations for Obtaining Pulse

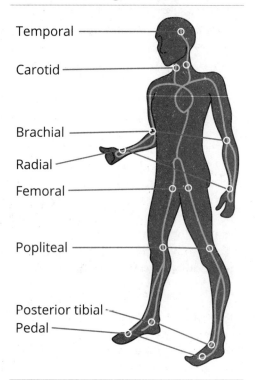

3.15 Vital Sign Ranges by Age

AGE	BLOOD PRESSURE (MM HG)	PULSE (BEATS/MIN)	RESPIRATIONS (BREATHS/MIN)
Older than 12 years	**Systolic:** 110 to 130 **Diastolic:** 65 to 80	60 to 100	12 to 20
6 to 12 years	**Systolic:** 100 to 120 **Diastolic:** 60 to 75	60 to 110	16 to 22
3 to 6 years	**Systolic:** 95 to 110 **Diastolic:** 60 to 75	70 to 120	20 to 24
1 to 3 years	**Systolic:** 90 to 105 **Diastolic:** 55 to 70	80 to 150	22 to 30

CHALLENGE

1. Place the steps in the correct order.
   A. Document the date, time, pulse, strength, and rhythm.
   B. Count the pulse for 30 seconds.
   C. Place two or three fingers on the radial pulse.
   D. Multiply the number of beats counted in 30 seconds by 2.
   E. The MA introduces themselves and explains the procedure to the patient.

   E, C, B, D, A
   Introduce oneself and explain the procedure to the patient. Place two or three fingers on the radial pulse. Count the pulse for 30 seconds. Multiply the number of beats counted in 30 seconds by 2. Document the date, time, pulse, strength, and rhythm.

2. Which of the following sites is most commonly used to check a pulse in children?
   A. Brachial
   B. Radial
   C. Carotid
   D. Temporal

   A is correct. The brachial pulse is most commonly used in children.

3. Which of the following are assessed when taking a pulse? (Select all that apply.)
   A. Rate
   B. Depth
   C. Rhythm
   D. Strength

   A, C, and D are correct. When assessing a patient's pulse, document the beats per minute (rate), rhythm (regular), and strength (strong, weak, thready).

Respiratory Rate

Respirations are evaluated on rate, rhythm, and depth. The respiratory rate also decreases with age and is affected by health conditions or environmental factors. The rate can be classified as fast (also referred to as tachypnea) or slow (bradypnea).

3.16 Take Note

One respiration includes one complete inhalation and exhalation (indicated by the rise and fall of the chest with each breath).

3.17 Types of Abnormal Breathing

TERM	DEFINITION	POSSIBLE CAUSES
Hyperventilation	Fast/rapid breathing	Intense pain Anxiety Panic attacks
Hyperpnea	Excessively deep breathing	Extreme pain or anxiety
Dyspnea	Difficult or painful breathing	Chronic obstructive pulmonary disease (COPD) Pneumonia Asthma High altitudes Physical exertion
Orthopnea	Difficulty breathing unless in the upright position	Congestive heart failure COPD
Wheezing	Whistling sound during breathing	Asthma
Rales	Small clicking, bubbling, or rattling sounds	Fluid in air sacs Pneumonia
Rhonchi	Large airway sounds	COPD Chronic bronchitis Pneumonia

Respiratory rhythm is the breathing pattern, and depth describes how much air is inhaled. For example, a patient might have a rate of 28/min with an irregular rhythm and shallow depth. This would indicate some respiratory distress, as all three notations are abnormal.

The normal average respiratory rate in a newborn is 30 to 50/min compared to an adult rate of 12 to 20/min. When observing the chest, the respiratory rate is counted. The provider may also identify abnormal breathing sounds during auscultation, including wheezing, rales, or rhonchi.

Most people can control their breathing to a certain extent. Therefore, the MA should not announce that they are counting the patient's respiration rate as the

3.18 Respiratory Rate Expected Reference Ranges

AGE	RATE (BREATHS/MIN)
Newborn	30 to 40
Infants	30 to 60
Toddler	26 to 32
Child	20 to 30
Adolescent	16 to 20
Adults	16 to 22

respiration. One complete inhalation and exhalation.

patient may alter their breathing pattern while being observed. It is common to count the respirations immediately following the measurement of the pulse rate. Without removing fingers from the pulse, shift eyes to the patient's chest and count the respiratory rate with the rise and fall of the chest. The MA may watch the rise and fall of the shoulders or back to determine the respiratory rate. Count for 30 seconds and multiply the number by two, or count for 1 full minute. Listen for wheezing, which is a whistling sound on expiration as the body attempts to expel trapped air. Also, listen for rales, which are clicking or crackling sounds that can sound like moist or dry rhonchi heard on inspiration. Common rattling snoring sounds are often associated with chronic lung diseases.

Pulse Oximetry

Although usually not considered a vital sign, pulse oximetry is a valuable tool and a simple procedure to ascertain the percentage of oxygen saturation in the blood. Many oximeters also display the heart rate, which is why it is termed pulse oximetry.

Obtaining a pulse oximetry reading is done by attaching a probe to the patient, usually on a finger. This probe incorporates infrared light to obtain the measurement of oxygen saturation. An alternate site is an earlobe, which can be used if a finger is not an option. Darker skin may also be impacted when the oxygen level is low (less than 80%). In this case, a pulse oximeter reading of 95% or higher is considered a normal result. Results are notated by using SpO_2 and the percentage reading. For example, SpO_2 equals 98%. Readings below 90% should be reported to the provider, and often, oxygen therapy for hypoxemia (decreased oxygen in the blood) may be ordered and initiated.

3.20 Pulse Oximeter

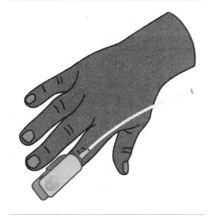

CHALLENGE

1. Match the term with the correct definition.

TERM	DEFINITION
A. Apnea	1. Rapid shallow breathing
B. Bradypnea	2. Abnormally slow breathing
C. Tachypnea	3. Difficulty breathing unless in the upright position
D. Dyspnea	4. Periodic cessation of breathing
E. Orthopnea	5. Difficulty breathing

A: 4, B: 2, C: 1, D: 5, E: 3
Apnea is a periodic cessation of breathing. Bradypnea is abnormally slow breathing. Tachypnea is rapid shallow breathing. Dyspnea is difficulty breathing. Orthopnea is difficulty breathing unless in upright position.

2. Which of the following is the respiratory expected reference range for an adult?
   A. 26 to 40/min
   B. 20 to 30/min
   C. 18 to 24/min
   D. 12 to 20/min
   E. 10 to 20/min

D is correct. The normal respiratory rate is 12 to 20/min for an adult.

3.19 Take Note

Nail polish and artificial nails block the infrared light of the oximeter and interfere with the results. They should be removed prior to the test, or an alternate site should be used to obtain a reading.

CHALLENGE

1. While observing pulse oximetry, the MA notices the reading is 89%. What should the medical assistant do, and why?

Notify the provider of the reading and await further instruction.

2. Which of the following does an oximeter measure?
   A. Oxygen saturation in the blood
   B. Oxygen saturation in the skin
   C. Electricity of the heart
   D. Blood pressure
   E. Heart rate

A is correct. An oximeter measures the oxygen saturation of the blood.

CHAPTER 3: PATIENT INTAKE AND VITALS
Measure Vital Signs

Temperature

Methods for Obtaining in Various Locations, Coordinating Ranges, Common Errors

Measuring temperature determines the relationship between heat production and heat loss in the body. The most common cause of *pyrexia*, or fever, is infection. Fever is the body's natural defense to fight invasive organisms and is a normal reaction to illness. Patients who have a fever can present with chills, loss of appetite, malaise, thirst, and generalized aching.

Temperature is usually measured orally via a digital thermometer, with a probe placed under the tongue on either side of the frenulum linguae. Body temperature can also be measured in the armpit for an axillary temperature or in the rectum for a rectal temperature. A tympanic thermometer can measure the temperature by being inserted into the ear. The tympanic thermometer is popular due to the speed of obtaining the temperature and its comfort. This site should not be used if the patient is complaining of pain in both ears when the ear is touched. Also, a tympanic thermometer will not provide an accurate reading if a patient has a history of impacted cerumen in both ears. The temporal artery scanner is moved across the forehead and behind the ear to produce a temperature reading. Many pediatricians prefer the temporal artery scanner. It has been identified that it is more accurate than the tympanic due to high user error rates with the tympanic.

When an oral temperature is measured, the MA does not have to indicate the site when documenting the reading in the patient's health record. If an alternative site was used, document the following identifiers after recording the temperature.

- (T) for tympanic or (AU) for aural
- (Ax) for axillary
- (R) for rectal
- (TA) for temporal artery

Axillary temperature (Ax) is approximately 1° F (0.6° C) lower than an oral reading because axillary readings are not taken in an enclosed body cavity, making them less accurate than the core body temperature. Tympanic, rectal, and temporal artery temperatures are approximately 1° F (0.6° C) higher than oral readings.

3.21 Take Note

Drinking hot or cold liquids, chewing gum, or smoking prior to taking an oral temperature can result in inaccurate results.

3.22 Types of Thermometer

Digital

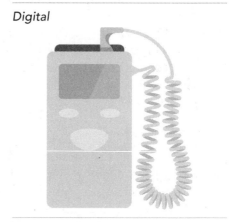

Rectal

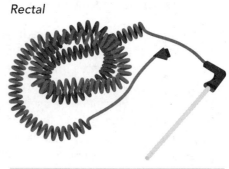

Temporal artery   *Tympanic*

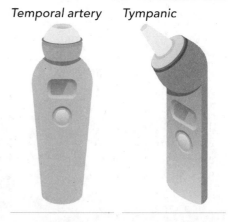

---

pyrexia. Fever greater than 100.4° F.

Take into consideration temperature results, patient history, and clinical appearance. Age influences body temperature. Infants' and children's body temperatures fluctuate in response to the external environment. Adults lose insulation and thermoregulatory control with age. External stressors such as exercise and emotional stress can elevate the body temperature. Genders influence body temperatures also. Female patients have more hormonal secretion, especially during the menstrual cycle. This can cause fluctuation in the body temperature. Overall, when evaluating a person's body temperature, you will find that their body temperature is lowest in the morning and highest in the late afternoon. If the medical assistant experiences erroneous results, retaking the temperature with a different type of thermometer would be appropriate to ensure the correct reading has been measured.

3.23 Age-Related Temperature Norms

AGE	FAHRENHEIT	CELSIUS
Newborn (axillary)	98.2°	36.8°
1 year (tympanic)	99.7°	37.6°
6 years to adult (oral)	98.6°	37°
Older adults over age 70 (oral)	96.8°	36°

Converting Temperatures

Temperatures are measured and recorded as degrees Fahrenheit or degrees Celsius. Many thermometers can switch between Celsius and Fahrenheit. However, medical assistants must know how to calculate the conversion between the two systems. The two formulas below will help you convert temperatures.

To convert Fahrenheit to Celsius: °C = (°F − 32) ÷ 1.8

To convert Celsius to Fahrenheit: °F = (°C × 1.8) + 32

Examples

Fahrenheit to Celsius: °C = (°F − 32) ÷ 1.8

99° F = X° C

Step 1: 99 − 32 = 67

Step 2: 67 ÷ 1.8 = 37.2° C

Celsius to Fahrenheit: °F = (°C × 1.8) + 32

38° C = X° F

Step 1: 38 × 1.8 = 68.4

Step 2: 68.4 + 32 = 100.4° F

CHALLENGE

1. List three factors that can affect a temperature reading.

   Drinking hot or cold liquids, smoking, chewing gum, cold weather, hot weather, age, and menstrual cycle can affect a temperature reading.

2. Which of the following temperature sites does not have to be indicated when documenting the reading in the patient's health record?
   A. Tympanic
   B. Oral
   C. Rectal
   D. Temporal artery

   B is correct. Oral temperatures obtained do not have to indicate the site when documented. The site of the temperature only has to be documented if the medical assistant uses an alternative site other than oral.

3. Match the site for temperatures to its abbreviation.

SITE		ABBREVIATION
A. Rectal	1.	A
B. Temporal artery	2.	R
C. Axillary	3.	T
D. Tympanic	4.	TA

A: 2, B: 4, C: 1, D: 3
The temperature sites with abbreviations are R for rectal, TA for temporal artery, A for axillary, and T for tympanic.

PAIN SCALE

Pain is subjective and therefore difficult to interpret. Observe the patient to gather clues about pain level, such as facial grimacing or holding or clutching areas of pain on the body.

Children's pain can be assessed using the Wong-Baker faces rating scale. Ask additional questions to determine the location, onset, duration, and other characteristics of the pain to get a more precise clinical picture. Ask whether methods used for relief have been effective. Report all verbal and nonverbal responses related to pain to the provider, who can conduct additional assessments as needed to ensure the patient is heard and understood about reporting their pain levels. Health care organizations require that patients are assessed for pain when indicated.

CHALLENGE

1. In addition to documenting the number for the pain level, which of the following characteristics of the patient's pain need to be documented? (Select all that apply.)
   A. Location
   B. Onset
   C. Duration
   D. Cause
   E. Characteristics

   A, B, C, and E are correct. Cause is a helpful characteristic but not required when documenting pain.

MENSTRUAL STATUS AND LAST MENSTRUAL PERIOD

Menstruation is the body's way to prepare for pregnancy or cleanse the uterine lining. Each month (approximately every 28 days), the endometrium, which lines the uterus, is shed a lining via vaginal bleeding. This is commonly known as a period. If the patient becomes pregnant, the endometrium will not shed, and they will miss a period. The hormonal changes of estrogen and progesterone stimulate a menstrual cycle.

Evaluate the last menstrual period (LMP), considered the first day of the previous menstrual cycle, at each visit to evaluate the potential of patient pregnancy. For example, at a yearly pelvic exam, the practitioner will ask about the patient's last menstrual period and possibly conduct a urine pregnancy test before any are ordered to ensure no active pregnancy. A patient needs to identify their menstrual period to aid the provider in identifying what diagnostic or laboratory tests must be ordered if issues arise. The LMP will help evaluate the estimated due date if the patient is pregnant.

3.24 Take Note

Ask the patient to rate pain on a scale of 1 to 10 (with 10 being the worst) to determine the pain level the patient is experiencing.

CHALLENGE

1. Which of the following indicates last menstrual period?
   A. Last day of the last menstrual period
   B. First day of the last menstrual period
   C. Late menstrual period
   D. Heaviest flow day of the last menstrual period

   B is correct. The first day of the last menstrual period is indicated as the LMP.

PEDIATRIC MEASUREMENTS AND GROWTH CHARTS

Pediatric measurements monitor growth. Height, weight, and head circumference are measured during a routine well-child visit during infancy and early toddler years. As children age, height and weight are the only *anthropometric* measurements obtained at each visit.

It can be challenging to measure a child's growth patterns due to a lack of cooperation from the child. The medical assistant may need to ask a parent or caregiver for assistance while obtaining measurements. Another option is giving the child a toy or something else that could distract them while the measurements are obtained.

If the child cannot stand erect, lay the child or infant flat on a paper-covered exam table to obtain a length measurement. Place a mark at the top of the head and the heel of the flexed foot. Measure the distance between the two lines and record this measurement in centimeters or inches, according to office protocol.

Infant scales are desirable when obtaining an infant's weight. Weigh infants without clothing or a diaper and record the weight using both pounds and ounces. Always keep one hand hovering over the infant to ensure their safety on the scale. The medical assistant should never turn their back to an infant on a scale or leave them unattended.

Using a tape measure, measure the head circumference at the widest area. This is usually done by placing the measuring tape directly above the eyebrows, around the side of the head, above the ears, and behind the back of the head at its widest point. The measurement is recorded in inches or centimeters, depending on office protocol.

Length, weight, and head circumference are tracked on growth charts from birth to 36 months. Head circumference is not recommended past 36 months (unless abnormal measurements are found), as the brain reaches 75% of its growth by this point, making continuous measurement and tracking unnecessary. Stature and weight are tracked on specific charts from 2 to 20 years. These measurements are plotted on a growth chart to represent growth visually. This alerts the provider to potential concerns. The growth chart also provides tangible data to have conversations with parents and guardians regarding concerns such as obesity or malnutrition. It may also be noted that many EHR systems will automatically plot the measurements on the appropriate growth charts using the EHR software and the information based on the age and gender of the child.

Measurements are plotted on the grid. The outcome of the plot identifies a standard growth percentile ranging from less than 5th percentile to greater than the 95th percentile. For example, a weight measured below the 5th percentile would be considered underweight. A normal or healthy weight on the grid would range between the 5th and 85th percentile. A child determined to be overweight would have a reading in the 85th to 95th percentile. Growth chart percentiles indicating obesity would be equal to or greater than the 95th percentile.

anthropometric. Related to measurement and proportion of the body.

3.25 Take Note

Growth charts compare the child's growth pattern with the national standard. The Centers for Disease Control and Prevention (CDC) developed growth charts that track growth continuously until age 20. These growth charts are sex-specific.

CHALLENGE

1. The circumference of a child's head should be measured at a well-child visit until which of the following ages?

   A. 1 year
   B. 2 years
   C. 3 years
   D. 5 years

   C is correct. The brain has completed 75% of its growth by the time a child has reached 3 years of age. Therefore, it is recommended that head circumferences are only measured until the age of 3.

2. An 18-month-old patient is in for a well visit. After the medical assistant weighs the infant and measures their length, the data gets transferred to the electronic health record, which plots the 18-month-old patient's measurements on the growth chart. The medical assistant shows the patient's parent that the infant is in the 90th percentile for their weight. The parent is shocked, thinks their baby is overweight, and asks what they should do. How should the medical assistant respond?

   Reassure the parent that this does not indicate that the infant is overweight. Explain that the measurements should stay within the grid and that the patient's weight is in the 90th percentile among other 18 month old patients of their sex.

OBTAIN ANTHROPOMETRIC MEASUREMENTS

Obtain Anthropometric Measurements

Anthropometric measurements involve the measurement of height, weight, and sometimes other parts of the human body. These measurements are documented along with the vital signs. Anthropometric measurements can play a significant role in providing a snapshot of the patient's health to the provider prior to physical examination. Many patients require their weight to be checked every visit, but height is usually only checked annually.

Weight

Measuring a patient's weight is performed at each office visit. Medication dosages are often determined based on weight. BMI, predisposition to medical conditions, eating disorders, and weight management are monitored in relation to a patient's overall general health.

Be alert to these concerns and display empathy and privacy while ensuring accuracy when obtaining measurements. Weight can be a sensitive issue; some patients may be embarrassed about their weight and resistant to having it measured. Measure a patient's weight in a private area and avoid stating the measured weight loud enough for others to hear. Additionally, the patient may request that you not share their weight with them—this is their right and should be respected. If a patient declines to be weighed, inform the provider. While patients can decline any medical assessment or treatment, weight is sometimes critical to monitoring certain diseases. The provider can help explain this to the patient if needed. Completing the task promptly and efficiently reduces patient anxiety regarding this part of the visit. Make sure the scale is balanced and review the patient's health record to determine a baseline weight before asking the patient to stand on the scale. Take precautions to protect the patient from injury and be alert to issues regarding limitations with mobility. A scale with built-in handrails is ideal for patients who cannot maintain balance. If a facility does not have this type of scale, a walker can be placed over the scale for the patient to use as hand support for getting up and off the scale and for balance.

3.26 Take Note

Assist the patient on and off the scale as needed. Patients should not wear shoes or heavy jackets when being weighed.

Weight is measured in pounds or kilograms. Document weight in the units approved by medical office protocol. Sometimes a medical assistant will have to convert weight from one unit of measurement to another. One pound equals 2.2 kilograms (1 lb equals 2.2 kg).

To convert pounds to kilograms, divide the weight in pounds by 2.2.

Example:

148 lb = X kg

148 ÷ 2.2 = 67.27

Round to the nearest tenth = 67.3 kg

To convert kilograms to pounds, multiply the weight in kilograms by 2.2.

Example:

87 kg = X lb

87 × 2.2 = 191.4 lb

Considerations Related to Weight Management

Some medical specialties and specific medical problems require continuous monitoring of weight. Hormone disorders (diabetes), growth patterns in children, and eating disorders (anorexia, bulimia) require accurate weight checks during every medical visit. Also, patients who are pregnant must have their weight measured every visit to monitor adequate weight gain and excessive weight, which may indicate fluid retention. Patients who have cardiovascular conditions and patients undergoing dialysis tend to retain fluid and should have their weight checked every visit.

Height

Height is a part of a routine physical to track normal development, monitor conditions such as scoliosis or osteoporosis, and assist in determining BMI.

Measurements are often obtained in inches, which can be converted to include feet. To convert height from inches to feet, divide the total number of inches by 12. The remainder is inches.

Example: 62 inches = 62 ÷ 12 = 5 feet, 2 inches

Measurements can also be recorded in centimeters depending on the provider's preference.

Body Mass Index

Body mass index (BMI) is a tool to screen patients and classify results based on a patient's height and weight. This classification can then correlate risk factors or predisposition for conditions such as heart disease or diabetes. A patient's BMI is a percentage used to represent body fat in relation to a person's height and weight. BMI is calculated using the following formula.

$$BMI = \frac{\text{weight in kg}}{\text{height in m}^2}$$

or

$$\frac{\text{weight in lb}}{\text{height in inches}^2} \times 703 = BMI$$

A BMI percentage of 18.5 to 24.9 is considered normal. Results less than 18.5 classify an individual as underweight. Greater than 24.9 leads to a classification of overweight, with obesity being 30.0 and greater. The MA may be responsible for calculating BMI using calculations and graphs or using a calculation program within the electronic health record.

CHALLENGE

1. Which of the following criteria is used to determine a patient's BMI?
   A. Height and age
   B. Weight and age
   C. Height and weight
   D. Age and birthday

   C is correct. BMI is calculated by weight (kg) divided by height (m²).

2. A patient has come for a routine office visit. The medical assistant is about to measure the patient's weight but sees that they use a cane to ambulate. What can the medical assistant do to help this patient balance on the scale if there are no handrails?

   Assist the patient up on the scale. Use a walker to assist the patient in stepping on and off the scale.

---

body mass index (BMI). An individual's weight divided by the square of their height, used to determine weight status.

IDENTIFY, DOCUMENT, AND REPORT ABNORMAL SIGNS AND SYMPTOMS

The MA is responsible for obtaining information from patients, documenting the information, and reporting any abnormal findings to the provider. This is mostly completed during the patient interview while preparing the patient for an examination by the provider. The usual process for obtaining information is first to record anthropometric measurements and vital signs and obtain the chief complaint. Clearly document intake information in the medical record and alert the provider of any abnormal results prior to them seeing the patient. See the table of vital signs below, outlining normal, abnormal, and emergent ranges for adults. Ranges for pediatric vital signs vary widely based on the child's specific age. Those working in pediatrics should have a validated reference guide easily accessible when measuring vital signs. The measurements are taken as a baseline for each visit. Remember that any abnormality or extreme change may indicate a disease or disorder that needs to be brought to the provider's attention.

3.27 Vital Sign Findings

VITAL SIGN	NORMAL RANGE (ADULTS)	ABNORMAL (ADULTS)	EMERGENT (ADULTS)
Blood pressure (mm Hg)	**Systolic:** less than 120 AND **Diastolic:** less than 80	**Systolic:** 120 to 179 OR **Diastolic:** 80 to 110	**Systolic:** greater than 180 OR **Diastolic:** greater than 110
Pulse (beats per minute)	60 to 100	**Bradycardia:** below 60 **Tachycardia:** above 100	Varies based on many factors
Temperature	97.6° to 99.6° F	99.6° to 104.0° F	**Dangerous:** 104° to 105° F **Fatal:** 106° F or higher
Respiratory rate (breaths per minute)	12 to 20	**Bradypnea:** less than 12 **Tachypnea:** greater than 20	Varies based on many factors

CHALLENGE

1. A 30-year-old patient's vital signs are temperature 98.2° F, heart rate 117/min, respirations 18/min, blood pressure 146/94 mm Hg. Which of the following vitals are outside the expected reference range? (Select all that apply.)
   A. Temperature
   B. Heart rate
   C. Respirations
   D. Blood pressure

   B and D are correct. Expected reference range for heart rate is 60 to 100/min. Expected reference range for blood pressure is less than 120/80 mm Hg.

2. Which of the following are abnormal vital signs in an adult? (Select all that apply.)
   A. Heart rate 88/min
   B. Respiratory rate 28/min
   C. Temperature 102° F
   D. Blood pressure 110/18 mm Hg
   E. Pulse oximetry 96%

   B and C are correct. The heart rate, blood pressure, and pulse oximeter are within normal ranges. The respiratory rate and temperature are elevated.

FACTORS AFFECTING VITAL SIGNS

Vital signs can be influenced by many physical and emotional factors. Some factors can influence more than one vital sign.

3.28 Factors Affecting Vital Signs

FACTOR	INFLUENCE ON VITAL SIGN
Consuming a hot beverage	Increased oral temperature reading
Consuming a cold beverage	Decreased oral temperature reading
Anxiety	Increased blood pressure
	Increased heart rate
Smoking	Increased blood pressure
	Increased heart rate
Exertion (such as a long walk to the exam room)	Increased blood pressure
	Increased heart rate
	Lower oxygen levels
Age	Increased temperature fluctuation in young children (inability to regulate)
	Decreased temperature in older adults (loss of insulation in the form of body fat)
Pain	Increased blood pressure
	Increased heart rate
Illness	Increased temperature
Beta-blocker medication	Decreased blood pressure
	Decreased heart rate

Consider all these influences and give time for the patient to rest and recover before taking vital signs. If a vital sign is abnormal, report it to the provider, along with any possible explanation. For example, the patient's temperature was high, but they drank hot coffee shortly before it was checked. Recheck one or several vital signs later in the visit if the provider believes external factors falsely influenced the initial readings.

CHALLENGE

1. An adult patient has started taking medication for hypertension since their last visit. Which of the following would the MA most likely expect at this visit?

   A. Blood pressure within normal range
   B. Blood pressure higher than normal
   C. Blood pressure lower than normal
   D. Blood pressure lower than it was on the previous visit

   D is correct. The medical assistant would expect the blood pressure to be lower than the previous visit. The patient just started the blood pressure medication, so it is not certain how the medication is working, but the medical assistant can anticipate the pressure being lower than the last visit.

2. A patient tells the medical assistant they smoke. What is an important question to ask before measuring the patient's vital signs?

   Find out when the patient last smoked a cigarette. If they just smoked, their temperature will be falsely elevated.

WRAP-UP

The medical assistant must be aware of normal growth and development as well as the patient's physical and medical status in determining the best method to obtain anthropometric measurements and accurate vital signs. Many influential factors can affect vital signs, and medical assistants have to understand those factors and be able to work around them or alleviate the factors that can influence false readings. Vital signs are the baseline for the patient to enable providers to see a snapshot of a patient's health and identify any potential disorders that may arise. Accuracy and communication are essential skills of the MA, and the knowledge they obtain from their patients across the lifespan related to vital signs is an integral part of their job.

CHAPTER 4
General Patient Care: Part 1

OVERVIEW

Medical assistants perform multiple duties in the ambulatory care setting, such as preparing the exam room before the patient encounter, obtaining vital signs and medical history, documenting information in the patient's medical record, positioning and draping the patient, assisting the health care provider during the examinations, cleaning the examination room, and maintaining instruments and equipment.

The MA will complete several tasks prior to the provider encounter with the patient in addition to assisting during the encounter. Although patient encounters are individualized, following a consistent intake procedure ensures patient safety and preparedness for the examination.

Preparing the exam room and patient, including assembling all the supplies and equipment required for a general or specialized examination, is important to have a successful patient encounter. There are several critical skills medical assistants must be competent to perform, such as preparing for minor surgical procedures, ear and eye irrigations, and delivering medication through the different routes of administration. It is important to be familiar with many of the advances in patient care, such as the use of electronic medical and health records systems, electronic prescribing, and telehealth.

Objectives

Upon completion of this chapter, you should be able to

- Prepare the examination/procedure room.
- Prepare the patient for procedures, including providing patient education.
- Assist the health care provider with general and specialty examinations and procedures, including positioning and draping.
- Prepare and administer medications using nonparenteral routes.
- Prepare and administer medications using parenteral routes, demonstrating patient safety.
- Manage supplies for injections and injection and medication logs, including controlled substances and immunizations.
- Perform ear and eye installation and irrigation.
- Operate basic functions of an electronic medical record/electronic health record (EMR/EHR) system.
- Enter orders using computerized physician order entry.
- Conduct telehealth or virtual screenings in the context of a telehealth/virtual visit.
- Follow guidelines for sending orders for electronic prescriptions and refills by telephone, fax, or email.

PREPARE EXAMINATION/PROCEDURE ROOM

General Physical Examinations

Review Schedule to Determine Reason for Visit

The medical assistant is often responsible for preparing the patient examination and procedure rooms, including assembling all the necessary supplies and equipment. Examination rooms in the medical practice and other facilities vary in size, layout, and type of equipment used. For example, an examination room that is used for general examinations can look very different than a room used specifically for minor surgical procedures. Review the schedule at the beginning of each day that identifies the patient's name and the reason for the visit. This can help in determining what room, supplies, or equipment will need to be prepared for the visit.

Examination Room Supplies and Equipment

A standard examination room is most often furnished with an examination table (with stirrups in a practice where pelvic exams are performed), a pillow, a footstool, a supply cupboard, a trash can, biohazardous waste and sharps containers, a rolling stool, and a chair. Oftentimes, a writing surface and a sink are present. For health care providers in specialty practices, diagnostic equipment specific to the practice may be present. Some clinics will have a dedicated exam room for specialized procedures and equipment, such as an EKG machine, nebulizer, and sigmoidoscope.

For routine physical examinations, ensure that all the necessary supplies and equipment are readily available. Supplies and equipment needed will vary depending on the patient's condition and disease.

Supplies are disposable items used for patient examination and treatment. Supplies include examination table paper, paper drapes and gowns, dressings and bandages, tongue depressors, disposable gloves (sterile and nonsterile), syringes and needles (stored securely locked), and alcohol pads.

Equipment is usually more durable and requires routine maintenance and cleaning between use. Equipment should be properly stored and not left on countertops or within reach of the patient. Proper storage both ensures patient safety and avoids the possibility of contaminating or damaging expensive medical equipment. The following are examples of equipment.

- **Thermometer:** Used to measure body temperature
- **Stethoscope:** Used to amplify sounds in the body, such as the beating of the heart, respirations in the lungs, and bowel sounds in the abdomen
- **Sphygmomanometer:** Used to measure blood pressure
- **Pulse oximeter:** Used to measure oxygen saturation in the blood
- **Reflex hammer:** Used for testing reflexes
- **Otoscope:** Used to examine the ears
- **Ophthalmoscope:** Used to examine the interior of the eye, especially the retina

---

otoscope. An instrument used for visual examination of the eardrum and ear canal, typically having a light for visibility.

ophthalmoscope. Instrument used to examine the interior of the eye.

CHAPTER 4: GENERAL PATIENT CARE: PART 1
Prepare Examination/Procedure Room

Maintaining a Clean Examination Area

At the beginning of the day, check that all the rooms are adequately stocked with supplies and have been properly cleaned and that the equipment is properly functioning. Anticipating items that might be needed for a visit and preparing the room in advance demonstrate a well-run, organized facility. Doing these things each day enhances patient confidence and assists in operational efficiency.

CHALLENGE

1. Match the vital sign with the equipment, supply, or instrument used.

VITAL SIGN	EQUIPMENT
A. Blood pressure	1. Stethoscope
B. Temperature	2. Pulse oximeter SpO$_2$
C. Pulse	3. Sphygmomanometer
D. Respiration sounds	4. Manually (fingers)
E. Oxygen level	5. Thermometer

A: 3, B: 5, C: 4, D: 1, E: 2
Vital signs include temperature, pulse, respiration, blood pressure, and, in some cases, oxygen levels. Medical assistants must be familiar with the specific equipment and techniques needed to obtain these vital signs.

2. Which of the following supplies and equipment are commonly in an examination room for a general patient exam? (Select all that apply.)
   A. Exam gowns
   B. Sigmoidoscope
   C. Exam table
   D. EKG machine
   E. Otoscope

A, C, and E are correct. Many supplies and equipment are needed for a general patient exam. Exam gowns, exam table, and an otoscope are common items found in the exam room. A sigmoidoscope is used to examine parts of the intestine and rectum and is not part of a standard exam room. An EKG machine should be available in the medical practice but is often located in a specific room for patients who have a history of or are experiencing angina (chest pain).

3. Match the instrument with the correct function it is used for.

INSTRUMENT	FUNCTION
A. Ophthalmoscope	1. Used to examine the ear canal and tympanic membrane
B. Otoscope	2. Used to test for reflexes
C. Reflex hammer	3. Used to view the interior of the eye

A: 3, B: 1, C: 2
An ophthalmoscope is used to view the interior of the eye. An otoscope consists of a light source, a magnifying lens, and an ear speculum to examine the inner ear. A reflex hammer is used to test for reflexes.

Surfaces, including counters, chairs, any reusable equipment, and exam tables, should be cleaned at the beginning and end of each day and between patients to reduce the risk of transmitting infectious agents. Clean the examination table with the proper disinfectant and allow it to dry before placing new paper on the table. The paper covering the exam table must be disposed of and replaced between each patient. If available, change pillow covers after each patient. Disposable equipment used during the previous examination must be discarded in the appropriate containers. Reusable equipment must be taken to the appropriate area for cleaning and disinfection, following standard precautions.

At the end of each day, disinfect the work area and stock the exam rooms. Stock routine items, such as gloves, paper towels, exam gowns, table paper, and sharps and biohazard waste containers, in each of the examination rooms. Other supplies and items may need to be added depending on the patient and procedure.

SPECIALTY EXAMINATIONS OR PROCEDURES

In addition to a wide range of general procedures and skills, medical assistants should also be familiar with and competent practicing within the scope of specialty care. Medical assistants must be aware of the various procedures and skills that are unique to medical specialties.

4.1 Medical Specialties

SPECIALTY	DESCRIPTION	COMMON SUPPLIES AND EQUIPMENT
Dermatology	A medical assistant may assist in minor surgical procedures to help obtain skin biopsies or in the debridement of wounds and collect specimens from wound cultures. Follow sterile procedures when assisting in minor surgical procedures and obtaining wound cultures.	Dermal punch biopsy Dermal cutter Scalpel Gauze Incision and drainage tray Specimen collection swabs and containers
Cardiology	A medical assistant may need to perform electrocardiograms (EKGs) and Holter monitoring on patients with cardiac symptoms or diseases. Both tests are used to monitor and record the heart's electric activity and are often used to diagnose heart disorders, especially regarding its rhythm and rate.	Three-channel electrocardiograph Electrodes EKG paper Holter monitor
Endocrinology	Endocrinology involves hormones. Medical assistants should be familiar with venipuncture and capillary punctures (fingersticks). Medical assistants will perform glucose monitoring and patient education related to proper use of glucose monitoring equipment.	Glucometers Alcohol pads Adhesive strips Test strips Lancets
Neurology	A neurological examination focuses on the patient's reflex response, motor response, muscle tone, speech patterns, coordination, sensory response, gait, and mental status and behavior. The MA may assist the provider throughout the exam, as directed.	Otoscope Ophthalmoscope Percussion hammer Penlight Tuning fork Cotton balls Safety pin Tongue depressor Small vials containing hot and cold liquids Vials with different scents Vials with different tasting liquids

4.1 Medical Specialties (continued)

SPECIALTY	DESCRIPTION	COMMON SUPPLIES AND EQUIPMENT
Obstetrics and gynecology	This specialty practice may assist in a number of procedures, including minor surgery. A common procedure is a Pap test. A Pap test is a screening procedure that collects and examines cells from the vaginal and cervical mucosa to check for precancerous or abnormal cells.	Vaginal speculums and retractors Cytology kits Stitch removal sets Dressing kits Exam tables with stirrups Ultrasound machine Handheld fetal Doppler machine
Pulmonology	A pulmonology practice may conduct different tests to assess respiratory function, to assist in the diagnosis of patients with suspected obstructive or restrictive pulmonary disease, and to assess the effectiveness of medication and other pulmonary therapies. One of the most common tests to evaluate lung function that a medical assistant may perform is a pulmonary function test (PFT). The most common tests and procedures performed are spirometry, peak flow meters, and pulse oximetry. Spirometers are small, handheld devices that provide digital readings, and there are portable meters with integrated printers. Advanced spirometry systems are computerized and can be configured to send results directly to a patient's electronic health record (EHR). All spirometers consist of a mouthpiece and tubing connected to a recording device. The peak flow meter is often used for patients who have asthma to monitor their daily respiratory function and condition. The peak flow meter measures the fastest rate at which the patient exhales after taking a maximum breath. Oxygen saturation is commonly measured by a pulse oximeter, which is a noninvasive device that is clipped on the fingertip, bridge of the nose, forehead, or earlobe.	Peak flow meter Spirometry machine Disposable mouthpieces and nose clips

CHAPTER 4: GENERAL PATIENT CARE: PART 1
Prepare Patient for Procedures

CHALLENGE

1. Match the equipment or instrument with the medical specialty for which it is commonly used.

EQUIPMENT	SPECIALITY
A. Holter monitor	1. Endocrinology
B. Percussion hammer	2. Gynecology
C. Glucometer	3. Cardiology
D. Spirometer	4. Neurology
E. Vaginal speculum	5. Pulmonology

   A: 3, B: 4, C: 1, D: 5, E: 2
   There are a variety of equipment and instruments commonly used in medical specialties, such as a glucometer in endocrinology (study of hormones and endocrine glands and organs), a Holter monitor in cardiology (study of the heart and cardiovascular system), a percussion hammer to test for reflexes in neurology (study of the nervous system), a vaginal speculum for pelvic exams in gynecology (study of the female reproductive system), and a spirometer in pulmonology (study of the respiratory system).

2. Which of the following equipment and instruments are commonly used during a gynecological exam? (Select all that apply.)
   A. Stirrups
   B. Scratch test
   C. Retractor
   D. Peak flow meters
   E. Speculum
   F. Cytology kit

   A, C, E, and F are correct. Common supplies for a routine gynecological exam are gloves, gown and drape, vaginal speculum and retractor, specimen collection equipment (cytology kit), and exam table with stirrups.

3. Which of the following equipment and instruments are commonly used in a pulmonology specialty? (Select all that apply.)
   A. Audiometer
   B. Peak flow meter
   C. Pulse oximeter
   D. Holter monitor
   E. Snellen chart
   F. Spirometer

   B, C, and F are correct. An audiometer is used to measure one's hearing. A Holter monitor is used to monitor a patient's cardiac electrical activity. A Snellen chart is a visual acuity screening test.

PREPARE PATIENT FOR PROCEDURES

Patient Instruction

Preparing for the Examination

Prior to the patient's arrival, review the patient's medical record, including the completed history and physical examination, to make sure you understand the procedure and what supplies and equipment will be needed in the exam room. There are several tests and procedures that require specific patient preparation prior to the procedure, such as a colonoscopy or a fasting glucose test. Explain and review the needed preparation with the patient and verify that all instructions were followed before the procedure. If the patient did not complete necessary preparation or they have any questions, direct them to the health care provider. Confirm that an informed consent has been signed and is in the patient's medical record.

4.2 Take Note

All procedures should begin with good hand hygiene and a routine introduction (identifying the patient and introducing yourself).

Before entering an examination room that is occupied by a patient, always knock, announce yourself, and ask for permission to enter. Do not enter the room until the patient has expressed consent. This will help reassure patients that their privacy is respected.

Explain the procedure and the importance of the procedure in an empathetic, simple, and direct manner. Avoid using overly technical terms and encourage the patient to ask questions and to express any anxiety or concerns.

Ask patients to empty their bladder before undressing. If a urine sample is required, give complete and detailed instructions. Patient gowns and drapes should be provided for the patient's comfort and privacy for all examinations. Explain to the patient which items of clothing should be removed for the exam and instruct them whether to put on the gown with the opening in the front or the back. For a problem-focused visit or exam, only some clothing items may need to be removed, such as all clothing above the waist. Assist patients with disrobing and with stepping up onto the examination table as needed. Ensure that gowns of all sizes are available for patients who are required to change clothing for an examination or a procedure. Inform patients where their personal clothing and belongings can be stored during the examination. Once the patient is ready, notify the health care provider.

After the procedure, assist the patient down from the examination table if needed. The patient may become lightheaded when sitting up if they were lying down for the procedure. Allow the patient privacy when getting dressed. Assist the patient with getting dressed as needed.

4.3 Take Note

If the patient has any discomfort or complications postprocedure, the patient should notify the health care provider or call 911 in case of an emergency or life-threatening situation.

Providing Patient Education

Provide the patient information about any follow-up appointments, additional exams, aftercare instructions, and referrals. Let the patient know when to expect results from lab, radiology, or any other diagnostic tests. Ask if the patient has any questions and direct appropriate questions to the health care provider to answer.

In some cases, it may be helpful to call the health care provider for advice on whether a situation is an emergency. If the provider is not immediately available, the patient may be recommended to call 911 or go to the nearest hospital.

CHALLENGE

1. Order the steps of preparing a patient for a procedure or examination into the correct sequence.
   A. Assist the patient with dressing, if requested.
   B. Prepare the exam room.
   C. Identify the patient and introduce yourself.
   D. Provide the patient a gown and drape.
   E. Review the patient's medical chart.

   E, B, C, D, A
   The correct sequence is the following: review the patient's medical chart, prepare the exam room with the necessary supplies and equipment, identify the patient and introduce yourself, provide the patient a gown and drape, and assist the patient with dressing, if requested, after the procedure.

2. Which of the following procedures will require specific preparation prior to the procedure?
   A. EKG test
   B. Snellen test
   C. Urinalysis
   D. Colonoscopy

   D is correct. Before a colonoscopy, the patient must prepare by eating a low-fiber diet, consuming clear liquids, and taking a laxative.

ACCOMMODATION FOR PATIENT NEEDS

Patient populations are diverse, and every patient will have different needs that must be met during the visit.

Older Adults

Consider ways to support older adults' physical and emotional needs during the medical visit. When an older adult patient is seen in the medical practice, it is often the medical assistant who is responsible for reviewing their medication list and verifying the dosages taken. Allot extra time for a patient who has an extensive medication history.

> **4.4 Take Note**
>
> Maintain a calm, relaxed, and respectful manner when interacting with older adult patients. Do not rush, speak clearly and slowly, and be prepared to repeat questions or instructions, if necessary.

Allow ample time for the patient to process or recall information. Avoid affectionate terms, such as "sweetie" or "honey," since it may be interpreted as condescending or patronizing even if that is not your intent.

Physical Disability

Observe the patient's overall physical ability to adhere to your requests as you progress with preparing the patient for the examination or procedure. Patients may have decreased mobility and instability. You may need to provide additional assistance while escorting patients to the examination room or provide extra care when assisting them on or off the examination table. Offer any assistance if it appears the patient needs it. However, allow the patient to do as much as possible independently and ask before you touch a patient. Do not leave the patient unattended if the patient is physically unstable or appears confused. If you are unable to remain in the room, a family member or another medical assistant should be asked to sit with the patient until the health care provider is ready to begin the examination.

If a patient arrives in a wheelchair, assist as needed. Communicate with the patient prior to touching them or their wheelchair. Respect the patient's wishes and expertise. If a transfer is necessary between a wheelchair to the exam table, request assistance from a team member. Remember to lock the wheels and to position the chair before trying to help the patient move from the chair to the exam table.

Children

Considerations must also be taken when providing patient care to infants and children. In almost every case, the child is accompanied by a parent or guardian. Although the child's medical information most likely will be provided by the parent or guardian, it is important to establish a positive rapport with the child. Smile and speak to the child at eye level. Speak gently and calmly with an even tone and avoid using "baby talk," especially to older or adolescent children. Depending on the child, role playing can be helpful, particularly when preparing a patient for a procedure or trying to get more information from the patient, for example, asking the child to point on a stuffed animal where the pain may be located.

During procedures, plan extra time to explain to the child what is being done and to provide a sense of calmness. Explain in simple, age-appropriate terms exactly what you want them to do. Holding or entertaining an uncooperative child may be necessary so that an examination or procedure can be safely performed. Once the child enters the medical practice, that child's safety is your primary concern. Children should never be left alone on an examination table, scale, toilet, or other place that could pose possible danger for falling or other injury. Always place a protective hand on infants to protect them from rolling or falling.

Environmental Considerations

Examination rooms must conform to the standards established by the Americans with Disabilities Act (ADA). These federal standards were designed to make sure that people who have disabilities are not discriminated against in public places because of a lack of proper accommodations. These standards address such things as the width of doorways and hallways; placement of door handles, grab bars, and handrails; spatial accommodations for patients in wheelchairs; and floor surfaces.

Clutter, spills, improperly stored equipment, and unsecured electrical cords or cables are unsafe for both patients and medical practice staff. Make sure all electrical cords and cables are secured to the floor or wall.

Routinely check all furniture in the examination room for proper maintenance. Immediately report items such as a broken drawer, a sharp edge on the countertop, or a broken hinge on a door. If it cannot be repaired right away, document the situation in the maintenance logbook or follow the facility's procedures related to maintenance requests.

4.5 Take Note

Address unsafe situations immediately. Unsafe situations might include clutter in the hallway or examination room, a spill on the floor, or equipment left lying around where a patient, especially a child, could get hold of it.

CHALLENGE

1. Which of the following considerations should be done when communicating with older patients?
   A. Speak loudly.
   B. Repeat questions or comments, if necessary.
   C. Direct questions to the accompanying family member about the patient.
   D. Show respect by referring to the patient as "sweetie" and "honey."

   B is correct. To ensure the patient understands any questions or instructions, it may be necessary to repeat questions or comments. Do not assume that patient cannot hear by speaking loudly or that the patient cannot answer questions by directing questions to family members. Do not use overly affectionate terms.

2. A child is scheduled to get an immunization and is very anxious and scared. What can you do to help calm the child?

   Be honest and calm and explain to the child that they will feel a small pinch and that the feeling will not last long. Distract or have the parent or guardian distract the child during the shot. Role play by pretending to administer a shot to a stuffed animal. Reward the child with a treat or toy afterward.

ASSIST THE PROVIDER WITH EXAMINATIONS

Positioning and Draping

As a medical assistant, you will assist the provider with the physical encounter by positioning and draping the patient based on the procedure or examination. Patients are not usually placed in specific examination positions until the exam is conducted. Some positions may not be comfortable for long periods of time, and patients should be placed in them only when necessary. A patient's comfort should be of utmost importance.

The following are the most common positions used for medical and surgical examinations and procedures.

Supine

In the supine position, also known as the horizontal recumbent position, patients lie flat on their back with hands at the sides. Be sure that the patient's feet are supported by extending the examination table. This position is used to examine anything on the anterior or ventral (front) surface of the body (head, chest, stomach) and for certain types of x-rays. The patient should be draped from the chest down to the feet. During the examination, expose areas as necessary and as indicated by the health care provider. The supine position may not be comfortable for patients who have difficulty breathing or who have lower back problems. For these patients, placing a pillow under the head and under the knees may help alleviate pain and provide more comfort.

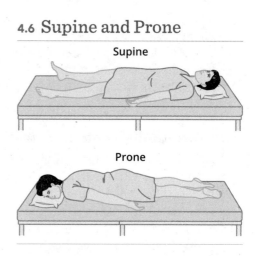

4.6 Supine and Prone

Prone

The prone position requires the patient to lie face down, flat on the stomach, with the head turned to one side, and arms either alongside the body or crossed under the head. This position is the opposite of the supine position. The drape should cover the patient from upper back to over the feet. This position is used for back exams and certain types of surgery.

4.7 Dorsal Recumbent

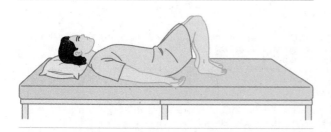

Dorsal Recumbent

In the dorsal recumbent position, the patient is lying flat on the back with knees bent and feet flat on the examination table. This position relieves strain on the lower back and relaxes abdominal muscles. The dorsal recumbent position is used to inspect the head, neck, chest, vaginal, rectal, and perineal areas. This position can be used for digital (using the gloved fingers) exams of the vagina and rectum. To drape the patient, place the drape at the patient's neck or underarms and cover the body down to the feet.

Lithotomy

The lithotomy position is similar to the dorsal recumbent position, except the patient's feet are placed in stirrups attached to the end and sides of the table. The stirrups must be locked in place to ensure patient safety. Provide additional assistance to patients who may have difficulty placing their feet in the stirrups. After the feet are in place in the stirrups, the patient is instructed to slide down until the buttocks are positioned at the edge of the table. The patient is draped from under the arms to the ankles. This position is used for vaginal examinations, often requiring the use of a vaginal speculum (an instrument used to hold open the walls of the vagina) and for obtaining cell samples of the cervix.

Fowler's

In the Fowler's position, the patient sits on the examination table with the head of the table raised to a 90-degree angle. If able, the patient may be seated on the edge of the table with feet over the edge in an upright position. This position is useful for examinations of the head, neck, and upper body. Patients who have difficulty breathing in the supine position may find this position more comfortable. The drape should be placed over the patient's lap and cover the legs.

Semi-Fowler's

The semi-Fowler's position is a modified Fowler's position with the head of the table at a 45-degree angle instead of a 90-degree angle. This position is used for postsurgical exams and patients with breathing difficulties or lower back injuries. The drape should be placed over the patient's lap and covering the legs.

Left Lateral

The left lateral position (also known as lateral semi-prone recumbent position and formerly known as Sims' position) requires the patient to be placed on the left side with the right leg sharply bent upward and the left leg slightly bent. The right arm is flexed next to the head for support. The patient is draped from under the arm or shoulders to below the knees at an angle. This allows the health care provider to raise a small section of the drape while keeping the rest of the patient covered. This position is used for rectal exams, taking rectal temperatures, enemas, and perineal and pelvic exams.

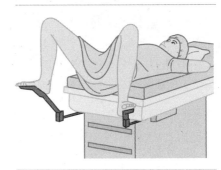
4.8 Lithotomy

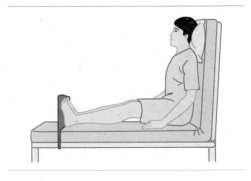
4.9 Fowler's

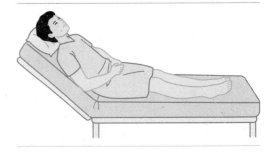
4.10 Semi-Fowler's

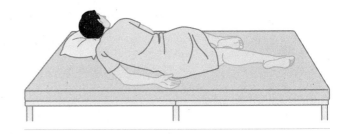
4.11 Left Lateral

CHAPTER 4: GENERAL PATIENT CARE: PART 1
Assist the Provider With Examinations

Knee–Chest

In the knee–chest position, the patient is placed in the prone position and then asked to pull the knees up to a kneeling position with thighs at a 90-degree angle to the table and buttocks in the air. The head is turned to one side, and the arms may be placed under the head or on either side of the head for comfort and support. This position is used for proctologic exams, sigmoidoscopy procedures, and rectal and vaginal exams.

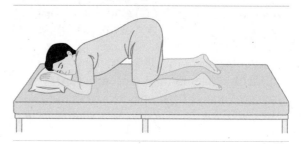

4.12 Knee–Chest

CHALLENGE

1. Match the position with its description.

POSITION	DESCRIPTION
A. Dorsal recumbent	1. Sitting position with back at 90° angle to exam table
B. Fowler's	2. Lying flat on the back with the arms down to the side
C. Semi-Fowler's	3. Laying on the left side with the left leg slightly flexed and the right leg flexed at 90° angle
D. Lithotomy	4. Sitting position with back at 45° angle to the exam table
E. Left lateral	5. Lying flat on the back with the knees bent
F. Supine	6. Lying flat on the table with feet resting on stirrups

   A: 5, B: 1, C: 4, D: 6, E: 3, F: 2
   The dorsal recumbent position is lying flat on the back with the knees bent. The Fowler's and semi-Fowler's positions are a sitting position with the back at 90-degree and 45-degrees angles to the exam table. The lithotomy position is lying flat on the table with feet resting on stirrups. The left lateral position is lying on the left side with the left leg slightly flexed and the right leg flexed at 90° angle. Supine is lying flat on the back with the arms down to the side.

2. Which of the following positions would be best for a patient that has dyspnea?
   A. Prone
   B. Lithotomy
   C. Semi-Fowler's
   D. Left lateral

   C is correct. In the semi-Fowler's position, the patient is seated, and the patient's back is at a 45-degree angle from the exam table. This allows for exams of the chest for patients who are unable to lie flat and for patients experiencing shortness of breath since it allows for expansion of the lungs.

3. A medical assistant is preparing a patient for a pelvic exam. Which of the following positions should the patient be placed in?
   A. Prone
   B. Lithotomy
   C. Semi-Fowler's
   D. Left lateral

   B is correct. The lithotomy position is when the patient is lying flat on the exam table with the buttocks at the end of the table and feet are resting in stirrups. This position is commonly used for pelvic exams and other gynecological exams and procedures.

PREPARE AND ADMINISTER NONPARENTERAL MEDICATIONS AND INJECTABLES

Dosage Calculations

Accurately administering medications is critical to preventing medical errors. The name of the medication, dosage, time, frequency, and route of administration direct the medical assistant in preparing medication for administration.

Parenteral medication administration is non-oral. Generally, the medication is injected directly into the body, bypassing the gastrointestinal tract.

Nonparenteral, or enteral, administration is oral medication given by the mouth delivered to the gastrointestinal tract.

> **4.13 Take Note**
>
> Medication can be administered in several different routes, which are dependent on how the medication should be taken and the medication form: parenteral and nonparenteral.

4.14 Parenteral routes

ROUTE	LOCATION
Subcutaneous	Injection administered below the skin layer into the adipose (fat) layer
Intradermal	Injection administered into the dermis
Intramuscular	Injection administered into the muscle
Intravenous	Injection administered directly into the vein

4.15 Other Routes of Administration

ROUTE	LOCATION
Oral	Taken by mouth
Sublingual	Placed under the tongue
Buccal	Between the cheek and gums resulting in rapid absorption
Inhalation	Inhaled through the mouth, passes through the trachea into the lungs; inhaled through the nose and absorbed through the nasal mucous membrane
Ocular or *otic*	Drops of medication are instilled directly into the eye (ocular) or ear (otic).
Transdermal	Applied to the skin and designed to release slowly and systemically into circulation. Administered in an adhesive patch in a single layer drug, multi-layer drug, drug in reservoir, or drug matrix.
Topical	Applied to the skin or mucous membrane (faster) and acts locally. Administered as creams, ointments, or emulsions.
Rectal	Inserted into rectum

---

parenteral. Administered or occurring in the body bypassing the gastrointestinal tract.

nonparenteral. Given by mouth, delivered to the gastrointestinal tract.

otic. Relating to the ear.

When administering medication, you must also know the dosage. Due to the importance of accurate dosage calculations, a quick review of calculations will be discussed again in the sections below.

Dosages can be in milligrams (mg) for tablets or capsules, grams (g) for creams or ointments, and milliliters (mL) for liquid medications. Some medications and supplements, such as insulin and vitamins, are listed as units (U).

When calculating an individual dose, we must have three pieces of information:

The desired dose (D)

- The dosage strength or supply on hand (H)
- The medication's unit of measurement or quantity of unit (Q)

4.16 Take Note

The dosage indicates the strength of the medication or how much of the medication a person should take. Only the dose stated in the prescription or medical order should be administered.

Once we know this information, we can then use the following dosage formula to calculate the medication.

$$X = \frac{D}{H} \times Q$$

X = the amount to administer

For example, you receive a medication order for 20 mg of a medication once a day. The dosage of the supply on hand is 10 mg per tablet. How many tablets should you administer to the patient?

Using the dosage formula, determine the three pieces of information.

$D = 20$ mg, $H = 10$ mg, $Q = 1$ tablet

$$X = \frac{D}{H} \times Q$$

$$X = \frac{20 \text{ mg}}{10 \text{ mg}} \times 1 \text{ tablet}$$

$X = 2$ tablets

Some medication dosages are based on the weight of the patient. For example, the dose of a medication for a patient who is 200 pounds might be higher than the dose for a patient who weighs 110 pounds. Weight-based dosage calculations are commonly done for pediatric medications. You will most likely have to convert the patient's weight from pounds into kilograms to perform a weight-based dosage calculation.

For example, a medication order is for 2 mg/kg of a medication. The patient weighs 77 lb. The medication is supplied as 100 mg/mL. How much should be administered to the patient?

CHAPTER 4: GENERAL PATIENT CARE: PART 1
Prepare and Administer Nonparenteral Medications and Injectables

To calculate this, there will be several steps.

1. Since the medication order is in kg, you will need to convert the patient's weight from lb to kg. You should know that 1 kg = 2.2 lb. This makes the patient 35 kg (77 lb ÷ 2.2).

2. You know that the medication order is 2 mg/kg. This means that for every kg, the patient should receive 2 mg of the medication: 35 kg × 2 mg = 70 mg of medication

3. You now know that the patient should receive 70 mg of the medication, which is supplied as 100 mg/mL. Use the dosage formula to calculate how much should be administered.

$$X = \frac{D}{H} \times Q$$

$$X = \frac{70 \text{ mg}}{100 \text{ mg}} \times 1 \text{ mL}$$

$$X = 0.70 \text{ mL}$$

CHALLENGE

1. Which of the following is a parenteral route of medication administration?
   A. Buccal
   B. Oral
   C. Subcutaneous
   D. Transdermal

   C is correct. Parenteral routes of medication administration include subcutaneous, intramuscular, intradermal, and intravenous.

2. A medication is prescribed to a patient at 25 mg tablets twice a day. Which of the following is the total milligrams prescribed to the patient each day?
   A. 2.5 mg
   B. 25 mg
   C. 50 mg
   D. 75 mg

   C is correct. If the patient takes two 25 mg tablets per day, the daily dosage is 50 mg, or 25 mg tablets × 2.

3. A patient is at prescribed 40 mg/day of a medication. The medication is dispensed as 10 mg tablets. How many tablets should the patient take a day?
   A. 1
   B. 4
   C. 10
   D. 40

   B is correct. If the patient is prescribed 40 mg of a medication per day, taking 4 tablets each day would equal 40 mg.

4. A medication is available at 160 mg per 5 mL. The patient is prescribed 240 mg of the medication. How much should be administered?
   A. 1.5 mL
   B. 3.3 mL
   C. 5 mL
   D. 7.5 mL

   D is correct. Using the basic formula for dosage calculations, the amount needed is 240 mL, the amount available is 160 mL, and the quantity on hand is 5 mL. The calculation would be 240 mL/160 mL × 5 mL = 7.5 mL.

COMMONLY USED ORAL AND PARENTERAL MEDICATIONS

Medications may be either prescription or nonprescription. Prescription medications require a medication order by an authorized health care provider to be dispensed to patients. Medication orders are directions provided by an authorized health care provider for a specific medication to be administered to an individual. Authorized health care providers include physicians, dentists, nurse practitioners, and, depending on the state, physician assistants. Nonprescription, also called over-the-counter (OTC), medications do not require a prescription.

Medications often have two names: brand name and generic name. The brand name (or trade name) is the name assigned by the medication manufacturer. The generic name is the standard or official name and assigned by the United States Adopted Names (USAN) Council and the World Health Organization (WHO). Every medication has a generic name that must be present on the medication label. However, there may be multiple brand names for the same medication, and it may not always be present on the medication label. For example, a common medication for hypertension (high blood pressure) is metoprolol, which is the generic name for Lopressor and Toprol XL—both the medication's brand names. Brand names are usually capitalized and are listed first, followed by the generic name, which is not capitalized, for example, Lopressor (metoprolol) and Toprol XL (metoprolol). Even OTC medications have brand and generic names, such as aspirin (Bayer), acetaminophen (Tylenol), and ibuprofen (Advil, Motrin).

Every medication label indicates the medication's form. The following are the different types of medication forms.

- Tablets
- Capsules
- Oral suspension
- Emulsions
- Lozenges
- Liquid

Medication Regulations and Best Practices

Checking the Medication Order

The name of the medication, dosage, time, and route of administration direct the MA in preparing medication for administration. Consent for administration of a medication should be obtained from the patient or guardian prior to preparing the medication. Tell the patient what the medication is, what it is given for, the dosage, and the route that will be used.

4.17 Take Note

Checking the medication three times helps prevent medication errors.

The first check is comparing the medication order to the medication. The second check occurs when preparing the medication for administration. The third check is completed when returning the medication back to the shelf.

Rights of Medication Administration

The rights of medication administration are a collection of safety checks that everyone who administers medications to patients must perform to avoid medication errors. Once the medication has been ordered, always follow the rules of medication administration.

These rules serve as safety checks to prevent medication errors.

4.18 Take Note

Ensure the right patient, right medication, right form, right dose, right route, right time, right technique, right education, and right documentation.

Right Patient

Use two patient identifiers, usually full name and date of birth, to verify the right patient. Then verify that data with the information on the medical record or medication administration record (MAR).

Right Medication

Check the label three times to verify the medication, strength, and dose—often referred to as the "three befores." The first time to check the medication label is when taking the medication container from the storage cabinet or drawer. The second is when taking the medication from its container to prepare to administer it. The third check is when putting the container back in storage or discarding it.

Right Form

Medications can come in several different forms. Some of these include liquid, tablet, capsules, suppositories, drops, and creams. The same medication can be available in several different forms. For example, amoxicillin can come in a capsule, tablet, chewable tablet, and liquid. Each form of medication has benefits in terms of effectiveness, ease of use, and safety. Checking the correct form of medication to be administered is essential when checking all rights of medication administration.

Right Dose

Compare the dosage on the prescription in the patient's MAR with the dosage on the medication's label and determine if medication calculations need to be performed to arrive at the prescribed dose.

Right Route

Compare the route on the prescription in the MAR with the administration route they are planning to use. Determine whether the route is appropriate for the patient and that the medication formulation is right for that route.

Right Time

In most office and clinic settings, MAs give medications right after the provider writes the order. Nevertheless, always confirm whether the medication has any timing specifications, such as the patient having an empty stomach or waiting several hours after taking another medication (such as an antacid) that might interact with the new medication.

Right Technique

MAs must know the correct techniques for administering every medication they give by every route, for example, taking an apical pulse prior to administering digoxin to ensure the patient's pulse is not less than 60.

CHAPTER 4: GENERAL PATIENT CARE: PART 1
Eye and Ear Medications

Right Education

Prior to administration of a medication, explain to the patient the name of the medication, the ordering provider, and the reason and intended effect of the medication; disclose any side effects; and confirm any allergies the patient may have.

Right Documentation

Always document administering a medication after the patient receives it, not before. If you do not administer a medication as prescribed, the documentation must include this and why the patient did not receive it. Proper documentation includes date, time, quantity, medication, strength, lot number, manufacturer, expiration date, consent obtained, and patient outcome.

CHALLENGE

1. Order the steps of performing a triple check for medication administration in the correct sequence.
   A. Returning the medication to the storage cabinet
   B. Preparing the medication
   C. Comparing the medication label to the medication order

   C, B, A
   The first check is comparing the medication to the medication order. The second check occurs when the medication is being prepared. The third check is completed when returning the medication to the storage shelf.

2. Which of the following are part of the nine rights of medication administration? (Select all that apply.)
   A. Right medication
   B. Right dose
   C. Right technique
   D. Right insurer
   E. Right documentation

   A, B, C, and E are correct. The eight rights of medication administration are right patient, right medication, right dose, right route, right time, right technique, right education, and right documentation.

EYE AND EAR MEDICATIONS

The most common form of medication is liquid solution in the form of drops that is applied directly to the eyes and ears. If you are approved to administer this form of medication, the same precautions and rules must be taken when instilling eye and ear medications. You may also be required to provide patient education and instructions on self-administration of eye and ear medication if a treatment is prescribed to the patient to administer at home.

Eye Instillation

Eye instillation (ocular or **ophthalmic** administration) is a common duty of a medical assistant. Only ophthalmic or optic medications should be used in the eye. All optic medications must be sterile, and sterile procedures must be followed before and during the administration.

4.19 Take Note

The patient should look toward the ceiling with both eyes open.

For eye instillation, the patient should be lying down or sitting back in a chair with the head tilted back. Clean any debris from the eye area. Provide a tissue to the patient to blot excess medication.

---

ophthalmic. Relating to the eye and its diseases.

With your nondominant hand, gently pull down the lower lid of the affected eye using the thumb or two fingers to expose the conjunctival sac. Gently rest the dominant hand on the patient's forehead and dispense a drop approximately ½ inch above the sac. If a cream or ointment is being administered, evenly apply a thick ribbon of the ointment along the inside edge of the lower eyelid on the conjunctiva, moving from the medial to lateral side. Release the eyelid and instruct the patient to close the eyes. Repeat if the other eye requires treatment. Remove any excess medication with a clean tissue. Ask whether the patient is feeling any discomfort or pain and observe for any adverse reactions. Apply a clean eye patch, if ordered.

Ear Instillation

A medical assistant may also be asked to perform an ear instillation (otic administration). Have the patient lie on one side with the affected ear facing up.

This will straighten the ear canal and allow for better medication distribution. Hold the applicator ½ inch above the ear canal and administer the number of prescribed drops. Have the patient remain in the position for at least 5 min. Ask whether the patient is feeling any discomfort or pain and observe for any adverse reactions. Loosely insert a small, clean wad of cotton, if ordered, before treating the other ear, if applicable.

4.20 Take Note

With your nondominant hand, pull the pinna of the auricle (outer ear) outward and upward for adults and outward and downward for infants and children.

CHALLENGE

1. When performing an ear instillation for a child, how should you adjust the auricle of the ear?
   A. Pulling the auricle outward and upward
   B. Pulling the auricle outward and downward
   C. Pulling the auricle inward and upward
   D. Pulling the auricle inward and downward

B is correct. The auricle should be gently pulled outward and downward for infants and children. This will straighten the ear canal and allow for better medication distribution.

ALLERGIC REACTIONS

Types of Allergic Reactions

An important part of the patient medical history is documenting any allergies or history of *allergic* reactions. An allergy is an abnormal or hypersensitive reaction to an allergen, or a substance that is capable of causing an allergic reaction. Patients can have an allergic reaction to a variety of things, such as dust, mold, pollen, animal dander, foods (peanuts, strawberries), insect bites, and medications.

Most allergic reactions are common and present with mild symptoms, such as hives, itching, rashes, watery eyes, and nasal congestion. Treatment usually includes an over-the-counter hydrocortisone cream and an antihistamine.

A severe allergic reaction can result in anaphylaxis or *anaphylactic shock*, which is a systemic allergic reaction that can be life threatening without immediate medical intervention. People can have initial symptoms of weakness, sweating, and dyspnea and can progress to hypotension, arrhythmia, difficulty in swallowing, and convulsions. Anaphylactic shock can occur within minutes after exposure to the allergen, or a delayed reaction could occur within a couple of hours.

4.21 Take Note

Moderate and severe allergic reactions may result in abdominal pain, coughing, diarrhea, dyspnea, dysphagia, swelling of the face, nausea and vomiting, convulsions, and unconsciousness.

allergic. A condition of sensitivity in which the immune system reacts abnormally to a foreign substance.

anaphylactic shock. A systemic allergic reaction that can be life-threatening without immediate medical intervention.

Responding to Allergic Reactions

Be prepared to manage or assist if a patient is experiencing anaphylactic shock, especially if you work in an allergist clinic. Most medical practices should have epinephrine or an epinephrine autoinjector (EpiPen) used to treat patients experiencing anaphylaxis. Epinephrine is considered the first line of treatment for a patient experiencing anaphylactic shock.

Massage the injection site for a few minutes. Immediately call 911. The autoinjector is for emergency supportive care and does not replace the patient seeking advanced medical care afterwards. If the patient loses consciousness and stops breathing, administer cardiopulmonary resuscitation (CPR).

> **4.22 Take Note**
>
> Epinephrine should be administered as an intramuscular (IM) injection. The upper thigh is a common site and, in an emergency, can be injected through the patient's clothes. Once injected, hold the injector or needle into the thigh for at least 10 seconds.

Patient's Allergy Status

A patient's medication allergy status should be checked and updated at every patient appointment. Although a patient might not have had an allergic reaction to a medication or allergen in the past, it is always possible to develop a reaction later. It is common practice for patients to complete a questionnaire about their allergy history, particularly as a new patient. This includes having patients list their current medications, any current allergies to any medication or food or if they have any environmental allergies, and what was the allergic reaction to the medication or allergen.

During the patient interview, confirm the patient's allergy history and document the allergy status in the patient's medical record. Ask details about the allergy, including what the reaction was and what the offending agent or allergen was.

For medication allergies, ask and document the following.

- Name of the suspected medication, prescribed (brand or generic) and non-prescribed (over-the-counter) medications
- Timeframe of the reaction from initiation of the medication
- Strength and formulation
- Description of the reaction
- Indication for the medication being taken (if there is no clinical diagnosis, describe the illness)
- Date and time of the reaction
- Number of doses taken or number of days on the medication before onset of the reaction
- Route of administration

The patient's medication allergy history must be taken and updated at all patient visits and whenever a medication is prescribed, dispensed, or administered. After administration of any medication, ask the patient to wait 20 to 30 minutes before leaving for observation of any possible adverse reactions or allergic reactions.

CHALLENGE

1. Which of the following is a sign of anaphylactic shock?
   A. Rash
   B. Watery eyes
   C. Hives
   D. Difficulty swallowing

   D is correct. People experiencing anaphylactic shock may have initial symptoms of weakness, sweating, and dyspnea and may progress to hypotension, arrhythmia, difficulty in swallowing, and convulsions.

2. A patient reports having a medication allergy. What questions should you ask? (Select all that apply.)
   A. Who is the medication manufacturer?
   B. What was the reaction?
   C. When did the reaction start after taking the medication?
   D. How many doses have you taken?
   E. Why are you prescribed this medication?

   B, C, D, and E are correct. For medication allergies, ask about and document the name of the medication, how many doses were taken, why it was prescribed, when the reaction started, and what was the patient's reaction.

PREPARE AND ADMINISTER MEDICATIONS – PARENTERAL ROUTES

Sterile Techniques

Whenever invasive procedures are to be performed, caution must be taken to maintain sterility. Some medical equipment is intended to be disposable while others are to be reused. Reusable equipment must be disinfected or sterilized accordingly prior to being used with each patient. Reusable equipment includes some surgical instruments (clamps, forceps, some scalpels, and endoscopes).

All reusable medical devices can be grouped into one of three categories according to the degree of risk of infection associated with the use of the device.

4.23 Take Note

Sterilization is required for all instruments and equipment that will penetrate a patient's skin, enter a patient's body, or come in contact with any other normally sterile areas of the body.

- Critical devices, such as surgical forceps, come in contact with blood or normally sterile tissue
- Semi-critical devices, such as endoscopes, come in contact with mucus membranes
- Non-critical devices, such as stethoscopes, come in contact with unbroken skin

Sterilization is also required for all instruments that will be used in a sterile field, even if they will not be used on a patient. An item is considered either sterile or unsterile. If in doubt, consider it unsterile. Equipment should be sterilized according to manufacturer's instructions.

To minimize risk of infection, some medical equipment and supplies are to be disposed of after a single use. This includes needles, syringes, sterile gloves, gowns, face masks, and suction catheters.

Since they will be entering the patient's body, needles must be sterile when used for injections. According to the Centers for Disease Control and Prevention (CDC), unsafe injection practices that have resulted in disease transmission have most commonly included the following.

- Using the same syringe to administer medication to more than one patient
- Accessing a medication vial with a syringe that has already been used to administer medication to a patient, then using the remaining contents from that vial or bag for another patient
- Using medications packaged as single-dose or single-use for more than one patient
- Failing to use aseptic technique when preparing and administering injections.

sterilization. The complete destruction of all micro-organisms through specific means.

CHAPTER 4: GENERAL PATIENT CARE: PART 1
Prepare and Administer Medications – Parenteral Routes

Needles come individually wrapped. Check the expiration date on the wrapper to make sure the needle is still in good quality. In rare cases, old needles may bend or break.

Take care to not place the exposed or uncapped needle on a tray or countertop. A clean needle may be recapped for protection prior to injection using a one-handed scoop method. However, caution should be used since contamination by an incidental stick is possible while recapping. Injection is an invasive procedure, and the medical assistant could be exposed to blood and body fluids, so nonsterile gloves and other appropriate PPE are required.

Alcohol swabs are necessary to wipe off vials or wrap around the neck of an *ampule*, as well as for skin preparation. The top of the vial stopper should be wiped with an alcohol swab each time it's used. Cleaning the vial stopper assists in preventing contamination or introduction of germs into the solution as well as keeping the needle sterile. Do not introduce the needle into the vial more than once. Each repuncture into a vial dulls the needle and predisposes the equipment to contamination. Allowing solutions to run down a needle also increases the likelihood of contamination. A gauze pad is used to apply pressure or hold at the site after administration. An adhesive bandage should be available if there is bleeding at the site.

Unsterile or used needles, which are those that have been used on a patient, should never be recapped. They should immediately be disposed of in the sharps waste container. Disposing of them in the regular trash bin or the biohazard waste container may result in a needlestick injury. A sharps container should be located nearby to avoid transporting contaminated needles from where the injection was administered. A biohazard container is necessary for disposal of other potentially contaminated items, such as contaminated gowns, blood-soaked gloves, and used specimen swabs.

As a safety feature, many needles now come with different safety devices. The most common safety features are resheathing devices. These are shields that cover the needle or retract the needle after use, such as a needle cap and safety lock. Resheathing covers, as well as other needle safety devices, prevent the repeated use of needles and do not penetrate, cut, or scratch during the disposal of the needles.

CHALLENGE

1. Used needles should be disposed of in which of the following ways?
   A. Recapped and placed in the trash bin
   B. Recapped and placed in the sharps container
   C. Uncapped and placed in the biohazard container
   D. Uncapped and placed in the sharps container

   D is correct. Used or unsterile needles should not be recapped to prevent needle stick injuries. They should immediately be disposed of in the sharps waste container.

2. Which of the following is considered a reusable equipment or supply?
   A. 5 mL syringe
   B. Surgical forceps
   C. Injection needle
   D. Medication ampule

   B is correct. Surgical forceps are reusable equipment and must be sterilized between patient use.

ampule. Sealed glass capsule containing a liquid.

TECHNIQUES AND INJECTION SITE

A common route of medication administration is the parenteral route. Parenteral is the administration of a substance, such as a medication or any kind of fluid, into the muscle, vein, or any means other than through the gastrointestinal tract (i.e., oral). Some medications may need to be injected for a variety of reasons: to allow for better absorption into the body, to administer a more precise level of medication, the patient needing a rapid effect, or the inability of the patient to receive the medication through a different route of administration, such as oral due to inability to swallow or the medication can be destroyed in the GI tract.

A needle and syringe are the items needed to perform an injection. Parts of a needle and syringe are outlined below. A syringe has two parts: a barrel and a plunger. The barrel is a cylinder that holds the medication and has volume marking on its side. The plunger forces the medication through the barrel and out the needle. Syringes come in many different volume sizes and different unit measurements, such as milliliter (mL) or cubic centimeter (cc). These measurements are equivalent, 1 mL = 1 cc. Syringes can be as small as 0.5 mL to 500 mL. Insulin syringes are calibrated in units (U), commonly either 50 U or 100 U. Insulin syringes are usually packaged with attached needles.

The needle consists of a hub, shaft, and bevel. The hub is what is twisted on to the syringe. The tip of the needle is beveled, or angled, to allow for better skin penetration. When inserting a needle, the bevel should be up. The lumen is the opening of the needle. The shaft is the length of the needle.

4.24 Parts of a Syringe and Needle

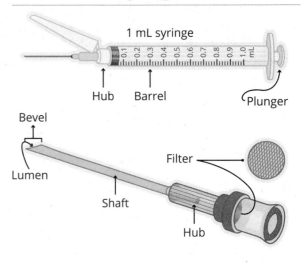

4.25 Take Note

When selecting a needle, select an appropriate length for the type of injection and size of the patient.

When selecting a needle, the gauge and the length need to be considered. A needle's gauge (G) refers to the size of the opening of the needle, or lumen. The higher the gauge, the smaller or narrower the lumen is. For example, a 25 G has a smaller lumen than an 18 G needle. The needle length is based on inches and can vary from 5/16 inch to 1 ½ inches. Syringes and needles may be individually packaged or packaged together. The volume, gauge, and length of the needle and syringe are labeled on the package. For example, a label showing 3 mL 22 G x 1 ½ indicates that the syringe can hold up to 3 mL, the needle gauge is 22, and its length is 1.5 inches.

The needle should be long enough to penetrate the layers of tissue appropriate to the injection without being too long. For example, if a patient is obese, a longer needle may be needed in order to penetrate the fat layer.

When preparing for an injection, only use a sterile needle and syringe that has been wrapped and not tampered with. If you did not remove the needle and syringe yourself, consider them unsterile, dispose of them in the sharps waste container, and start over. All needles should come with a cap.

Injection Sites

The most commonly used routes of parenteral administration are subcutaneous (SC), intradermal (ID), and intramuscular (IM). Another route is intravenous (IV), which is administering medication directly into the vein. This route is more commonly done in the hospital setting or in the emergency setting. In most cases, medical assistants will not perform an IV administration.

Subcutaneous

SC injections are administered beneath the skin and into the adipose (fat) tissue. This allows for slow, sustained release of a medication with long duration of effect. SC injections are used to administer smaller doses of medication, usually less than 1.5 mL. Common medications that are injected SC are insulin, heparin, immunizations, and allergy medications.

SC injections may be administered in many sites, with the most common being the upper, outer arm; abdominal region; and the upper thigh. Lesser common areas are the scapula (upper back area) and lower back/upper buttocks. When performing a SC injection, ensure that you can pinch at least 1 inch of skin in order to inject below it. Since SC administration is to be delivered in the adipose tissue, the injection is 45 degrees from the surface of the skin to penetrate the layers of the skin but not deep enough to enter any muscle tissue.

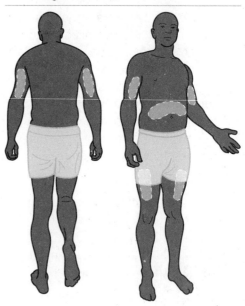

4.26 Subcutaneous (SC) Injection Sites

Intradermal

ID injections are administered between the upper layers of the skin, between the epidermis and dermis. The most common site for ID injections is the mid forearm. In rare cases, the upper chest and scapula (upper back) regions may be used. When using the forearm, measure using one hand width above the wrist and one hand width from the elbow or antecubital space. Any area within the anterior forearm visible is acceptable for the injection. The forearm is often used to administer a tuberculosis (TB) test. The upper chest and scapula may be used for skin tests, such as allergy testing.

4.27 Intradermal (ID) Injection Sites

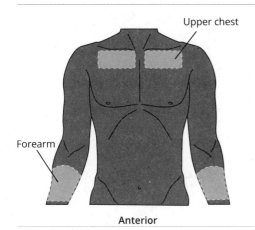
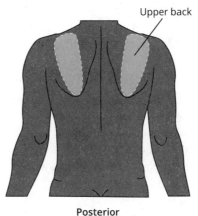

4.28 Wheal in a TB Test

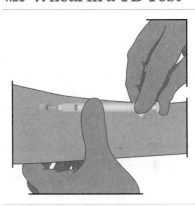

With ID injections, a very small amount of a medication may be injected, often 0.1 mL or less. Since the medication is administered between the skin, the angle of the needle is almost parallel to the skin, or 5 to 15 degrees. In a TB test, a wheal, or a bubble, below the skin must be formed with the ID injection. Do not massage or apply pressure or a bandage to the site after injection.

Intramuscular

IM injections are administered into the muscle of the patient. Common sites are the deltoid (shoulder), ventrogluteal (outer hip), and vastus lateralis (upper, outer thigh) muscles. IM injections generally allow for larger administration of medication than SC and ID injections. However, the amount varies with injections sites.

4.29 Take Note

In general, up to 3 mL of a medication may be administered into the ventrogluteal and vastus lateralis for adults. Older adults and thin patients may only tolerate up to 2 mL in a single injection. No more than 1 mL should be given in the deltoid.

Common medications that are administered via IM injections are antibiotics (penicillin), hormones (testosterone), and some vaccines. Since an IM injection is to deliver a medication to the muscle, the needle should be at a 90-degree angle to the skin to ensure penetration past the skin and adipose tissue to reach the muscle.

The deltoid muscle is the most common injection site since it is the easiest to access, with patients only having to lift their sleeve. It should be avoided for infants or children younger than 3 years of age. The site of injection on the deltoid should be 1 to 2 inches below the acromion process. The deltoid muscle can only hold up to 1 mL of medication.

The ventrogluteal site involves the gluteus medius and minimus muscles and is a safe injection site for adults, children, and infants. This site provides the greatest thickness of muscle that is free of nerves and blood vessels, and it has a narrower layer of fat. This is also the preferred site for all oily and irritating solutions for patients of any age. To locate the site, place the heel of your hand on the greater trochanter (right hand placed on left hip and left hand placed on right hip), the middle finger is placed on the iliac crest, and your fingers are spread. Give the injection where the V is made between your index finger and middle finger (position the thumb pointing towards the groin). This injection site can hold up to 3 mL of medication.

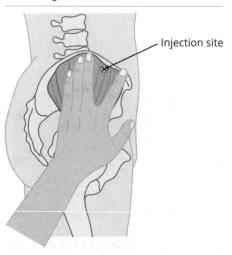

4.30 **Site for Ventrogluteal Injection**

The vastus lateralis muscle is located on the lateral side of the thigh. The injection site is halfway down the muscle, between the greater trochanter and the lateral femoral condyle. This site is recommended for children younger than 3 years of age. This muscle is located on the anterior lateral aspect of the thigh and extends from one hand's breadth above the knee to one hand's breadth below the greater trochanter. The outer middle third of the muscle is used for injections. Before giving an IM injection, make sure to avoid injuring nerves and blood vessels. Injecting into a vein may result in faster absorption of the medication than prescribed.

4.31 **Intramuscular (IM) Injection Sites**

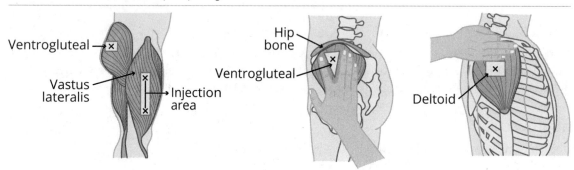

Each injection type must deliver the medication to the appropriate tissue. To do so, identify the following.

- Needle size
- Syringe/barrel size
- Site for injection
- Angle of injection

4.32 **Angle of Injections**

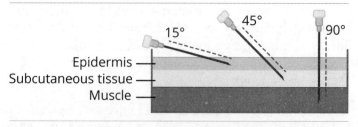

4.33 Site, Angle, and Needle Selection for Injections

TYPE	COMMON SITES OF INJECTIONS	ANGLE OF INJECTION	NEEDLE SIZE	NEEDLE LENGTH
Subcutaneous (SC)	Upper, outer arm; abdominal region; and the upper thigh	45 degrees	25 to 31 G	⅝ to ¾ inch
Intradermal (ID)	Forearm	5 to 15 degrees	25 to 26 G	⅜ to ½ inch
Intramuscular (IM)	Deltoid, ventrogluteal, vastus lateralis	90 degrees	18 to 25 G	⅝ to 3 inches

Don nonsterile gloves. Clean the site with an alcohol swab for 30 seconds using firm, concentric circles. Allow the site to dry to prevent introducing alcohol into the tissue, which can be irritating and uncomfortable. Remove the guard cap from the needle by pulling it off in a straight motion. A straight motion helps prevent needlestick injury.

For an SC injection, gently grasp and pinch the area selected as an injection site using your nondominant hand. Hold the syringe in the dominant hand between the thumb and forefinger like a dart and insert the needle quickly at a 45-degree angle. After the needle is in place, release the tissue with your nondominant hand. With your dominant hand, inject the medication. Avoid moving the syringe. Withdraw the needle quickly at the same angle at which it was inserted. Using gauze, apply gentle pressure at the site after the needle is withdrawn. Do not massage the site.

Insulin is considered a high-alert medication requiring special care to prevent medication errors. Care must be taken to ensure the correct type and amount of insulin are administered at the correct time. Only insulin syringes should be used to administer an insulin injection. Insulin syringes are supplied in 30-, 50-, or 100-unit measurements, so read the barrel increments (calibration) carefully. Insulin is always ordered and administered in unit dosage. One anatomic region should be selected for a patient's insulin injections to maintain consistent absorption, and then sites should be rotated within that region. The abdomen absorbs insulin the fastest, followed by the arms, thighs, and buttocks. If regular SC injections need to be given, as in the case of insulin, rotate the injection site and avoid using a site that is edematous (swollen) and has too much scar tissue or adipose (fat) tissue.

For an ID injection, use your nondominant hand, spread the skin taut over the injection site. Taut skin provides easy entrance for the needle and is also important to do for older adults, whose skin is less elastic. Hold the syringe in the dominant hand between the thumb and forefinger, with the bevel of the needle up at a 5- to 15-degree angle at the selected site. Place the needle almost flat against the patient's skin, bevel side up, and insert the needle into the skin. Keeping the bevel side up allows for smooth piercing of the skin and induction of the medication into the dermis. Advance the needle no more than an eighth of an inch to cover the bevel. Once the syringe is in place, use the thumb of the nondominant hand to push on the plunger to slowly inject the medication. Carefully withdraw the needle out of the insertion site using the same angle it was placed.

For an IM injection, stabilize the skin around the injection site by pulling the skin taut with the forefinger and thumb of your nondominant hand. With your dominant hand, hold the syringe like a dart and insert the needle quickly into the muscle at a 90-degree angle using a steady and smooth motion. After the needle pierces the skin, use the thumb and forefinger of the nondominant hand to hold the syringe and inject the medication. Remove the needle at the same angle at which it was inserted. Cover the injection site with sterile gauze using gentle pressure and apply a bandage if needed.

CHAPTER 4: GENERAL PATIENT CARE: PART 1
Techniques and Injection Site

Although it may depend on the policy of your medical practice, the CDC no longer recommends aspirating before an IM injection. Aspiration is meant to ensure that the needle tip is located at the desired site and has not accidentally punctured a blood vessel. However, this practice has not been evaluated scientifically. As long as the appropriate site has been located, the veins and arteries within reach of a needle in these sites for injections are too small to allow an intravenous entry without blowing out the vessel.

After administration of any medication, ask the patient to wait 20 to 30 min before leaving for observation of any possible adverse reactions or allergic reactions. Inform patients they may experience mild discomfort after an injection. However, certain symptoms may be a sign of a more serious complication. Immediately notify the health care provider if patients are experiencing any of the following.

- Severe pain at the injection site
- Tingling or numbness
- Redness, swelling, or warmth at the injection site
- Prolonged bleeding
- Signs of an allergic reaction, such as difficulty breathing or facial swelling

CHALLENGE

1. Match the injection site with the type of injection.

TYPE OF INJECTION	INJECTION SITE
A. Abdominal region	1. Intradermal
B. Deltoid	2. Intramuscular
C. Upper, outer arm	3. Subcutaneous
D. Anterior forearm	
E. Vastus lateralis	

1: D; 2: B, E; 3: A, C

2. Which of the following needle size would you select for a tuberculin (TB) test?
   A. 31 G 1
   B. 26 G ½
   C. 25 G 1 ½
   D. 18 G 1 ½

B is correct. A tuberculin test is performed as an intradermal injection. The appropriate needle and syringe size would be 26 gauge and ½ inch long.

3. Match the site of injection with the angle of injection.

INJECTION SITE	ANGLE OF INJECTION
A. Abdominal region	1. 15 degrees
B. Upper, outer arm	2. 45 degrees
C. Anterior forearm	3. 90 degrees
D. Deltoid	
E. Ventrogluteal	

1: C; 2: A, B; 3: D, E

INJECTION SUPPLIES AND EQUIPMENT

Vials

Parenteral medications come packaged in vials, ampules, and premeasured syringes and cartridges. Vials are the most common packaging for medication that is administered parenterally. A vial is a plastic or glass container that has a rubber stopper (diaphragm) on the top. The rubber stopper is covered with a metal lid or plastic cover to maintain sterility until the vial is used for the first time. Some manufacturers do not guarantee a sterile top even though it is covered, and therefore it is necessary to wipe the top with alcohol pad with first use and any use after. Vials are available in different sizes. Multidose vials contain more than one dosage of the medication. The label on the vial will specify the amount of medication in a certain amount of solution, for example, 60 mg per mL or 0.2 mg per 0.5 mL. Multidose vials usually expire after 28 days unless the manufacturer states otherwise. Make sure you write the expiration date on the vial upon opening. Single-dose vials contain a single dosage of medication for injection. Many vials are single dose because it is safer. Even if medication is in a single-dosage vial, it should still be measured and drawn up according to the prescribed amount. The medication in a vial may be in liquid (solution) form, or it may contain a powder that must be reconstituted before administration. Reconstitution requires the adding a liquid diluent to a dry ingredient to make a specific concentration of a medication.

Withdrawal from a Vial Technique

Before withdrawing medication from a vial, wipe the top with alcohol and allow it to dry. A vial is a closed system, and air must be injected into it to allow for withdrawal of the medication. If air is not injected into the vial before the medication is withdrawn, a vacuum remains in the vial that makes the withdrawal of medication difficult. Inject air equal to the amount of solution being withdrawn into the air space between the solution and the rubber stopper, invert the vial, and the withdraw the desired volume of medication.

Ampule

An ampule is a sealed glass container designed to hold a single dose of medication. Ampules have a particular shape with a constricted neck. They are designed to snap open. The neck of the ampule may be scored or have a darkened line or ring around it to indicate where it should be broken to withdraw medication.

Withdrawal from an Ampule Technique

When withdrawing medication from an ampule, snap the neck off by grasping it with an alcohol wipe, sterile gauze, or ampule protector. Aspiration of the medication into a syringe occurs easily and may be accomplished with a filter needle, if required by the medical practice's policy. A filter needle prevents withdrawal of glass or rubber particulate. When the needle is inserted into an ampule, take care to prevent the shaft and tip of the needle from touching the rim of the ampule. Withdraw medication into the syringe by gently pulling back on the plunger, which creates a negative pressure and allows the medication to be pulled into the syringe. Discard the needle used to withdraw the medication and replace it with a new needle.

CHAPTER 4: GENERAL PATIENT CARE: PART 1
Injection Supplies and Equipment

Syringes

Premeasured Syringes

Premeasured syringes and cartridges are prefilled syringes that are single dosed and packaged with the needle that is provided by the manufacturer. These syringes are disposable and supplied already loaded with the substance to be injected. Premeasured syringes are convenient and help ease the administration process. They allow for convenience and efficiency, accuracy in dosing, reduced risk of infection and contamination, and reduced waste. You do not have to worry about the transfer of a medication from a vial to a syringe or about leaving a small percentage of the dose behind. Common prefilled syringes are often used for immunizations and for emergency administration, such as naloxone for overdoses and sodium bicarbonate for shock and cardiac arrests.

Hypodermic Syringe

There are generally three types of syringes: hypodermic, tuberculin, and insulin. Hypodermic syringes come in a variety of sizes from 0.5 to 60 mL and even larger. Syringes are calibrated or marked in milliliters but hold varying capacities. Of the small-capacity syringes, the 3 mL syringe is used most often for the administration of medication. Although many syringes are labeled in milliliters, a few syringes are still labeled with cubic centimeters (cc). Milliliter (mL) is the correct unit. The milliliter is a measure of volume, the cubic centimeter is a three-dimensional measure of space and represents the space that a milliliter occupies. The terms, although sometimes used interchangeably, are not the same. Many institutions are now purchasing syringes that indicate mL as opposed to cc, but either is acceptable for use.

Tuberculin Syringe

A tuberculin syringe is a narrow syringe that has a capacity of 0.5 mL or 1 mL. The 1-mL size is used most often. The volume of a tuberculin syringe can be measured on the milliliter scale. On the milliliter side of the syringe, the syringe is calibrated in hundredths (0.01 mL) and tenths (0.1 mL) of a milliliter. Tuberculin syringes are used to accurately measure medications given in very small volumes (e.g., heparin). This syringe is also often used in pediatrics and for diagnostic purposes (e.g., skin testing for tuberculosis). It is recommended that dosages less than 0.5 mL be measured with a tuberculin syringe to make certain that the correct dosage is administered to a patient. Dosages such as 0.42 mL and 0.37 mL can be measured accurately with a tuberculin syringe. When using a tuberculin syringe, read the markings carefully to avoid error.

Insulin Syringe

Insulin syringes are designed for the administration of insulin only. Insulin dosages are measured in units. Insulin syringes are calibrated to match the dosage strength of the insulin being used. They are marked U-100 and are designed to be used with insulin that is marked U-100. U-100 insulin should be measured only in a U-100 insulin syringe. It is important to note that for U-100 insulin, 100 units = 1 mL. Insulin syringes do not have detachable needles. The needle, hub, and barrel are inseparable.

CHALLENGE

1. Which of the following syringes would best be used to administer 0.1 mL?
   A. 2 mL hypodermic
   B. Insulin
   C. Tuberculin
   D. 3 mL hypodermic

   C is correct. The best syringe used to administer 0.1 mL is a tuberculin.

2. Which of the following items should be disposed of in the trash and not the sharps container? (Select all that apply.)
   A. Alcohol pad
   B. Gloves
   C. Bandages
   D. Needle and syringe
   E. Gauze

   A, B, C, and E are correct. All sharps must be disposed of in the sharps container to prevent needlestick or sharps injuries.

STORAGE OF INJECTABLES

Some common injectable medications are controlled substances, and there are strict guidelines on storing them in the medical practice. A controlled substance is any medication, whether prescription or illegal, that has the potential for abuse or addiction. The Drug Enforcement Administration (DEA) maintains oversight for legally prescribed and used narcotic drugs and for containment of illegal drugs. Controlled substances and the records of their prescribing and dispensing must be protected from misuse by storing them under double lock, such as a combination of two keys.

Check labels, directions, and package inserts to determine the proper method of storage for all products because storage requirements can vary. Medications kept for patient administration must not be stored in the same refrigerator with food or other items.

Some medications may require being stored in the freezer. Follow the storage guidelines per the manufacturer to maintain efficiency and efficacy of the medication. Daily temperature logs for both refrigerators and freezers where medications are stored are required to ensure that the necessary temperatures are maintained and the medical practice is in compliance with Safety Data Sheet (SDS) regulations.

Some injectable medications, such as vaccines, should be refrigerated and must be stored immediately upon arrival at the medical practice. Store all medications at the recommended temperature. Store refrigerated medications between 2° and 8° C (35° and 46° F). Frozen medications must be stored between −50° and −15° C (−58° and 5° F). The temperatures of the refrigerators and freezers must be checked daily.

Expiration dates on medications and all supplies for injection should be routinely checked. Medications must be rotated according to their expiration dates. The supply of medications should be rotated to use the ones with the shortest or soonest expiration date. They may be stored and organized alphabetically or based on their classification, according to the Controlled Substance schedule.

Disposing of medication is also regulated by states and often follow guidelines from the *Food and Drug Administration (FDA)* and the Environmental Protection Agency (EPA). It is important for medical practices and other health care organizations to check with their local municipal governments.

CHALLENGE

1. Many medications require storage in the refrigerator or freezer. How often should the temperatures be checked?
   A. Annually
   B. Daily
   C. Monthly
   D. Weekly

   B is correct. Medications, such as vaccines, must be stored at recommended temperatures. The temperatures of the refrigerators and freezers need to be checked daily.

2. Refrigerated medications must be stored at which of the following temperature ranges?
   A. 58° to 5° F
   B. 35° to 46° F
   C. −58° to 5° C
   D. 35° to 46° C

   B is correct. Store refrigerated medications between 35° and 46° F (2° and 8° C). Frozen medications must be stored between −58° and 5° F (−50° and −15° C). The temperatures of the refrigerators and freezers need to be checked daily.

Food and Drug Administration. Organization responsible for protecting the public health by ensuring safety, efficacy, and security of human medications.

MANAGE INJECTION LOGS

When any procedure is performed on a patient, it must be documented in the patient's medical record. As the saying goes, "If it wasn't documented, it wasn't done."

Administered medications, including injections, are to be documented by law. A MAR, or medication administration record, is a report that serves as a legal record of the medications administered to a patient at a facility by a health care provider or professional. It should include key information about the patient's medication, including the medication name, dose taken, date and time, route given, special instructions, and any reaction to the medication. A MAR must be filled out each time a patient is administered a medication. Accurately completing a MAR can help reduce the risk of medication errors and ensure the patient receives the correct treatment. The MAR should be kept in a safe location close to where the medications are stored.

Some medical practices will use a MAR form provided by the pharmacy or will document medication in the *electronic medical record (EMR)* system. Regardless, the captured information and elements should be the same.

Sample Medication Administration Record

Taking the information from a medical provider's order and transferring it to the MAR is known as "transcribing." Sometimes the pharmacy provides completed MARs, but if a new medication is started and a pharmacy-generated MAR is not available, you will need to transcribe that order onto the MAR. This ensures that others know that a new medication has been prescribed. Changes to the MAR should also be made if the dose of a medication is changed. If your facility does not use paper MARs, orders are updated and released through the EHR.

The following information must be documented in the MAR about the medication.

- Any allergies or history of allergies
- What medication is being administered
- Medication dosage
- Administration route
- When is it being administered—what time, how often, how long
- The name of the health care provider who prescribed the medication

As previously stated, some injectable medications are controlled substances, and there are strict requirements on how they are stored. In addition to a double-lock system for storage, a logbook or electronic sign-off and a daily count by two people are required for controlled substances kept in the practice. Daily counts ensure that all medications are accounted for. Records, whether in a logbook or electronic, are required to be maintained for controlled substances administered to patients.

CHALLENGE

1. Which of the following must be included in a MAR? (Select all that apply.)
   A. Name of the medication
   B. Dosage of medication
   C. Any allergies
   D. Name of the pharmacy
   E. Name of the prescriber

A, B, C, and E are correct. MARs should include any allergies or history of allergies, name of the medication, the dosage, route, when it should be administered, and the name of the prescriber.

electronic medical record (EMR). Record in a medical practice or clinic to document the patient's demographic information, care, progress, and treatment.

STORAGE, LABELING, EXPIRATION DATES, AND MEDICATION LOGS

Medications must be stored in the proper environment where temperature, light, and moisture are kept at appropriate levels. Different medications require different storage temperatures. Most medications' temperature requirements will fall into one of the following categories.

- Room temperature is 20° to 25° C (68° to 77°F).
- Refrigeration means 2° to 8° C (35° to 46° F). As mentioned previously, these medications must be stored in a refrigerator that is not used for any other purpose. It must have a thermometer so that staff can regularly monitor its storage temperature. Check the temperature daily when storing regular medications and twice daily for stored vaccines.

Storage areas must be clean, well lit, clutter-free, and locked at all times. Only authorized personnel should have access to your storage areas.

When storing medication, be sure to clearly separate topical medications, such as creams and ointments, from other medications. These medications must be clearly labeled as topical and stored separately from medications that are administered orally, for example. Cleaning products, urine test reagent tablets, disinfectants, household poisons, and any other substances that are potentially harmful should be clearly labeled and stored in their own locked area far from all medications.

Medications must be removed and disposed of immediately if they are discontinued, expired, contaminated, deteriorated, unlabeled, or in cracked, soiled, or unsecured containers. Any time you remove a medication from storage to dispose of, document the disposal on the Medication Disposition Record.

Medication expiration dates do not always mean that a medication has been found to be unstable after the date of expiration. The expiration date is the date that the manufacture has determined a medication to be stable in the original sealed container based on stability testing and accelerated degradation studies. Once the seal on the medication's original container has been broken, the expiration date may not apply because all expiration dates are related to the storage conditions stated on the labeling.

CHALLENGE

1. A patient has been prescribed two 200 mg tablets of ibuprofen. At which point should you initial or sign the MAR during the medication administration process?

   A. After you confirm the medical order
   B. After administering the medication to the patient
   C. After you verify the medication order with the MAR
   D. After preparing the medication

B is correct. Place your initials on the MAR or sign the eMAR only after you observe that the person has swallowed the medication or if the medication was applied or otherwise given as directed. Do not initial or sign that a medication was given before it is administered.

PERFORM EAR AND EYE IRRIGATION

Irrigation Instruments, Supplies, and Techniques

Irrigations (or lavage) of the eye and ear are done for a variety of reasons. The eye can be irrigated to remove a foreign body or chemical irritants. The ear can be irrigated to remove a foreign body or remove wax that prevents the health care provider from seeing the tympanic membrane through the otoscope.

Eye Irrigation

Eye irrigation is the process of using a sterile solution to flush the eyes of any foreign bodies or any toxic chemicals. Eye irrigation requires *sterile technique* and equipment. As with all procedures, review the patient's medical record and the health care provider's order. Introduce yourself and identify the patient. Explain the procedure to the patient and reason why it needs to be performed.

Assemble the equipment and two sets of the supplies and equipment if both eyes are to be irrigated. This may include a sterile basin, a return basin, sterile solution, a sterile irrigating syringe, sterile gauze, tissues, towel, a waterproof drape, and nonsterile gloves. Perform a triple check of the medication and provider's order and the rights of administration and check for expiration dates on the medication and all supplies.

Warm the irrigation solution to normal body temperature by placing the solution in a basin of warm water. Place the patient in a supine or sitting position and place a waterproof drape on the patient's shoulder to absorb any solution if any spills. Perform hand hygiene.

4.34 Take Note

Continue the flow until the irrigation solution is empty and the desired results are achieved, such as removal of debris. Repeat if the other eye requires treatment.

Cleanse the eyelid with a gauze pad moistened with the sterile solution, making sure to maintain sterility at all times. Clean from the inner to outer canthus (corner) of the eye, where the upper and lower lids meet. Repeat with a newly moistened gauze pad until the eyelid is free of dirt and other debris. Instruct the patient to tilt the head toward the side that is being irrigated, to hold the return basin below the affected eye, and to look straight ahead on a fixed object while keeping both eyes open.

4.35 Take Note

Take the return ear basin from the patient, observing for any debris, and instruct them to lie on the side that was irrigated for 15 minutes.

Using the thumb and index finger of your nondominant hand, pull upward on the patient's upper lid and downward on the patient's lower lid—hold the eye open and maintain this position throughout the irrigation. With the dominant hand, hold the irrigating bottle of solution on or near the bridge of the nose and hold the tip of the solution about an inch above the eye. Do not to touch any part of the eye or skin with the tip of the solution applicator. Start squeezing the bottle so that the solution flows from the inner canthus to the outer canthus in a steady stream directed toward the lower conjunctiva.

Take the collection basin from the patient and dry the eyelid with gauze, once again moving from the inner to outer canthus. Provide the patient with a towel to dry any skin that may have gotten wet during the procedure and help the patient to a comfortable position. Examine and take note of any visible debris in the return basin. Discard the solution from the return basin, throw away disposable items, remove gloves, and wash hands.

sterile technique. A group of strategies used to reduce exposure to micro-organisms and keep the patient as safe as possible.

Ear Irrigation

Ear irrigation is necessary to remove impacted cerumen, or earwax, or a foreign matter from the ear. It will be important for you to explain the procedure to the patient and prepare them for possible mild discomfort. Patient preparation will be similar to the eye irrigation procedure. Supplies you will need are an ear syringe, sterile basin, return basin, warmed irrigation solution, a waterproof drape, towel, and gauze or cotton balls.

For ear irrigation, have the patient sitting or lying on the side with the affected ear facing up. Place a waterproof drape over the shoulder on the side that is being irrigated. Using an otoscope, examine the affected ear, taking note of any cerumen or foreign bodies (if allowed by practice policy). Cleanse the outer ear with a gauze pad moistened with the irrigating solution. Instruct the patient to tilt their head toward the side that is being irrigated and to hold the ear wash basin tightly below the affected ear. Gently insert the disposable tip into the ear so that it is positioned toward the top of the ear canal. Start spraying the solution by pushing the trigger on the spray bottle, checking to be sure the tubing remains straight. Continue to spray until you have used up the solution, the maximum time has been reached, or you have obtained the desired results (cleared the ear of cerumen).

Remove the tip from the patient's ear, allow any residual solution to drain out, and place a loose cotton ball in the canal.

Dry the outside of the ear. If policy allows, examine the ear with an otoscope to see if all cerumen has been removed. (If not, check with provider about proceeding.) Have the provider check the ear and follow any additional orders. Dispose of the supplies in a waste can and clean the area. Remove gloves and wash your hands.

CHALLENGE

1. Order the steps for ear irrigation into the correct sequence.
   A. Examine the affected ear with an otoscope.
   B. Position the patient.
   C. Warm the solution.
   D. Hold the wash basin tightly below the affected ear.
   E. Insert the tip of the syringe pointed toward the top of the ear canal and spray the solution.

C, B, A, D, E
The correct sequence is warm the solution, position the patient, examine the affected ear with an otoscope, hold the ear wash basin tightly below the affected ear, insert the tip of the syringe, and spray the solution.

SEND ORDERS FOR PRESCRIPTIONS AND REFILLS

Legal Requirements for Content and Transmission of Prescriptions

Medication orders, or prescriptions, may be written, electronic, or verbal. These orders may be transmitted electronically, faxed, or delivered by hand to the pharmacy by the patient. Regardless of the method, it is important to follow the policies and procedures identified by the facility.

Most prescriptions are created electronically. EHRs in the ambulatory care setting allow prescriptions to be ordered and transmitted to a pharmacy selected by the patient. E-prescribing applications streamline communications between pharmacies and prescribers. The e-prescribing tool can automatically send the prescription to the pharmacy via a fax server or through secure electronic transmission of prescriptions. In addition, pharmacies have the capability to request refills electronically or to pose routine questions to the health care provider via the e-prescribing system rather than through a phone call to the provider. This process is more efficient because refill requests can be queued up and reviewed at the health care provider's convenience. The provider will be able to review those requests anywhere using a hand-held device (PDA) or a remote computer. This results in increased efficiency and fewer pharmacy calls to the provider.

Written orders may be created and transmitted in different ways as well. Instead of manually being created on a paper form (such as a prescription pad), they may be computer-generated paper prescriptions. The preparation of the prescription is carried out on a computer, typically in an EHR, and then printed on paper. The advantage here is that the printed-paper copy eliminates issues caused by poor penmanship and the EHR software can perform a number of edits to reduce the occurrence of clinical errors. The software can also check the prescription against a list of known allergies and against a list of the patient's other medications for contraindications. Once the prescription is printed on paper and manually signed, it is still a written paper prescription. The patient will need to deliver the prescription to the pharmacy to fill the order. The written order on a prescription form or computer-generated paper prescription may be scanned and transmitted via email or fax.

> **CHALLENGE**
>
> 1. Which of the following process is considered the most convenient and efficient when prescribing?
>   A. Computer-generated order provided to the patient to bring directly to the pharmacy
>   B. Computer-generated order by EHR faxed to the pharmacy
>   C. Written order that is faxed
>   D. Electronic order by EHR that is transmitted to the pharmacy
>
> *D is correct. The most efficient, electronic process is a medication order created by e-prescription tool in the EHR software that is automatically sent to the pharmacy through a secure electronic transmission.*

ELECTRONIC PRESCRIBING SOFTWARE

With the advances in health information software, electronic creation and transmission of prescriptions has made the process fast, efficient, and more secure. Using the medical practice's EMR software, health care providers can enter prescription information into a computer device (tablet, laptop, desktop computer) and securely transmit the prescription to pharmacies using a special software program and connectivity to a transmission network. When a pharmacy receives a request, it can begin filling the medication right away. Electronic prescribing (e-prescribing) can also reduce opportunities for diversion of controlled substances by eliminating the use of paper forms, which can be lost, stolen, and used illegally.

For e-prescribing, the EHR system that has been implemented in the medical practice must have a prescribing software that has been approved or authorized to transmit electronic prescriptions, especially for controlled substances. In some cases, a medical practice or health care organization may choose to adopt a standalone prescribing software instead of a software application associated with an EHR system. Regardless of the system, the software or application must meet DEA approval for transmission of a prescription.

On June 1, 2010, DEA's rule on Electronic Prescriptions for Controlled Substances (EPCS) became effective. The rule provided health care providers with the option of writing prescriptions for controlled substances electronically. The regulations also permitted pharmacies to receive, dispense, and archive these electronic prescriptions. In order for any pharmacy to receive an electronic prescription for a controlled substance from a prescribing health care provider, the pharmacy must use software that has been approved through a third-party audit and certification process to attest the software is DEA EPCS compliant. If either the pharmacy or health care provider does not use the approved or verified software to transmit the prescription, the electronic prescription will be considered invalid.

Many states require health care providers to use e-prescriptions for both controlled and noncontrolled substances with very few exceptions. Paper prescriptions will no longer be allowed in some states due to potential to alter the prescription written on paper. All pharmacies across the state must be capable of accepting those prescriptions as well.

When creating an electronic prescription, medical practices will be able to select the prescribed medication based on a list of medications, strength, dosage, quantity, route of administration, and refills from a drop-down menu. The medical practice can securely transmit the prescription to a pharmacy of the patient's preference. When a pharmacy receives a request, it can begin filling the medication right away, with the medication ready for pickup when the patient arrives.

In addition to the elements required on all prescriptions, electronically generated prescriptions must also have the following.

- A DEA number of the prescribing health care provider if the prescription is for a controlled substance
- The telephone number of the health care provider
- The time and date of the transmission
- The name of the pharmacy to which the prescription is sent

CHALLENGE

1. Which of the following is an advantage of electronic prescriptions?
   A. Controlled substances cannot be prescribed
   B. Can be transmitted with any EHR software
   C. Reduces the risk of prescriptions being lost, stolen, or altered
   D. Electronic prescriptions being valid once transmitted

   C is correct. Controlled substances may be transmitted via an electronic prescription, but it must be sent using software approved by the DEA. If it is not, the prescription is considered invalid. An advantage is that it makes it harder for electronic prescriptions to be stolen, lost, or altered.

2. Which of the following is true when transmitting an e-prescription? (Select all that apply.)
   A. Pharmacy must use approved software.
   B. Provider must use software as a part of an EHR system.
   C. Provider must use approved software.
   D. Provider must have DEA number for controlled substances.
   E. Prescribing software must be DEA EPCS approved.

   A, C, D, and E are correct. Both the pharmacy and the health care provider must use software that is DEA Electronic Prescription for Controlled Substances (EPCS) approved. The software may be either a standalone product or a part of the EHR software.

SPECIALTY PHARMACIES

Specialty pharmacies have similar functions to other pharmacies in that they dispense medications as prescribed by a health care provider to treat patients' conditions and diseases. However, these pharmacies prepare and dispense intricate medications for more complex, chronic, and rare health conditions (such as cancer, HIV/AIDS, immune diseases, hormone deficiencies, and bleeding disorders). They will stock many of the medications that are not usually found in your community or retail pharmacy.

Specialty pharmacies provide services that include training in how to use these medications, comprehensive treatment assessment, patient monitoring, and frequent communication with caregivers and the patient's health care providers. In addition, specialty pharmacies are able to manage special storage, handling, and administration requirements; perform ongoing monitoring of patient safety and medication efficacy; and prepare and deliver high-cost treatments, some exceeding $10,000.

4.36 Compounding

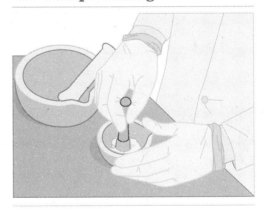

CHAPTER 4: GENERAL PATIENT CARE: PART 1
Specialty Pharmacies

Specialty pharmacies may serve specific purposes. For example, nuclear pharmacies are a specialty area of pharmacy practice dedicated to the compounding and dispensing of radioactive materials for use in nuclear medicine procedures. Radioactive materials used in pharmaceuticals (radiopharmaceutical) may be used for diagnostic imaging and therapeutic procedures. For example, a radiopharmaceutical can be administered orally, by injection, or via other routes to diagnose cancer, kidney disease, urinary bladder disease, and liver disease.

CHALLENGE

1. Which of the following patients would require a specialty pharmacy?
   A. A patient needing a urinalysis test to diagnose a urinary tract infection
   B. A young patient needing a weight-based dosage of a medication for leukemia
   C. A young patient with a prescription for diabetes supplies.
   D. An older adult patient needing a prescription for a laxative

   B is correct. A specialty pharmacy prepares and dispenses medication for complex, chronic, and rare diseases. It can also create a medication specific to the needs of a specific patient, such as weight.

2. Which of the following describes a compounding medication?
   A. A medication from a mixture of two or more ingredients
   B. A medication that is a liquid and must be infused
   C. A medication that does not need to be refrigerated
   D. A medication that can be prescribed without a prescription

   A is correct. A compounding medication is one created by combining, mixing, or altering two or more drugs or ingredients to create a medication tailored to the needs of a specific patient. It may be in many forms, including capsules, injectables, syrups, and creams. It may be prepared by a licensed pharmacist or physician.

Specialty medications have complex profiles that require intensive patient management and, in some cases, special handling. Although some are taken orally, many of these medications need to be injected or infused, at times in a medical practice or hospital. Some medications and treatments are required by the FDA to be prescribed and dispensed only by certified physicians and pharmacists. Specialty pharmacies may provide these medications, along with required education and monitoring.

Specialty medications can be taken in many routes of administration, including oral, injection, inhalation, or by infusion. Many specialty pharmacies must compound, which is the process of combining, mixing, or altering two or more drugs or ingredients to create a medication tailored to the needs of a specific patient. A drug may be compounded for a patient who cannot be treated with a regularly prepared medication. This may include a patient that is allergic to a certain dye and needs a medication made without it or an older adult patient requiring a liquid form of a medication that the drug manufacturer only makes as a tablet. Although capsules may be compounded, other forms of compounded drugs may include injectables, syrups, creams, serums ointments, supplements, elixirs, and gels.

Compounding medications may be prepared by a licensed pharmacist in a state-licensed pharmacy, or federal facility, or by a physician, and by or under the direct supervision of a licensed pharmacist in an outsourcing facility.

DOCUMENT CARE IN THE PATIENT RECORD

Required Components of Medical Records

Whether the medical practice uses an electronic or paper record, there are specific sections and components that are required of all patients' medical records.

Administrative Sections

Demographic Data
- Name
- Address
- Birthdate
- Sex
- Gender
- Social Security number
- Phone number
- Employment information

Administrative Data
- Notice of privacy practices form
- Advance directives
- Consent forms
- Medical records release form

Correspondence: Any correspondence related to the patient (e.g., from patient's insurance company, attorney, or the patient themselves)

Schedule, Financial, and Billing Information: Information regarding any appointments, insurance information, balances

Clinical Section

Health History
- Chief complaints
- Present illness
- Past medical history
- Family history
- Social history
- Review of systems

Physical Examination: Assessment of each body part

Allergies: All known patient allergies

Medication Record: Detailed information related to patient's medication

Problem List: Problems identified, updated each visit

Progress Notes: New information each time the patient visits or telephones the office

Laboratory Data: Any laboratory reports obtained on the patient

Diagnostic Procedures
- Electrocardiogram report
- Holter monitor report
- Spirometry report
- Radiology report
- Diagnostic imaging report

Continuity of Care
- Consultation report
- Home health care report
- Therapeutic service documents
- Hospital documents

CHALLENGE

1. Where can you find an advance directive in a patient's medical record?
   A. Demographic data
   B. Administrative data
   C. Correspondence
   D. Financial information

   B is correct. An advance directive would be found in the administrative data section of a patient's medical record.

OPERATE AN EMR/EHR SYSTEM

Implement Updates in an EMR/EHR

Although EMR and EHR are often used interchangeably, there are differences. An EMR is an electronic version of a patient's medical history. It is used within a single organization. An EHR also contains the patient's EMR, except it can be incorporated across more than one health care organization. EHRs are designed to reach out beyond the health organization that originally collects and compiles the information. They are built to share information with other health care providers, such as laboratories and specialists, so they contain information from all the clinicians involved in the patient's care.

Health care providers and organizations are required to report statistics on communicable and infectious diseases (HIV/AIDS, tuberculosis, sexually transmitted infections) to local and state government agencies. These agencies will also collect this data and report it to the federal government and agencies, such as the CDC.

Since health care providers are required to report cases of births, deaths, and communicable diseases, this information can be collected and provides the vital records or statistics that are maintained by state and local governments. Vital records are useful because they offer detailed information that includes the incidence (new cases) and prevalence (existing cases) that can inform public health decisions. For example, increased incidences of deaths and head injuries from motorcycle accidents led to helmet laws.

Federal and state governments and agencies often use health information in medical records when making decisions related to health care. Their decisions may be related to new and existing policies and legislation that govern health care and other areas as well. Health information may be used to determine the type of coverage that Medicare or Medicaid patients receive. For example, the Centers for Medicare & Medicaid Services, the federal agency that oversees these programs, reviews the history of care provided to its beneficiaries and determines the cost and quality of care to decide on reimbursements and enact legislation. These decisions and the legislation affect future coverage, reimbursement, and availability of services for Medicare and Medicaid beneficiaries.

CHALLENGE

1. Which of the following patient conditions is required to be reported to local and state government agencies?
   A. Confirmed tuberculosis
   B. A broken arm
   C. A new diagnosis of breast cancer
   D. Pneumonia

A is correct. Health care providers and organizations are required to report statistics on communicable and infectious diseases to local and state government agencies, such as HIV/AIDS, tuberculosis, and sexually transmitted infections.

ENTER ORDERS USING COMPUTERIZED PHYSICIAN ORDER ENTRY

As a part of EHR adoption, many state and federal laws were created to enforce health care providers to use a *computerized provider order entry (CPOE)* system, which helped to make health care delivery safer and more efficient. CPOE is an electronic process that allows a health care provider to enter medical orders electronically into a system instead of the more traditional order methods of paper, verbal, telephone, and fax. Once you have electronically entered an order for lab tests, prescription medications, radiology tests, and referrals, the CPOE system interfaces or integrates with other EHR components, such as the pharmacy or laboratory system, to process the order. By reducing the use of written orders, this reduced medical and medication errors since it prevented transcription errors, misplaced decimals, and illegible handwriting. The following is an overview of the benefits of a CPOE system.

- Reducing the potential for human error
- Reducing time to care delivery
- Improving order accuracy
- Decreasing time for order confirmation and turnaround
- Improving clinical decision support at the point of care
- Making crucial information more readily available
- Improving communication among health care providers and professionals and patients

By enabling health care providers to submit orders electronically, CPOE can help get medication, laboratory, and radiology orders to pharmacies, laboratories, and radiology facilities faster, saving time and improving efficiency. CPOE can improve workflow processes by eliminating lost orders and ambiguities caused by illegible handwriting, generating related orders automatically, monitoring for duplicate orders, and reducing the time required to fill orders. It can also help to reduce errors by ensuring health care providers produce standardized, legible, and complete orders.

In many cases, a CPOE is either paired with or has a built-in clinical decision support system (CDSS). A CDSS helps patient care by enhancing medical decisions with targeted clinical knowledge, patient information, and other health information. For example, a CDSS can automatically check for medication interactions, medication allergies, and errors in medication dosage and frequency. More advanced CDSSs can prevent the prescription that has been ordered at too high of a dose, alert when a medication needs to be prescribed for or after a procedure, prevent over prescribing due to abuse, and even assist in prescribing the correct treatment.

A CPOE system may be a standalone system, but now most EHR software includes a CPOE system that allows health care providers and professionals to enter patient data electronically into text boxes and drop-down menus. The use of CPOE with an EHR can also improve clinical productivity. For example, when integrated with an EHR system, a CPOE can flag orders that require pre-approval, helping to reduce denied insurance claims.

---

computerized provider order entry (CPOE). Process in which providers enter and send treatment instructions, including medications, laboratory, and radiology orders, via a computer application rather than paper, fax, or phone.

Many CPOE systems work by the following six-step process.

1. A provider will log into an EMR.
2. Once logged in, the provider will see a list of patients on the screen.
3. The provider can select a patient and use the system to order prescriptions, lab work, and medical scans.
4. The system automatically validates the order against a patient's medical history, health insurance plan, and other relevant data that has been stored in the system.
5. If no error is detected, the order will be sent to a product or service provider, typically a pharmacy or lab.
6. Finally, this order is added to the patient's permanent records, expediting future reviews, orders, and access for care providers.

The use of CPOE allows entering orders electronically rather than on paper and will result in faster turnaround times for patients and reduce life-threatening errors. Although medical assistants are not authorized to submit an order, you may be required to enter the information for an order before requesting the health care provider to authorize it.

CHALLENGE

1. Which of the following are advantages of an order in the CPOE compared to a written order? (Select all that apply.)
   A. Corrects misplaced decimals
   B. Prevents incorrect dosage
   C. Identifies medication interactions
   D. Recommends treatment options

   B, C, and D are correct. CPOE systems can improve the order process by reducing medication errors (such as incorrect dosing and medication allergies) and assist in recommending treatment options for diseases. Regardless of how the order is submitted, only authorized health care providers may approve and submit an order.

2. You are on a committee to select a new EHR software for your medical practice. How would you describe the advantages of adding a CPOE with a CDSS?

   CPOE systems are generally paired with some form of clinical decision support system (CDSS), which can help prevent errors of medication ordering and suggest recommendations for medication dosage, routes of administration, and frequency. More sophisticated CDSSs may have medication safety features, such as checking for medication allergies or drug-drug or even drug-laboratory. This would improve not only efficiency in the medical practice but also patient safety.

CONDUCT TELEHEALTH OR VIRTUAL SCREENINGS

Patient Conditions Appropriate for Telehealth/Virtual Visit

Telehealth has a broad definition. It is generally a type of service that uses video calling and other technologies to help health care providers provide patient care to a remote location, such as the patient's home, instead of at a medical facility.

Although often used interchangeably, telehealth and telemedicine are different types of online health care services. Telemedicine refers specifically to online health care provider visits and remote clinical services, while telehealth is more expansive and includes health-related education services like diabetes management or nutrition courses and health-related training. Telehealth may also refer to remote nonclinical services, such as provider training, administrative meetings, and continuing medical education.

Insurance coverage for telehealth varies widely from state to state, with differences in how telehealth is defined and reimbursed for. For example, some states may reimburse for telemedicine but only specific telehealth services.

Telehealth most closely resembles a real visit to a health care provider, enabling two-sided communication. The provider can check on patients, inquire about the state of their health, and then prescribe an appropriate treatment. It requires interoperability across various devices to make such a visit possible, such as a web-camera, a phone, a computer audio system, or chat capabilities.

The use of telehealth has increased over the last decade due to willingness of both patients and health care providers to use it, regulatory changes enabling greater access and reimbursements, and the need for health care during pandemics. The types of care that you can get using telehealth may include the following.

- General health care, like wellness visits
- Prescriptions for routine medicine
- Dermatology (skin care)
- Eye exams
- Nutrition counseling
- Mental health counseling
- Urgent care conditions, such as sinusitis, urinary tract infections, and common rashes

One of the most common forms of telehealth is virtual visits. Patients are able to see a health care provider or a nurse via online or phone chats. Virtual visits can offer care for many conditions, such as migraines, skin conditions, diabetes, depression, anxiety, colds, coughs, and COVID-19. In addition, health care providers may use virtual consultations where one health care provider can get input from specialists in other locations if there are questions about a diagnosis or treatment options. The health care provider can send exam notes, history, lab results, x-rays, or other images to the specialist to review.

Telehealth may include remote patient monitoring, which allows health care providers to monitor measurements from a device the patient may be wearing, such as heart rate and blood glucose levels, and that sends that information to them. Some surgical procedures may be performed remotely from a different location using robotic technology. A health care provider may also send a patient an online video to watch on proper inhaler use.

CHALLENGE

1. Which of the following is a type of telehealth but not telemedicine?
   A. Patient being evaluated for a cough
   B. An irregular mole being checked on a patient
   C. Continuing education for a medical assistant
   D. Medical assistant demonstrating how to use a blood glucose meter

   C is correct. Telehealth and telemedicine comprise many of the same remote services. Telehealth also includes non-patient and nonclinical services, such as team meetings and professional development training for the health care team.

2. Which patients do you think would most benefit from telehealth?

   Patients who have difficulty with transportation and getting to an in-person medical visit, such as older adult patients, those who have disabilities, those who are bed- or homebound, and those in rural areas

MODIFICATIONS FOR TELEHEALTH/VIRTUAL HEALTH CARE

In many cases, health care providers' encounters with patients via telehealth are as effective as standard face-to-face visits held in a medical practice. There are preparations that need to be made prior and after the medical visit for the patient and health care team.

For health care providers and professionals, the use of technology does not alter their standard of practice, ethics, or scope of practice or the laws that protect patients and health care providers.

Before the visit, request the patient to send information or forms to fill out online and return them. You may have to send instructions and information on technology requirements for any telehealth services, such as for a virtual visit. The instructions should include how the patient should sign on to join the video chat for the visit and how to use the microphone, camera, and text chat. The patient will need a smartphone, tablet, or computer with internet access to join the virtual visit. The patient should also make sure to update or install any software or applications needed. Both the patient and health care provider should find a comfortable, quiet, private spot to sit during the visit.

CHALLENGE

1. Which of the following criteria are appropriate for a telehealth visit with a health care provider? (Select all that apply.)
   A. Patient has a wound that won't stop bleeding.
   B. Private area is needed.
   C. Patient meets the technology requirements.
   D. Patient is self-reporting blood pressure readings.

   B, C, and D are correct. Although there are many benefits to telehealth, it may not be appropriate for every patient, such as a patient with a severe or rare condition that should be seen by a health care provider in-person.

With advancing technology, some medical practices are able to perform remote physical examinations through viewing images and hearing sounds. As a result, health care providers can assess and treat a variety of diseases and conditions, such as cardiac and respiratory illnesses, by listening to digital heart and lung sounds live by sending the data over by a video conferencing system. The health care provider can even use video scopes to conduct eye, ear, nose, and throat examinations. In some cases, patients may also self-report vital signs and other biometric data, such as height, weight, and blood pressure. Many patients with conditions such as hypertension, obesity, and diabetes may be experienced at measuring glucose and blood pressure, and the health care provider may be comfortable with the patient self-reporting. The medical assistant should remind patients to have those measurements ready prior to the appointment.

WRAP-UP

Patient care encompasses many broad functions in a medical practice or health care organization. This includes the patient examination; preparing the patient for the examination, such as positioning them for a procedure; preparing the appropriate supplies and equipment for the procedure; explaining the purpose of the procedure; and answering questions and gaining consent. The medical assistant may be involved in more advanced procedures, such as preparing medications and administering injections.

Advances in technology have allowed patient care to be more efficient and better at meeting patient's needs. EHRs have made patient data collection more efficient and effective and allow more secure and confidential sharing of patient information. Electronic prescribing, computerized provider order entry (CPOE), and telehealth improve access to care and give health care providers new methods to provide patient care.

CHAPTER 5
General Patient Care: Part 2

OVERVIEW

In addition to providing general patient care, such as obtaining vital signs and administering medications, medical assistants can perform other advanced skills, such as assisting in office-based minor surgeries and procedures. This includes assembling the appropriate supplies and equipment for minor office procedures, preparing and maintaining a sterile field, and performing aseptic procedures. The medical assistant can be responsible for educating the patient and providing home-care instructions, including knowing when to notify the health care provider if certain conditions or symptoms are present.

Emergencies can occur at any time, and medical assistants must prepare themselves and the medical office for different *emergency* situations. The proper ways to identify and respond to medical emergencies—such as shock, *seizures*, *strains* and *sprains*, choking, hemorrhaging wounds, and burns—are also a part of the MA's foundational knowledge. The MA should be skilled in *first aid* and *cardiopulmonary resuscitation (CPR)* and be able to support the health care provider during medical emergencies.

Objectives

Upon completion of this chapter, you should be able to

- Prepare and maintain a sterile field.
- Perform staple and suture removal.
- Assist with surgical interventions and discharge instructions.
- Administer first aid and basic wound care.
- Identify and respond to emergency/priority situations.
- Assist provider with patients presenting with minor and traumatic injury.
- Order and identify durable medical equipment, prosthetics, orthotics, and supplies (DMEPOS) as well as obtain prior authorization.

PREPARE AND MAINTAIN A STERILE FIELD

Many office-based surgical procedures can be performed effectively and safely in the medical office. Minor office surgeries consist of procedures that can be performed without the need for anesthesia. Medical assistants assist with many duties related to minor surgical procedures. Strict adherence to aseptic or sterile technique is necessary when assisting with these procedures.

Surgical asepsis, or sterile technique, is used when sterility of supplies and the immediate environment is required, as in surgical procedures. Surgical asepsis requires surgical handwashing or scrub, sterile gloves, and sterile technique when handling materials. Sterile technique is necessary during any invasive procedure (a procedure in which the body is entered), such as making a surgical incision or an open wound.

emergency. Unforeseen circumstance that requires immediate attention.

seizure. Uncontrolled muscle activity that can be caused by high body temperature, head injuries, drugs, and epilepsy.

strain. A stretched or torn muscle or tendon.

sprain. A stretched or torn ligament.

first aid. Immediate care given to the victim of injury or sudden illness to sustain life and prevent death.

cardiopulmonary resuscitation (CPR). Lifesaving technique that consists of chest compressions combined with artificial ventilation.

surgical asepsis. Techniques to eliminate pathogenic and other potentially harmful microbes related to invasive procedures.

Before the procedure, the health care provider will expect the medical assistant to assemble all the necessary supplies and equipment and set up the sterile field for the procedure being performed. During the procedure, the health care provider can ask the medical assistant to add items to the sterile field and, if properly scrubbed and wearing sterile gloves, hand sterile instruments to the provider. A sterile field is an area free of micro-organisms and is used as a work area during a surgical procedure. The sterile field must be maintained before and during the procedure.

5.1 Autoclaved and Dated Instrument Packets

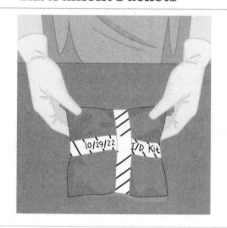

Guidelines for Establishing a Sterile Field

Sterile packets (packages) are prepared for use in surgical procedures. Each one can contain either a single instrument, a piece of equipment, or several items packed together. These instrument packets can be purchased from a medical supply company or packaged by the medical assistant in the office. These packets are autoclaved and have sterilization indicators (tape) and are dated with the date of sterilization. The primary method of sterilization of instruments and equipment is autoclaving, which is the process of using high-temperature steam to kill any micro-organisms.

All items and packets to be autoclaved must have autoclave indicators to confirm if the item has been properly sterilized. Before using an instrument packet, check for the sterilization indicator and confirm the date. If the instrument packet has either not been autoclaved or was improperly autoclaved, the tape would not show the change of color of the indicator marks.

5.2 Before and After Indicator of Autoclave Tape

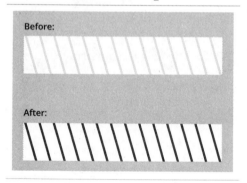

A sterile field is often set up on a Mayo stand, which is a movable, stainless steel instrument tray on a stand. The tray should be disinfected and allowed to dry. Adjust the stand to slightly above the waist and position it at least 12 inches from the body.

If a prepackaged sterile kit is used, the packet will be placed on the Mayo stand to be opened. If creating the sterile field with individually wrapped items, a sterile drape is placed carefully on the Mayo stand to create the sterile field.

5.3 Mayo Stand

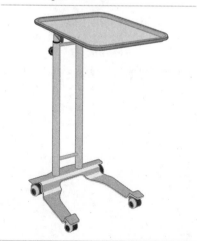

When opening a sterile packet on the Mayo stand, the flap farthest away from the MA should be opened first, followed by the sides. Then the flap closest to the MA should be opened last without reaching over. Keep in mind that the inside area of the drape is sterile and that only sterile items should be placed on the drape.

A border of at least 1 inch around the sterile drape is considered nonsterile. Therefore, do not place items in this area.

Once a sterile field is created, only sterile objects and health care professionals and providers (who have enacted sterilization procedures) can be allowed within the sterile field. The sterile area must be within the field of vision and above the waist. Do not leave a sterile field unattended, reach over a sterile field, or turn away from a sterile field. If items within this field must be rearranged, use sterile forceps. If a sterile item must be opened within the instrument setup, then someone wearing sterile gloves must open it. If the health care provider wants an additional instrument while performing a procedure, open a sterile packet and drop the instrument carefully onto the sterile field. Open packages so that they can easily drop onto the sterile field or be grasped by the health care provider without touching the outer wrapper.

5.4 Sterile Field

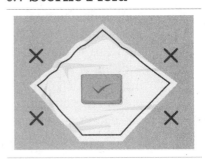

If there is any chance of contamination, remove the contaminated item or correct the error and open a new packet. Always remember that an item is either sterile or nonsterile. When in doubt, assume the item is nonsterile.

CHALLENGE

1. Place the steps below into the correct sequence for creating a sterile field.
   A. Open the flap closest to the MA.
   B. Pull both of the side flaps open.
   C. Open the flap farthest away from the MA.
   D. Place the packet on the Mayo stand
   E. Disinfect the Mayo stand.

   E, D, C, B, A
   The correct sequence is disinfect the Mayo stand, place the packet on the Mayo stand, open the flap farthest away from the MA, open the sides, pull the two flaps to each side, and open the flap closet to the MA.

2. Which of the following would result in contamination of the sterile field?
   A. Placing the Mayo stand above the MA's waist
   B. Forceps that are placed on the 1-inch border
   C. Touching the inner area of the wrapper with a sterile glove
   D. Placing the Mayo stand 12 inches away from the MA

   B is correct. Once a sterile field is set up, the border of 1 inch at the edge of the sterile drape is considered nonsterile. Place all objects inside the sterile field and away from the 1-inch border.

ASSIST WITH SURGICAL INTERVENTIONS

Many minor surgical procedures can be performed in a medical office. There are advantages to office-based surgeries, such as saving the patient the time and expense of having to go into an ambulatory surgical facility or a hospital. The basic surgical setup is the standard setup with the addition of specific instruments for each procedure. Some minor procedures performed in the medical office include *biopsy*, removal of foreign bodies, *endoscopy*, *colposcopy*, cryosurgery, and incision and drainage.

5.5 Splinter Forceps

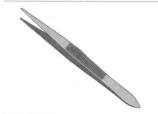

5.6 Endoscopy of the Colon

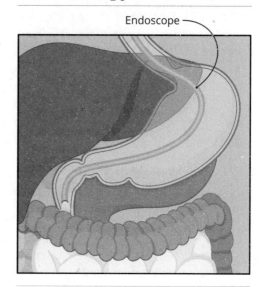

5.7 Commonly Occurring Types of Surgical Interventions

PROCEDURE	DESCRIPTION	PURPOSE
Biopsy	The surgical removal of tissue for later microscopic examination.	Diagnose cancer, skin conditions, or other diseases of the body.
Removal of a foreign object	Surgical removal of an object, such as a small splinter, or a larger object, such as a piece of wood or metal that is embedded in tissue. Splinter forceps are commonly used with this procedure.	Remove a foreign object to relieve pain and prevent infection.
Removal of a small growth (cyst, wart, mole)	Surgical removal of a small growth from the body.	Conduct further examination of the growth, prevent future growth.
Endoscopy	Procedure that uses an endoscope to view a hollow organ or body cavity, such as the larynx, bladder, colon, sigmoid colon, stomach, abdomen, and some joints.	Evaluate a patient having stomach pain, difficulty swallowing, gastrointestinal bleeding, diarrhea or constipation, and colon polyps.

biopsy. The surgical removal of tissue for later microscopic examination.

endoscopy. Procedure that uses an endoscope to view a hollow organ or body cavity, such as the larynx, bladder, colon, sigmoid colon, stomach, abdomen, and some joints.

colposcopy. Examination of the vagina and cervix performed using a colposcope, which is a specialized type of endoscope.

5.7 Commonly Occurring Types of Surgical Interventions *(continued)*

PROCEDURE	DESCRIPTION	PURPOSE
Colposcopy	Examination of the vagina and cervix performed using a colposcope, which is a specialized type of endoscope. With the patient in the lithotomy position, the colposcope allows the health care provider to observe the tissues of this area in detail through light and magnification.	Examine abnormal tissue development during a routine pelvic examination, when a Papanicolaou (Pap) smear result is abnormal, and to obtain a biopsy specimen. Abnormal areas of tissue or cells can then be removed for biopsy to detect cancer.
Cryosurgery	Procedure using local application of intense cold liquid or special instrument called a cryoprobe to destroy unwanted tissue.	Can be used to destroy abnormal cells and tissues, which uses extremely cold liquid such as liquid nitrogen and an instrument called a cryoprobe. Cryosurgery can be used in conjunction with other procedures, such as a colposcopy as a treatment of cervical erosion and chronic cervicitis.
Incision and drainage (I&D)	Lancing a pressure buildup caused by pus or other fluid under the skin.	A procedure is performed to relieve the buildup of purulent (pus) material as a result of infection, such as from an abscess. The purulent discharge can be cultured to determine what micro-organism is causing the infection and what antibiotic would be effective in treating it.

CHALLENGE

1. Match the condition or action match with the correct diagnostic procedure.

PROCEDURE	CONDITION
A. Biopsy	1. Viewing of the stomach for ulcers
B. Cryosurgery	2. Treating an abscess located in the underarm
C. Colposcopy	3. Destruction of abnormal tissue in the cervix
D. Endoscopy	4. Further testing of a suspicious lump on the breast
E. Incision and drainage	5. Viewing of abnormal tissue located in the cervix

A: 4, B: 3, C: 5, D: 1, E: 2

A biopsy should be performed in the case of a suspicious lump on the breast, for example, in the case of cancer. Cryosurgery uses cold liquid to destroy abnormal tissue. Colposcopy is the process of viewing inside the vagina and cervix. Endoscopy is viewing into hollow organs or body cavities, such as the stomach. Incision and drainage (I & D) is a procedure to relieve abscesses.

incision and drainage (I&D). Lancing a fluid or pressure build up under the skin to allow it to drain and relieve pressure.

TECHNIQUES AND INSTRUMENTS FOR SUTURE AND STAPLE REMOVAL

Wound closure is often necessary in emergency situations and after office-based surgical procedures. Properly closing an exposed area of the body prevents infection and other complications, aids in the healing process, and minimizes scarring. There are many different types of wound closure and materials, such as sutures, surgical staples, skin closure tapes, and adhesives. The selection of which types to use when closing a wound or incision depends on the wound, how much soft tissue is exposed, how clean the wound is, and the assessment of the health care provider.

5.8 Sutures

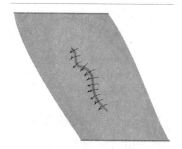

Suturing is the use of any device to close or sew together tissue after an injury or surgery. The most common method in suturing is the use of specialized thread, or sutures. Sutures are inserted by the health care provider at the end of a procedure to hold tissues in alignment during the healing process. There are a number of different types of sutures based on size, materials, and absorbability. Sutures can be made of many different materials and can be absorbable or nonabsorbable.

Types and Sizes of Sutures

Absorbable sutures do not need to be removed and are digested by tissue enzymes and absorbed by the body tissues. Sutures used to attach tissues beneath the skin are often made of an absorbable material that disappears in several days. Absorption usually occurs 5 to 20 days after insertion.

Nonabsorbable sutures are used on skin surfaces where they can easily be removed after an incision heals. Sutures generally remain in place five or six days and then must be removed if they are nonabsorbable and include materials such as nylon, silk, polyester fiber, and even stainless steel. If sutures remain in the body too long, they can cause skin irritation and infection. Suture removal times differ depending on the site.

5.9 Suture Package Label

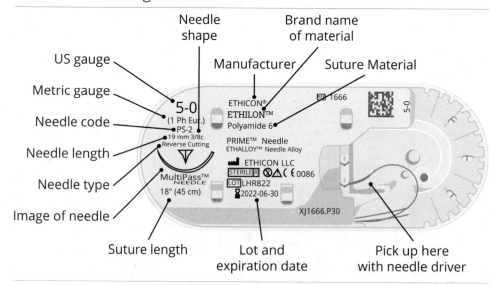

The size of the suture material, which is measured by the gauge or diameter, is stated in terms of "0"—the more 0s, the smaller the gauge. For example, 0 is thicker or larger than 6-0 (000000). Sizes 2-0 through 6-0 are the most used. Delicate tissue, such as areas on the face and neck, would be sutured with 5-0 to 6-0 suture sizes because these finer sutures would leave less scarring. Heavier sutures, such as 2-0, would be used for the chest or abdomen. The health care provider will determine the type and gauge of sutures to be used. The suture package label will indicate type, size, length of the suture material, and if it is absorbable or nonabsorbable.

5.10 Surgical Staples

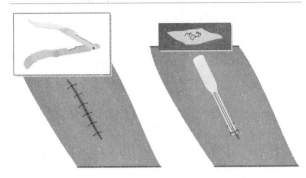

Another common type of wound closures are staples. Staples are made of stainless steel and applied with a surgical stapler. Staples allow for the closure of wounds under high tension, such as on the trunk, extremities, and scalp. They are not generally used in delicate tissues or wounds in finely contoured areas, over bony prominences, or in highly mobile areas. Staples can shorten the closure time and are used to rapidly close an incision, which helps decrease risk of infection. Using a specialized set of extractors, staples need to be removed within 4 to 14 days.

Other materials used for wound closure include sterile tapes and skin adhesives. Sterile tapes are nonallergenic and available in a variety of widths. They are used instead of sutures when not much tension will be applied to a wound, such as on a small facial cut. Skin adhesives are composed of cyanoacrylate adhesives that react with water to create an instant, strong, flexible bond.

Perform Suture and Staple Removal

Medical assistants, generally, can remove sutures and staples under the delegation of a provider. As with all procedures, explain the procedure to the patient, reminding the patient that there can be a pulling sensation. Thorough inspection of the wound to approximate the edges and the absence or presence of drainage is necessary. Wounds that have crusting blood or exudate will usually need soaking with saline prior to removal of the sutures or staples. If there are any problems, have the health care provider inspect the wound before starting the procedure.

5.11 Surgical Staple Remover

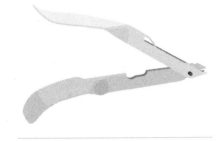

In most cases, a disposable suture removal kit will be used that includes suture scissors and forceps, or a staple removal kit will be used that includes a removal device along with sterile gauze, forceps, sterile gloves, and antiseptic. After proper hand hygiene, open the kit and create a sterile field with the wrapper. Thoroughly cleanse the skin with an antiseptic, such as alcohol or povidone-iodine solution, and allow to dry.

CHAPTER 5: GENERAL PATIENT CARE: PART 2
Techniques and Instruments for Suture and Staple Removal

To remove the sutures, cut the suture with suture scissors below the knot and as close to the skin as possible. Remove every other suture and then go back and remove the remaining sutures until all sutures have been removed, observing the incision line for separation. Remove the suture by pulling the long remaining suture out. Never pull suture material that is outside the skin through the skin.

If at any time there is gaping, bleeding, or presence of an exudate, stop and notify the health care provider. Once all the sutures and staples have been removed, clean the wound with antiseptic, allow to dry, and dress the wound as ordered. Prior to disposal, count the number of staples or sutures that were removed. This number must be documented in the patient's health record. Dispose of sutures in the biohazard waste container and staples in the sharps waste container. Butterfly closures can be used to provide reinforcement of the wound after removal of the sutures or staples depending on the condition and location of the wound.

5.12 Take Note

To remove staples, begin with the second staple of the wound and carefully place the lower tip of the sterile staple remover under the staple. Advance the lower jaw of the staple remover under the staple to be removed. Squeeze the handle together until they are completely closed. This will bend the staple in the middle and pull the edges of the staple out of the skin. Do not lift the staple remover when squeezing the handles. Remove every other staple until all staples have been removed and while observing the site.

CHALLENGE

1. A patient has a deep wound on their scalp. Which of the following types of wound closures should be used?
   A. Absorbable sutures
   B. Non-absorbable sutures
   C. Sterile tape
   D. Surgical staples

   D is correct. Surgical staples allow for the closure of wounds under high tension, such as on the trunk, extremities, and scalp.

2. Which of the following are benefits of wound closure? (Select all that apply.)
   A. Allows for frequent irrigation of the wound bed
   B. Helps minimize scarring
   C. Is a painless procedure
   D. Prevents infection
   E. Aids in healing

   B, D, and E are correct. Once the wound is closed, it is not feasible to irrigate the wound bed. Wound closure can be quite painful, and in some instances, anesthesia should be provided. Wound closure helps reduce the risk of infection and other complications, aids in the healing process, and minimizes scarring.

REVIEW PROVIDER'S DISCHARGE INSTRUCTIONS/PLAN OF CARE WITH PATIENTS

Patients should have a clear understanding of what to expect during recovery, how to care for the surgical incision at home, and what to do in case of complications from the surgery. Patients can be anxious and have difficulty remembering instructions following a procedure. Provide verbal and written instructions for follow-up care. Clear instructions about postoperative medications should be given in writing as well as verbally to the patient and possibly to family members, if appropriate. Review all instructions with patients and answer questions prior to their departure. Furthermore, the patient should be instructed about whether a follow-up appointment to the office will be necessary and when that should be scheduled.

Most medical offices will have a standard set of printed instructions to send home with the patient. These instructions can include keeping the site clean and dry, not placing stress on the area, drinking plenty of fluids, getting proper rest, and returning for their follow-up appointment. Depending on the surgery or procedure, additional postsurgical or discharge instructions can include the following.

- Activity restrictions: This includes bathing and exercising.
- Diet restrictions: It is unlikely to have dietary restrictions following minor ambulatory surgery. However, in cases of abdominal pain, diarrhea, or vomiting, a liquid diet with progress as tolerated may be recommended by the provider.
- Wound care: This includes instructions such as changing the dressing, applying medications to the wound, and observing for signs of infection.
- Medications: If the patient has prescriptions for medications such as antibiotics, instruct the patient on how and when to take the medication, how it should be stored, and possible side effects.

If the patient is unable to drive after the procedure, this should be discussed with the patient prior to the surgery and again at the time of the procedure. In some cases, if the patient did not make appropriate transportation arrangements, the procedure may need to be rescheduled.

Explain when the patient should notify the health care provider of possible postoperative problems, such as fever, bleeding, swelling, or other symptoms. The medical assistant is often responsible for patient education regarding the healing process of a wound. Making sure the patient understands the importance of notifying the provider if infection is suspected is a crucial part of this education. The patient should notify the health care provider in the case of the following.

- Unusual pain or burning
- Swelling, redness, or other discoloration in the area
- Bleeding or other drainage, including unpleasant odor
- Fever of 100° F or greater (37.7° C)
- Nausea and vomiting

CHALLENGE

1. Which of the following are postsurgical discharge instructions for a patient who had a biopsy of the breast? (Select all that apply.)
   A. Change the dressing.
   B. Observe signs of infection.
   C. Eat a balanced diet.
   D. Apply medication to the wound.
   E. Refrain from working for 14 days.

   A, B, and D are correct. Postsurgical instructions for a biopsy should include basic wound care, such as applying any medication to the incision, changing the dressing, and observing for any signs of infection, such as redness or swelling.

2. Several days after an office-based surgery, a patient experiences nausea and abdominal pain. Based on postsurgical instructions, which of the following should the patient do?
   A. Call 911.
   B. Immediately go to the emergency department.
   C. Contact the medical office to speak with the health care provider.
   D. Go to an urgent care center.

   C is correct. The patient should immediately notify the health care provider if nausea or abdominal pain occurs. The patient should call 911 or go to the emergency department in case of life-threatening situations. Although an urgent care center can be helpful, the health care provider should be contacted first because the provider is more aware of the patient's medical history and the surgery performed.

IDENTIFY AND RESPOND TO EMERGENCY/PRIORITY SITUATIONS

The goal of providing care in an emergency is to help stabilize the patient and prevent further injury. Although medical offices and ambulatory clinics generally do not see emergency or life-threatening situations, they always need to be prepared, alert, and ready to respond to potential threats or emergencies in the clinical setting. An emergency is any condition that leads to cardiac or respiratory failure and mandates rapid implementation of life-saving measures, including calling 911 and cardiopulmonary resuscitation (CPR). Medical assistants should be able to handle emergencies outside and inside the medical office and on the phone.

When severe injury or sudden critical illness occurs, the patient should receive emergency care as soon as possible. The first hour after the time of injury or appearance of symptoms is considered the most critical. In fact, the first hour is often coined the "golden hour" and correlates with prognosis and the possibility of recovery. There has been no evidence to suggest survival rate declines after 60 min; however, rapid intervention in trauma and emergency situations must be provided as soon as possible for the best outcome for the patient.

The medical assistant must be able to identify emergency and life-threatening situations. Examples of life-threatening situations are cardiac arrest (heart attacks), respiratory arrest, uncontrolled bleeding, head injury, poisoning, open chest or abdominal wound, shock, and third- and fourth-degree burns.

In an emergency, the medical assistant should be able respond to the emergency and support the health care provider during this time. Evaluate the situation and provide appropriate care as directed. Every medical office should have a policy manual and an emergency preparedness plan. All staff members should be familiar with them. As a part of the preparedness and training, the MA should be trained and certified in CPR, the use of the automated emergency device, what to do if an airway is obstructed, bandaging, splinting, and managing wounds and bleeding.

When a patient or a patient's family member calls the medical office stating they are experiencing an emergency, the medical assistant must be able to listen attentively and quickly determine how to proceed. The MA's first step in an emergency situation on the phone is to obtain critical information. This includes the following.

- The patient's name, contact information, and location
- What the situation is and when did it start
- The status of the patient—conscious, breathing, presence of pulse

If the patient is not breathing, has no pulse, or is unconscious, follow the medical office's policy. Some medical offices will require the MA or a nearby staff member to contact 911 immediately on the patient's behalf while remaining on the phone with them.

Regardless of who calls, gather information on the nature of the situation and the location of the patient. This information will need to be reported to the *emergency medical services (EMS)* when calling 911 and to document it into the patient's medical record.

---

emergency medical services (EMS). System that provides urgent pre-hospital treatment and care.

Remain on the phone until EMS arrives and provide appropriate instructions depending on the injury, such as not moving the patient in case of spinal injury, not removing an object that has pierced or penetrated the patient, and applying pressure and elevating the body part if there is bleeding. Stay calm and support the person on the phone until EMS arrives and assures that the patient is being cared for.

5.13 Signs and Symptoms Related to Urgent and Emergency Situations

EMERGENCY SITUATION	DESCRIPTION	SIGN AND SYMPTOMS	TREATMENT/PROGNOSIS
Severe hypoglycemia	Low blood glucose levels are a serious heath risk for patients with diabetes. Also called insulin reaction or insulin shock, it can occur when there is an imbalance between insulin levels and blood glucose in the body.	Mild case: irritability, moodiness or change in behavior, hunger, sweating, and rapid heart rate. Moderate to severe: fainting, seizures, confusion, headache, coma, and potentially death.	For mild or moderate hypoglycemia, the patient's blood glucose level needs to be raised by consuming foods or liquid high in glucose. In cases of severe hypoglycemia, glucagon (a prescription medication) is administered.
Hypovolemic shock	This occurs when a patient loses an excessive amount of body fluids or blood. It can result from internal or external hemorrhaging (hemorrhagic shock), prolonged vomiting or diarrhea, or severe dehydration.	Thirst, muscle cramping, and lightheadedness—symptoms can progress to chest pain, confusion, lethargy, and death if left untreated.	Control of blood loss, blood transfusion, and IV fluid replacement.
Heat exhaustion or heat stroke	When the body temperature varies too much over its normal range.	Muscle cramping, which results from an electrolyte imbalance caused by loss of sodium from sweating, perspiration, and pale and clammy skin.	The individual will need to be removed from warm temperatures. Apply any available cold compresses such as ice pack. Death can result from heat stroke if it is not treated quickly.
Hypothermia or frostbite	Exposure to cold temperatures. Frostbite occurs when the skin and tissue are exposed to freezing temperatures. Tissues are not able to get oxygen supply due to the freezing, causing the tissue to die. The tissues of the nose, ears, fingers, and toes are the most susceptible.	Frostbite includes redness and tingling. As damage progresses, the tissue becomes pale and numb. Hypothermia is an abnormal lowering of body temperature, usually resulting from immersion in cold water or being stranded in subzero weather. Signs and symptoms include shivering, numbness, confusion, paleness, and eventual loss of consciousness.	Individual will need to be removed from cold temperatures. Remove any wet clothing. Cover the individual with a blanket. Provide any available warm/dry compresses and any warm beverages. Death can result if not treated.

5.13 Signs and Symptoms Related to Urgent and Emergency Situations (continued)

EMERGENCY SITUATION	DESCRIPTION	SIGN AND SYMPTOMS	TREATMENT/PROGNOSIS
Obstructed airway, or choking	Food aspiration while eating. This occurs when partially chewed food enters the trachea when talking, laughing, or coughing when eating. In children, small objects that obstruct airway include toys, toy parts, buttons, or candy.	A patient who is choking usually places their hand at their throat. This is often called "conscious choking." The patient may not be able to cough or speak.	Abdominal thrusts are effective for forcing an obstruction for the airway for adults and children older than 1 year of age. A combination of chest thrusts and back slaps are effective for infants younger than 1 year old.
Syncope, or fainting	A brief episode of unconsciousness. Syncope is not a disease but the result of an underlying condition or disease.	Pale, perspiring, and complain of nausea or dizziness.	Aromatic spirits of ammonia capsules, which can be easily broken and used to wake the patient. These should not be held directly under the patient's nose but moved back and forth at least 6 inches away.

Commonly Occurring Types of Injuries and Treatment

Sprains and Strains

Sprains are caused by a stretched or torn ligament, which are tissues that connect bones to a joint. Falling, twisting, or landing on an uneven surface can all cause a sprain. Ankle and wrist sprains are common. Symptoms include pain, swelling, bruising, and being unable to move the joint. The patient can feel a pop or tear when the injury happens.

A strain is a stretched or torn muscle or tendon. Tendons are tissues that connect muscle to bone. Trauma to the tissue, such as excessive twisting or pulling these tissues, can cause a strain. Strains can happen suddenly or develop over time. Back and hamstring muscle strains are common. Strains are common when playing sports. Symptoms include pain, muscle spasms, swelling, and trouble moving the muscle.

Treatment of both sprains and strains usually involves resting and elevating the injured area, applying cold compresses, wearing a bandage or brace, and the use of anti-inflammatory medications. Later treatment might include exercise and physical therapy depending upon the severity of the injury.

---

syncope. Fainting; a brief episode of unconsciousness.

Dislocations

Dislocations occur when a bone end slips out of the socket or when the capsule surrounding a joint is stretched or torn. Dislocations occur usually at any freely moving joint, with the shoulder being the most common. Other dislocations can occur at the ankles, knees, hips, elbows, jaw, and finger. Dislocated joints often are swollen, very painful, and visibly out of place. The patient may not be able to move it.

A dislocated joint is an emergency, and the patient should seek medical attention. Treatment depends on which joint is dislocated and the severity of the injury. It might include manipulations to reposition the bones, medication, a splint or sling, and rehabilitation. When properly repositioned, a joint will usually function and move normally again in a few weeks. However, once a shoulder or kneecap is dislocated, it is more likely to dislocate again. Wearing protective gear during sports can help prevent dislocations.

Fractures

Fractures can be broadly classified as closed or open. Simple, or closed, fractures do not penetrate the skin. In open (compound) fractures, the bone breaks through the skin and is exposed. Open fractures present a greater chance of infection.

A patient with a suspected fracture will need advanced medical care. Immediate care can include stopping any bleeding by elevating the body part and applying pressure. Immobilize the injured area and apply localized cold to the area, such as an ice pack in cloth.

5.14 Types of Bone Fractures

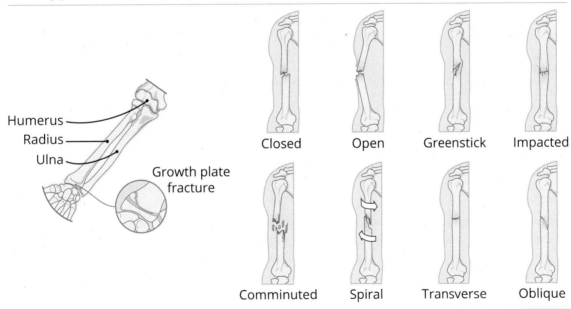

Administer First Aid and Basic Wound Care

First aid is the immediate care given to the victim of injury or sudden illness. The purpose of first aid is to sustain life and prevent death. It includes the prevention of permanent disability and the reduction of time needed for recovery. First aid includes basic life support and maintenance of vital functions. The most common need for first aid is for the treatment of shock, seizures, burns, poisoning, fractures, temperature alterations, and wounds.

Shock

The response of the cardiovascular system to the presence of adrenaline, resulting in capillary constriction. This causes inadequate circulation of blood to the body tissues, lowered blood pressure, and decreased kidney function. Shock can result from trauma, electrical injury, insulin shock, *hemorrhage* (excessive bleeding), or as a reaction to drugs. It can occur in conjunction with other injuries or illness such as respiratory distress, fever, heart attack, and poisoning.

Anaphylactic Shock

The response of the body to an allergen such as a medication or an insect bite or sting. Early signs and symptoms of shock include pale and clammy skin, weakness, and restlessness. The pulse and respiratory rate are rapid, and vomiting can occur. Late signs of shock include apathy, unresponsiveness, dilated pupils, mottled skin, and loss of consciousness, the state of being alert and aware. Shock can result in death if the condition is not reversed. An EpiPen, a preloaded pen filled with epinephrine, is the first line of defense for an anaphylactic shock if it is readily available.

If a patient is going into shock, emergency medical care is critical, and 911 should be contacted. Then, lay the patient down and elevate the legs and feet slightly, unless this can cause the patient pain or further injury, and try to keep the patient still. Continue monitoring the patient's pulse regularly until emergency services arrive. If the patient stops breathing, begin CPR.

Seizure

Uncontrolled muscle activity, seizures can be caused by high body temperature, head injuries, drugs, and epilepsy. During the seizure, steps should be taken to prevent injury to the patient. Help them to the floor if they are sitting or standing. Do not try to restrain them. Move objects out of their way and turn them to the side to prevent aspiration or choking. After the seizure, or the postictal phase, the patient can be confused, complain of headache, and be exhausted. Allow the patient to rest.

Poisoning

This can occur in several ways, and most poisoning occurs in the home. Poison can be ingested, inhaled, absorbed, injected, or obtained by radiation. Ingestion is the taking in of a substance by eating or drinking. Signs and symptoms of poisoning include discoloration or burns on the lips, unusual odor, emesis (vomiting), or presence of a suspicious container. Emergency care or 911 is needed if the patient presents as drowsy or unconscious, is having difficulty breathing or has stopped breathing, or is having seizures. While waiting for emergency care, try to remove any poison present on the patient, such as in the mouth, on the skin, or in the eye. Be cautious of aspiration or choking if the patient vomits and continue to monitor the patient's vital signs in the case CPR is needed.

---

hemorrhage. Escape of blood from a ruptured blood vessel.

Open Wound

Any break in the skin, whether from injury or a surgical incision, is referred to as an open wound. When applying or changing a dressing, the medical assistant should perform proper hand hygiene prior to donning sterile or nonsterile gloves. The use of sterile gloves is needed when performing a sterile dressing change. A surgical mask worn by the medical assistant can be recommended to avoid exposure of the wound to micro-organisms.

Wounds

Any break in the skin, whether from injury or a surgical incision, is referred to as a wound. Wounds can be open or closed, intentional through surgical intervention, or accidental through trauma. Wounds heal based on location, mode of injury, available blood supply, and the patient's general health status. There are four types of wound classification.

- **Abrasion:** outer layers of skin are rubbed away because of scraping; will generally heal without scarring.
- **Incision:** smooth cut resulting from a surgical scalpel or sharp material, such as razor or glass; can result in excessive bleeding and scarring if deep.
- **Laceration:** edges are torn in an irregular shape; can cause profuse bleeding and scarring.
- **Puncture:** made by a sharp, pointed instrument such as a bullet, needle, nail, or splinter; external bleeding is usually minimal, but infection can occur because of penetration with a contaminated object, and there can be scarring.

Treatments for wounds include managing bleeding by applying pressure, proper wound cleaning, and bandaging. Deep wounds can require a suture or staple insertion.

5.15 Wound Types

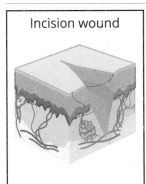 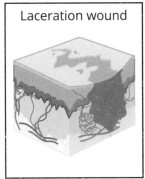 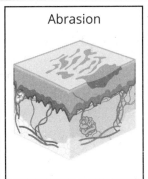 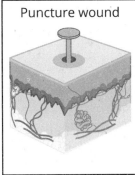

Wound Care

When providing first aid for a wound, controlling hemorrhage—or excessive, uncontrolled bleeding—is often necessary. There are generally three types of hemorrhaging based on the blood vessels affected: arterial, venous, and capillary. Identify the specific type of bleeding in order to provide the appropriate first aid and care to minimize the hemorrhage.

- Arterial bleeding is the most severe and urgent type of bleeding. It can result from a penetrating injury, blunt trauma, or damage to organs or blood vessels. Arterial bleeding is high pressure, and, thus, the bleeding is bright red in spurts. If a large artery, such as the aorta, is ruptured or bleeding has occurred for several minutes, this is a potentially life-threatening situation and can lead to death. This type of bleeding can be hard to control because of the pressure in the blood vessels. The first step should be to put pressure on the wound with sterile gauze. Elevate the site of the bleeding. In some cases, a tourniquet will need to be applied, above the site of the bleed, if the bleeding continues. The health care provider should be notified and should advise if a tourniquet should be used.

- Venous bleeding produces a steady flow of dark red blood. Similar to an arterial bleed, the site of the wound should be covered with a clean cloth or gauze, pressure should be exerted on the wound, and the area should be elevated. Capillaries are the smallest blood vessels, and bleeding is minimal. There will be a small and steady flow of blood from the site, but it will clot on its own within minutes.

- After the bleeding has been controlled, clean and dress the wound. A wound must be cleaned before a sterile dressing can be applied. The health care provider should inspect the wound site and indicate what should be used to clean the wound, such as an antiseptic cleanser. Cleanse the center of the incision line or wound from the top to the bottom and discard swab. Repeat this step for both sides of the wound. Apply sterile gloves and remove sterile dressing from package. Apply over wound, avoiding dragging the bandage. This will prevent dragging more micro-organisms into the wound. Wrap bandage material over wound and securely fasten the bandage with hypoallergenic tape and check circulation. Discard all waste contaminated with body fluids in a biohazard container.

- Once the wound has been cleaned, apply a new sterile dressing. After the wound is dressed, the health care provider can instruct the MA to apply a bandage to hold the dressing in place. Bandages can be gauze, fabric, or elasticized and are usually unsterile but clean. Patients should also be asked about allergies to any adhesives. Instruct the patient on dressing care and to schedule a follow-up appointment to see the health care provider.

- When changing a bandage and dressing, the wound must be cleaned before a sterile dressing can be applied. Using a set of bandage scissors, cut the bandage material, to the side of both the wound and dressing. Remove the bandage without removing the dressing, if possible. Then, carefully remove the dressing by pulling the corners toward the center of the wound. When changing dressings that are stuck to the wound, soak the dressing in sterile saline or sterile water prior to removal. Always take precautions to prevent further contamination of the wound when conducting a dressing change. Once the bandage has been removed, dispose of the bandages, used gauze, and gloves into the biohazard waste container.

5.16 Take Note

Remember that dressings are sterile and that bandages are nonsterile. Dressings cover wounds, and bandages cover dressings. Care must be taken not to bandage too tightly and restrict circulation.

Signs and Symptoms of Wound Infection and Wound Stages

Wounds pass through various stages of healing, including inflammation, as the body starts to fight off potential infection. Inflammation is the body's protective response to trauma and invasion by micro-organisms; it is generally localized around the site of trauma or infection. Signs of inflammation are redness (*erythema*), swelling, warmth, and pain. The three phases of wound healing or restoration of structure and function are the following.

- **Inflammatory phase (3 to 4 days):** Marked by pain, swelling, and loss of function at the site of the wound. Blood clot forms to stop bleeding and plug the opening of a wound.
- **Proliferating phase (4 to 21 days):** Fibrin threads extend across the opening of a wound and pull edges together; cells multiply to repair the wound, and eschar or scab begins to form to keep out micro-organisms.
- **Maturation phase (21 days to 2 years):** Tissue cells strengthen and tighten the wound closure, forming a scar; scar eventually fades and thins.

5.17 Three Phases of Wound Healing

Inflammatory phase	Proliferative phase	Maturation phase
• Starts when wound occurs. • Immune system prevents infection.	• Wound begins to heal. • New cells form around damaged tissue.	• New tissues cover wound. • Scar tissue forms.

If the wound is not properly healing or staying clean, micro-organisms can enter the wound, and complications can occur. Wound complications include the following.

- Infection (signs of inflammation, swelling, purulent or puslike drainage, fever)
- Hemorrhage or bleeding
- *Dehiscence* (separation of wound edges)
- *Evisceration* (separation of wound edges and protrusion of abdominal organs)

---

erythema. Superficial reddening of the skin.

dehiscence. Partial or total separation of a wound's edges.

evisceration. Separation of wound edges and protrusion of abdominal organs.

Burns

Burns can result from exposure to heat, chemicals, or radiation. The severity of a burn is determined by the location, depth, and size. Injury to the face, arms, legs, and genitals are the most critical. Burns that cover more than 10% of the body surface generally require hospitalization. Burns are classified into four degrees according to their depth.

A first-degree (superficial) burn affects only the outer layer of skin tissue. The skin becomes red and discolored, and some slight swelling can occur. Healing of first-degree burns is generally rapid. Examples of a first-degree burn are sunburn and a burn caused by immersing part of the body briefly into hot water.

A second-degree (partial-thickness) burn is one that breaks the surface of the skin and injures the underlying tissue. Second-degree burns can result from a severe sunburn and exposure to hot liquids or heat. The appearance of blisters commonly indicates a second-degree burn. The skin is red or mottled in appearance. The skin can become wet when plasma is lost through the damaged skin. This type of burn causes greater pain and swelling.

5.18 Classification of Burns

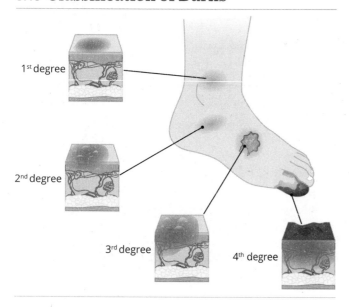

A third-degree (deep-thickness) burn is deep enough to damage the nerves and bones. Tissue burned to the third degree is charred and white. A third-degree burn can cause less pain because the nerves are damaged. Third-degree burns can result from exposure to fire, hot water, hot objects, or electricity.

A fourth-degree (deep full-thickness) burn goes through both layers of the skin and underlying tissue as well as deeper tissue, possibly involving muscle and bone. There is no feeling in the area because the nerve endings are destroyed. Fourth-degree burns are often caused by flames and chemicals, such as from a hot iron or stove, fireplace, and a building fire.

Treatment of Burns

For minor burns, cool the burn by holding the area under cool (but not cold) running water for about 10 min. If the burn is on the face, apply a cool, wet cloth until the pain eases. For a mouth burn from hot food or drink, put a piece of ice in the mouth for a few minutes. After the burn is cooled, apply a lotion, such as one with aloe vera or cocoa butter. This helps prevent drying and provides relief. If a blister appears, do not break it, because this can increase the risk of infection. If a blister does break, gently clean the area with water and apply an antibiotic ointment. Cover the burn with a clean bandage. Wrap it loosely to avoid putting pressure on burned skin. Bandaging keeps air off the area, reduces pain, and protects blistered skin. A minor burn might need emergency care if it affects the eyes, mouth, hands, or genital areas. Infants and older adults might need emergency care for minor burns as well.

When treating a major burn, emergency care is needed. Call 911 or seek immediate care. Until help arrives, protect the patient from further harm. Do not try to remove clothing stuck in the burn. Remove jewelry, belts, and other tight items, especially from the burned area and the neck. Burned areas swell quickly, so ensure the patient does not choke. Make certain that the person burned is breathing. If needed, begin CPR. Cover the burn. Loosely cover the area with gauze or a clean cloth. Raise the burned area. Lift the wound above heart level if possible. Watch for signs of shock, such as cool, clammy skin; weak pulse; and shallow breathing.

Assist Provider with Patients Presenting with Minor and Traumatic Injury

When a patient presents to the office with minor or traumatic injuries, the medical assistant can be responsible for obtaining the chief complaint, obtaining vital signs, and assisting the provider as necessary. This can also include cleaning wounds, preparing sterile fields for minor surgical interventions, bandaging wounds, administering injections, instructing patients on the signs of infections, providing wound care, and scheduling follow-up appointments. Minor and traumatic injuries include strains and sprains, dislocations, fractures, burns, lacerations, and abrasions.

CHALLENGE

1. Which of the following burns would result in no pain but the tissue is whitish?
   A. First degree
   B. Second degree
   C. Third degree
   D. Fourth degree

   C is correct. Third-degree burns are deep enough to damage the nerves and bones. Tissue burned to the third degree is charred and white. A third-degree burn can cause less pain because the nerves are damaged.

2. Match the description of the wound with the type of wound.

TYPE	DESCRIPTION
A. Abrasion	1. Smooth cut
B. Incision	2. Outer layers of skin rubbed away because of scraping
C. Laceration	3. Penetrating, made by a sharp, pointed instrument
D. Puncture	4. Edges torn in an irregular shape

   A: 2, B: 1, C: 4, D: 3
   The four main types of wounds are abrasion (outer layers of skin are rubbed away because of scraping), incision (smooth cut resulting from a surgical scalpel or sharp material, such as a razor or glass), laceration (edges are torn in an irregular shape), and puncture (penetrating from sharp, pointed instrument).

3. An MA is caring for a bleeding wound. The blood is bright red, and the bleeding is fast and profuse. Which of the following kinds of hemorrhage is this?
   A. Arterial
   B. Capillary
   C. Cauterized
   D. Venous

   A is correct. Arterial bleeding is high pressure and, thus, the bleeding is bright red in spurts. If a large artery, such as the aorta, is ruptured or bleeding has occurred for several minutes, this is a potentially life-threatening situation and can lead to death.

4. Which of the following should a medical assistant do when caring for hemorrhage? The blood is dark red and has a steady flow. (Select all that apply.)
   A. The site should be elevated.
   B. A tourniquet should be applied.
   C. The site should be covered with a clean gauze.
   D. The blood vessel should be cauterized to stop the bleeding.
   E. Pressure should be exerted on the site.

   A, C, and E are correct. For venous bleeding (dark red blood and steady flow), the site of the hemorrhage should be covered with a clean cloth or gauze, pressure should be exerted on the wound, and the area elevated.

5. Which of the following should a medical assistant do in the case of a patient having a seizure? (Select all that apply.)
   A. Move objects out of the way to prevent injury.
   B. Restrain the patient to minimize moving.
   C. If the patient is sitting, support the patient from falling.
   D. Help patient to the floor if standing.
   E. Turn the patient to the side to prevent choking.

   A, D, and E are correct. During a seizure, help patients to the floor if they are sitting or standing. Do not try to restrain them. Move objects out of their way and turn them to the side to prevent aspiration or choking.

EMERGENCY ACTION PLANS

Preparation for emergencies should include a preparedness plan, or an emergency action plan, that has a detailed emergency protocol that outlines the steps to be followed in the event of an office emergency. In addition to medical emergencies, this can also include other emergencies, such as earthquakes, tornadoes, floods, fires, shootings, and bioterrorism.

The emergency action plan can include the following.

- Identifying patients who have life-threatening conditions and need immediate care
- Identifying when and who should contact emergency medical services during a crisis situation
- The location of fire extinguishers and emergency evacuation routes
- Identifying an individual to make sure all needed equipment and supplies are ready for the provider during an emergent situation

Every medical office must have an emergency kit that contains supplies needed during an emergency. The emergency kit is commonly referred to as a *crash cart*, but it can be a bag or a container of emergency supplies. Many emergency kits can be purchased with all the necessary items, and some states have specific requirements for emergency kits. The health care provider can also determine what items and emergency medication should be included. Equipment and medication choice should reflect each medical office's patient population and specialty. For example, a pediatric specialty should have more medication appropriately dosed for children, and an allergy specialty practice can increase the number of epinephrine auto-injectors in the emergency kit.

Most emergency kits contain surgical instruments, such as forceps; oxygen supply; airway and suction device; bag valve mask (Ambu bag); heart monitor-defibrillator; and emergency medications.

The medical office should have several automated external defibrillators (AEDs)—one in the emergency kit or at least accessible, usually within 3 min from any location. *Automated external defibrillators (AEDs)* are lightweight, battery-operated, portable devices that check the heart's rhythm and send a shock to the heart to restore normal rhythm. Electrodes are attached to the patient who is experiencing cardiac arrest. The electrodes send information about the patient's heart rhythm to a computer in the AED. The computer analyzes the heart rhythm to find out whether an electric shock is needed. If it is needed, the electrodes deliver the shock. Most states have requirements on AEDs.

Emergency medications are often delivered as injectables or rectal suppositories for faster absorption. Some of the emergency medications that can be included are the following.

- Epinephrine auto-injector: treatment for anaphylactic shock
- Naloxone: rapidly reverses an opioid overdose
- Morphine: treatment for pain
- Nitroglycerin, sublingual or spray: treatment for chest pain
- Albuterol nebulizer: treatment for difficulty breathing, shortness of breath, wheezing
- Lidocaine: to treat or prevent localized pain
- Atropine: treatment for bradycardia
- Normal saline for IV administration: treatment for dehydration
- Prochlorperazine suppositories: for nausea and vomiting

crash cart. Portable cart stocked with emergency supplies; emergency kit.

automated external defibrillator (AED). Device that provides electrical shock to restore a normal heartbeat.

In the emergency kit, medications should be arranged so that they are easy to locate and the names are clearly visible. Clearly label pediatric medications and place them in plastic bags to separate them from other medications.

The emergency kit must be checked regularly, such as once a month, and maintained so that its contents are there when needed. Create a process for restocking, conducting inventory, and replacing the contents of the cart. Expiration dates on medications should also be checked routinely per facility policy. Expired medications should be promptly removed and replaced. The defibrillation pads on the AED or the defibrillator should be checked for expiration date. The battery charge on the monitor and/or AED should be checked and documented. The emergency kit should be in a location easily accessible to the examination rooms and that all staff members know where it is located.

All staff members should receive training on emergency preparedness and how to respond in the case of medical emergencies. To maintain a level of preparedness, the medical office should routinely conduct an emergency simulation in which an emergency situation is created and responses are practiced by health care professionals. These practice drills allow the health care team the opportunity to practice all steps in the emergency protocol as well as individual lifesaving skills. Often, unanticipated problems with the protocol or medical equipment can be identified and corrected during these practice emergency drills.

5.19 Automated External Defibrillator (AED)

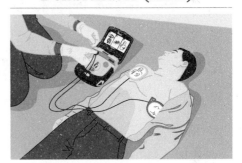

Procedures to Perform CPR, Basic Life Support, and Automated External Defibrillator (AED)

One of the most common medical emergencies inside and outside of the medical office is a *myocardial infarction*, or heart attack. A myocardial infarction (MI) happens when the flow of blood that brings oxygen to the heart muscle suddenly becomes blocked. The heart does not get enough oxygen. If blood flow is not restored quickly, the heart muscle will begin to die, and sudden cardiac arrest can occur, which is when the heart stops beating. An MI and cardiac arrest are life-threatening medical emergencies that require immediate treatment. The longer the patient's heart is without oxygen, the more damage is done to the heart muscle. Symptoms of an MI can vary, although common symptoms are the following.

- Chest pain, heaviness, or discomfort in the center or left side of the chest
- Pain or discomfort in one or both arms, the back, shoulders, neck, or jaw or above the belly button
- Shortness of breath when resting or doing a little bit of physical activity
- Excessive sweating for no reason
- Feeling unusually tired for no reason, sometimes for days
- Nausea (feeling sick to the stomach) and vomiting
- Lightheadedness or sudden dizziness
- Rapid or irregular heartbeat

5.20 Take Note

Compress the chest at least 2 inches (adults and children) and allowing it to recoil completely. Compress about 1 ½ inches in infants, using two fingers. Perform compressions at a rate of at least 100/minute.

myocardial infarction. The flow of blood that brings oxygen to the heart muscle suddenly becomes blocked. If not restored quickly, the heart muscle will begin to die and cardiac arrest can occur.

CHAPTER 5: GENERAL PATIENT CARE: PART 2
Emergency Action Plans

If a patient is experiencing an MI or cardiac arrest, immediately activate the emergency response team. If the patient is still conscious, the health care provider can administer emergency medication, such as aspirin, nitroglycerin, or thrombolytics to dissolve blood clots that can be blocking the coronary arteries in the heart. In addition, the health care provider can ask to administer oxygen to the patient via the nasal cannula or face mask.

Cardiac arrest occurs when the heart suddenly and unexpectedly stops pumping. If this happens, blood stops flowing to the brain and other vital organs. Cardiac arrest is a medical emergency and a common cause of death.

A patient experiencing a cardiac arrest can collapse suddenly and lose consciousness, stop breathing or gasp for air, not respond to shouting or shaking, and not have a pulse. Check for breathing and a pulse. Palpate for a pulse for no more than 10 seconds. If there is no pulse, use an automated external defibrillator (AED). If an AED is not available, cardiopulmonary resuscitation (CPR) should be initiated.

When using an AED, make sure the area around the patient is clear. Touching the patient could interfere with the AED's reading of the person's heart. Listen for voice prompts that tell when and how to give an electric pulse or shock if one is needed to restore a normal rhythm. Electrodes deliver the shock, and some deliver more than one shock. Start CPR after the shock is delivered and if the device instructs to do so.

If an AED is not available or in between AED use, initiate chest compressions and CPR. To perform CPR, perform the following.

- Begin chest compressions by placing the heel of one hand in the middle of the patient's sternum and the other hand on top of the base hand.
- Give 30 chest compressions.
- Use the head-tilt, chin-lift method to open the airway.
- Pinch the nose closed and give two slow mouth-to-mouth breaths. The chest should rise and fall with each breath administered.
- Continue giving sets of 30 chest compressions and two breaths.
- If the patient recovers and there are no other signs of injury to the back or neck, turn the victim to their side.

Medical assistants should be certified in basic life support and CPR (BLS/CPR) and maintain the certification. Although AEDs can be safely used by people with no medical training, medical assistants should complete a course on proper usage of an AED. Certification is also offered for AED training. Certification is often required to renew every two years.

CHALLENGE

1. An MA observes a patient in the waiting room clutch their chest and collapse. Which of the following should be done first?
   A. Call 911.
   B. Begin CPR.
   C. Use an AED.
   D. Administer epinephrine auto injector.

   A is correct. If the MA suspects a heart attack or cardiac arrest, immediately contact 911.

2. Which of the following are common signs and symptoms in a heart attack? (Select all that apply.)
   A. Dilated pupils
   B. Shortness of breath
   C. Chest pain
   D. Difficulty in coughing and speaking
   E. Muscle convulsions

   B and C are correct. Common signs and symptoms of a heart attack (myocardial infarction) are chest pain, pain or discomfort in different parts of the body, shortness of breath when resting or doing a little bit of physical activity, excessive sweating for no reason, nausea, dizziness, and rapid or irregular heartbeat.

3. Place the steps of performing CPR in the order they should be performed.
   A. Tilt the head back.
   B. Give 30 chest compressions.
   C. Continue giving sets of 30 chest compressions and two breaths.
   D. Give two slow breaths mouth-to-mouth.
   E. Pinch the nose.

   *B, A, E, D, C
   The correct sequence is give 30 chest compressions, tilt the head back, pinch the nose, give two slow mouth-to-mouth breaths, and continue giving sets of 30 chest compressions and 2 breaths.*

ORDER AND OBTAIN DURABLE MEDICAL EQUIPMENT (DME) AND SUPPLIES

Durable medical equipment (DME) includes medical devices and supplies that can be used repeatedly. The most common examples of durable medical equipment used outside of a hospital are dialysis machines, continuous positive airway pressure (CPAP) machines, oxygen concentrators and ventilators, orthotics and prostheses, bed equipment (hospital beds, lift beds), mobility aids (wheelchairs, crutches), and personal care aids (bath chairs, commodes). Oftentimes, DME can be written as DMEPOS for durable medical equipment, prosthetics, orthotics, and supplies. The following is necessary to qualify as a DMEPOS.

- Primarily serve a medical purpose
- Be prescribed by or ordered by a health care provider
- Be able to be used repeatedly
- Have an expected lifetime of at least three years
- Be used in the home
- Only be useful to patients who have an injury or disability

In a medical office or ambulatory care setting, the medical assistant will assist the health care provider with these devices and will provide education and support for the patient. In some cases, the MA will teach the patient how to use specific DMEPOS, such as crutches and canes.

DMEPOS items can be kept in some medical offices as inventory. If the medical office purchased the item, it is allowed to bill patients and/or their insurance company for it. In other cases, the health care provider will prescribe the DME item for the patient. As with any prescriptions or treatment, the health care provider must document the patient's diagnosis and the medical necessity for the patient to have the DMEPOS.

Prior Authorizations for Medication Durable Medical Equipment

What is considered DMEPOS is defined by Medicare, Medicaid, and other insurance companies—at least for reimbursement purposes. For example, compression leggings, incontinence pads, and ramps installed in the home are not considered DMEPOS.

For a patient to be eligible for DMEPOS, the health care provider must order the item through a prescription or medical order form to be submitted to a supplier. The health care provider must state that the DMEPOS is needed for the patient's medical condition or injury and is for home use. Some DMEPOS items, such a power wheelchair, require a face-to-face encounter, where a visit to the health care provider is required within 6 months before the order. The face-to-face encounter must be documented in the patient's medical record. The supporting documentation must include subjective and objective information and information used for diagnosing, treating, and managing the patient's condition for which the DMEPOS is ordered.

For some DMEPOS items, prior authorization may be required. Centers for Medicare & Medicaid Services (CMS) established a list of items that are considered DMEPOS, called the Master List. In addition, CMS created a subset list of items requiring prior authorization, the "Required Prior Authorization List." Prior authorization is a process through which a request for provisional affirmation or approval of coverage is submitted for review before a DMEPOS item is furnished to a

durable medical equipment. Medical devices and supplies that can be used repeatedly outside of a hospital.

beneficiary and before a claim is submitted for payment. Items that require prior authorization can include power wheelchairs, powered air flotation beds, powered pressure-reducing air mattresses and more.

To submit a DMEPOS item for prior authorization, the health care provider will submit the necessary forms and information to the Durable Medical Equipment Medicare Administrative Contractor (DME MAC) for review. If the DME MAC denies prior authorization for the patient's equipment, the health care provider can appeal but must provide more reasons and additional documentation related to why the patient needs the DMEPOS.

CHALLENGE

1. Which of the following DMEPOS requires prior authorization? (Select all that apply.)
   A. CPAP machines
   B. Thermometer
   C. Power wheelchairs
   D. Pressure-reducing air mattresses

   A, C, and D are correct. Items that require prior authorization are power wheelchairs, powered air flotation beds, and powered pressure-reducing air mattresses.

2. Which of the following would qualify an item as a DMEPOS? (Select all that apply.)
   A. Used in a facility
   B. Prescribed by a health care provider
   C. Last for at least one year
   D. Can be repeatedly used
   E. Used by a patient with a disability

   B, D, and E are correct. To qualify as a DMEPOS, the item must primarily serve a medical purpose, be prescribed by or ordered by a health care provider, be able to be used again and again, have an expected lifetime of at least three years, be used in the home, and only be useful to patients who have an injury or disability.

WRAP-UP

This chapter introduced many advanced skills and concepts for medical assistants, including how to assist in office-based surgical procedures. The chapter explored how to maintain sterile procedures, how to set up and maintain a sterile field, and how to assist with and perform different surgical procedures. This includes removing sutures and staples and, depending on the medical practice, assisting in endoscopies, cryosurgeries, and incisions and drainages.

This chapter additionally discussed how to identify various emergencies in the medical setting and how to prepare for them. Knowing how to prepare an emergency preparedness kit and how to stabilize and treat patients during medical emergencies are crucial skills for when an emergency situation arises. Common medical emergencies include heart attacks, cardiac arrest, wounds, burns, sprains and strains, dislocations, and fractures. Providing postsurgical care and understanding the processes involved in ordering and obtaining prior authorization for durable medical equipment are imperative to the medical assistant role.

CHAPTER 6
Infection Control and Safety

OVERVIEW

The purpose of infection control is to minimize and remove a variety of disease-causing *micro-organisms* from the health care environment. These pathogens need to be minimized at every opportunity. Effective infection control helps to ensure the safety of patients and health care staff. As a member of the health care team, the medical assistant plays a vital role in the implementation of infection control procedures. From basic handwashing to the appropriate disposal of biohazardous materials, the medical assistant can break the cycle of infection, resulting in fewer *pathogenic* transmissions and, as a result, illnesses.

COMMUNICABLE DISEASES AND TRANSMISSION

Having a medical facility that is clean and safe for both the health care team and patient is very important. Ensure that infection control practices are always being implemented, as well as that everyone completes *medical asepsis* when necessary. For the transmission of a disease to occur, there must be a pathogen or infectious agent present.

Transmission can occur in various ways but mainly from direct contact with the pathogen. Below is a table of some of the common *communicable diseases* and their means of transmission.

Objectives

Upon completion of this chapter, you should be able to

- Adhere to standard and universal precautions and guidelines related to infection control.
- Adhere to regulations and guidelines related to infectious diseases.
- Follow guidelines related to use of personal protective equipment (PPE), including donning and doffing.
- Adhere to guidelines regarding hand hygiene.
- Perform disinfection/sanitization.
- Perform sterilization of medical equipment.
- Perform appropriate aseptic techniques for various clinical situations.
- Dispose of biohazardous materials as dictated by Occupational Safety and Health Administration (OSHA) (sharps containers, biohazard bags).
- Follow post-exposure guidelines (needle safety guidelines, use of eyewash stations).

6.1 Communicable Diseases and Transmission

DISEASE	TRANSMISSION
Varicella (chicken pox)	Direct or indirect contact from infected droplets or airborne secretions
Viral meningitis	Direct contact, respiratory secretions, and oral-fecal route
Bacterial meningitis	Direct contact and infected droplets from respiratory tract

micro-organism. A microscopic organism that cannot be seen by the naked eye.

pathogenic. Causes disease.

medical asepsis. Clean technique that includes frequent hand hygiene, proper use of gloves, cleaning and sterilizing medical equipment, and sanitizing surfaces.

communicable disease. Illness caused by an infectious agent that occurs through direct or indirect contact.

6.1 Communicable Diseases and Transmission (continued)

DISEASE	TRANSMISSION
Conjunctivitis (pinkeye)	Direct or indirect contact with eye discharge or discharge from upper respiratory tract of infected patient
Rhinovirus (common cold)	Direct or indirect contact from airborne or respiratory secretion droplets
Strep throat	Direct contact with infected individual, respiratory secretions
Pertussis (whooping cough)	Direct contact with respiratory secretion droplets
Influenza (flu)	Direct contact with respiratory secretion droplets

Organisms and Micro-Organisms

Disease-causing micro-organisms are most often in the form of viruses, bacteria, fungi, or parasites. Parasites can be further classified as protozoa, helminths, ectoparasite, and rickettsia.

Common Pathogens and Nonpathogens

There are certain requirements for pathogens to grow and multiply. If this process is interrupted, disease prevention can be reduced. Not all micro-organisms are pathogenic. Some micro-organisms are *nonpathogens* that are considered *normal flora* and provide balance in the body. Normal flora are micro-organisms that live on or within the body without causing disease. Normal flora are responsible for many important functions, such as synthesizing and excreting vitamins as well as preventing colonization of pathogens.

6.2 Common Pathogens

PATHOGEN	EXAMPLES	PATHOGEN	EXAMPLES
Viruses	Rhinovirus (common cold)	Fungi	Histoplasmosis (lung infection passed on by certain bird/bat droppings)
	Varicella (chicken pox)		
	HIV/AIDS		*Tinea pedis* (athlete's foot)
	Hepatitis		*Candida albicans* (yeast infection)
	Coronavirus		
Bacteria	*Escherichia coli* (urinary tract infections)	Parasites	Toxoplasmosis
			Pinworm
	Vibrio cholerae (cholera)		Tapeworm
	Bordetella pertussis (whooping cough)		Scabies
			Lice
			Lyme disease

nonpathogenic. Harmless and does not cause disease.

normal flora. Micro-organisms that live on or within the body without causing disease.

Infectious Agents, Chain of Infection, Modes of Transmission, and Conditions for Growth

For the transmission of a pathogen to spread, certain links are required, and there must be a pathogen or infectious agent present. An environment conducive to pathogen survival is known as a reservoir. In a clinical setting, the reservoir is often the patient but can also be an inanimate object such as an exam table or a piece of medical equipment. The human body makes an ideal reservoir for microbial growth because of the presence of nutrients, moisture, and ideal temperature and pH levels. The portal of exit is the passageway that the pathogen uses to exit the reservoir. This can be via the infected body fluids of an individual in a patient care setting. Once the pathogen exits the reservoir, a mode of transmission is necessary for the cycle to continue. A direct transmission takes place when there is contact with the infected person or body fluid that is carrying the pathogen. Indirect transmissions occur when there is an intermediate step between the portal of exit and portal of entry. Once the pathogen has a means of transmission, it will need a new portal of entry to continue the infectious cycle. Pathogens often enter a host via an open wound or through the mouth, nose, eye, intestines, urinary tract, or reproductive system. The final step in the cycle is the presence of a susceptible host. Several variables make the human body—especially of a compromised patient—the ideal susceptible host. Factors such as overall health, age, and the condition of a person's immune system affect the chances of them becoming a host for a disease transmission. If one of the links in the infection is broken, the transmission is halted. It is the responsibility of all health care professionals to take the necessary steps to break this cycle of infection.

Each pathogen has specific routes in which transmission can occur. Clinical facilities issue a variety of isolation practices according to the identified pathogen. If one is not identified, the most restrictive isolation practices are implemented.

For the transmission of a pathogen to occur, the following links in the cycle of infection must be connected.

- Infectious agent
- Reservoir/source
- Portal of exit
- Mode of transmission
- Portal of entry to host
- Susceptible host

If this chain is interrupted, it can break the infection process, thus preventing the continuation of the cycle and halting infection.

6.3 Chain of Infection

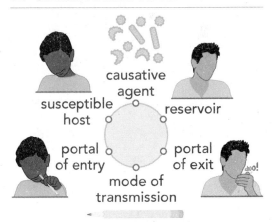

CHAPTER 6: INFECTION CONTROL AND SAFETY
Communicable Diseases and Transmission

Signs and Symptoms of Infectious Diseases

There can be many different signs and symptoms depending on the type of infectious disease. A sign is a manifestation that can be perceived. A symptom is a manifestation of something that is only apparent or felt by patient. Some of the most common signs and symptoms are the following.

6.4 Signs and Symptoms of Infectious Diseases

SIGNS	SYMPTOMS
Fever	Chills
Swollen lymph nodes	Pain and aching
Tachycardia	Nausea
Septicemia	Fatigue/malaise
Chest sounds	Headache
Skin eruptions	Sore throat
Leukopenia	Chest tightness

CHALLENGE

1. Which of the following would be considered a direct mode of transmission?
   A. Contact with a mosquito
   B. Contact with an infected person
   C. Contact with a pencil
   D. Contact with a contaminated table

   B is correct. Direct transmission takes place when there is contact with an infected person or body fluid that is carrying the pathogen. Contact with a mosquito, pencil, or contaminated table would be considered indirect transmission, which provides an intermediate step between the portal of exit and portal of entry.

2. Which of the following affects the chance of a patient becoming a host for disease transmission?
   A. Age
   B. Race
   C. Geography
   D. Occupation

   A is correct. Overall health, age, and the condition of a person's immune system all affect the chances of the patient becoming a host for disease transmission.

3. Which of the following pathogens would the common cold fall under?
   A. Bacteria
   B. Fungi
   C. Virus
   D. Parasite

   C is correct. The common cold is caused by various viruses, some of which are rhinovirus, parainfluenza, or a seasonal coronavirus.

4. Order the chain of infection in the correct sequence.
   A. Mode of transportation
   B. Portal of exit
   C. Portal of entry
   D. Infectious agent
   E. Reservoir/source
   F. Susceptible host

   D, E, B, A, C, F
   The correct sequence is infectious agent, reservoir/source, portal of exit, mode of transportation, portal of entry, and susceptible host.

INFECTION CONTROL GUIDELINES

Adhere to Standard and Universal Precautions and Guidelines Related to Infection Control

Universal precautions and guidelines are set in place to prevent health care professionals from exposure to infections when providing first aid or health care. These guidelines include considering each patient potentially infectious for blood-borne pathogens including but not limited to human immunodeficiency virus (HIV) and the hepatitis B virus.

Universal Precautions

Universal precautions apply when in possible contact with any of the following.

- Blood products
- Human tissue
- Body fluids such as cerebrospinal fluid, amniotic fluid, and pleural fluid
- Any body fluid visibly contaminated with blood
- Vaginal secretions and semen

Standard Precautions

Health care professionals are responsible not only for protecting their patients but also for protecting themselves from blood-borne pathogens. The Centers for Disease Control and Prevention has been recommending *standard precautions* since 1987. Protecting the health care professional against exposure to blood and other body fluids is essential when the status of infection is unknown in a patient.

Some general guidelines are as follows.

- Wash hands before and after every procedure.
- Use gloves with encountering patient blood/body fluids, handling anything contaminated with blood, performing venipuncture, handling blood specimens, and cleaning up body fluids or blood.
- Cover any scratches or breaks in the skin.
- Refrain from eating, drinking, or chewing gum while working.
- Wear appropriate *personal protective equipment* (PPE) if blood or body fluid splatter could occur.
- Clean all spills immediately with appropriate cleaning supplies.
- Dispose of sharps immediately.
- Place sharps or broken glass in a puncture-proof container.
- Dispose of all *biohazard waste* in appropriate biohazard container.

---

universal precautions. Precautions that apply when it is possible to come into contact with human blood, tissue, body fluids or secretions, regardless of patient infection status.

standard precautions. Guidelines recommended by the Centers for Disease Control and Prevention (CDC) to ensure the safety and welfare of health care workers and the public.

personal protective equipment. Gear worn when there is a chance of coming in contact with blood or body fluids. In the health care setting, this includes gloves, gowns/aprons, shoe covers, lab coats, masks and respirators, protective eyewear, and face shields.

biohazard waste. Materials that present a potential or actual risk to the health of humans, animals, or the environment.

Adhere to Regulations and Guidelines Related to Infectious Diseases

There are three categories for job tasks and the potential for exposure to blood borne pathogens. They are determined by how much exposure to potential infectious agents you would likely encounter.

6.5 Task Categories

CATEGORY	EXAMPLE
Category I	Tasks that have a chance of body fluids or blood spilling or splashing, or tasks that can cause exposure to blood or body fluids such as a minor surgical procedure
Category II	Tasks that do not usually involve chance of exposure, such as CPR; precautions must still be taken
Category III	Tasks that do not require any PPE, such as taking a patient's vital signs

CDC Guidelines for Infectious Disease (Prevention, Reporting)

If a health care professional has a fever or feels sick, refrain from contact with patients to reduce the risk of spread. Stay home and only return to work if the MA has been fever-free for at least 24 hours without the use of any fever-reducing medications. OSHA also outlines standard safeguards to take when performing specific medical tasks.

The *Needle Safety and Prevention Act* was signed into law in November 2000. Health care professionals must implement the use of devices that help reduce the risk of needlestick injuries such as needle safety devices. Facilities must also maintain a detailed logbook of any needlestick or sharps injuries from dirty or contaminated sharps. Health care facilities must also implement work practice controls to help reduce the risk of injury at work by altering the way a task is performed.

Approaches for the Control of Infectious Diseases, Epidemics, and Pandemics

Additional precautions may need to occur when working with a patient with a suspected infection. These guidelines are known as transmission-based precautions. This is broken down into three categories.

- Contact precautions: Transmission through direct and indirect touching; using proper PPE such as gloves and gown, washing hands before and after working with the patient, and disinfecting the exam room are all precautions that should be taken.

- Droplet precautions: Transmission by contact of secretions and usually occurs when an infected person coughs or sneezes; get the patient to an exam room as quickly as possible, have the patient put on a face mask, and have the health care professional use appropriate PPE such as mask and gloves.

- Airborne precautions: Transmission by infectious agents floating in the air, which can expose anyone around the patient; allow the patient to enter the facility by a different route, place the patient in an isolation room, have the patient place a face mask on, and have the health care working use appropriate PPE such as mask, gloves, and gown.

Needle Safety and Prevention Act. Law signed in November 2000 that requires safety measures in workplaces where there is an occupational exposure to blood or other potentially infectious materials.

Guidelines for Exposure to Bloodborne Pathogens (OSHA, American Hospital Association [AHA])

The *Occupational Safety and Health Administration (OSHA)* established a blood-borne pathogen standard to reduce the risk of occupational exposure to infectious disease. Exposure can occur in several ways: needlesticks; cuts; or blood or bodily fluid coming into contact with the eyes, nose, mouth, or other non-intact skin. One component of this standard requires employers to have a written exposure control plan to protect their employees who have the potential for exposure based on their job duties and responsibilities. The Centers for Disease Control and Prevention has outlined health care personnel that are considered "at risk" for occupational exposure to bloodborne pathogens including hepatitis B and C virus as well as human immunodeficiency virus (HIV).

Employers are required to update their exposure control plan annually to align with changes that help reduce the potential for exposure. The following must be detailed in the employer's exposure control plan.

Engineering Controls
Devices used to isolate or remove the blood-borne pathogen hazard from the workplace.

Workplace Controls
Practices in the workplace that reduce the chances of exposure by changing or mandating the way a task is performed.

PPE
Employers must provide personal protective equipment to employees.

Hepatitis B Vaccinations
Employers must provide hepatitis B vaccinations to all employees with a risk of exposure within 10 days of employment, at no cost to the employee. Documentation of the offer or a vaccination record for the employee must be kept on file.

Post-Exposure Follow-Up
Employers must follow up with any professional who had an exposure incident at no cost to the employee. All employee diagnoses must remain confidential.

Labels and Signs to Communicate Hazards
Labels are required to be on all regulated waste and storage containers containing potentially infectious materials.

Information and Training to Employees
Employers must provide regular training that covers the dangers of blood-borne pathogens, preventive practices, and post-exposure procedures. This training must be provided on initial hire and annually thereafter.

Documented Employee Medical Training Records
Medical training and records must be maintained for each employee, in addition to a log of occupational injuries and illnesses and a sharps injury log.

CHALLENGE

1. What are the three types of transmission-based precautions?

   Contact precautions, droplet precautions, and airborne precautions.

2. Match the category of exposure with the correct task.

CATEGORY	TASK
A. Category I	1. CPR
B. Category II	2. Minor surgical procedure
C. Category III	3. Taking a patient's blood pressure

   A: 2, B: 1, C: 3
   Category I = assisting in a minor surgical procedure. Category II = CPR. Category III = taking a patient's vital signs (blood pressure).

Occupational Safety and Health Administration (OSHA). Agency that creates regulations that employers must follow for employees to remain safe while working.

FOLLOW GUIDELINES RELATED TO USE OF PPE

Following specific guidelines on how to don (put on) and doff (remove) various PPE helps stop the spread of infectious agents. Gloves are the most used PPE in a health care setting.

Donning Nonsterile Gloves
- Perform handwash.
- Select appropriate size of nonsterile gloves.
- Place hand through opening and pull glove up to wrist.
- Repeat on other hand.
- Adjust gloves as necessary.

6.6 Removing Gloves

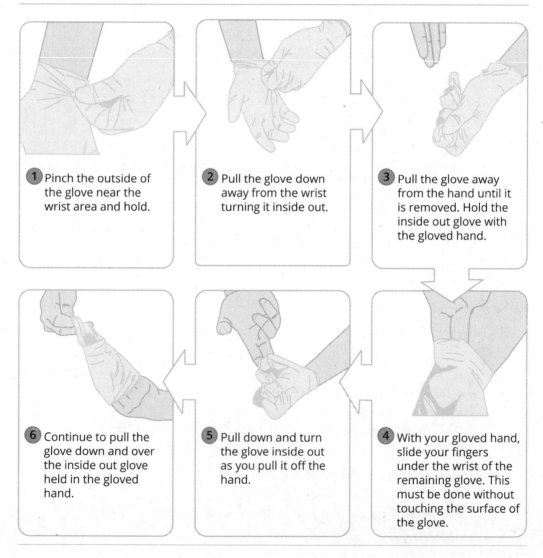

1. Pinch the outside of the glove near the wrist area and hold.
2. Pull the glove down away from the wrist turning it inside out.
3. Pull the glove away from the hand until it is removed. Hold the inside out glove with the gloved hand.
4. With your gloved hand, slide your fingers under the wrist of the remaining glove. This must be done without touching the surface of the glove.
5. Pull down and turn the glove inside out as you pull it off the hand.
6. Continue to pull the glove down and over the inside out glove held in the gloved hand.

Doffing Nonsterile, Contaminated Gloves

- Grasp palm of glove of nondominant hand with dominant hand.
- Pull glove off the nondominant hand in a downward motion while turning the glove inside out. Hold in dominant hand.
- Roll the glove up into the dominant hand.
- Place two fingers of the ungloved hand under the cuff of the other gloved, dominant hand, making sure not to touch the outside of the glove.
- Pull the glove over the hand, turning it inside out over the other glove.
- Throw away the gloves in the appropriate container.
- Wash hands.

ASEPSIS

Aseptic Techniques for Various Clinical Situations

Asepsis is the state of being free from disease-causing micro-organisms. Keeping the front office, back office, and reception areas clean is an important step in achieving asepsis by slowing the spread of infectious agents in the medical facility. Below are a few simple yet effective steps to initiate these methods.

- Clean and disinfect the office daily. Be sure to focus on all high-traffic areas, (for example, examination rooms, restrooms, height/weight scale area, patient check in/out areas) and inspect office surfaces or objects that can be contaminated or require frequent *disinfection*.
- Remove trash.
- Move sick and contagious patients from the reception area to an exam room or separate them from well patients upon arrival to a medical facility.
- Provide appropriate personal protective equipment including gloves, gowns, masks, and eye protection as needed for each situation.
- Do not allow eating or drinking in lab, clinical, or patient areas.
- Post reminder signs regarding good hand hygiene and covering coughs or sneezes.

CHALLENGE

1. Place the following steps of removing contaminated gloves below into the correct sequence.
   A. Wash hands
   B. Pull glove off the nondominant hand.
   C. Place two fingers of the ungloved hand under the cuff of the other glove, making sure not to touch the outside of the glove.
   D. Roll the glove up into the dominant hand.
   E. Throw away the gloves in the appropriate container.
   F. Pull the glove over the hand, turning it inside out over the other glove.
   G. Grasp palm of glove of nondominant hand with dominant hand.

   G, B, D, C, F, E, A
   The correct sequence is grasp palm of glove of nondominant hand with dominant hand, pull glove off the nondominant hand, roll the glove up into the dominant hand, place two fingers of the ungloved hand under the cuff of the other glove, making sure not to touch the outside of the glove, pull the glove over the hand, turning it inside out over the other glove, throw away the gloves in the appropriate container, and wash hands.

2. Which of the following PPE is the most widely used in a health care setting?
   A. Mask
   B. Gown
   C. Gloves
   D. Goggles

   C is correct. Gloves are the most widely used PPE in a health care setting.

---

disinfection. Process of killing disease-producing micro-organisms but not spores.

Techniques for Medical and Surgical Asepsis

Medical asepsis, or clean technique, is used daily in every clinical setting. The goal of medical asepsis is to reduce the number of pathogenic micro-organisms and prohibit their growth. Handwashing is a medical aseptic technique that is routinely used. This type of asepsis does not provide for a complete pathogen-free environment, but it greatly reduces their numbers and their ability to multiply and continue the chain of infection. Gloves, gowns, and masks can be used during medical asepsis. These items, considered personal protective equipment (PPE), are primarily used to protect the health care professional.

Medical assistants use clean or medical aseptic techniques on a daily basis. Below are a few examples.

- Washing hands prior to and after each patient encounter
- Assuring the workspace has been wiped down with sanitizing wipes between patient encounters
- Using proper PPE, such as gloves and masks, when in contact with bodily fluids
- Proper cleaning of supplies
- Setting up the laboratory area with a "clean" side and "dirty" side
- Properly covering coughs or sneezes and washing hands afterward

Surgical asepsis is the complete removal of all micro-organisms and must be used during invasive procedures. The goal of surgical asepsis is to eliminate micro-organisms from entering the body. During procedures such as invasive procedures, wound care, endoscopies, and insertion of urinary catheters, all PPE and instruments used should be sterile. Supplies used during these procedures would consist of the use of sterile gloves, gowns, and drapes.

Medical assistants need to know when to use medical versus surgical aseptic techniques. For most noninvasive procedures and if the skin and mucous membranes are intact, medical asepsis can be used. Surgical asepsis is used for invasive procedures and wound care. There are several actions that medical assistants can take to reduce the chances of pathogen transmission.

CHALLENGE

1. Which of the following helps slow down the spread of infectious agents?
   A. Provide sterile gown and gloves for every patient visit.
   B. Refrain from eating in laboratory areas, but eating and drinking in patient areas is fine.
   C. Move sick patients to exam rooms as soon as they enter the office.
   D. Clean only areas that look contaminated.

   C is correct. Moving sick patients away from others ensures that well patients are not exposed to infectious agents. Gowns and gloves are necessary for patient visits, but sterile gloves and gowns are not needed for each visit. Eating and drinking should not be allowed in patient areas, as the areas could be contaminated. Cleaning daily is necessary, and focus should be on high-traffic areas even if they do not appear contaminated.

2. When should surgical asepsis be used?

   Strategies include using surgical asepsis during invasive procedures, wound care, endoscopies, and insertion of urinary catheters.

ADHERE TO GUIDELINES REGARDING HAND HYGIENE

Good hand hygiene can be a major contributor that stops the cycle of infection in both clinical and nonclinical settings and is the single most important factor in preventing the spread of pathogens. Both medical professionals and patients benefit from this essential and simple safety practice. Clinical staff are discouraged from wearing excess jewelry such as rings and bracelets; a single plain band is often the exception. These items can harbor pathogens, which makes asepsis difficult to achieve. Artificial nails should also not be worn in a clinical setting. Research has shown that health care professionals who wear artificial nails have more bacteria on their nails than those with natural nails. Alcohol-based hand sanitizers can be used in certain situations to help stop the infectious cycle—for example, if a sink is not available. Health care professionals should wash hands with soap and water when hands are visibly contaminated or dirty. Alcohol-based sanitizer can be used on hands that are not visibly soiled.

CDC Hand Hygiene Recommendations

Proper hand hygiene must be used in the following situations even if disposable gloves are used.

6.7 CDC Hand Hygiene Recommendations

TASK	PROPER HANDWASHING REQUIRED	ALCOHOL-BASED HAND SANITIZER OR PROPER HANDWASHING ALLOWED
Before and after patient contact	✓	✓
After contact with contaminated surfaces	✓	✓
Contact with blood or body fluids	✓	
Before performing an aseptic procedure, such as blood draws and medication administration	✓	
Before and after contact with supplies or equipment near patients	✓	✓
After contact with contaminated body site prior to contact with a clean body site	✓	✓
After glove removal	✓	
Hands are visibly soiled	✓	

Additional times to use hand hygiene include the following.

- After using the restroom (soap and water)
- Before and after eating (soap and water)
- When arriving and before leaving work (soap and water)

CHAPTER 6: INFECTION CONTROL AND SAFETY
Adhere to Guidelines Regarding Hand Hygiene

Handwashing Techniques

Remove all jewelry except a plain ring or band. Turn on the faucet and regulate the water temperature to lukewarm. Wet the hands, apply approximately 3 milliliters or 3 pumps of soap, and lather using a circular motion with friction while holding the fingertips downward. The friction that is created with this step helps to lift debris from the skin. Rub hands well while interlacing fingers together to create friction and use circular motions around wrist. This process should be continued for at least 15 seconds (preferably 20 seconds).. Microbes tend to concentrate near and under the nails, so pay special attention to those areas, ensuring the water is flowing down from the wrist to the fingertips. Rinse the hands a second time, always keeping fingers lower than the wrist. Dry both hands with paper towels. Do not touch the paper towel dispenser when obtaining the towels. If an automated paper towel dispenser is not available, make sure to have paper towels ready prior to beginning handwashing. If the faucets are not foot operated, turn them off with a dry paper towel. Discard the paper towel in a covered waste container.

CHALLENGE

1. When using soap and water, which of the following is the minimum amount of time that hands should be rubbed together?
   A. At least 5 seconds
   B. At least 10 seconds
   C. At least 15 seconds
   D. At least 20 seconds

   C is correct. Apply the soap into a lather and rub hands in a vigorous circular motion for 15 to 20 seconds.

2. Which of the following is the minimum alcohol content in an alcohol-based sanitizer that can be used in a health care setting?
   A. 40%
   B. 50%
   C. 60%
   D. 75%

   C is correct. Washing hands is the most effective way to clean the hands, but if clean water and soap are not available or hands are not visibly soiled, an alcohol-based sanitizer with a minimum of 60% alcohol can be used.

Alcohol-Based Rubs/Sanitizer

In certain circumstances and when hands are not visibly soiled, an alcohol-based sanitizer with a minimum of 60% alcohol can be used. Start by pushing watch and uniform sleeves above wrists and removing rings. When using an alcohol-based sanitizer, dispense proper amount per manufacturer's recommendations into the palm of one hand. Rub both hands together, creating friction, making sure to cover all surfaces, including palms, backs of hands, fingers, and between fingers. Continue rubbing until the solution has dried. Keep in mind that sanitizers can be a good solution in specific circumstances, but they cannot be used to replace washing hands when they are visibly dirty. In this situation, soap and water must be used to remove the debris and wash the hands.

PERFORM DISINFECTION/SANITIZATION

Infection control can be managed through proper *sanitization*, disinfection, and sterilization of supplies. These techniques and skills should be done on a routine basis to ensure they become an unbreakable habit. Infection control includes ensuring that the equipment and supplies used in the clinical setting are free from disease-causing micro-organisms, which also helps protect the patient and the employee. The type of cleaning depends on the piece of equipment and the type of procedure in which it will be used. Surgical instruments are handled differently than patient assessment tools found in an examination room.

Sanitization is the cleaning process that is often the first step in assuring that medical equipment and instruments are as clean as possible. This process reduces the number of microbes to a lower level so that they are ready to undergo the sterilization or disinfection process. Sanitization helps to remove debris such as body fluids and blood that is present on the instruments and equipment. Gloves must always be worn during the sanitization process. If there are sharp instruments needing sanitization, wear thick utility gloves to avoid injury. Follow manufacturer's instructions regarding water temperatures and types of detergent to use during this process. Keep the work area separated into dirty and clean areas to avoid cross-contamination of equipment. For facilities that work with very delicate instruments, ultrasonic sanitization is used to avoid damage to the equipment. Rather than using friction to remove the debris, the sound waves loosen the debris so the object is free from excess material going into the disinfection or sterilization phase. Ultrasonic sanitization also reduces the risk of potential sharps injury for the health care professional. If sanitization cannot be completed directly after the use of the instrument, items should be immediately rinsed under cold water and placed in a detergent solution.

Disinfection is the process of destroying pathogens or rendering them inactive on surfaces and items, such as countertops and surgical instruments. Even though it does not destroy all the microbial spores or certain viruses, it greatly reduces the spread of infection by destroying or limiting microbial activity. The solutions used in disinfection are effective when used correctly. The process can often require lengthy submersion of instruments in a chemical solution that must touch every surface area of the instrument. Glutaraldehyde is a disinfectant used in the clinical setting but usually requires a long submersion time to be fully effective and can be costly. A cheaper and effective alternative is a 1:10 bleach solution. Chemical disinfectants cannot be used on patients and are reserved for medical supplies, equipment, clinical surroundings, and surfaces. A medical assistant is usually responsible for disinfecting the exam table, sink, countertop, computer keyboard, and other high-traffic surface areas.

---

sanitization. The cleaning process that reduces the number of micro-organisms to a safe level.

6.8 Types of Low- and Intermediate-Level Disinfectants

TYPE AND LEVEL	TYPICAL USE	ADVANTAGE	DISADVANTAGE
Alcohol: Intermediate	Fixed equipment Patient care items Drying agent	Fast-acting No residue Non-staining	Wet contact time a minimum of 5 min Flammable Inactivated by organic material Can dissolve lens mounting Tends to harden and swell plastic Alcohol is a fixative, increasing the difficulty of residual soil removal.
Chlorine (Chlorinated compounds): Low or Intermediate	Dialysis machines Bleach for laundry Bathtubs A 1:10 dilution recommended for cleaning blood spills	Fast-acting (minimum contact time 2.5 min)	Inactivated by organic matter Corrosive Stains fabric, plastics Relatively unstable
Iodophors: Low	Patient care equipment	Fast-acting (less than 2 min)	Corrosive to metals Detrimental to some plastics Stains fabrics and other materials Requires a longer contact time to kill fungi
Phenols: Low or Intermediate	Housekeeping for walls and floors	For housekeeping use; residual activity that can be reactivated when moisture is applied	For patient care items; residual activity can harm patients. Corrosive to some plastics
Quaternary ammonium (Quats): Low or Intermediate	Housekeeping for walls and floors Can be used on certain instruments if thoroughly rinsed	Wetting agents with built-in detergent properties	Typical contact time 6 to 10 min Can be inactivated by cotton or charcoal Not compatible with soap

Order of Cleaning and Types of Cleaning Products

Follow infection control protocols at work to help prevent the spread of infection. It is suggested to clean according to the following order to ensure best infection control practices.

- Hand hygiene: Complete aseptic handwashing or use an alcohol-based sanitizer. Use a clean paper towel to handle doorknobs or faucets to help avoid contaminating clean hands with microorganisms.

- Examination table: Remove disposable paper covering over examination table by tightly rolling it up to ensure the contaminated side is on the inside.

- Surfaces: Disinfect work surfaces beginning with the examination table, sink, countertop, and computer keyboard.

There are three levels of disinfectants.

6.9 Order of Cleaning and Types of Cleaning Products

LEVEL	USED FOR	EXAMPLE DISINFECTANT
Low-level disinfection kills most vegetative bacteria and some viruses and fungi.	Exam tables and countertops	Hydrogen peroxide
Intermediate-level disinfection kills vegetative bacteria and most viruses and fungi but does not kill spores.	Stethoscopes, percussion hammers, blood pressure cuffs	Isopropyl alcohol
High-level disinfection kills all microorganisms except for a small number of bacterial spores.	Instruments that do not penetrate soft tissues or bone but contact mucous membranes, such as endoscopes	Cidex OPA

Safety Data Sheets (SDSs)

OSHA requires that all employers provide SDSs to their employees. Any time a new chemical is brought into the work environment, SDS information must accompany the chemical. Each SDS is in the same format so professionals can find information quickly in case of an accidental exposure or emergency. Many employers can keep a hard copy in a binder located in a central location or have it available on accessible computers. Medical assistants work with a variety of solutions ranging from mild detergents to toxic chemicals. The following information must be included on the SDS to communicate the hazards and actions necessary if exposure to the chemical occurs.

- **Identification:** Product identifier, manufacturer information, recommended use, restrictions on use
- **Hazard identification:** All hazards related to the chemical, including hazard classification (combustible) and label requirements
- **Composition/ingredients:** Chemical ingredients contained in the product
- **First-aid measures:** Initial treatment from exposure, including symptoms and routes of exposure
- **Fire-fighting measures:** Appropriate extinguishing methods and chemical hazards from fire, including proper extinguishing equipment and special protective equipment
- **Accidental release measures:** Emergency procedures, PPE, containment, and cleanup in case of spills
- **Handling and storage:** Safe handling and appropriate storage requirements
- **Exposure controls/personal protection:** Recommended exposure limits and PPE necessary to reduce exposure
- **Physical and chemical properties:** Chemical characteristics such as appearance, odor, and pH
- **Stability and reactivity:** Chemical stability and potential reactions
- **Toxicological information:** Routes of exposure, effects of exposure, and symptoms
- **Other nonmandatory content:** Ecological information, disposal considerations, transport information, and regulatory information

CHALLENGE

1. Which of the following must be included in the SDS? (Select all that apply.)
   A. Disposal considerations
   B. First-aid measures
   C. Regulatory information
   D. Handling and storage
   E. Composition/ingredients

   B, D, and E are correct. First-aid measures, handling and storage, and composition/ingredients are all required to be included on the SDS. Disposal considerations and regulatory information are nonmandatory information for the SDS.

2. Match the level of disinfectant with the example disinfectant.

LEVEL	DISINFECTANT
A. Low level	1. Isopropyl alcohol
B. Intermediate level	2. Cidex OPA
C. High level	3. Hydrogen peroxide

   *A: 3, B: 1, C: 2
   An example of a low-level disinfectant is hydrogen peroxide, intermediate level is isopropyl alcohol, and high level is Cidex OPA.*

PERFORM STERILIZATION OF MEDICAL EQUIPMENT

The destruction of all living organisms, including pathogens and their spores, can be achieved with sterilization. Prior to sterilization, sanitizing and disinfecting must occur. These steps are necessary to perform on any instruments used in surgical procedures or used in a sterile field. The use of dry heat, gas, chemicals, ultraviolet radiation, ionizing radiation, chemicals, or steam under pressure in an autoclave are all methods that can be used in the sterilization of medical equipment. Autoclaves are the primary method medical facilities use to sterilize equipment. This process uses moist heat and pressure to achieve sterilization. Medical facilities can purchase supplies and equipment from manufacturers already sterilized and packaged, or they can establish a sterilization space in the facility. Although medical assistants might not perform this task every day, MAs must perform sterilization of supplies and equipment used in surgical and other invasive procedures. Once an item is sterilized, specific handling must occur so the item is not contaminated. If completed properly, the items are generally considered sterile for 30 days if packaging stays intact and kept dry.

Sterilization Techniques and Maintaining Sterilization Equipment

Autoclaving is the most widely accepted method to achieve sterilization. To ensure all equipment is sterilized, the recommended temperature an autoclave must reach is between 250° and 270° F. The amount of time necessary to establish sterility fluctuates depending on what items are being sterilized and how they are wrapped. It is always suggested to follow the manufacturer's guidelines. Generally, unwrapped items are sterilized for 20 min and wrapped items for 30 min. The most widely used cycle is the gravity cycle in ambulatory health care facilities. This is used to sterilize stainless steel instruments.

Instruments should be wrapped prior to autoclaving. Wrapping can be performed using disposable double-ply autoclave paper or peel-apart polypropylene pouches. When using autoclave paper, it is recommended to use at least two layers to maintain sterilization.

Guidelines when wrapping instruments are the following.

- Discard any autoclave paper that is torn or has holes.
- Wrap hinged instruments in open position by placing a gauze between the tip.
- When using pouches, place the handle of the instrument into the end of the bag that will be opened first.
- When using autoclave paper, use specialized autoclave tape to seal the package, in addition to placing an indicator strip inside with the instrument.
- Label the outside with the date, the time, initials, and the instrument that it contains.

Sterilization indicators change colors only when sterilization is achieved by steam reaching its optimum temperature for the required length of time. Two types of sterilization indicators are chemical and biologic. Lines on autoclave tape will turn black when sterilization is achieved. Autoclave pouches have indicator arrows that change colors to indicate sterilization is achieved.

Chemical sterilization can also be used but is not considered practical in an ambulatory health care facility. This is used for instruments that cannot tolerate the high temperatures of the autoclave. The chemicals used must be mixed precisely to the instructions on the bottle and marked with a preparation and expiration date. Contents requiring sterilization must be submerged in the chemical bath for 8 hours with a closed lid. Once completed, the items are removed with forceps and rinsed with water until all chemicals are removed. These items cannot be wrapped and are no longer considered sterile once out of the chemical fluid. This process is good for items such as endoscopes, which would be damaged if autoclaved.

Once an item is sterilized, specific handling must occur so the item is not contaminated.

To ensure equipment sterility:

- The CDC no longer identifies a specific timeframe to use sterilized items, but most facilities have specific protocols to follow, such as using oldest to newest sterilized items. As a rule, double-layer fabric or paper-wrapped packages are considered sterile for 30 days.
- Packages should be stored in a dry, covered area, and confirm the item does not show signs of watermarks.
- Packages should be inspected, after they are completely dry, to ensure they are intact and do not have any tears or punctures.

CHALLENGE

1. To ensure all equipment is sterilized, which of the following is the recommended temperature for the autoclave?
   A. 200° F
   B. 212° F
   C. 220° F
   D. 250° F

   D is correct. To ensure sterilization of equipment has occurred, the autoclave must be at 250 to 270° F. This guarantees destruction of all organisms.

2. What two things need to be completed prior to sterilization?

   Sanitization and disinfection

BIOHAZARD MATERIALS

Dispose of Biohazardous Materials

To make sure certain biohazardous materials do not harm the environment or individuals, OSHA has set specific laws to specify how you must handle infectious waste according to the OSHA Bloodborne Pathogens Standard of 1991. Although OSHA enforces these laws, it is up to the medical facility to guarantee the laws are being followed. The use of PPE and *Safety Data Sheets* (SDSs) provides the health care professional with the tools and resources to maintain a safe clinical work environment. The proper identification of any potentially infectious waste materials and disposal of contaminated material is another step in preventing the spread of infectious material.

Cautions Related to Chemicals

The medical assistant must be familiar with all chemicals used in the office and proper precautions when using them. Some general precautions to keep in mind include wearing protective eyewear and other PPE to prevent damage to skin. Also, be careful when carrying chemicals by using both hands and working in a well-ventilated area. An eye wash station should be accessible in the lab. It is recommended that staff knows the location of the eyewash station and how to properly use it. Eyewash stations should be inspected monthly to ensure they are in proper working order.

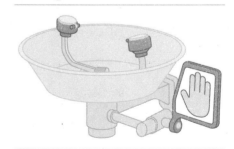

6.10 Eye Wash Station

Safety Data Sheets. Sheets that provide information on the hazards and actions necessary when working with specific chemicals.

Disposal Methods

Any item that likely contains infectious waste material must be disposed of properly in a biohazard waste container. Some examples of items are blood products, bodily fluids, sharp instruments, gauze containing body fluids, and contaminated gloves. There are a variety of biohazard waste containers that are used for different infectious waste materials.

6.11 Disposal Methods

BIOHAZARD WASTE CONTAINER	USE
Biohazard waste bag	Items contaminated with blood/bodily fluids such as gloves, gauze, and dressings
Biohazard waste box	Items contaminated with blood/bodily fluids such as table covers and disposable gowns
Biohazard sharps container	Needles, lancets, and sharp objects

The following guidelines must be followed when handling biohazard materials.

- Wear proper PPE, including gloves.
- Immediately place biohazard materials in appropriate receptacle.
- Keep containers upright and closed.
- Drop items into sharps containers and avoid pushing them in.
- Discard of disposable sharps container when it has reached the fill line.

Never recap needles. Rather, place them in a sharps container immediately after use on a patient. Any item that has sharp edges or blades, such as a scalpel, should also be disposed of in a sharps container. Sharps containers must be made of a puncture-proof, leak-proof material and be labeled with the biohazard symbol. When a sharps container is two-thirds full, the container should be sealed and placed in the designated area for disposal. Gloves, gauze, bandages, and other items that do not have sharp edges or contain needles should be placed in a biohazard bag, which is leak-proof and labeled with the biohazard symbol. If biohazardous waste contaminates the outside of the biohazard bag or the integrity of the bag is compromised, it must be double bagged.

6.12 Biohazard Symbol

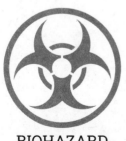

6.13 Sharps Container

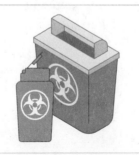

6.14 Biohazard Container

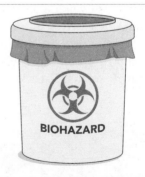

All biohazard waste must be identified with the biohazard symbol and must be contained. All bags used to collect infectious material must be made of an impermeable polyethylene or polypropylene material. A lid must be present on all boxes or receptacles and replaced after each use. A specialized waste management company is often used for the pick-up and disposal of biohazard material from medical facilities. These agencies also must abide by OSHA standards regarding biohazard material handling and disposal.

Personal Protective Equipment

Employers must provide PPE to all employees when there is a potential for exposure to blood or body fluids. It is the employee's responsibility to use the PPE when contact with blood or body fluids is anticipated. This helps reduce the risk of contact with blood or body fluids and helps break the cycle of infection. Examples of PPE include gloves, goggles, face shields, and gowns. Gloves should be worn in the following medical office tasks.

- Encountering blood, body fluids, or other potentially infectious materials (OPIM)
- Handling anything contaminated with blood or body fluids
- Performing injections or venipuncture
- Assisting a provider with a surgical procedure
- Handling blood specimens or any body fluids
- Cleaning up body fluids or blood

If an employee is allergic to latex or the powder used in the gloves provided, the employer must provide hypoallergenic or powder-free gloves at no expense to the employee. However, most organizations have replaced all latex gloves and use nitrile, powder-free gloves.

CHALLENGE

1. Match the contaminated item with the correct biohazard waste container.

ITEM	WASTE CONTAINER
A. Venipuncture needle	1. Biohazard waste bag
B. Contaminated gauze	2. Biohazard waste box
C. Contaminated disposable gown	3. Biohazard sharps container

A: 3, B: 1, C: 2
All sharp objects, including venipuncture needles, must be disposed of in a sharps container to minimize the risk of a needlestick. Contaminated gauze must be placed in a biohazard waste bag, and disposable gowns must be placed in a biohazard waste box.

FOLLOW POST-EXPOSURE GUIDELINES (NEEDLE SAFETY GUIDELINES, USE OF EYEWASH STATIONS)

Exposure Control Plan

It is the responsibility of the employer to have an exposure control plan in place and available for all employees. The exposure control plan needs to be updated annually and whenever procedures that require exposure to potentially contaminated material are added or changed. The plan should be reviewed with each employee upon hiring and annually thereafter. All employees and OSHA authorities should have access to the exposure control plans. The exposure control plan covers all scenarios regarding emergency procedures specific to their practice.

Some items included in the plan are the following.

6.15 Exposure Control Plan

ITEM	EXAMPLE
Engineering controls	Needles with safety devices, sharps disposable containers, and needless systems
Workplace controls	Handwashing procedures, disposal of sharps, and packaging lab specimens
PPE	Proper PPE such as gloves, gowns, face masks, and goggles
Hepatitis B vaccinations	Provided to employees that may have exposure to bloodborne pathogens within 10 days of employment at no cost
Post-exposure follow-up	Provided post-exposure follow-up for any employee who encounters an exposure incident at work at no cost
Labels and signs to communicate hazards	Warning labels posted to containers, refrigerators, and freezers used to store blood or other infectious materials
Information and training to employees	Regular training to cover bloodborne pathogens and post-exposure procedures
Documented employee medical training and records	Logged and maintained medical and training records of each employee

Each employer should have a system in place for reporting any exposures and assess the exposure risk. With exposure to blood, the CDC recommends to immediately wash the area that was cut or punctured by a needle with soap and water, flush any splashes to the face with water, or irrigate the eyes with an eye wash station or clean water. Next, the exposure needs to be reported to the immediate supervisor, and an incident exposure form must be filled out.

It is estimated that half a million exposures occur each year when handling contaminated sharps. To help prevent this, needles should never be recapped, and needles with safety devices should be used. Once finished with a needle, it should be immediately placed in a puncture-proof biohazard container.

---

engineering controls. Devices used to isolate or remove the bloodborne pathogen hazard from the workplace.

workplace controls. Practices in the workplace that reduce the chances of exposure by changing or mandating the way a task is performed.

Steps to follow after an exposure include the following.

- Wash or flush exposed area with water. For needlesticks, wash with soap and water.
- Report immediately to supervisor.
- Employee involved in the incident must receive a medical evaluation. All information must remain confidential, and documentation must be kept for the duration of employment plus 30 years.
- Complete an incident exposure form.
- Vaccination is offered for hepatitis B.
- Health care provider provides copy of written opinion within 15 days of evaluation.
- Employee receives health counseling.

The CDC has developed a checklist to ensure that facilities have proper policies and procedures in place and have adequate PPE and supplies to prevent infection or accidental exposure.

Logs (Maintenance, Equipment Servicing, Temperature, Quality Control)

The MA must complete and maintain various logs in a medical office. Some of those would be for maintenance of equipment, equipment servicing, temperature logs of refrigerator and freezers, and any additional *quality control (QC)* measures.

Refrigerator temperatures should always be maintained between 36° F and 46° F. This guarantees test kits, blood specimens, vaccinations, and other stored materials are not out of date. Daily temperatures for both refrigerators and freezers must be measured and logged where medications and vaccinations are stored to verify the required temperatures are maintained.

Quality control is performed to ensure accuracy of tests being performed. A laboratory must follow certain procedures to stay in compliance with quality control standards.

- Calibration: In accordance with the manufacturer's guidelines, equipment used to test patient specimens must be calibrated regularly.
- Control samples: Used to ensure accuracy of a test prior to running a patient sample. Depending on the test, it can be used before each patient sample is processed or every time a new test package is opened.
- Reagent control: Run every time new testing products or supplies are opened. This can include staining materials and reagents such as urinalysis test strips.
- Maintenance: In accordance with the manufacturer's guidelines, equipment should be routinely maintained, and any work performed should be logged.
- Documentation: Document all procedures with quality control log, equipment maintenance log, reagent control log, and temperature log.

quality control (QC). Steps performed to ensure the reliability of test results through detecting and eliminating error.

CHALLENGE

1. Which of the following are when an exposure control plan should be reviewed with an employee? (Select all that apply.)
   A. Every 4 years
   B. Annually
   C. Semi-annually
   D. Upon hire

   B and D are correct. Exposure control plans should be reviewed when an employee is hired and annually.

2. Order the steps following an exposure to a needlestick in the correct sequence.
   A. Employee receives health counseling.
   B. Employee receives medical evaluation.
   C. Report incident immediately to supervisor.
   D. Complete an incident exposure form.
   E. Wash affected area with soap and water.

   *E, C, B, D, A
   The correct sequence is wash affected area with soap and water, report the incident immediately to supervisor, employee receives medical evaluation, complete an incident exposure form, and employee receives health counseling.*

WRAP-UP

From handwashing to equipment sterilization, medical assistants play a vital role in successful infection control within the clinical setting. Breaking the cycle of infection is key to reducing the number of pathogenic transmissions. The main goal of infection control is to reduce and eliminate the transmission of infectious agents. By accomplishing this goal, patients, staff, and the community are safer. Each employer needs to ensure its employees are given the necessary training and tools to carry out the goal of infection control in the workplace. However, it is the employee's responsibility to take appropriate action to assure the best practices are carried out in each situation.

CHAPTER 7
Point-of-Care Testing and Laboratory Procedures

OVERVIEW

Laboratory testing is the science that applies *clinical laboratory testing* science to the care and diagnosis of patients. Patient specimens are collected and processed in either a laboratory or an ambulatory care facility. A specimen can include a sample obtained from body fluid, a waste product, or tissue collected for analysis. Once the specimen has reached the laboratory, it will be processed and directed to the correct department. Each department in the laboratory will analyze and evaluate the specimen based on a specific test ordered by the provider. The tests that are ordered can be performed manually (by hand) or by a variety of specialized automated instruments. Once the tests are completed, the results will be reported to the provider.

Point-of-care testing, specimen collection, and performance of screening procedures are other important aspects of the medical assisting scope of practice. Patient education and preparation, as well as proper specimen handling, are imperative to ensure accurate results. This chapter focuses on testing and other screening procedures classified as "waived testing" by the *Clinical Laboratory Improvement Amendments (CLIA)*.

Objectives

Upon completion of this chapter, you should be able to

- Collect nonblood specimens (for example, urine, stool, cultures, sputum).
- Perform CLIA-waived testing.
- Recognize, document, and report in-range and out-of-range laboratory and test values.
- Match and label specimen to patient and completed requisition.
- Process, handle, and transport collected specimens.
- Perform vision and hearing tests.
- Perform allergy testing.
- Perform spirometry/pulmonary function tests (electronic or manual).
- Identify common testing errors leading to testing discrepancies or inaccurate results.

LABORATORY PROCEDURES

Medical laboratories are found in hospitals, ambulatory care facilities, public health departments, health maintenance organizations, and referral laboratories. These clinical laboratories are often staffed by a director, certified medical technologists (MTs), certified medical laboratory technicians (MLTs), medical laboratory assistants (MLAs), certified clinical medical assistants (CCMAs), and phlebotomists. In ambulatory medical laboratories, medical assistants (MAs) are trained to properly collect specimens that are sent to outside reference laboratories for testing. These tests are used to document the health of the patients, screen patients for disease and conditions, help diagnose a medical disease, and help the provider decide the most appropriate treatment to monitor the effects of a treatment or medication and progression of a disease.

clinical laboratory testing. Testing used in conjunction with health history and physical examination to provide essential data for the diagnosis and management of a patient's condition.

Clinical Laboratory Improvement Amendments (CLIA). A 1988 amendment that regulates federal standards that apply to all clinical laboratory testing performed on humans in the United States.

Laboratory Requisitions and Documenting Specimen Collection

Lab requisitions are required whenever sending specimens to be tested at an outside laboratory. Requisitions that are not accurately completed can result in a rejected specimen, which causes patient dissatisfaction and possible delays in treatments.

Properly label all collected specimens and ensure the specimens are matched with the correct lab requisition and placed in a specimen collection pouch for transport. Incorrect specimen labeling contributes to laboratory error more than any other factor. Label specimen containers with the patient's name and date of birth, date and time of collection, and medical assistant's initials. Label the container of a specimen and not a lid, which could mistakenly be put on another specimen container. Verify the labels against the patient's health record and the lab order before sending the specimen to the lab for processing.

Information Required on Completed Requisition

Whether the laboratory requisition form is electronic or paper, there are specific parts included. The first part of the requisition includes patient demographic information. If the requisition is computer-generated, this information should populate automatically. A provider's signature or authentication that the provider ordered the lab work is also present on all requisitions. The specific tests ordered by the provider must be identified and marked. These are often organized on the laboratory requisition based on the clinical laboratory department that will perform the test. The source of the specimen, as well as the date and time of specimen collection and diagnosis code related to the medical necessity of the test ordered, is also required on the requisition.

Departments in Clinical Laboratory

- Urinalysis: Includes the physical, chemical, and microscopic examination of urine
- *Hematology*: Blood cell counts that determine RBCs, WBCs, and platelets of a blood specimen
- Chemistry: Chemicals found in blood, cerebrospinal fluid, urine, joint fluid, lipid profiles (such as triglycerides, total **cholesterol**, HDL, and LDL), and fasting glucose
- *Microbiology*: Studying bacteria, fungi, parasites, yeasts, and viruses; specimens can include urine, blood, sputum, cerebrospinal fluid, stool, and wound material
- *Cytology*: Microscope examination of cells for diagnostic purposes
- Blood bank: Processes and stores blood and blood products for transfusion and blood disorder treatments

Select the appropriate laboratory tests on the laboratory requisition based on the provider's orders. Some urine screenings require documentation of the urine temperature at the time of specimen collection. Always confirm with the patient if they have fasted (not consumed food or liquids) when required for specific blood tests.

---

hematology. Study of cause, prognosis, treatment, and prevention of diseases related to blood.

cholesterol. A waxy, fatlike substance made by the liver.

microbiology. Study of all living organisms that are too small to be visible by the naked eye.

cytology. Microscope examination of cells to identify a diagnosis.

Demographic Information

Demographic accuracy on the requisition form is important for billing purposes and patient identification. Requisition information can vary based on the organization, but typical demographic information found on a requisition includes the following.

- Patient name
- Address
- Date of birth
- Sex
- Telephone number
- Insurance information
- Provider information
- Diagnosis code or indications for testing
- Order date

CHALLENGE

1. Identify items that must be included on a specimen container label.

   Specimen containers should be labeled with the patient's name and date of birth, date and time of collection, and medical assistant's initials.

2. Match the laboratory test to the correct laboratory department.

TEST	DEPARTMENT
A. Fasting glucose	1. Urinalysis
B. White blood cell count	2. Chemistry
C. Identifying bacteria in a specimen	3. Microbiology
D. Physical and chemical examination of specimen	4. Blood bank
E. Typing and screening of blood sample	5. Hematology

A: 2; B; 5; C: 3; D: 1; E: 4.
Fasting glucose is tested in the chemistry department. White blood cell count is tested in hematology. Identifying bacteria in a specimen is performed in microbiology. A physical and chemical examination of a specimen is tested in urinalysis. Blood typing and screening are tested in the blood bank.

SPECIMEN COLLECTION

Point-of-Care Testing

Various tests related to chemistry, immunology, microbiology, and hematology are identified as CLIA-waived and easily performed in provider office laboratories. The following are common point-of-care tests.

Pregnancy Testing

Urine or blood is screened for the presence of **human chorionic gonadotropin (hCG)** antibodies. For the purpose of point-of-care testing, a urine sample is obtained to evaluate for the presence of hCG.

7.1 Pregnancy Test Results

1. Place test strip into sample for 5-10 seconds.

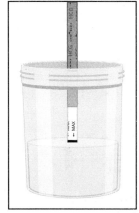

2. Place test strip on flat, dry surface and wait 5 minutes.

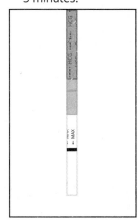

3. Read as:
   1 line – not pregnant,
   2 lines – pregnant

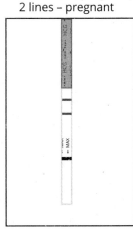

human chorionic gonadotropin (hCG). Hormone secreted by the placenta during pregnancy.

CHAPTER 7: POINT-OF-CARE TESTING AND LABORATORY PROCEDURES
Specimen Collection

Rapid Streptococcus Testing

Throat swabs are obtained to screen for group A streptococcus. Both sides of the posterior throat/tonsil area are swabbed and tested for the presence of the group A antigen.

Dipstick, Tablet, or Multi-Stick Urinalysis

The urinalysis is a screening tool for *analytes* that are excreted in the urine. The urine sample is performed and tested with a reagent strip.

Hemoglobin

A machine is used to screen for the oxygen-carrying protein in whole blood, performed using capillary blood from a fingerstick (capillary puncture).

Spun Hematocrit

Fingerstick (capillary puncture) collection of blood is obtained in microcapillary tubes, which are centrifuged and evaluated for the percentage of red blood cells.

Blood Glucose

Whole blood is analyzed in a glucometer for a quantitative glucose level and is a screening test for diabetes, performed using capillary blood from a fingerstick.

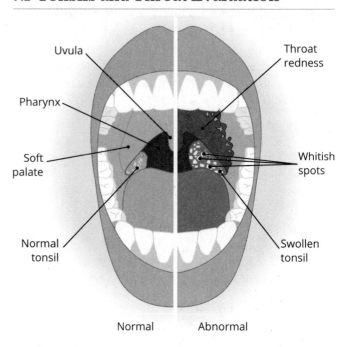

7.2 Tonsils and Throat Evaluation

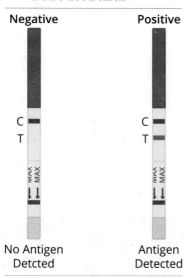

7.3 Streptococcus Test Results

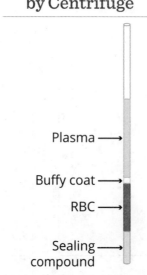

7.4 Components of Blood Separated by Centrifuge

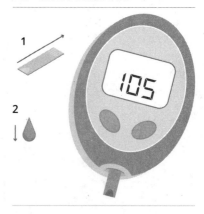

7.5 Glucometer

analytes. A substance or chemical that is being identified and measured.

Hemoglobin A1C

This capillary blood test determines the approximate control of blood glucose levels over a 3-month period.

Cholesterol Testing

Lipids are evaluated from a capillary blood sample. The sample is placed on a reagent strip and analyzed in a cholesterol testing machine.

Helicobacter Pylori

A whole blood sample can screen for the presence of *H. pylori* antibodies.

Mononucleosis Screening

This screening tool tests for the presence of the Epstein-Barr virus in a capillary blood sample.

7.6 Capillary Puncture

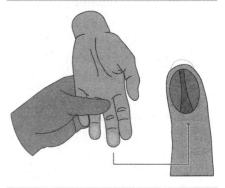

7.7 Results of H. Pylori Screening

7.8 Screening for Epstein-Barr Virus

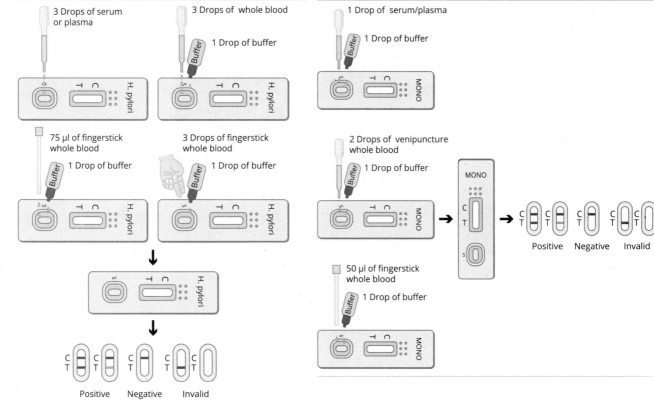

Helicobacter pylori. Type of bacteria that infects the digestive tract.

mononucleosis. Contagious virus that is spread through saliva, also known as mono, most commonly caused by the Epstein-Barr virus.

Nasal Swab Specimen for Influenza Types A and B

This screening is a *qualitative* test for multiple influenza antigens using a swab that is inserted into the nostril to obtain the sample specimen.

Drug Testing

Substances such as recreational drugs and medications can be detected in urine and blood samples.

Fecal Occult Blood

This test is performed to screen for hidden blood in the stool. This test is performed with a fecal occult blood testing kit using the patient's stool specimen.

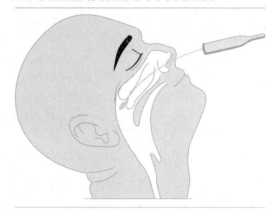

7.9 Nasal Swab Procedure

CLIA-Waived Testing

The Food and Drug Administration (FDA) requires that all testing performed in all testing facilities meet federal guidelines. It also determines the complexity of the tests performed in the laboratory. Ambulatory care centers typically perform CLIA-waived testing, which is the simplest form of testing of all laboratory procedures. Medical assistants are trained in CLIA-waived testing and may perform these tests per the provider's request.

CLIA-Waived Testing Regulations

CLIA was established in 1988 to ensure the quality of diagnostic testing through laboratory regulations. There are three designations for laboratory testing based on complexity.

- CLIA-waived is the most common designation for ambulatory care and is the lowest level of complexity. These tests could be performed in the home environment or easily conducted in the medical office with minimal risk of incorrect results. They pose no reasonable risk of harm to the patient if the tests are performed incorrectly.

- Moderate- and high-complexity tests are considered nonwaived. Labs performing these tests must have a CLIA certificate and undergo inspections to ensure standards are being met. These tests are typically performed in a reference or hospital laboratory.

Some providers in the ambulatory care setting choose to view some specimens microscopically. Although this is considered a form of moderate-complexity testing, CLIA approves provider-performed microscopy procedures for microscopic screening of some specimens, such as urine or body excretions. This allows the provider to develop a preliminary diagnosis and begin treatment as warranted.

---

qualitative. Identifying or measuring by the quality of something rather than its quantity.

Quality Controls

The importance of quality cannot be understated in maximizing accuracy and patient safety. *Quality assurance (QA)* is comprehensive and relates to policies and procedures that must be implemented for the reliability of test results.

For example, reviewing the expiration date of urine reagent strips is a means of quality control, whereas policies related to rotating stock to put the newest containers in the back of the storage area is a quality assurance measure.

Also, checking the temperature of the laboratory refrigerator and documenting it on a log is a quality control measure. The policy of checking the temperature and maintaining it between 2° C and 8° C (35° F and 46° F) is a quality assurance measure.

Specimen Collection Techniques and Requirements

Remember the following when collecting specimens.

- Collect the specimen at the appropriate time.
- Collect the specimen from the site of suspected infection.
- Minimize transport time to a reference lab.
- Collect the appropriate quantity.
- Use the appropriate containers and label them accordingly.

Match and Label Specimen to Patient and Completed Requisition

It is the responsibility of the medical assistant to properly confirm that all collected specimens match the correct lab requisition or order prior to transport to the laboratory. Sending specimen containers that do not coincide with the same patient's laboratory request form contributes to delayed patient diagnosis and treatment and also laboratory errors.

Collect Nonblood Specimens

Collection of Urine Specimens

Urine is the most commonly tested specimen in an ambulatory care setting. There are various means of collecting urine specimens.

Random Urine

This sample can be collected at any time of the day and is used for screening purposes. The patient urinates in a clean, nonsterile container.

First Morning Specimen

The patient collects their first urine specimen of the morning in a clean container. This specimen is more concentrated and is often used for pregnancy testing or when other analytes (protein, nitrites) need to be evaluated.

7.10 Take Note

Quality control (QC) is included in quality assurance but is more specific; it is related to test reliability and accuracy while attempting to uncover errors and eliminate them.

---

quality assurance (QA). Maintenance of a desired level of quality related to a service or piece of equipment.

quality control (QC). Steps performed to ensure the reliability of test results through detecting and eliminating error.

Clean-Catch Midstream

The patient cleanses the genitalia area using three moist antiseptic wipes. Females will cleanse each side and the middle of the urinary meatus from front to back using a separate wipe for each passage. Males will cleanse each side of the glans penis and across the middle using a separate wipe for each passage. The patient will begin by urinating in the toilet, then pause and collect the rest of the urine specimen in a sterile container or until it is adequately filled. This specimen is used for cultures or when a noncontaminated specimen is required.

24-Hour Sample

This method uses a large container with preservatives. The patient discards their first morning urine specimen and collects all remaining urination specimens for the next 24 hours, including the first morning void of the second day. This type of collection is important in the *quantitative* analysis of components such as protein when analyzing kidney function. It is also used to analyze substances that are sporadically released into the urine over a 24-hour period.

Catheterized Collection

This method is used when a sterile urine sample is needed or if patients are unable to provide a specimen on their own. It involves insertion of a sterile tube (catheter) through the urethra into the bladder. The provider or nurse performs this procedure, with the medical assistant prepping the patient and assisting, if needed.

Collection of Stool Specimens

A fecal occult blood test requires a stool specimen collection to screen for the presence of hidden blood, which can indicate the presence of disease or gastrointestinal bleeding.

Instruct the patient on medications and foods to avoid for three days prior to obtaining the specimen. Patients should avoid red meats or dyes, aspirin or aspirin products, vitamin C, and iron supplements because these could create false-positive *fecal occult blood tests (FOBT)*.

Collecting Specimens for Cultures

Specimens for cultures are always collected in sterile containers. Take precautions to avoid touching the insides of lids, swabs, or containers, which could contaminate the specimen. If the specimen is not properly collected, the identification of the causative agent might not occur, and proper treatment cannot be started.

7.11 Take Note

Correct patient instructions are imperative to ensure that false positives do not occur.

7.12 Fecal Occult Blood Testing

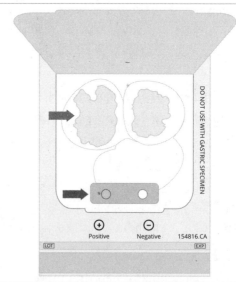

---

quantitative. Related to measuring the amount of something.

fecal occult blood test (FOBT). A lab test used to check stool samples for hidden (occult) blood.

CHAPTER 7: POINT-OF-CARE TESTING AND LABORATORY PROCEDURES
Specimen Processing and Transportation

CHALLENGE

1. Which of the following category of tests is most often offered in a laboratory at a provider's office?
   A. Waived
   B. Moderate complexity
   C. High complexity
   D. Nonwaived

   A is correct. CLIA-waived is the most common designation for ambulatory care and is the lowest level of complexity. These tests could be performed in the home environment or easily conducted in the medical office.

2. Which of the following number of antiseptic wipes will be provided for a female patient when instructing them to obtain a clean catch, midstream urine specimen?
   A. One
   B. Two
   C. Three
   D. Four

   C is correct. Female patients use three antiseptic towelettes to clean the perineal area by spreading the labia and wiping front to back. Wipe with the first towelette on one side and discard it. Wipe with the second towelette on the other side and discard it. Wipe with the third towelette down the middle and discard it.

3. Based on your understanding of CLIA-waived test, summarize at least five examples an MA would commonly perform, along with their function.

   Pregnancy testing: Urine is screened for the presence of human chorionic gonadotropin (hCG) antibodies. Rapid strep testing: Throat swabs are obtained to screen for group B streptococcus. Dipstick, tablet, or multi-stick urinalysis: The urinalysis is a screening tool for analytes that are excreted in the urine. Hemoglobin: A machine is used to screen for the oxygen-carrying protein in whole blood, performed using capillary blood from a fingerstick (capillary puncture). Spun hematocrit: Fingerstick collection of blood in microcapillary tubes is centrifuged and evaluated for the percentage of red blood cells. Blood glucose: Whole blood is analyzed in a glucometer for a quantitative glucose level and is a screening test for diabetes, performed using capillary blood from a fingerstick (capillary puncture). Hemoglobin A1C: This capillary blood test shows blood sugar control over an approximate 3-month period. Cholesterol testing: Lipids are evaluated using capillary blood. Helicobacter pylori: A blood sample screens for H. pylori, which is the main cause of gastric ulcers. Mononucleosis screening: This screening tool tests for the presence of the Epstein-Barr virus in capillary blood. Nasal smear for influenza types A and B: This screening is a qualitative test for influenza antigens using a swab that is inserted into the nostril. Drug testing: Substances can be detected in urine and blood samples. Fecal occult blood: This test is performed to screen for hidden blood in the stool.

SPECIMEN PROCESSING AND TRANSPORTATION

The role of the medical assistant is to obtain, process, and prepare the specimen for transportation. When obtaining and processing a specimen, consider all specimens as potentially infectious. Take precautions to protect yourself, the patient, and others in the environment from exposure to disease-causing micro-organisms. Follow standard precautions when handling, processing, and transporting specimens.

Requirements for Transportation, Diagnosis, Storage, and Disposal of Specimens

Proper preservation and storage need to be identified when handling specimens.

Process, Handle, and Transport Collected Specimens

Take precautions to avoid contamination of specimens that are being prepared for transport and testing. Proper processing, handling, and transporting of specimens are also necessary for testing validity and accuracy of results. Patient identifiers are crucial for proper identification of patients to ensure accurate and integral testing. The following are examples of patient identifiers.

- Name
- Assigned identification number (e.g., medical record number)
- Date of birth
- Phone number
- Address

Handwashing is the most effective means of preventing the spread of infection, and personal protective equipment should be used based on the specimen being handled. The most common types of specimens in the ambulatory care setting are blood, urine, and swab samples.

Specimens might need to be processed prior to transport to maintain the integrity of the specimen. Something as simple as making sure that a swabbed specimen is moist by breaking the fluid chamber within the specimen container is an example of a processing technique to achieve accurate results. Urine specimens for microscopic analysis can require centrifuging prior to transport with the supernatant fluid removed. Centrifuging is also done to some blood samples based on the test that is ordered.

7.13 Biohazard Transport Bag

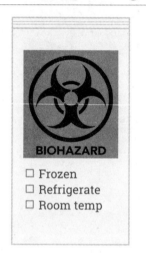

- ☐ Frozen
- ☐ Refrigerate
- ☐ Room temp

Always follow proper office procedure and reference the lab manual for proper handling of specimens. For example, a urine sample that requires testing for bilirubin needs special handling to protect the specimen from light, which would affect the accuracy of the testing. For this situation, a dark container is required for the specimen. Urine samples also need to be tested within one hour of collection, and if not tested, the specimen must be refrigerated. When urine is left sitting out longer than an hour, it can allow bacteria to grow and cause the test to have inaccurate results. Refrigerating helps prevent the bacteria from growing.

Appropriate packaging for specimen transport is imperative. Each specimen must have a clear plastic bag with a zip closure and dual pockets, which allows for the separation of the specimen and lab requisition. If the container has the potential to break or crack, padding and protection from leakage must occur. Wrapping the container in absorbent material and placing the item in a biohazard bag are added safety measures to ensure that the outside of the package does not get contaminated. Whenever specimens are transported via mail, biohazard identification on the outside of the package alerts handlers of a potentially infectious agent within the package.

Chain of Custody

Occasionally, a medical assistant may need to obtain a urine specimen for drug and alcohol analysis. These are considered legal specimens because they may be used in a court of law and must be handled carefully. The specimen has to be placed into a specimen bag that is permanently sealed until it is opened for analysis. The seal will ensure that there has been no tampering with the bag's contents prior to reaching the lab for testing.

7.14 Take Note

A chain of custody must be established to document the handling of the specimen. Everyone who handles the specimen, including the patient being tested, must sign the chain of custody form.

Supplying the specimen for a drug or alcohol test could be incriminating to the patient; therefore, the procedure needs to be explained thoroughly to the donor, and they need to sign a consent form. The consent form can be part of the chain of custody form. The consent will state the purpose of the test and gives you permission to collect the specimen, prepare it for transport to the laboratory for analysis, and release the results to the agency requesting the test. Copies of the chain of custody form will be distributed to the medical review officer, laboratory, patient, collector, and employer or requesting party.

The donor needs to be aware and informed that medications (both prescription and nonprescription), drugs, and alcohol could show in the test results. Encourage the donor to list any substances that may have been consumed within the last 30 days, indicating the name and amount of what was taken.

The chain of custody form will indicate the source of the specimen. The patient's signature on the consent form states, officially, that they are the same person that provided the sealed specimen to send for laboratory analysis.

Specimens need to be properly disposed of to prevent the spread of infection. Red biohazard waste bags are sufficient for specimen containers that are not breakable. Use sharps containers for anything that could break or splinter. A designated sink is often adequate for the disposal of urine specimens.

Always follow the policies and procedures outlined by the facility and adhere to OSHA standards.

CHALLENGE

1. How should the MA prepare a blood sample for transport to an outside lab?

   Prepare it for transport in the proper container for that type of specimen, according to OSHA regulations. Place the container in a clear plastic bag with a zip closure and dual pockets, with the international biohazard label imprinted in red or orange. The requisition form should be placed in the outside pocket of the bag.

2. The laboratory courier cannot pick up the patient's urine sample for another 4 hr. Which of the following methods will ensure specimen preservation?
   A. Storing the urine at room temperature
   B. Storing the urine in the refrigerator
   C. Storing the urine away from the lights
   D. Storing the urine in the incubator

   B is correct. Storing the urine in the refrigerator will preserve the specimen because it will inhibit the growth of bacteria.

LABORATORY RESULTS

When performing office laboratory testing, the medical assistant should be familiar with the expected values and normal ranges of test results. There can be times when the provider needs to be notified immediately of abnormal results in order to provide immediate patient care or intervention. Even if laboratory testing is not done in the office, a general knowledge of normal values for commonly performed laboratory tests is important. This knowledge will allow the MA to alert the provider of abnormalities and provide education to the patient as directed.

Recognize, Document, and Report Laboratory and Test Values

With the implementation of electronic medical records (EMRs), communication of laboratory tests is expedited through the provider portal. This eliminates the need for the laboratory to deliver a hard copy of the results, often done using a fax machine or a printer system setup with direct access to the laboratory.

In today's health care environment, those offices that do not have a lab interface with their electronic health record systems will need to scan or upload results to the portal.

When providers review results, note the date of the review and the action to be taken. If possible, results should be made accessible to patients for viewing in their EHR. The MA might need to call the patient or mail the results. Ensure the correct address for the patient and verify identity when communicating information over the phone to maintain HIPAA compliance. Do not release any lab results to patients without the provider reviewing and signing off on them first. Miscommunication of laboratory results can have a significant and adverse effect on patients.

CHAPTER 7: POINT-OF-CARE TESTING AND LABORATORY PROCEDURES
Laboratory Results

CLIA requires rapid communication of critical laboratory values. Electronic technology allows laboratories to send electronic alerts to the provider for rapid review. When taking a call from the laboratory with a *critical value*, ensure accuracy of the information by repeating the test results back to the laboratory personnel. After obtaining the information, notify the provider immediately and accurately document the communication and actions taken in the medical record.

7.15 Recognize, Document, and Report Laboratory and Test Values

LABORATORY TEST	SPECIMEN TYPE	TEST INCLUDED	REFERENCE RANGE/RESULTS
Hemoglobin (Hgb)	Hematology Blood specimen	Hgb	Male: 13.5 to 17.5 g/dL Female: 12 to 16 g/dL
Hematocrit (Hct)	Hematology Blood specimen	Hct	Male: 41% to 53% Female: 36% to 46%
Complete Blood Count (CBC)	Hematology Blood specimen	White blood cell count	4,500 to 1,1000/mm^3
		Red blood cell count	Male: 4.5 to 5.9 million/mm^3 Female: 4 to 5.5 million/mm^3
		Platelet count	150,000 to 400,000/mm^3
		Granulocyte ratio	50% to 70% (of all white blood cells)
		Hgb	(See above)
		Hct	(See above)
		MCV	A value score of 80 to 95
Glucose	Chemistry Blood specimen	Glucose	70 to 100 mg/dL (fasting)
Hemoglobin A1C	Hematology Blood	Hemoglobin A1C	Below 5.7%
Cholesterol Cholesterol Panel/Lipid Profile	Chemistry Blood	Total Cholesterol	130 to 200 mg/dL
		LDL	Less than 100 mg/dL
		HDL	Greater than 60 mg/dL
		Triglycerides	40 to 150 mg/dL

critical values. Laboratory results at such variance to the normal value range that a potential life-threatening, pathophysiologic state is occurring. Action must be taken as soon as possible.

hemoglobin (Hgb). Iron-containing oxygen-transport in red blood cells that is responsible for carrying oxygen from the respiratory organs to the rest of the body.

hematocrit (Hct). Volume percentage of red blood cells in blood.

hemoglobin A1c. Identifies blood glucose levels over approximately 3-month period.

Common Testing Errors

Human error is common. Make sure to follow the proper steps to obtaining a specimen to avoid errors that can lead to testing discrepancies and inaccurate results. Mislabeled specimens are a common error impacting laboratory testing.

The following are other errors that often occur.

- Improper instructions for clean-catch urine samples. This could alter the results of the test due to excessive bacteria presence and may result in the need for the patient to provide a new sample.

- Lack of patient adherence. A patient who has not completed proper testing preparation may need to delay their testing, such as when a patient has not fasted for bloodwork requiring fasting.

Preanalytical and Postanalytical Errors

The overall process required for quality assurance in the laboratory is divided into three stages. These three stages must be applied to each test or procedure that is performed in the laboratory. If any of these steps are missed or not performed correctly, quality assurance is broken.

Preanalytical Phase

- The provider orders a test to screen, monitor, or diagnose a patient's condition.
- A written or electronic requisition is filled out, showing the requested tests to be ordered, the specimen required, and where the specimen will be tested.
- The specimen is collected, labeled, and processed.
- The specimen is transported to the laboratory or properly prepared for off-site laboratory pickup.

Errors That Affect the Results

- Inappropriate test request
- Order entry error
- Misidentification of the patient
- Inappropriate container
- Improperly labeling of specimen
- Inadequate sample collection
- Inadequate sample/anticoagulation ratio

Analytic Phase

- Instruments are maintained and calibrated.
- Controls are run and analyzed for each testing method.
- The specimen is tested, and the results are compared with reference ranges.
- The test results are logged and documented in the patient's health record.

Errors That Affect the Results

- Equipment malfunctions (Personnel are required to perform calibration on laboratory equipment. Preventive maintenance schedules must be followed and documented.)
- Sample mix-up
- Unindicated failure of quality controls
- Procedures not properly followed

Postanalytical Phase

- Specimens are properly discarded.
- Analyses of control results are compared over time.
- Patient reports from outside laboratories are logged or documented.
- The provider interprets and signs all lab reports.
- The patient is notified of the results in the office or is contacted by laboratory personnel.
- The final report and all communication with the patient are documented in the patient's health record.

Errors That Affect the Results

- Failure to report
- Improper data entry (Accurate recording is a key responsibility of the medical assistant.)
- Excessive turnaround time

CHALLENGE

1. Documenting control sample results when performing certain laboratory tests on a log is referred to as which of the following?
   A. Quality assurance
   B. CLIA testing
   C. Quality control
   D. Proficiency testing

C is correct. The CLIA mandates documentation as part of the quality control guidelines. Documentation of quality control is performed on laboratory logs and patient charting and includes control sample results.

SPECIALTY TESTING

Tests performed in the medical office that do not fall under point-of-care testing or CLIA-waived tests are considered specialty tests. A medical assistant may be responsible for conducting hearing and vision screening tests or performing respiratory or peak flow testing to aid the provider in assessing pulmonary function. Specialty exams and procedures vary based on the provider and the medical specialty in which they practice.

7.16 Take Note

Adult patients stand 20 feet and identify letters on the Snellen chart, with each row of letters getting progressively smaller in size.

Vision and Hearing Tests

Screening tests are frequently conducted in ambulatory care and provide guidance for treatments or referrals. Vision and hearing screenings are affordable, as well as easily and efficiently conducted.

Vision testing is performed as a noninvasive screening to detect visual abnormalities of the eye. Distance vision is easily tested by using a Snellen chart to evaluate for myopia (nearsightedness).

Children stand 10 feet away from a chart at eye level and identify letters, shapes, or the direction an "E" is pointing. Each eye is tested individually, and then both are tested together. Patients are allowed to wear corrective lenses during the test (which should be documented in the patient's EHR). The last line at which the patient can clearly read the letters or pictures with accuracy is their screening result. Most facilities state that a patient can miss one item and still pass that line. Once the patient misses two items in a single line, the test is complete, using the previous line read without error as the final result.

Vision is recorded as a fraction. The numerator in the fraction represents the distance at which the test is performed (20 feet away from the chart). The denominator represents the distance at which patients with typical vision can read the line. For example, a patient with *20/20 vision* represents typical vision.

Near vision testing screens for presbyopia (a refractive disorder that occurs with the aging eye) or hyperopia (farsightedness) by using the Jaeger eye chart. The patient is asked to read words from various-sized prints on cards that are held 14 to 16 inches away from the eyes (without corrective lenses). Similar to distance vision, each eye is tested individually and then together. The level at which the patient can read the smallest printing clearly and accurately is the final result.

Color Vision Testing

The most common type of color deficiency is a red-green deficiency. Screening is done by testing the patient using 11 color plates within an *Ishihara test* color-plate book. If the patient misses four or more plates, there might be a color deficiency, and further testing is warranted.

Hearing Tests Performed in Ambulatory Care

Hearing screenings can be a valuable tool in detecting hearing loss. These tests use an audiometer to measure hearing acuity at different frequencies. Sound amplitude is measured in decibels (dB), and sound frequency is measured in hertz (Hz).

Tympanometry

Tympanometry records movement of the tympanic membrane, which can be affected by increased pressure in the middle ear. Using a small earbud, eardrum movement can be measured by changing the amount of air pressure applied. This test is valuable for determining the presence of fluid and potential infections in the middle ear. A normal tympanogram produces a peak on the graph, whereas an abnormal tympanogram will produce a flat line.

7.17 Snellen Chart

Line	Acuity
1	20/200
2	20/100
3	20/70
4	20/50
5	20/40
6	20/30
7	20/25
8	20/20
9	
10	
11	

20/20 vision. The ability to see at 20 feet what the average person sees at 20 feet.

Ishihara test. Vision test to assess for color deficiency.

Speech, Tone, and Word Recognition Information

Medical assistants can perform audiometry if patients (especially children) can respond to directions. The patient will wear a set of headphones, and various tones will be played. The patient will be directed to push a button or raise their hand to indicate they hear the tone.

7.18 Scratch Testing (Allergy)

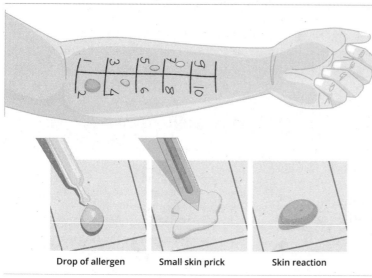

Drop of allergen | Small skin prick | Skin reaction

7.19 Take Note

Generally, the larger the wheal, the more significant the allergy. If a wheal is evaluated less than 15 minutes from time of application, it may not have had enough time to develop a reaction.

7.20 Intradermal Allergy Testing

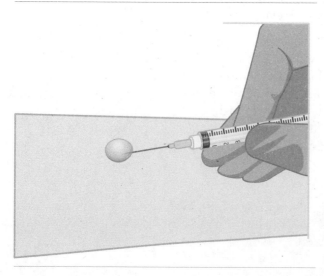

The level of hearing is documented in decibels and the frequency in hertz. An adult who has normal hearing should be able to hear tones below 25 decibels, and a child should be able to hear below 15 decibels.

Allergy Testing

A medical assistant who works in an allergist's office will likely perform allergy testing. Medical assistants in other ambulatory care settings can be responsible for scheduling the referral appointment and need to be aware of how the tests are performed and what the patient should expect in preparation for the testing. Patient education is important to ensure accuracy of skin testing results. Instruct the patient to discontinue the use of antihistamines three days prior to allergy skin testing. Antihistamines block histamine's response time, inhibiting skin testing reactions and possibly producing a false-negative result.

Scratch Test and Intradermal Allergy Test

A diluted allergen is applied to a scratch or prick that has been made on the surface of the patient's skin. The testing is usually conducted on the forearm or upper back. If a wheal occurs in the first 15 minutes, the allergist can identify the substance as a possible allergen and consider further allergy testing to be conducted intradermally.

Intradermal Testing

A diluted allergen is injected intradermally, and the patient is observed. An initial wheal is expected. If the wheal becomes inflamed with induration (raised, hard area), the substance can be identified and confirmed as an allergen.

Spirometry/Pulmonary Function Tests

Spirometry, or *pulmonary function test*, is a noninvasive test that detects the lung's ability to function. It is an automated test that produces a graphic result by measuring how "fast" a patient can move air into and out of the lungs and how "much" air is moved into and out of the lungs.

The patient's demographic factors (age, gender, weight, and height) are used to calculate the predicted respiratory values for a healthy patient. These values are then compared to three measured values that are obtained while the patient is performing the test. Prepare the patient for the procedure, facilitate and document the procedure, and provide results to the provider for interpretation.

The patient should wear loose clothing, be in an upright sitting or standing position, and breathe through the mouth, pursing the lips around the mouthpiece. The medical assistant will likely apply a clip to the patient's nose to avoid nose-breathing during the procedure. The patient should lift the chin slightly and extend the neck a little during the test to reduce breathing resistance. Instruct the patient to "Take the deepest breath possible. Seal your lips around the mouthpiece. Blow as hard and as fast as you can, blowing until you empty the air from your lungs." Proper coaching is essential for yielding the best results from the patient. The procedure is repeated until there are three acceptable maneuvers or attempts.

Patients require pretest preparation for spirometry. This prep includes the following.

- No large meals 2 hours before the test
- No smoking 1 hour before the test
- Discontinuation of the use of bronchodilators or other breathing therapies (inhalers, nebulizers) for at least 6 hours before the test

7.21 Spirometry

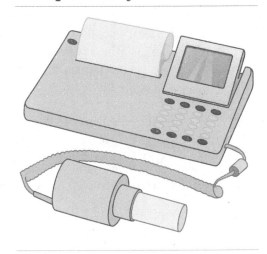

7.22 Spirometry Norms

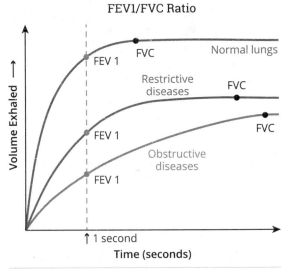

7.23 Expected Values of Pulmonary Function Tests

TEST	EXPECTED VALUE (95% CONFIDENCE INTERVAL)
FEV_1	80% to 120%
FVC	80% to 120%
Absolute FEV_1/FVC ratio	Within 5% of the predicted ratio
TLC	80% to 120%
FRC	75% to 120%
RV	75% to 120%

pulmonary function test. Test to assess lung functioning, which will help assist in the detection and evaluation of pulmonary disease.

CHAPTER 7: POINT-OF-CARE TESTING AND LABORATORY PROCEDURES
Specialty Testing

Peak Flow Rates

This test can be used to monitor lung function at home by the patient. This is especially helpful for patients who have chronic respiratory diseases such as asthma or chronic obstructive pulmonary disease (COPD). The *peak flow meter* measures the forced expiratory volume, which indicates the effectiveness of airflow out of the lungs. A peak flow rating of 80% or better is considered well-controlled and does not require treatment.

Peak flow meters can vary in size and shape depending on the manufacturer, but most are inexpensive.

Patient instructions are the same across models.

- Wear nonrestrictive clothing.
- Begin with the marker at the bottom of the scale on the meter.
- In an upright sitting or standing position, take a deep breath and forcefully blow out of the mouth, which is secure around the mouthpiece of the machine.
- Record the number where the marker is located at the end of the test.
- Repeat the test two to three times and record the results.

Assist the patient by providing instructions, demonstrating the technique, and allowing the patient to practice several times before completing the procedure.

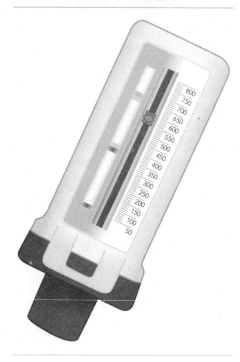

7.24 Peak Flow Meter

CHALLENGE

1. How far from the Snellen eye chart should an adult patient be placed for a visual acuity distance test?
   A. 5 feet
   B. 10 feet
   C. 20 feet
   D. 30 feet

   C is correct. The Snellen chart is placed 20 feet from the patient.

2. To obtain accurate results on spirometry, a patient should be advised to do which of the following?
   A. Lean against the wall.
   B. Use a bronchodilator inhaler prior to the test.
   C. Apply a nose clip.
   D. Exhale until the examiner instructs the patient to inhale.

   C is correct. A nose clip will be applied to provide a more accurate reading to prevent air from coming out the nose.

peak flow meter. Device that measures the amount of air exhaled upon forceful exhalation.

WRAP-UP

The medical assistant performs many diagnostic screenings and laboratory tests as ordered by a provider. Quality assurance is safeguarded through monitoring the quality of patient care that is provided in the medical office. A thorough knowledge of the tests and proper specimen handling requirements, as well as skill in assisting with or performing these tests, is imperative to obtain accurate results and minimize errors. A medical assistant must also have the knowledge of abnormal lab values so that the provider can be informed of abnormalities. Documentation is essential for providing quality patient care, and it is recognized through recording patient records, tracking specimens that leave the medical office, completing laboratory requisition forms, and inventory control. Accuracy in performing screenings and laboratory tests allows the medical assistant to demonstrate competency to the provider and gain the trust and cooperation of the patient. Patient education is imperative, and the patient's understanding of what is expected of them prior to a test is an essential part of a medical assistant's job.

CHAPTER 8
Phlebotomy

OVERVIEW

Phlebotomy is the process of withdrawing blood from a vein for laboratory testing. It is used to assist the provider in the proper diagnosis of disease, as well as monitor a patient's condition, treatment, and/or medication levels. Medical Assistants who complete additional training in this skill can increase their career opportunities. Even for medical assistants who do not intend to perform this procedure, it is important to review and be familiar with phlebotomy techniques as well as the handling and processing of specimens as they apply to the medical assistant's responsibilities and overall scope of work related to health care facilities.

Phlebotomy, typically performed by medical assistants in the ambulatory care setting, requires professionalism, the ability to multi-task, and utilizing appropriate procedure techniques. The provider will rely on the medical assistant to perform this procedure according to laboratory guidelines, including adhering to OSHA bloodborne pathogen standards and sharps safety protocols. Performing phlebotomy procedures effectively and processing specimens correctly ensures the provider receives accurate results to aid in diagnosis, treatment, and maintenance of the patient's condition.

Objectives

Upon completion of this chapter, you should be able to

- Verify order details, identify the patient, and determine whether the patient followed testing preparation instructions.
- Follow procedures for collecting special testing samples (timed specimens, drug levels, blood cultures).
- Recognize preanalytical factors and how to address them.
- Select appropriate supplies for the tests ordered.
- State tube top colors used for chemistry, hematology, coagulation, and microbiology testing; list additives in each tube; and state the order of draw that should be used when drawing multiple tubes.
- Explain how tubes should be positioned following a blood draw, the number of inversions necessary for each tube, and the importance of fill/level ratios.
- Determine the venipuncture method to be used (evacuated tube method, syringe method, butterfly method) and perform the steps of a venipuncture.
- Perform a capillary puncture and determine the proper order of draw when using microcapillary tubes.
- Perform postprocedure care including bandaging procedures and providing discharge instructions.
- Match and label specimen to patient and completed requisition.
- Handle, process, and store blood samples as required for diagnostic purposes.
- Prepare samples for transportation to a reference (outside) laboratory.

PATIENT PREPARATION

Patient preparation instructions are essential for accurate test values. **Fasting** is the most common patient preparation instruction. If a patient is required to fast prior to a procedure, they need to be instructed not to eat or drink anything but water for a certain period of time prior to having their blood drawn. Most fasting blood tests require a 12-hour fast. Presence of certain substances in the blood can be affected by fluid intake and food. For example, patients should fast prior to having a lipid panel. If the patient ate a meal prior to having blood drawn, the test values would likely detect fats from the food and the results would indicate elevated lipid levels. Another possible patient preparation requirement is medication restrictions. Therefore, verify that all preparation guidelines were followed by the patient prior to all phlebotomy procedures. The *laboratory directory* will indicate if any patient preparation is required prior to blood collection. Patients must be asked upon arrival if they have completed the required preparations (if any). If they have not, the MA must explain to the patient that the procedure cannot be performed.

The MA should introduce themselves and approach each patient with a pleasant, warm demeanor. Some patients have little or no issue with the process of blood collection. Other patients have a great deal of anxiety when having blood drawn. In addition to performing the procedure correctly, make patients as comfortable as possible and be sensitive to their needs.

In preparation for the venipuncture, seat the patient in a comfortable, well-lit area. Position the patient with their arm extended out. If a phlebotomy chair with an extended arm rest is not available, have the patient make a fist with the opposite hand and place it behind the elbow of the arm being used for the procedure. This ensures the arm will stay straight and stable during the procedure. There could be difficulty when obtaining blood from children and infants. For pediatric patients, a support person could assist in holding the patient's arm still to avoid injury. Effective communication and accurate skills are necessary when dealing with children.

Question patients about previous blood draws and what, if any, reactions they have had. This can prepare the MA for a possible adverse reaction to a phlebotomy procedure, allowing them to make adjustments or accommodations as needed. For example, if a patient reports that they often faint while having their blood drawn, have the patient in semi-Fowler's position or supine during the procedure to eliminate the risk of a fall.

Explain the procedure and safety precautions to the patient. Be sensitive to verbal and nonverbal communication. If the patient is in obvious distress during the procedure, it may need to be stopped.

---

fasting. The absence of eating food and sometimes drinking.

laboratory directory. A catalog of information regarding laboratory tests with up-to-date test menus; testing information; specimen collection requirements; and storage, preservation, and transportation guidelines.

CHALLENGE

1. Which of the following instructions is often provided to patients that require fasting prior to blood work?
   A. Nothing to eat or drink the morning of blood work
   B. Nothing to eat or drink besides water for 12 hours prior to blood work
   C. Nothing to eat or drink besides water the morning of blood work
   D. Nothing to eat or drink besides water for 24 hours prior to blood work

   B is correct. Fasting is the most common patient preparation instruction. If a patient is required to fast prior to a procedure, they need to be instructed not to eat or drink anything but water for at least 12 hours before having their blood taken. The presence of certain substances in the blood can be affected by fluid intake and food.

2. When having blood work for a lipid panel, how can eating a meal prior to having blood drawn affect blood test results?

   If a patient is required to fast prior to a procedure, they need to be instructed not to eat or drink anything but water for at least 12 hours before having their blood taken. For example, patients should fast prior to having a lipid panel. If the patient just ate a meal prior to having blood drawn, the test values would detect fats from the food and the results would indicate elevated lipid levels.

3. Which of the following would be most appropriate in preparing a patient for phlebotomy?
   A. Ask the patient how they have responded to blood draws previously.
   B. Ask the patient to lie down on the exam table for the procedure.
   C. Inform the patient that the procedure causes pain, but it will be worth it to get the information provided by the tests.
   D. Ask the provider to determine which vein to use.

   A is correct. Asking the patient how they have responded to blood draws in the past will provide valuable information in terms of what to expect. This allows the medical assistant to make accommodations prior to starting the procedure that will help ensure a successful draw and positive patient experience. Typically, patients can remain seated for a blood draw. Asking the patient to lie down is unnecessary unless the patient has a history or concern of fainting during the procedure. Setting expectations prior to beginning the procedure is important, but this should be done in a supportive and warm manner. Telling the patient that their pain does not matter due to the need for the results can instill more fear and anxiety in the patient, which is not helpful. The MA will be responsible for vein selection.

VERIFY ORDER DETAILS

Obtaining the provider's order for laboratory testing is the first step to beginning any phlebotomy procedure. Review the provider's order for blood work to determine what tests need to be completed. Venipuncture procedures should not be performed on patients without a provider's order.

Patient Identifiers, Content of Requisition

Review the laboratory order and complete the laboratory requisition form. If you are unfamiliar with a laboratory test, check the laboratory directory. A laboratory directory manual will identify an up-to-date list of orderable tests and provide information on specimen requirements, patient preparation requirements needed, container type needed, and transport and/or processing requirements. A hard copy can be found in most laboratories, or a digital copy can be found online.

When identifying the patient, use two patient identifiers. These are usually the patient's full name and date of birth.

CHAPTER 8: PHLEBOTOMY
Select Appropriate Supplies for Test(s) Ordered

Each laboratory test will require a laboratory requisition form. Information included on the laboratory requisition form includes the following.

- Ordering provider's name and contact information
- Test and test code (unique to each lab, usually on the requisition or in the laboratory reference manual)
- Diagnosis code that correlates with the tests being ordered (ICD-10)
- Special specimen requirements, such as fasting
- Patient demographics
- Insurance or other billing information

SELECT APPROPRIATE SUPPLIES FOR TEST(S) ORDERED

Supplies and equipment needed for blood draws vary depending on what type of venipuncture procedure is being performed.

In general, supplies needed include the following.

- Alcohol wipes
- Gauze
- Adhesive bandages
- Biohazard sharps container
- PPE, including disposable gloves
- Tourniquet
- Collection tubes
- Needle system

When preparing the needle system, there are three standard options.

Evacuated System

This system consists of a double-pointed needle, a plastic needle holder/adapter, and collection tubes. The collection tube system creates a slight vacuum that helps transport the blood from the vein into the collection tube when penetrated. Using this method helps to obtain multiple tubes of blood with one venipuncture stick. Vacutainer needles are typically 20 to 22 gauge with a needle length of ¾ inch to 1 ½ inches. The length and gauge of the needle will depend on perceived depth of the vein and the size of the patient. This is the most commonly used system.

CHALLENGE

1. While reading the order form, the MA does not recognize one of the tests that needs to be performed. What should the MA do in this situation?

   Always check the laboratory reference manual to determine which tube to use, how many tubes to draw, and other specifics about the test.

2. Which of the following should be included on the lab requisition form?
   A. Insurance information
   B. Visit note
   C. Previous lab values
   D. Signature of medical assistant

   A is correct. Insurance information needs to be included on a lab requisition for the lab to bill the patient appropriately. A visit note and previous lab values are not included on a lab requisition, as it would not provide value. The signature of the medical assistant is not required or included on the lab requisition.

Winged Infusion Set, or Butterfly System

The winged infusion set consists of flexible wings attached to a needle with 5 to 12 inches of flexible tubing that connects the needle to the collection device. This method is best used for patients who have small or fragile veins. This technique tends to cause less trauma or bruising to the patient. Butterfly needles are typically 21 to 23 gauge with a needle length of ½ to ¾ inch. The length of the needle will depend on the size of the patient.

Needle Syringe System

A needle and syringe can be used to draw blood from a vein. This is not ideal because only a small amount of blood can be obtained with this method. One advantage is the amount of suction can be controlled by the plunger of the syringe instead of the vacuum method. Generally, a 16-gauge injection needle and syringe are used with this method.

Parts of the Needle

- *Lumen*: hollow space inside the needle. Also referred to as the gauge. The larger the gauge number, the smaller the diameter.

- *Bevel*: shaft at the end of the needle that creates a point.

Arranging Supplies

All necessary phlebotomy supplies, including the sharps container for needle disposal, should be within reach. During the procedure, hold the needle in the dominant hand and avoid switching hands once the skin has been penetrated. This will require the remaining supplies be set up on the opposite side of the dominant hand.

Arrange the supplies in the order needed to use them, including placing the tubes in the correct order of draw (more information on this later in the chapter).

Whenever possible, place the sharps container on the dominant side as well. This allows the needle to be disposed of properly without the need for crossing the contaminated needle across the body. Always engage needle safety devices immediately after withdrawal from the vein and promptly dispose of the needle in the sharps container.

lumen. Open space in the needle.

bevel. Area around the surface of the needle point.

8.1 Evacuated Tube

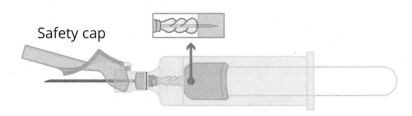

Safety cap

8.2 Winged Blood Collection Set

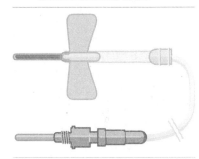

CHALLENGE

1. Match the needle system with the correct attribute.

SYSTEM	ATTRIBUTE
A. Evacuated needle system	1. Allows control over suction
B. Butterfly system	2. Best for drawing from small, fragile veins
C. Syringe needle system	3. Most commonly used system in adults

A: 3; B: 2; C: 1. The evacuated needle system is the most commonly used system in adults. It allows for multiple tubes to be filled in an effective time frame. The butterfly system should be selected when drawing from small, fragile veins. The needles are smaller, and the system is more stable. The syringe needle system should only be used for drawing lesser amounts of blood, as there is greater risk of damage to the vein, but it does allow the phlebotomist more control over the suction when needed.

BLOOD COMPONENTS

Blood is composed of four main components: *plasma*, white cells, red cells, and platelets. Blood plasma contains water, waste products, gases, proteins, and nutrients. White blood cells are responsible for defending the body against bacteria and viruses. Red blood cells are responsible for carrying oxygen to the tissues throughout the body and carbon dioxide from the body to the lungs. Platelets are responsible for limiting the loss of blood when a blood vessel is damaged or leaking.

Types of blood specimens include the following.

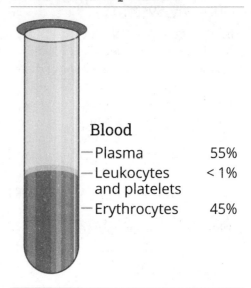

8.3 Blood components

Blood
- Plasma — 55%
- Leukocytes and platelets — < 1%
- Erythrocytes — 45%

Serum

The liquid portion of the blood obtained after a serum sample tube has clotted and centrifuged.

Plasma

The liquid portion of the blood obtained after centrifuging. The blood specimen must be collected in a tube containing anticoagulant. There will be three layers after the sample has been centrifuged: plasma (top layer), buffy coat (middle layer), and red blood cells (bottom layer).

Clotted Blood

This is obtained when blood is drawn in a tube that does not contain an anticoagulant.

Whole Blood

Whole blood is obtained when a tube is used with an anticoagulant, which inhibits blood clotting.

CHALLENGE

1. Which of the following components of blood is responsible for preventing excessive blood loss when a vessel is damaged?
   A. Platelets
   B. Red blood cells
   C. White blood cells
   D. Plasma

   A is correct. Platelets are responsible for limiting the loss of blood when a blood vessel is damaged by creating clots to control bleeding.

---

plasma. The liquid portion of the blood; mainly made of water; contains proteins, electrolytes, gases, some nutrients, and waste products; is required to recover from injury, distribute nutrients, and remove waste from the body.

whole blood. Blood obtained when drawn in a tube that contains an anticoagulant.

DETERMINE ORDER OF DRAW

Vacuum stopper tubes are identified by the color of the top of the tube, which also identifies any additive within the tube. The tubes must be drawn in the proper order to avoid cross-contamination of the additives. If the tubes are not drawn in the correct order, the additives could inadvertently affect laboratory results.

8.4 Take Note
The order of blood tube draw is critically important to avoid errors. During the blood draw process, the additive from one tube can carry over to another and affect test results.

Types of Tubes, Number of Tube Inversions, and Fill Level/Ratios

Vacuum tubes that contain an additive require gentle inversion for mixing of the blood and the additive after they are filled. While inverting the tubes, completely turn the tube upside down and return it to its upright position. The number of required inversions will depend upon the vacuum tube additive. Do not shake or forcefully invert tubes due to the risk of hemolysis.

Tubes should be filled completely. Best practice is to allow blood to fill the tube until blood flow stops. The light blue top tube contains a minimum fill indicator line indicating the minimum amount of blood required for accurate test results. During the collection process, allow blood to fill the tube until the tube has the full, required amount of blood.

Order of Draw for Venipuncture

The commonly used color-top tubes are listed below in the order in which they should be filled. Other color-top tubes are available but are not routinely used in collection. Adhere to the correct order of draw, as it impacts the ability of the specimens to produce accurate results and provide reliable data to aid in diagnosis and management of medical conditions.

8.5 Order of Draw

VACUUM TUBE COLOR	ADDITIVE	LABORATORY USE	NUMBER OF INVERSIONS
Yellow top tube or blood culture bottles	Sodium polyanethol sulfonate; prevents blood from clotting and stabilizes bacterial growth	Blood or body fluid cultures	N/A
Light blue	Sodium citrate; removes calcium to prevent blood from clotting	Coagulation testing	3 to 4
Red	None	Serum test; chemistry studies; blood bank; immunology	5
Red/gray marbled	No anticoagulant but contains silica particles to enhance clot formation; use for serum separation	Serum test; chemistry studies; immunology	5
Green	Heparin: inhibits thrombin formation to prevent clotting	Chemistry test	8
Green/gray marble	Lithium heparin and gel; for plasma separation	Plasma determinations in chemistry studies	8
Lavender	Ethylenediaminetetraacetic acid (EDTA); removes calcium to prevent blood from clotting	Hematology test	8
Gray	Potassium oxalate and sodium fluoride; removes calcium to prevent blood from clotting; fluoride inhibits glycolysis	Chemistry testing, especially glucose and alcohol levels	8 to 10

CHAPTER 8: PHLEBOTOMY
Determine Venipuncture Site Accessibility

CHALLENGE

1. Place the blood tubes below in the correct order of draw.
   A. Red
   B. Green
   C. Lavender
   D. Light Blue

   D, A, B, C. The correct sequence is light blue, red, green, and lavender.

2. How many times should a light blue tube be inverted following blood draw?
   A. 8 to 10
   B. 5 to 6
   C. 3 to 4
   D. 1 to 2

   C is correct. Light blue top tubes should be inverted three to four times.

DETERMINE VENIPUNCTURE SITE ACCESSIBILITY

Selecting a phlebotomy method is based on the condition of the patient's veins, age, skin conditions, and overall health, as well as the professional experience and judgment of the medical assistant. The method chosen should be the one that is most appropriate for each patient while providing the greatest chance for successful blood collection and limiting patient discomfort during and following the procedure.

The preferred vein within the *antecubital* space is the median cubital vein, as this area tends to cause less pain and this vein is the least likely to roll during the procedure. If the median cubital vein is not easily palpated or is covered with scar tissue, the cephalic vein and basilic veins—found on either side of the median cubital vein—are often strong alternatives. Note that these veins have a higher risk of rolling, so the medical assistant must take extra care to anchor the vein during the procedure.

8.6 Veins in the lower arm

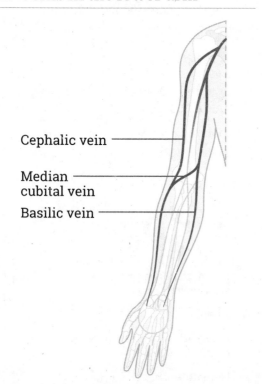

Cephalic vein

Median cubital vein

Basilic vein

If these veins within the antecubital space are inaccessible, the back of the hand, wrist, and foot are also options. Blood draws from the foot should only be performed under the supervision of a provider due to the risk of deep vein thrombosis (DVT). When drawing from the hand, be aware that these veins are the most likely to roll. Additionally, the back of the hand contains many nerves, which can lead to more discomfort for the patient. Reasons for looking at these alternative sites include circumstances in which both antecubital spaces have scars, bruises, or burns or are swollen.

For most healthy adults, the evacuated needle system is best. When drawing from the hand or small/thin veins in the antecubital space, the butterfly method is optimal. When only a small amount of blood is needed from a patient with limited options for draw site, the needle syringe system can be best.

antecubital. The inner or front surface of the forearm at the elbow.

To begin site selection, have the patient extend an arm out and straighten the elbow. Always inspect both arms. Palpate the antecubital area by pushing up and down on the patient's skin. Veins have a bouncy feel. The size, depth, and direction of the vein should be determined. Veins that are highly visible but do not have bounce to them should be avoided, as a successful draw is unlikely.

Tourniquet Application

A tourniquet should be applied to the patient's arm about 3 to 4 inches above the draw site to make the vein easier to palpate and more readily accessible for the blood draw. This is because it impairs blood flow. While the impaired blood flow does promote successful phlebotomy, tourniquets must be used properly to avoid unintended side effects. They should be placed snuggly, but not so tightly that blood flow is completely stopped or severe pain is caused. A tourniquet should not be left in place for longer than 1 minute. The tourniquet should be placed while the phlebotomist is palpating and selecting a site, but then should be removed until it is time to begin the procedure.

Site Restrictions

During site selection, check with the patient regarding possible restrictions due to fistulas, ports, or mastectomy. Avoid drawing blood from the same side of the body in which any of these conditions are present. Each of these medical conditions can require specific blood draw procedures to prevent complications and obtain the best specimen for blood testing. Guidance for phlebotomy procedures should come from the provider and the laboratory that will perform the tests. Exercise caution with patients who have these medical conditions and proceed only within scope of practice and experience level.

Additionally, avoid selecting site locations with scar tissue, injuries, burns, or wounds.

8.7 Take Note

Leaving the tourniquet on longer than 1 min can cause *hemoconcentration* and alter test results.

8.8 Applying a Tourniquet

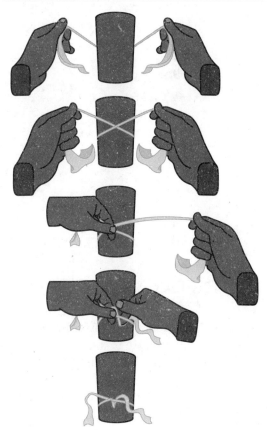

---

hemoconcentration. An increase of formed elements of the blood and a decrease of fluid content.

CHAPTER 8: PHLEBOTOMY
Prepare Site for Venipuncture

Skin Integrity and Venous Sufficiency

Older adult patients have concerns due to physiological changes including muscular atrophy, which changes the integrity of the skin; veins that have lost their elasticity; and venous insufficiency. With loss of venous sufficiency, veins are prone to roll, meaning the needle pushes the vein over rather than puncturing it as intended. When veins lose elasticity, they are fragile and easily damaged by venipuncture. The need to draw blood from the hand increases with older adults.

CHALLENGE

1. What can happen if the tourniquet is left on the patient's arm too long?

   Hemoconcentration can result if the tourniquet is left on the patient's arm for too long. This can affect the results of the test, making them inaccurate.

2. Which of the following is the maximum amount of time a tourniquet should be left in place?
   A. 1 min
   B. 2 min
   C. 5 min
   D. 30 seconds

   A is correct. The tourniquet should not be left on the patient's arm longer than 1 min.

3. The MA is preparing to perform phlebotomy and is assessing the patient for site selection. Based on the findings below, which of the following sites would be the best choice for vein selection?
   A. The basilic vein—found to bounce when palpated
   B. The right median cubital vein—the patient has had a unilateral mastectomy on the right side
   C. The cephalic vein—found to be highly visible; difficult to palpate
   D. The hand—the patient shared that they are extremely sensitive to the pain of blood draws

   A is correct. The best choice for draw site on this patient is the basilic vein due to the bouncy feel with palpation and given the concerns associated with the other sites. Given the patient's mastectomy, the right arm is not able to be considered for site selection. The cephalic vein is not a good option, as it is not easily palpated. Veins that can be seen but not felt are not likely to lead to an effective blood draw. Drawing blood from the hand should only be considered if there are not viable options in the antecubital space or if the patient has a strong preference for the hand to be used. In this case, there is a better option within the antecubital space, and the patient has expressed concerns about pain, which is more severe in the hand.

PREPARE SITE FOR VENIPUNCTURE

Cleanse the site with antiseptic, wiping in an upward-and-downward motion with friction. Allow the site to air-dry, and the tourniquet will be reapplied after the site is dry. Avoid touching the site again after cleansing, even with gloves on. Avoid blowing on the area or waving hands over it to dry the alcohol faster, as this can contaminate the skin.

CHALLENGE

1. Which of the following is an appropriate technique when cleansing the venipuncture site with an antiseptic wipe?
   A. Circular motion from outside to in
   B. Starting at the top, zigzagging down the area
   C. Circular motion from inside to out
   D. Upward and downward motions with friction

   D is correct. Cleanse the site with an antiseptic wipe using upward and downward motions with friction.

PERFORM VENIPUNCTURE

To begin the procedure, anchor the vein by grasping the skin firmly about 2 to 3 inches below the puncture location, holding the skin taut. This ensures the vein is stabilized. When drawing from the arm, insert the needle smoothly and quickly at about a 15- to 30-degree angle depending on the depth and position of the vein. When drawing from the patient's hand, the correct angle of insertion is lower, about 10 to 15 degrees, as the veins in the hand are smaller and thinner. The bevel of the needle should be facing upward.

Once the needle is in place, with the nondominant hand, insert the evacuated stopper tube into the needle holder until blood flow is established. Watch the needle and avoid any additional movement of the needle. Once proper blood flow is established, release the tourniquet with the nondominant hand. When the tube has exhausted the vacuum and the tube is full, remove the tube, gently inverting as necessary. If more than one tube is required, fill up the remaining tubes using the correct order of draw.

Once all needed tubes are full and inverted as needed, apply the gauze over the needle with the nondominant hand, not applying pressure until the needle is out of the patient's arm. With the dominant hand, close the needle safety guard and dispose of the needle in the biohazard sharps container.

CHALLENGE

1. At which of the following angles should the needle be inserted into the patient's arm?
   A. 5 degrees
   B. 15 degrees
   C. 45 degrees
   D. 60 degrees

   B is correct. The needle should be inserted into the skin at a 15- to 30-degree angle for phlebotomy.

2. Of the following sites, where should the vein be anchored on the patient?
   A. 2 to 3 inches above the puncture site
   B. 2 to 3 inches below the puncture site
   C. 1 inch below the puncture site
   D. 1 inch above the puncture site

   B is correct. To begin the procedure, anchor the vein by grasping the skin firmly about 2 to 3 inches below the puncture location, holding the skin taut. This ensures the vein is stabilized.

PERFORM CAPILLARY PUNCTURE

Capillary punctures are performed when only a small amount of blood is needed for testing or when immediate results can be acquired. It is the preferred method of blood collection for infants and young children, but it can also be utilized with adults. Capillary blood is a mixture of blood from arterioles, venules, capillaries, and intracellular and interstitial fluids. Due to this mixed composition, not all testing should be performed using capillary blood.

8.9 Capillary Puncture Supplies

- Gloves
- Automatic retractable lancet
- Disinfectant pads, such as 70% isopropyl alcohol
- Clean gauze pads
- Bandage
- Capillary tube sealer (when capillary tubes are used)
- Biohazard sharps container
- Blood collection device appropriate for the test such as:
  - Micropipette
  - Small glass tube (capillary tube)
  - *Micro-collection devices*
  - Glucometer and testing strip
  - Screening card or paper
  - Plastic testing cartridge or cassette

capillary puncture. The method of acquiring blood from a fingertip or heel.

micro-collection devices. Small plastic tubes designed to collect capillary blood.

Location of Capillary Punctures for Adults and Infants

The preferred puncture site for obtaining a capillary puncture in adults and children is the middle or ring finger of the nondominant hand. This procedure is also commonly referred to as a fingerstick. Perform the puncture slightly off-center, avoiding the central fleshy part of the fingertip, fingernail, and nail bed.

Infant capillary puncture will be performed on the outer edge of the underside of the heel.

Preparing the Site

For the procedure to be successful, the capillaries must have good blood flow. If the patient's hands are cold, the capillaries are somewhat constricted, and it can be difficult to collect enough blood. Warm the patient's hands prior to the procedure by having the patient rub them together or run them under warm water. For infants, heel warmers can be used on the infant's heel prior to performing the puncture.

> **8.10 Take Note**
>
> Never perform capillary puncture on the finger of an infant, as risk of damage to the bone is high.

Cleanse the area with a 70% isopropyl alcohol pad and allow the site to air-dry completely. Avoid touching the site after cleaning.

Performing the Puncture

Hold the patient's finger between your thumb and forefinger firmly but gently. Hold the **lancet** device in your dominant hand and at a right angle to the desired puncture site on the patient's finger or heel. Activate the spring or trigger system on the lancet and discard the used lancet into a sharps container immediately.

Wipe away the first drop of blood unless performing a prothrombin time (PT) test. This is to obtain a clean sample without any tissue or fluid contaminants. Collect the required amount of blood. If the blood is slow to flow, a gentle pressure and rubbing can be applied to the patient's finger.

Once the specimen has been collected, place a clean gauze pad over the puncture site and ask the patient to apply pressure to the area. Properly handle the collection container. Once the specimen and container are intact, remove the gauze from the patient's finger to assess hemostasis. If blood flow has slowed or stopped, a bandage can be applied. If blood flow is still considerable, apply additional gauze and pressure. For excessive blood flow from the puncture site, elevate the arm over the level of the heart to aid in hemostasis.

---

lancet. A small blade with sharp point.

CHAPTER 8: PHLEBOTOMY
Perform Postprocedure Care

Order of Draw for Microcapillary Tubes

The recommended order of draw for capillary blood collection is different from blood specimens drawn by venipuncture. The Clinical and Laboratory Standards Institute recommends the following order of draw for skin puncture.

- Blood gases
- EDTA tubes
- Other additive tubes
- *Serum* tubes

CHALLENGE

1. Which of the following areas of the foot should be used for capillary blood collection in infants?
    A. Underside of the heels
    B. Soles of the feet
    C. Sides of the toes
    D. Soles of the toes

    A is correct. The sides of the heels should be used when drawing capillary blood in infants.

2. Which of the following is a preferred capillary puncture site for an adult?
    A. Thumb
    B. Ring finger
    C. Pinkie finger
    D. Index finger

    B is correct. The preferred puncture site for obtaining a capillary puncture in adults and children is the middle or ring finger of the nondominant hand.

PERFORM POSTPROCEDURE CARE

The care after any phlebotomy procedure is just as important as the care during the procedure. Patients can have an extreme reaction to a phlebotomy procedure, most commonly fainting or vasovagal syncope. Check the patient for any unusual signs or symptoms prior to the patient standing. If there is any concern, bring in a nurse or provider to assess the patient before they stand up.

Bandaging Procedures

Following phlebotomy or capillary puncture, apply a gauze pad over the puncture site with pressure until the bleeding stops. The arm should be extended and elevated above the level of the heart if needed. Once bleeding has stopped, apply a clean gauze pad and bandage to the area.

Instruct patients to leave the bandaging in place for a minimum of 15 min.

CHALLENGE

1. How long should patients leave the bandage in place after phlebotomy?
    A. 5 min
    B. 15 min
    C. 30 min
    D. 45 min

    B is correct. Patients should leave bandages on for 15 min following phlebotomy.

2. Which of the following is the most common extreme reaction to phlebotomy?
    A. Fainting
    B. Vomiting
    C. Arterial bleeding
    D. Infection

    A is correct. Fainting is the most common extreme reaction to phlebotomy.

serum. Liquid portion of the blood obtained after a serum sample tube has clotted and has been centrifuged.

SPECIMEN INSTRUCTIONS

Match and Label Specimen to Patient and Completed Requisition

Labeling of specimen containers is another key step in proper specimen handling. Laboratory errors can occur due to mislabeling of specimens. Blood collection tubes should be labeled immediately after the procedure is completed—before the tubes are moved away from the area where the procedure takes place.

If the office does not have printed labels for specimens, the specimen label will need to be handwritten using permanent marker, labeling the patient's full name, date of birth, date and time of collection, and the MA's initials. Many lab requisitions come with adhesive numbered labels that can be affixed to all specimen containers associated with the requisition. This is another verification step to help avoid errors.

Match each specimen tube with the laboratory requisition form when placing it in a biohazard transport bag.

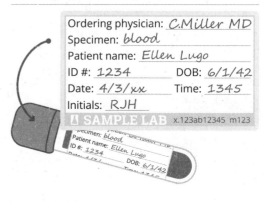

8.11 Specimen Tube

Processing and Labeling Requirements

Some specimen tubes require processing prior to being transported to the laboratory. Ensure all specimen tubes are labeled prior to processing. Check blood processing requirements in the laboratory directory if needed.

- Serum must be allowed to stand upright at room temperature for 30 to 45 min before being centrifuged. This allows the blood to clot, which produces more serum from the specimen. However, blood specimens should not be allowed to stand for longer than 1 hour. This will cause leaching of substance changes and changes to the integrity of the serum.

- *Clotted blood* must stand upright at room temperature for 30 to 45 min.

CHALLENGE

1. Why is it crucial to accurately label specimen containers?

   Providers rely on test results to make decisions in patient care. Improper labeling can result in missed or misdiagnosis of disease, which can harm the patient.

clotted blood. Blood obtained when drawn in a tube that does not contain an anticoagulant.

HANDLE BLOOD SAMPLES AS REQUIRED FOR DIAGNOSTIC PURPOSES

Each specimen has specific handling instructions, including whether the tube should be centrifuged, proper storage temperature (room air, refrigerated, or frozen), and guidelines regarding exposure to light. Consult the laboratory directory if there is any question regarding the required handling of a specimen or if the test is unfamiliar. The reference laboratory where the specimen will be sent for testing can also be called for assistance with specimen handling guidelines. Time management in the processing of specimens is crucial to accuracy of testing.

There are some blood tests that require specific timing, specific patient preparation, or handling of the blood specimens.

Preanalytical and Postanalytical Considerations Pertaining to Specimen Quality and Consistency

Preanalytical error considerations consist of errors that can occur prior, during, or immediately after performing the venipuncture procedures. Examples of preanalytical errors include mislabeling of specimens, errors in patient identification, mislabeling of specimen tubes, sample collection errors, insufficient quantity for testing, and incorrect handling or transporting processes.

Postanalytical errors can occur after the specimen has been processed. This can include failure in reporting results, improper data entry, or misinterpretation of results.

If there is any question about the integrity of the specimen or completed tests, the provider should be informed immediately. Medical judgment based on incorrect specimens and results can be extremely dangerous to the patient, as the results of lab testing often have a direct impact on the plan of care given.

Special Collections

If the provider has ordered a specimen collection at a specific time, the medical assistant is responsible for making sure that the procedure and specimen collection are performed at the correct time. Timed specimens are crucial for therapeutic drug level monitoring to confirm the patient's medication dosage and adherence. Another example of a timed specimen is the oral *glucose tolerance test (GTT)*, which evaluates glucose levels over time to assess for diabetes. If a patient arrives early or has not followed the test instructions, contact the ordering provider for direction.

Blood cultures require specific preparation of the skin, as well as multiple tubes and specific specimen labeling. Failure to adhere to any of these requirements will render a specimen unsuitable for testing and could compromise the integrity of the test results. Consult the laboratory reference manual if performing a blood draw for an unfamiliar test.

For specimens needed as evidence in court cases or for other circumstances, certain procedures must be followed. Specimens should be collected, handled, and stored with guidelines established by law often requiring a chain of custody. Blood alcohol levels and drug screening also require chain of custody documentation. Chain of custody requires documented signatures of every individual that has any contact with the specimen from the time of collection to the time results are reported.

CHALLENGE

1. Who is responsible for ensuring that specimen collection is performed at the ordered time?

The medical assistant is responsible for ensuring that specimen collection is performed at the ordered time.

---

glucose tolerance test (GTT). Test process that evaluates glucose levels over time to assess for diabetes by measuring the body's response to sugar.

PROCESS BLOOD SPECIMENS FOR LABORATORY

Proper handling of blood specimens is essential to preserve the viability of the sample. If the sample is mishandled or compromised, the testing might not be able to be performed and the results can be unreliable. In addition to performing blood collection procedures correctly, medical assistants are responsible for familiarizing themselves with proper specimen handling and storage techniques.

Centrifuge and Aliquot

During centrifugation of blood specimens, the blood collection tubes rotate at a high rate of speed. This causes heavier elements within the specimen to be pulled to the bottom of the tube, separating from the lighter specimen elements at the top.

Many centrifuge machines have speed control options because distinct types of specimens must centrifuge at different speeds (blood versus urine). The amount of time a specimen needs to be centrifuged varies; confirm prior to starting the machine (laboratory reference manual). Allow serum specimens to clot prior to centrifugation.

8.12 Centrifuge

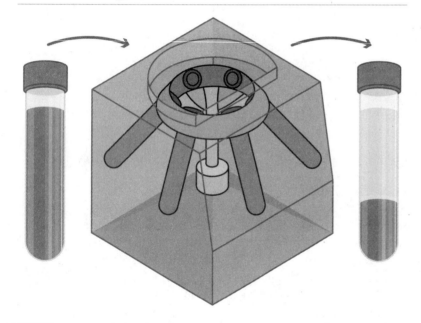

The weight in the centrifuge must always be balanced. If the MA has multiple tubes of blood to be spun, place tubes of the same size and containing similar amounts of blood across from one another. If there is only one specimen tube to spin or there are differences in the size and/or fill of the tubes to be spun, balance can be achieved by filling empty tubes with water and placing them across from the specimen tubes in the centrifuge. This ensures balanced weight distribution while the centrifuge is in motion.

Aliquot Samples

Use a single-use pipette for transfer of the serum from one tube to another. When transferring blood in the physician's office laboratory (POL) between containers, wear face and eye protection and use a tube rack for holding the tubes upright during the transfer. Never pour blood specimens from one container to another. Always use a disposable pipette to avoid splashing and spills. Label the tubes appropriately.

8.13 Take Note

Aliquot occurs when a single specimen must be divided into multiple tubes for testing on different equipment.

aliquot. A whole portion of something must be divided up into equal parts.

Calibration

Medical equipment can require calibration depending on use, working order, or manufacturer requirements. Avoid using equipment that is overdue for calibration to prevent errors or accidents. If a piece of equipment is overdue for calibration, notify the office manager or lab supervisor and place the unit out of service until it has been calibrated.

CHALLENGE

1. What should be worn when transferring blood into multiple test tubes?

Face and eye protection should always be worn when transferring blood into multiple test tubes.

PREPARE SAMPLES FOR TRANSPORTATION TO A REFERENCE (OUTSIDE) LABORATORY

Arrange transportation of the samples as soon as possible after collection. Many reference (outside) labs use a courier service to pick up specimens from clinics. Depending on the frequency of specimen collection, the laboratory transport service can have a daily scheduled pickup from a clinic. Other times, the transport service will need to be scheduled for a pickup. Have all specimens labeled, requisitions completed, and everything packaged together in anticipation of the laboratory transport arrival. If the specimens are not ready, the delay in processing could compromise the specimen. Confirm specimen pickup before leaving the clinic each day.

Storage Conditions Related to Sensitivity to Light and Temperature

All specimens should be placed into a clearly marked biohazard bag. Specimens that are to be stored and transported at room air temperature do not typically require any special management. Extra care should be taken for these specimens if they will be left in a lockbox outside the clinic for pickup by the lab when the outdoor temperature is extremely high or low. Accommodations can include waiting to place the labs in the lockbox until just before the pickup time, insulating the lockbox during cold weather, and adding ice packs to the lockbox during times of high heat. Specimens that are to be refrigerated should be kept in a medical-grade refrigerator that is not used for anything other than specimens. They should be packaged according to lab instructions for transport. Specimens needing to be stored frozen should be kept in a medical-grade lab freezer used only for specimens until the time of transport. Most labs provide small cooler bags that the specimen can be stored in, along with ice packs, to keep them frozen for transport. Note that a specimen should never be moved to the cooler bag until it is already completely frozen.

Specimens for certain tests must be protected from light to avoid changes to the specimen that could impact results. When processing these samples, keep the lights in the lab low or off. Once the specimen has been processed, it should be wrapped in foil to block out light or moved to a special amber transport tube designed for light protection. Always store specimens following their specific handling requirements while awaiting retrieval by the laboratory transportation service.

Requirements for Transportation

Specimen bags should be leakproof and free from punctures or tears to ensure the safety of the transporter while handling the specimen bags. Each tube must be labeled with the appropriate laboratory requisition with the patient's name and identification information and contained within the same biohazard bag to process the specimens. Use a separate biohazard bag for each patient's specimens.

CHALLENGE

1. How should multiple patient specimens be packaged for transport?

   A separate biohazard bag should be used to package each patient's specimens prior to transport.

FOLLOW GUIDELINES IN DISTRIBUTING LABORATORY RESULTS

Laboratories can send patient laboratory report results via email, fax, or directly to the electronic medical record. Providers are required to review and acknowledge all results prior to their inclusion in the medical record. Ensure the provider reviews the lab reports in a timely manner and patients are contacted accordingly. The role of the medical assistant often includes notifying patients of their results as directed by the provider, instructing or educating patients on any changes due to laboratory results, and scheduling follow-up appointments for patients to review the results with the provider.

When interacting with patients regarding lab preparation or results, be sure to confirm their understanding of the information by asking them to repeat it back and address any questions they have. Questions should be reviewed by the provider—the medical assistant should never provide medical information or advice to a patient based on what the provider directed in previous situations for another patient. This is because, while many patient encounters seem similar, there can be additional considerations individualized to each situation that the medical assistant is unaware of. Over time, medical assistants can learn to anticipate what questions can come up based on previous experiences or by thinking about the patient's perspective. It can be helpful to proactively discuss anticipated questions with the provider, allowing the medical assistant to be better prepared for the conversation with the patient and allowing the patient to have their questions answered in a more efficient way.

CHALLENGE

1. What should be done when lab results are received at the clinic?

   Laboratory results should be forwarded to the ordering provider for review.

RECOGNIZE AND RESPOND APPROPRIATELY TO OUT-OF-RANGE TEST RESULTS

When reporting abnormal or out-of-range laboratory results, some circumstances require immediate notification of the ordering provider and documentation that the provider was notified. The provider should review all laboratory reports and be notified of out-of-range results. Many laboratories have abnormal results flagged or highlighted. In most cases, an out-of-range result indicates a need for action, but the required intervention does not need to occur immediately. Emergent results can be referred to as critical lab results or critical lab values. The Joint Commission has determined that each organization can determine what is considered critical and how soon it must be reported. In general, critical results are those that indicate a life-threatening emergency for the patient if immediate intervention does not occur. For this reason, the office of the ordering provider is typically notified via a phone call from the lab as soon as the value is discovered. Who can receive this information is dependent upon the policies of both the lab and the ordering provider's office. In many cases, it is within the scope of the medical assistant to receive this information and report it to the provider. The medical assistant must always follow their organization's policy on how to receive and report critical lab values. Understanding the impact on the patient should there be any delay in the process is crucial for effective time management and prioritization of the patient.

CHALLENGE

1. What steps should be taken when a critical lab value is received at the clinic?

Immediately notify the ordering provider of the critical lab value and document the notification.

WRAP-UP

Performing phlebotomy and other blood collection procedures is a vital role for the medical assistant. Using correct venipuncture techniques is essential in maintaining the integrity of the blood specimen. Correct handling and transport are essential in the medical assistant's responsibilities when performing venipuncture.

Providers rely on medical assistants to be knowledgeable in specimen collection and handling processes to ensure the accuracy of the tests they have ordered. By performing these skills correctly, the medical assistant helps provide the best care possible to patients.

CHAPTER 9
EKG and Cardiovascular Testing

OVERVIEW

The *electrocardiogram (EKG)* is a commonly performed procedure in ambulatory health care. EKGs record the electrical activity of the heart. The electrocardiograph is the instrument used to record the heart's electrical activity. The electrocardiogram is the representation of the results. The cardiac cycle represents one complete heartbeat; it is the contraction of the atria and ventricles and the relaxation of the entire heart.

The MA must be knowledgeable and skilled with the EKG and other noninvasive tests used to diagnose cardiovascular conditions. The MA must understand the cardiac cycle and its relationship to the electrical conduction system. In the clinical setting, the MA will be expected to prepare patients for cardiovascular testing, perform cardiac monitoring, understand and use equipment, and recognize and respond to abnormalities.

Objectives

Upon completion of this chapter, you should be able to

- Describe preparing patients for EKG or ambulatory cardiac monitoring procedures.
- Identify the types of leads and proper anatomical electrode placement.
- Identify the steps in performing EKG tests.
- Recognize abnormal or emergent EKG results (dysrhythmia, arrhythmia, artifact).
- Describe assisting the provider with ambulatory cardiac monitoring (stress test, Holter monitoring, event monitoring).
- Characterize transmitting results or reports to the patient's electronic medical record, paper chart, and provider.
- Describe the proper functioning and storage of EKG equipment.

---

electrocardiogram (EKG). A cardiac test that records electrical activity of the heart, provides information about heart rate and rhythm, and can show evidence of a previous heart attack.

ELECTROCARDIOGRAPH

Cardiology

The MA plays a vital role in cardiovascular testing. This includes preparing patients for procedures, providing post-procedure assistance, accurately and efficiently performing testing, noting obvious abnormalities that need immediate intervention, and preparing testing materials for provider interpretation. Medical assistants must practice effective communication with patients and families to gain the trust and cooperation necessary to get an accurate reading.

9.1 Cardiac Cycle

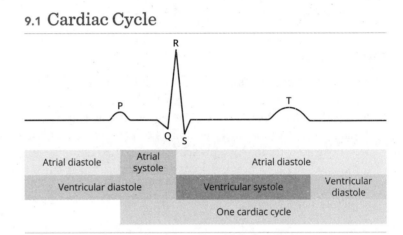

Waveforms, Intervals, and Segments

Each waveform, interval, and segment has significant meaning on the EKG. The MA does not diagnose conditions but must be aware of obvious normal vs. abnormal tracings.

- **P wave:** Represents atrial depolarization, contraction of the atria.
- **QRS wave:** Represents ventricular depolarization, contraction of the ventricles. (Atrial repolarization is not visible but occurs during this phase.)
- **T wave:** Represents ventricular repolarization, relaxation of the ventricles.
- **U wave:** Not always visible but represents a repolarization of the bundle of His and Purkinje fibers.

9.2 Waveforms, Intervals, and Segments

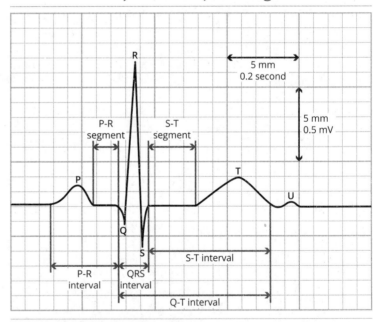

- **PR interval:** Starts at the beginning of the P wave and ends at the beginning of the Q wave. Represents the time from the beginning of atrial depolarization to the beginning of ventricular depolarization.
- **QT interval:** Starts at the beginning of the Q wave and ends at the end of the T wave. Represents the time from the beginning of ventricular depolarization to the end of ventricular repolarization.
- **ST segment:** Starts at the end of the S wave and ends at the beginning of the T wave. Represents the time from the end of ventricular depolarization to the beginning of ventricular repolarization.

Abnormal Rhythms

Abnormal Sinus Rhythms

Sinus rhythms are normal rhythms that originate from the firing of the sinoatrial (SA) node and are characterized by the presence of one P wave for each QRS interval on the EKG. Sinus dysrhythmias, also known as arrhythmias, can arise when the SA node fires too slowly or too quickly.

Sinus dysrhythmia is characterized by slight irregularity in the QRS complexes in an otherwise normal EKG. Sinus dysrhythmia is frequently seen in children and is caused by changes in vagal tone during normal breathing.

Sinus bradycardia is a dysrhythmia characterized by a heart rate less than 60/min

Sinus tachycardia is a dysrhythmia with a heart rate greater than 100/min and one P wave preceding each QRS complex.

A break in the normal EKG is sinus arrest. In this condition, the SA node failed to fire; it is not significant unless the person experiences symptoms such as shortness of breath, fainting, or chest pain, or if the periods of arrest last longer than 6 seconds.

Abnormal Atrial Rhythms

Atrial rhythms originate from the atrial tissue but outside the SA node and are characterized by the absence of P waves on the EKG. Commonly encountered atrial rhythms include atrial flutter, atrial fibrillation, and *premature atrial contractions* (PACs).

In *atrial flutter*, a single area within the atrial tissue is firing at a rate faster than the rate the ventricles are responding to. The result is multiple flutter waves for each QRS complex on the EKG. Atrial flutter can be treated with medication to control the rate.

9.3 Sinus Bradycardia

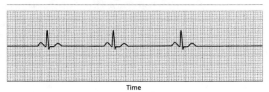

9.4 Sinus Tachycardia

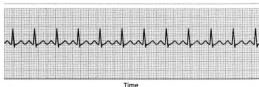

9.5 Sinus Arrest

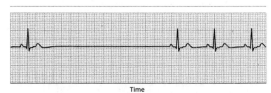

9.6 Atrial Flutter

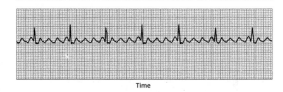

9.7 Atrial Fibrillation

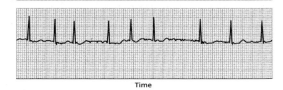

9.8 Premature Atrial Contraction

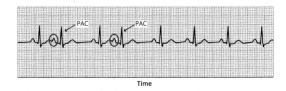

---

sinus rhythm. Rhythm that originates from the sinus (SA) node and describes the characteristic rhythm of the human heart.

premature atrial contraction. A premature contraction that results when the atria are triggered to contract earlier than they should.

atrial flutter. A single area within the atrial tissue firing at a faster rate than the rate the ventricles are responding to.

In atrial fibrillation, there is rapid, disorganized firing of multiple sites within the atrial tissue. This results in lots of fibrillatory waves between QRS complexes. It also results in an irregular QRS rhythm (the distance is different between any two QRS complexes on the EKG). Patients who have atrial fibrillation are at increased risk of developing blood clots, making recognition of dysrhythmia extremely important. Blood thinners may be prescribed to decrease the risk of stroke.

9.9 Premature Ventricular Contraction

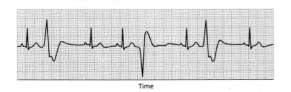

Premature Contractions

PACs occur when the atria are triggered to contract earlier than they should, resulting in a premature contraction. Premature contractions in the ventricles are called **premature ventricular contractions** (PVCs). Patients may experience an occasional PAC or PVC (ectopic beat). However, more than 6 per minute is an abnormal finding.

Abnormal or Emergent EKG Results

The MA should be able to recognize obvious abnormal rhythms or waves that need immediate attention. Ventricular arrhythmias typically need immediate intervention and include **ventricular tachycardia**, **ventricular fibrillation**, and asystole.

9.10 Ventricular Tachycardia

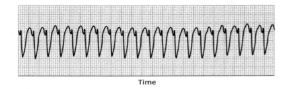

Ventricular tachycardia (V-tach) is a regular, fast rhythm characterized by large, irregular, wide QRS complexes on the EKG. Typically, P waves are absent, not visible, or occur randomly throughout the tracing. This dysrhythmia is caused by a single area in the ventricles firing outside the normal conduction pathway. Patients who experience ventricular tachycardia frequently do not have a pulse, although it is possible to have a pulse with this rhythm. Ventricular tachycardia is life-threatening and should be reported immediately. V-tach can be treated with medication and/or cardioversion. Without reversal, V-tach can progress to ventricular fibrillation.

9.11 Ventricular Fibrillation

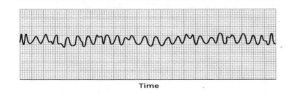

Ventricular fibrillation is a type of abnormal heart rhythm where the ventricles twitch or quiver, not pumping blood to the rest of the body. Ventricular fibrillation does not produce a pulse, as the ventricles cannot pump any blood, and patients typically become unconscious within seconds.

9.12 Asystole Fibrillation

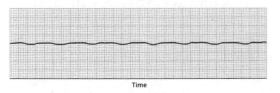

Asystole is the complete absence of any waves on the EKG tracing. Immediately check that the patient is awake and alert. If so, the likely cause of the arrhythmia is a disconnected electrode. If the patient is not awake, call 911 and begin CPR.

premature ventricular contractions. Premature contractions in the ventricles.

ventricular tachycardia. A regular, fast rhythm characterized by large, irregular, wide QRS complexes on the EKG.

ventricular fibrillation. A type of abnormal heart rhythm in which ventricles twitch or quiver, not pumping blood to the rest of the body.

Artifacts, Signal Distortions, and Electrical Interference

External interferences can occur and lead to *artifacts* within the EKG tracing. The MA must be able to detect artifacts and then determine the cause to reduce or eliminate them. EKG machines have software designed to filter out external interference. Be sure the equipment is serviced by manufacturer recommendations to ensure proper functioning.

Somatic tremor is characterized by irregular spikes throughout the tracing and is related to muscle movement. For example, shivering can occur when the patient is cold, causing an irregular tracing. Medical conditions such as Parkinson's disease can also result in somatic tremors. Somatic tremors can be reduced by decreasing patient anxiety and providing warmth and comfort as needed. If patients have conditions that lead to uncontrolled muscle movement, have them lay their hands palms-down under their buttocks to reduce somatic interference.

AC interference, or 60-cycle interference, is characterized by regular spikes in the EKG tracing. It is related to poor grounding or external electricity interfering with the tracing. Nearby electrical equipment such as lights, computers, and other items plugged into wall sockets can result in AC interference. Ensure proper grounding of the machine by using a three-prong plug, avoiding crossed lead wires, moving the bed away from the wall, and turning off unnecessary electronic devices.

A wandering baseline results from movement associated with breathing or poor electrode connection. The baseline will wander away from the center of the paper, causing difficulty in tracing interpretation. Clean the skin before attaching the electrodes. Instruct the patient to avoid using creams and lotions.

An interrupted baseline is obvious when there is a break in the tracing. It is usually related to a disconnected or broken lead wire. In an interrupted baseline, a flat, horizontal line will print on the EKG tracing. Regular cleaning, maintenance, and inspection of the lead wires will alert the MA to potential lead wire concerns.

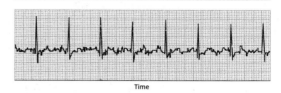
9.13 Somatic Tremor

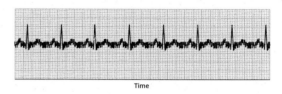
9.14 AC Interference

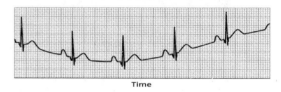
9.15 Wandering Baseline

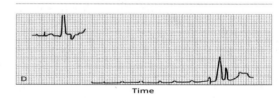
9.16 Interrupted Baseline

artifact. Alteration or interference on the EKG that is not related to cardiac electrical activity; appears as distorted lines or waves.

CHAPTER 9: EKG AND CARDIOVASCULAR TESTING
Patient Preparation

CHALLENGE

1. Which of the following terms describes a fast heart rate, greater than 100 beats per minute?
   A. Tachycardia
   B. Bradycardia
   C. Flutter
   D. Fibrillation

   A is correct. Tachycardia means "fast heart" and describes a heart rate greater than 100 beats per minute.

2. Which artifact is most likely caused by other electrical equipment in the room?
   A. Wandering baseline
   B. Somatic tremor
   C. Interrupted baseline
   D. 60-cycle interference

   D is correct. Sixty-cycle interference, or AC interference, is caused by lead wires not following body contours; other electrical equipment in the room; wiring in the walls, ceilings, or floors; and improper grounding of the EKG machine.

3. Which of the following represents ventricular depolarization, or contraction?
   A. PR interval
   B. QRS wave
   C. ST segment
   D. T wave

   B is correct. The QRS wave represents ventricular depolarization, or contraction.

4. Which of the following dysrhythmias does not produce a pulse?
   A. Atrial flutter
   B. Ventricular fibrillation
   C. Sinus tachycardia
   D. Atrial fibrillation

   B is correct. Ventricular fibrillation does not produce a pulse, as the ventricles cannot pump any blood. Patients typically become unconscious within seconds.

PATIENT PREPARATION

Prepare Patient for EKG or Ambulatory Cardiac Monitoring Procedure

Helping to ensure a pleasant experience during an electrocardiogram can reduce patient anxiety, which will aid in completing the EKG correctly and producing an accurate tracing. In addition to a patient-centered approach, consider the room and equipment preparation.

Use a minimum of two identifiers to confirm a patient's identity. Identifiers such as full name and date of birth are the most used.

Preparation, Positioning, and Draping of Patient

Protect the patient's privacy and make them feel as comfortable as possible. The patient will undress from the waist up and have lower legs or ankles accessible for lead placement.

- Instruct patients to remove pantyhose, tights, socks, or anything covering the feet or lower legs. A drape or gown should be worn with the opening in the front. Always ask patients if they want an additional cover for added privacy or comfort.

- Remove jewelry (bracelets, necklaces), which can interfere with lead placement or touch the lead wires during the procedure.

- Turn off all electronic devices, such as cell phones, and remove them from the patient. These items could lead to artifacts on the EKG tracing.

9.17 Take Note

Chest hair can interfere with electrode adherence to the skin. If the MA cannot properly place the electrodes with normal skin prep, the next step is to clip the hair using surgical clippers, if available. Use regular razors only if surgical clippers are not an option, as they often cause microabrasions and tears of the skin.

- Place patients in the supine position, lying flat on their back, for the EKG. If a patient cannot lie flat on their back, elevate the head of the bed to a 45-degree angle in semi-Fowler's position.

- If possible, instruct patients to avoid applying any substance to the skin (lotions, powders, oils, ointments) prior to the procedure. Help ensure the skin is clean by using alcohol wipes, soap, and water at the attachment or electrode sites. Some facilities have electrolyte pads to prep the sites of electrode placement.

Supplies Needed

EKG machines vary in size and shape, but all have basic identifiable parts.

The multichannel EKG machine monitors all 12 leads at once. It can record three, four, or six leads at a time and print the recording on a single sheet of paper. The three-channel EKG unit is typically found in the ambulatory care setting and records three leads at once. A single-channel EKG machine records one lead at a time and produces a running strip.

Electrodes are placed on 10 areas of the body to record heart activity from 12 angles and planes. Each electrode has an electrolyte gel that serves as a conductor of the impulses (or a gel is applied, and then an electrode and lead wire are attached). Both the electrodes and electrolyte gel are needed to transmit the impulses. Poor-quality or expired electrodes or gel can result in an artifact and interfere with the ability to produce a clean and accurate tracing.

9.18 **EKG machine**

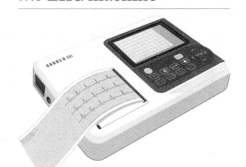

9.19 **Electrodes**

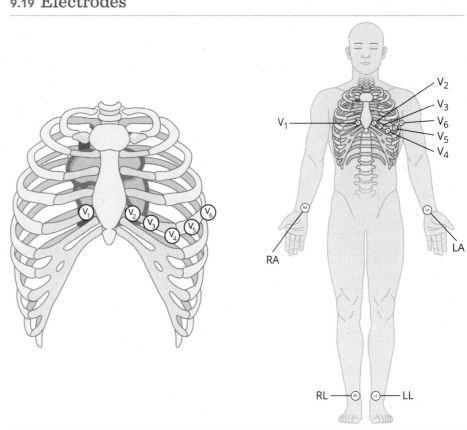

The EKG graph paper is heat- and pressure-sensitive. Waveforms are burned onto the paper via a stylus that heats when the machine is turned on. Avoid additional pressure contact via fingernails or other instruments when the EKG is being prepared for the provider. Electrocardiograph paper can be displayed in graph or dot matrix format, with vertical and horizontal lines or dots at 1 mm intervals. The vertical axis represents gain or amplitude. Each small horizontal square represents 0.04 seconds. Large squares are identified by darker lines and include five small boxes horizontally and vertically. The paper should run at the normal speed of 25 mm/second. Normal amplitude is 10 mm or 1 mv.

For hair located in areas of electrode placement, the area may need to be trimmed for the electrode to stick properly. In these instances, surgical clippers or a razor will be needed. Paper tape can help secure electrodes on oily skin.

9.20 **EKG Paper**

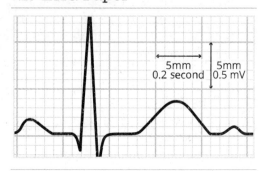

9.21 **EKG Grid**

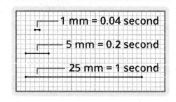

CHALLENGE

1. Which of the following is the standard EKG paper speed?
   A. 12.5 mm/second
   B. 25 mm/second
   C. 50 mm/second
   D. 100 mm/second

   B is correct. Standard EKG paper speed is 25 mm/second.

2. Which of the following time periods is captured by one large square containing five small boxes on the EKG?
   A. 0.04 seconds
   B. 0.08 seconds
   C. 0.12 seconds
   D. 0.20 seconds

   A is correct. Each small horizontal square represents 0.04 seconds. Large squares are identified by darker lines and include five small boxes horizontally and vertically.

3. Describe the steps for recording an EKG tracing on a patient with a very hairy chest.

   The electrode gel needs to make maximal contact with the patient's skin. In a patient with a hairy chest, use surgical clippers to remove enough hair to expose the chest.

PERFORM ELECTROCARDIOGRAPH

Lead Placement

Correct lead placement is critical to ensure EKG accuracy. Altering the location of electrodes on the body will produce an EKG, but the tracing may not reflect the actual electrical activity of the heart. It may lead to a missed or incorrect diagnosis. Always place the electrodes in the specified location and notify the provider if the electrode location has to be altered for any reason.

Types of Leads and Anatomical Electrode Placement

Placement of Limb and Chest Electrodes

Once the patient has been prepped for the procedure, attach the electrodes and leads. Place limb electrodes on fleshy areas of the skin and within the same general vicinity on each limb. For instance, if the left lower leg has been amputated, place the electrode on the left upper thigh. Then, place the right lower leg electrode on the right upper thigh and the arm electrodes on the upper arms. The first six recorded leads originate from the arms and legs.

Leads I, II, and III are bipolar and record impulses that travel from a negative to a positive pole at specific positions in the heart. Lead I records impulses between the right and left arms. Lead II records impulses between the right arm and left leg. Lead III records impulses between the left arm and left leg.

Leads aVL, aVR, and aVF are unipolar. Due to poor illustration of the waveforms, they must be augmented and therefore get assistance from two poles to enhance the tracing. In aVL, the left leg and right arm assist with the left arm tracing. In aVR, the left arm and left leg assist with the right arm tracing. In aVF, the right and left arms assist with the left leg tracing.

9.22 Bipolar Lead Placement

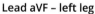

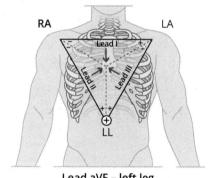

9.23 Unipolar Lead Placement

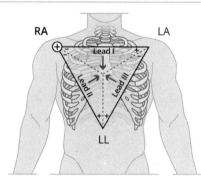

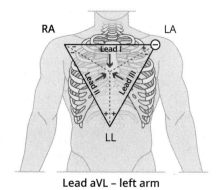

Once the electrodes are in place, connect the precordial (front of the heart or the chest) lead wires following the body's contour. Avoid excessive tension or crossing of the wires, which could lead to artifacts within the tracing.

The MA should be familiar with the universal lead wire colors in case markings are not clearly visible.

- White: right arm
- Black: left arm
- Red: left leg
- Green: right leg

Precordial leads can be all brown or can be individually colored.

- V1: red
- V2: yellow
- V3: green
- V4: blue
- V5: orange
- V6: purple

Using anatomical landmarks, place the six chest leads in a systematic order, avoiding placing electrodes over bone. All precordial leads are unipolar and record electrical activity from different parts of the heart.

9.24 Limb Lead Placement

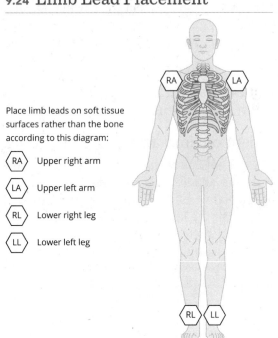

Place limb leads on soft tissue surfaces rather than the bone according to this diagram:

- RA Upper right arm
- LA Upper left arm
- RL Lower right leg
- LL Lower left leg

9.25 Chest Lead Placement

- V_1 Right of the sternum, 4th intercostal space
- V_2 Left of sternum, 4th intercostal space
- V_3 Between leads V_2 and V_4
- V_4 Midclavicular line, 5th intercostal space
- V_5 Left anterior axillary line, level with V_4
- V_6 Midaxillary line, level with V_5

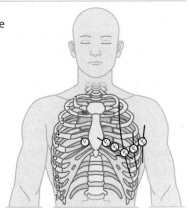

- V1: right side of the sternum at the fourth intercostal space
- V2: left side of the sternum, directly across from V1 at the fourth intercostal space
- V4: left side of the chest, fifth intercostal space, midclavicular line
- V3: left side of the chest, midway between V2 and V4*
- V5: left side of the chest, fifth intercostal space, anterior axillary line
- V6: left side of the chest, fifth intercostal space, midaxillary line
- * V4 is placed before V3 because of this.

CHALLENGE

1. The red limb lead should be placed on which of the following?
   A. Left leg
   B. Right leg
   C. Right arm
   D. Left arm

   A is correct. The red limb lead should be placed on the patient's left leg.

2. The electrode for lead V6 should be placed on which of the following?
   A. Left side of chest, fifth intercostal space, midaxillary line
   B. Left side of chest, fifth intercostal space, anterior axillary line
   C. Left side of chest, fifth intercostal space, midclavicular line
   D. Left side of sternum, directly across from V1 at fourth intercostal space

   A is correct. The electrode for lead V6 is placed on the left side of the chest, fifth intercostal space, and midaxillary line.

3. A medical assistant is placing electrodes for an EKG on a patient's left upper arm due to a left below-the-elbow amputation. On which of the following should the MA place the leg leads?
   A. Lower legs, proximal to the ankle
   B. Upper thighs
   C. Over kneecaps
   D. On hips

   B is correct. The limb electrodes should be placed on fleshy areas of the skin and within the same general vicinity on each limb.

PERFORM EKG TEST

The MA must be familiar with the electrocardiograph machine and be able to troubleshoot if it is not properly functioning. Efficient equipment care and proper patient preparation can reduce the need to troubleshoot.

After preparing the patient, applying electrodes, and attaching leads, it will be time to conduct the test. Instruct the patient to relax. Explain that they must lie still, breathe normally, and not talk while the EKG is being recorded.

Position the electrocardiograph so the power cord points away from the patient and does not pass under the table. Plug the lead cable into the EKG machine. Turn the EKG machine on. Enter patient data (typically, the patient's name, patient identification number, age, sex, weight, and height). With most machines you will press the AUTO button when the patient is ready and run the recording. This automatically inserts a standardization mark at the beginning of each EKG strip, followed by recording the 12-lead EKG in a three-channel format. It is important to follow the manufacturer's instructions when operating the EKG.

After the EKG has been recorded, check the printout to ensure the following.

- Make sure the standardization mark is 10 mm high.
- Check the direction of the R wave in lead I. The R wave on lead I should have a positive deflection. If it has a negative deflection, the limb leads are not attached correctly. Reattach leads and run the EKG again.
- Observe and check for artifacts.

Inform the patient that the EKG is completed and they can talk or move as needed.

Techniques and Methods for EKGs

The MA is responsible for connecting the electrodes and lead wires for the EKG. Preparing the patient often takes longer than the actual test.

- Explaining the procedure to the patient helps reassure apprehensive patients. Heavy breathing or sighing can cause a wandering baseline artifact.
- The chest, upper arms, and lower legs must be uncovered to allow proper placement of the electrodes.
- Proper positioning of the electrocardiograph machine reduces 60-cycle interference artifacts.
- After the use of the electrodes, close the sealable pouch to preserve moisture and prevent the remaining electrodes from drying out.
- Positioning the chest electrodes downward prevents the lead wires from pulling and causing artifacts.

Monitor the tracing as it is being recorded to ensure that leads are connected correctly and that artifacts do not appear. Items that should be visible include a universal standardization mark; a baseline tracking through the middle of the tracing; no abnormal spikes in the baseline; and visible P, QRS, and T waves. Unless there is cardiac pathology, waveforms should also be positively deflected.

Signs of an Adverse Reaction During Testing

The procedure is quick and noninvasive, but constant monitoring is required. Take any reports of chest pain seriously and immediately notify the provider.

Patients can experience syncope upon rising from the testing position. This can be minimized by having the patient sit for a short while before standing.

Patients can experience dyspnea when lying flat if they have COPD or other pulmonary disorders. Minimize this by elevating the head of the bed to a semi-Fowler's position when completing the EKG.

Once electrocardiography is completed, detach all leads from the electrodes, and remove and discard the electrodes. Inspect the skin for irritation at the connection sites. Thank the patient for cooperating, and provide privacy for redressing.

In patients undergoing *stress testing*, notify the provider immediately if blood pressure is elevated or if the patient reports shortness of breath or chest pain.

stress testing. Monitoring the heart during exercise on a treadmill or stationary bike to evaluate how the heart responds to stress.

CHALLENGE

1. Which of the following should the medical assistant instruct the patient to do while recording the EKG?
   A. Hold their breath.
   B. Lie still.
   C. Cross their legs.
   D. Count aloud to 10.

   B is correct. The MA should instruct the patient to relax and explain that they must lie still, breathe normally, and not talk while the EKG is being recorded.

2. Which of the following should the MA check for after the EKG has been recorded to ensure validity?
   A. R wave on lead one with a negative deflection
   B. Multiple regular spikes in the baseline
   C. Baseline on the bottom of the EKG page
   D. Standardization mark that is 10 mm high

   D is correct. After the EKG has been recorded, check the printout to ensure the standardization mark is 10 mm high. Check the direction of the R wave in lead I. The R wave on lead I should have a positive deflection. If it has a negative deflection, the limb leads are not attached correctly. Items that should be visible include a baseline tracking through the middle of the tracing and no abnormal spikes in the baseline.

3. What should the MA do first if a patient develops shortness of breath while they are recording an EKG?
   A. Notify the provider.
   B. Finish recording the EKG.
   C. Administer oxygen.
   D. Have someone call 911.

   A is correct. Immediately notify the provider anytime a patient reports feeling ill during the EKG.

TRANSMIT RESULTS OR REPORT

Transmit Results or Report to Patient's Electronic Medical Record or Paper Chart and Provider

Most EKG machines can both print a hard copy of the EKG tracing and save the tracing electronically. Once an EKG is acquired, the ordering provider will need to view the tracing for interpretation. Some EKG machines are integrated with the facility's EHR, and providers can view the image electronically. Other times, the tracing must be printed and handed to the clinician for interpretation. After the provider has reviewed the tracing, add it to the patient's chart by scanning it into the EHR or placing it in the patient's paper chart. Follow facility policies for uploading, archiving, and storing information.

As technology advances, more opportunities are available to record and transmit EKGs. Digital technology allows rapid data collection and distribution across the health care system. This facilitates effective patient care, whereas fax machines were once necessary to transmit results from one facility or provider to another.

Computer-based monitoring, such as telemetry, is typically conducted in a hospital setting. In these situations, the patient is constantly monitored for any irregularities. Emergency equipment is readily available if interventions are needed.

Other computer-based monitoring systems in the ambulatory care setting provide multiple capabilities, including transmission, storage, and retrieval of EKG information.

Regardless of the method used to compile the results, the EKG becomes part of the legal medical record.

CHALLENGE

1. Which of the following actions should the medical assistant take first after recording an EKG?
   A. Give it to the provider for interpretation
   B. Make a copy and leave it with the patient
   C. Make a copy and place it in the patient's chart
   D. Write their interpretation at the top of the EKG

   A is correct. The first thing to do after recording an EKG is to give it to the provider for interpretation.

FUNCTIONING AND STORAGE OF EKG EQUIPMENT

The electrocardiograph must be serviced according to manufacturer recommendations. However, the MA is responsible for day-to-day care and maintenance to ensure proper functioning.

The settings on EKG machines vary depending on the make and model. Many machines have features that can filter disturbances and help create a clear tracing. Refer to the machine's operation manual when changing any settings. Any changes to default settings will affect the measurements.

Some EKG machines have a self-test feature to check the battery level and memory.

Calibration of Equipment

All EKG devices are self-calibrating. When the machine is turned on, the software performs a self-check to ensure the system is working properly. Devices typically reset to default settings every time they are turned off and back on. However, it can help to check a few things every time a new EKG is acquired.

Two main settings can be adjusted: gain and paper speed. The gain refers to the amplitude or height of the EKG waves. Paper speed refers to the speed at which the EKG paper comes out of the machine. Devices print a calibration box at the beginning of the EKG tracing, enabling the MA to determine the calibration setting. The calibration box should measure 10 mm tall by 5 mm wide at the standard setting.

> **CHALLENGE**
>
> 1. Which of the following is the size of a standard calibration box on the EKG?
>   A. 10 mm tall by 5 mm wide
>   B. 5 mm tall by 10 mm wide
>   C. 20 mm tall by 10 mm wide
>   D. 5 mm tall by 5 mm wide
>
> A is correct. The size of a standard calibration box on the EKG is 10 mm tall by 5 mm wide.

AMBULATORY CARDIAC MONITORING

Besides a resting EKG, other noninvasive procedures can evaluate heart function. This includes stress testing and Holter or ambulatory monitoring. Echocardiograms can be done in a specialist's office to assess the cardiac structures and their movements, such as the heart's valves and blood flow from the heart.

Stress Testing

Stress testing is typically completed in hospital environments where thorough monitoring and emergency equipment are available. One of the greatest risks associated with this testing is cardiac arrest. However, stress testing can be conducted in a specialty setting, such as a cardiology practice. Patients are typically attached to heart monitoring equipment and exercise on a treadmill or stationary bike to see how the heart handles stress. They might receive thallium, a dye that provides additional information on blood flow within the heart. Patients who cannot run on a treadmill or ride a stationary bike may receive a non-exercise stress test that involves a medication that mimics the stress placed on the heart during activity.

The MA can assist the provider by attaching leads and monitoring vital signs throughout the procedure. The MA can be responsible for patient education, including pre- and post-procedure instructions.

Holter Monitoring/Event Monitoring

Ambulatory cardiac monitoring is common in cardiology practice and sometimes in family practice. It is commonly called *Holter monitoring*. The MA is responsible for attaching electrodes to the patient's chest and providing patient education, which is essential for acquiring accurate results. Before placing electrodes for ambulatory monitoring, review the manufacturer's guidelines.

Instruct patients to assume their normal activities and keep a diary of those activities while wearing the monitoring device. The diary activities should include the time of the activity and details pertaining to the activity. Patients should also press the "event" button on the monitor if they experience any cardiac symptoms (such as palpitations) or neurological symptoms (such as syncope) and record a description of the activity surrounding the symptoms. Patients should not move the electrodes. They should avoid showers until the electrodes are removed. Exposure to electrical forces such as metal detectors should also be avoided. Typically, patients will wear a Holter monitor for 24 to 72 hours, based on the provider's orders.

CHALLENGE

1. Which of the following should the MA instruct the patient to do if they experience palpitations while wearing a Holter monitor?
    A. Call the provider.
    B. Remove the Holter monitor.
    C. Change the electrodes.
    D. Press the event button.

D is correct. Patients should assume their normal activities and keep a diary of those activities. They should press the event monitor if they experience cardiac symptoms (such as palpitations) or neurological symptoms (such as syncope). Patients should not move the electrodes.

WRAP-UP

The most common cardiac diagnostic procedure performed in ambulatory care is the EKG. The MA may be responsible for assisting the provider with other cardiac monitoring and should be familiar with using the equipment, conducting the test, and preparing the patient properly. The MA ensures that the test is completed accurately. The MA is also responsible for properly preparing the patient, maintaining equipment, and troubleshooting when necessary. A thorough knowledge of the anatomy and physiology of the heart and the electrical conduction system aids the MA in identifying obvious abnormalities in a recording that could affect patient outcomes.

Holter monitor. A portable device for cardiac monitoring that is worn for at least 24 hours.

CHAPTER 10
Patient Care Coordination and Education

OVERVIEW

The medical assistant's role has evolved along with the changing demands of health care. Medical assistants play an active role in coordinating care between medical professionals and allied health personnel to provide the best outcome for patients. Education to promote active participation with patients and their families or caregivers is a key component of effective medical interventions and treatments. The MA is part of a team providing quality care, promoting health, providing education, and assisting with medical adherence.

Objectives

Upon completion of this chapter, you should be able to

- Review patient records prior to visit to ensure health care is comprehensively addressed.
- Ensure that documentation of preventive maintenance and screenings is included in the patient record.
- Identify timelines and track recommendations for screenings and preventive maintenance.
- Assist the provider with researching and supplying information on community resources for clinical and non-clinical services.
- Coordinate with health care providers and community-based organizations for continuity of care.
- Facilitate patient adherence to optimize health outcomes.
- Participate in team-based patient care (patient-centered medical home [PCMH], accountable care organization [ACO]).
- Participate in the transition of care for patients.
- Provide patient education via telehealth/virtual visit systems and processes.

PATIENT CARE

Team-Based Patient Care

Team-based health care creates a partnership between providers and patients to ensure that patients are educated and actively involved in their care. Every team member is accountable for providing quality care with the shared goal of patients receiving the right care from the right person at the right time. This approach requires communication among all members of the team.

Roles and Responsibilities

Implementing payment models such as "pay for performance" requires a specific mindset for those delivering health care. The patient's health is everyone's responsibility. In organizations that practice team-based care, team members work collaboratively to provide seamless care. This allows patients to obtain the best care possible without interruptions. Everyone works at the top of their license or credential by aligning staff responsibilities to their credentials. For team-based care to be effective, multiple clinicians are needed to address all needs of the patient. Primary care providers include a provider, nurse practitioner, or physician assistant. Other health care providers include mental health specialists; physical, occupational, and speech therapists; pharmacists; nutritionists; and dentists. Patients who have chronic

10.1 Take Note

Two common health care delivery models that practice team-based patient care include the patient-centered medical home (PCMH) and accountable care organization (ACO). In both models, the patient is the focus, with all members of the team working to provide the best outcome for the patient using the holistic health care approach.

conditions usually have a nurse case manager to follow their health care progress, treatment, and specific needs. Support staff (medical assistants, administrative staff members) also provide valuable and essential services.

Patient-Centered Medical Home

The patient-centered medical home (PCMH) care delivery model coordinates patient treatment through the primary care provider to ensure the patient receives the necessary care as they need it. The goal of a PCMH is to have a centralized setting that facilitates partnerships between the patient, provider, and patient's family (when appropriate). The long-term goal of PCMH is to improve patient outcomes and reduce costs.

There are five core functions and attributes of the PCMH.

- *Comprehensive care* is an approach that includes care for the patient's needs—that is, the whole patient and not just certain medical and physical concerns. This involves the providers as well as the entire health care team.

- Patient-centered care positions patients and their families as core members of the team. The focus is on the individual needs and preferences of the patient throughout various stages of life.

- Coordinated care means the provider-directed medical practice oversees all specialty care, hospital, home health care, and community services. The PCMH works to create and maintain open communication between the patient and other members of the team. This is aided by information technology, such as electronic health records (EHRs).

- Accessible services include tools (open scheduling, extended hours, communication with providers) provided through patient information web portals.

- Quality and safety commitments include delivering quality health care. This is met by delivering evidence-based medicine assessed by collecting safety data and measuring and responding to patient experiences and satisfaction.

PCMHs improve the patient experience through focused care and increased patient participation related to issues concerning their health care. PCMHs also save money by reducing emergency department visits, hospital admissions, and readmissions and thus provide an overall improvement in patient health.

Accountable Care Organizations

Accountable care organizations (ACOs) are made of providers associated with a defined patient population. The providers are accountable for the quality and cost of care delivered to those patients. They are at the delivery system level in response to payment reforms instigated by the Affordable Care Act. As with PCMHs, the focus is on care coordination but with many practices within one organization. This includes multiple providers, hospitals, and specialty clinics. ACOs can also have ambulatory, inpatient, or emergency care services. Because the focus of care extends beyond the patients in medical practice, there is a relationship to the community in which the organization is located and an emphasis on public health issues to prevent illness. The ACO might have outreach programs (smoking cessation, weight loss, nutrition, online education) available to the public to promote wellness.

---

comprehensive care. Care designed for the patient's physical and mental health needs using a team-based approach.

accountable care organizations (ACOs). Group of medical professionals associated with a defined patient population that are accountable for the quality and cost of care delivered to those patients.

Specific Roles of Team Members

Many medical providers can be part of the health care team providing services to a patient.

Primary Care Provider

The primary care provider (PCP) is the first provider from whom a patient will seek care and services. One of the PCP's main goals is coordinating preventive health care services (regular check-ups, screening, tests, immunizations, health coaching). PCPs can be family practitioners, internal medicine physicians, medical doctors (MDs), doctors of osteopathy (DOs), or pediatricians. Pediatricians offer preventive care services and treat common pediatric conditions such as viral infections or minor injuries from birth through age 18 or 21.

Specialist

A specialist is a provider that diagnoses and treats conditions that require a specific area of expertise and knowledge. Primary care providers may refer patients to specialists to diagnose or treat a specific short-term condition. Patients may work with specialists for an ongoing period for chronic diseases. Examples of specialists include dermatologists, oncologists, cardiologists, or gynecologists.

Physician Assistant/Physician Associate

Physician assistants (PAs) have similar training to physicians and are licensed to practice medicine as long as a licensed doctor (MD, DO) supervises them. PAs can conduct physical exams, provide preventive care, prescribe diagnostic tests, assist with surgical procedures, diagnose illnesses, and prescribe medicine.

Advance Practice Nurse

Advanced practice nurses (APNs) have more education and experience than RNs and can usually perform many of the same tasks as a physician assistant. Clinical nurse specialists, nurse anesthetists, nurse practitioners (NPs), and nurse midwives are common APNs.

Registered Nurse

Registered nurses (RNs) are licensed by individual states and have an associate or bachelor's degree in nursing. RNs can perform more complicated clinical tasks and usually oversee the case management of patients who have complex chronic conditions.

Licensed Practical Nurse

Licensed practical nurses (LPNs)—sometimes referred to as vocational nurses—are licensed by individual states. LPNs usually train for approximately 1 year at a community college or vocational school, receiving a diploma or associate degree. These health care professionals often triage phone calls, administer medications, and assist with other clinical duties in the clinical setting.

Pharmacist

Pharmacists prepare and dispense medications prescribed by authorized providers. They must be knowledgeable of individual and various combinations of medicines to educate patients on their use and answer questions about side effects.

Dentist
Dentists diagnose and treat issues relating to the teeth and mouth. Dentists also educate patients on ways to prevent problems associated with oral health. Many community health centers include oral health services to patients that are free or on a sliding scale based on patient income.

Therapist
Some clinics offer rehabilitation services. Therapy services within the clinic are an added convenience for many patients and improve the communication process between providers and therapists.

- Occupational therapists assist and educate patients on performing everyday tasks after a physical, mental, or developmental disability or injury.

- Physical therapists assess a patient's pain, strength, and mobility and then develop a treatment plan to improve movement and pain management. They are trained to use hands-on therapy, exercises, electrical stimulation, ultrasound, and other techniques to help improve patient movement.

- Speech therapists or speech-language pathologists work with patients who have problems with speech and swallowing due to an injury, cancer, or stroke. They focus on helping a person work toward improving, regaining, and maintaining the ability to communicate, chew, and swallow. They also assess and treat patients who have speech, language, voice, and fluency disorders.

Psychiatrist
Psychiatrists are physicians who diagnose, prescribe medications for, and treat mental, behavioral, and emotional disorders.

Psychologist
Psychologists are not physicians but have a Doctor of Psychology (PsyD) or a Doctor of Philosophy (PhD) degree. They work with patients experiencing mental health challenges, such as bipolar and personality disorders.

Social Worker
Social workers assist patients and families in times of transition or crisis. They assist patients in a clinical or hospital setting with physical, emotional, and financial issues related to an illness or injury. Social workers often coordinate additional services (transportation, housing, access to meals, financial resources, long-term care, hospice services). Providers on the mental health team that work in the PCMH or ACO usually contract with the facility to work a specific number of hours per week. Clinics with a large census can include a full-time social worker as part of their permanent staff.

Dietitian
A registered dietitian nutritionist (RDN) is an expert in diet and nutrition. RDNs educate patients on the connection between chronic disease and nutrition, assist with menu planning, and help low-income patients obtain healthier foods at lower prices.

Support Staff

Administrative and clinical staff professionals are also key players in providing the best possible experience for health care consumers. Common job titles for support staff include the following.

- Clinic coordinator
- Medical administrative assistant
- Clinical medical assistant
- Medical records specialist
- Medical billing specialist
- Financial counselor
- Scheduler

Patients and Family Members

The role of the patient and family members is more essential in patient-centered health care than the traditional delivery of health care. The patient's and family's wants and needs are the focus areas in this type of delivery. The patient decides how they receive treatment, what those treatments will be, the desired outcome, and education and counseling to achieve these goals. Include family members and caregivers in the process if they are involved and have the patient's approval. Effective communication is key to achieving the full participation of patients and their families. When this is successful, patients report improved symptoms and overall better outcomes. When patients feel like they are in partnership with their medical provider, they have increased satisfaction with their overall care. Fewer hospitalizations, less testing, and fewer treatments are also achieved with successful patient-family-centered health care. As a result, health care costs are also decreased.

10.2 Administrative and Clinical Support Staff Responsibilities

- Scheduling appointments
- Answering phones
- Greeting patients
- Maintaining medical record
- Assisting providers during exams and procedures
- Performing measurements
- Processing billing
- Completing insurance forms
- Performing laboratory or other diagnostic services
- Managing financial records

CHALLENGE

1. Team-based patient care provides a partnership between which of the following?
   A. Providers and nurses
   B. Providers and patients
   C. Insurance and specialists
   D. Patients and insurance

   B is correct. Team-based patient care between providers and patients ensures that patients are educated and involved in their care at all times.

2. Which of the following is the key to achieving full participation of families and patients?
   A. Communicating effectively
   B. Requiring participation
   C. Limiting choices
   D. Providing instructions and assuming patients are following them

   A is correct. Effective communication is essential for all parties to participate and work together.

PARTICIPATE IN THE TRANSITION OF CARE FOR PATIENTS

Successful transitional care occurs when there is appropriate coordination and continued quality in health care as a patient moves from one care provider to another. Lack of communication between providers regarding patient histories, medication therapies, and overall patient needs is directly associated with an increased risk of rehospitalizations, adverse clinical events, increased spending, and poor quality of care. To overcome these shortfalls, communicate effectively with the referring provider, other providers, and the patient. Educating patients regarding managing their own care and encouraging the patient and their family members to take an active role in health care decisions is empowering and leads to more adherence. The key is excellent communication between the primary care provider, patient, and new or additional providers associated with the patient's care.

Resources and Procedures to Coordinate Care and Outpatient Services
Coordinating Care With Community Agencies

Many services within the community can benefit patients. Be cognizant of what services are offered and provide contact information for those services to patients who will benefit from them. Brochures from organizations are usually free and available to hand out. Keep a list of community resources in an easily accessible location so that information can be provided to patients without any delays. Depending on the specialty of the practice, lists can be organized according to patient condition, age, or socioeconomic status. The Centers for Disease Control and Prevention (CDC) website has resources that provide services within specified geographic locations. Local hospital websites also provide information regarding outreach programs offered in the community. Document all information provided to the patient in the health record to promote continuity of care.

CHALLENGE

1. Which of the following are requirements for receiving resources from the CDC?
   A. Specified geographical locations
   B. Paying an annual fee
   C. Receiving federal resources
   D. 5-mile radius

A is correct. The CDC offers resources to those within a specified geographical location and does not require a fee or someone to receive federal or local resources to be eligible.

PREVENTIVE CARE

Preventive Medicine, Preventive Screenings, and Wellness Care

Approved educational tools can inform patients of the importance of preventive measures. Prevention of illness, injury, and disease is a common goal in health care. Educate patients on the importance of maintaining a healthy lifestyle such as preventive wellness and screenings, cancer screenings, counseling on healthy eating, treating mental health issues, and reducing alcohol use.

10.3 Take Note

Early detection of many illnesses and diseases leads to the best possible prognosis and a proactive health care outcome.

Reinforce the medical provider's recommendations with education that will increase the patient's willingness to adhere to the advice they are given. Knowledge empowers patients in their own health care choices, which can have lasting effects.

Timelines and Recommendations for Screenings and Preventive Maintenance

Routine preventive maintenance is critical. Inform patients when screenings are recommended based on age. The MA needs to be knowledgeable about recommended screenings for different diseases. Suggested screening times are based on adults who have an average risk. However, an increased risk for the disease might be indicated if there is a family history of the disease.

10.4 Suggested Regular Screenings

SCREENING	DESCRIPTION
Blood pressure	Risk factors include African American race, being overweight, family history, and previously recorded higher than normal blood pressure.
Breast cancer	A mammogram is an x-ray of the breast to help identify cancer. The American Cancer Society recommends that screening starts at age 40.
Cervical cancer	A Pap test is used to help identify cervical cancer. Recommendations include every 3 years from age 21 to 29 years. For patients age 30 to 65 years, recommend screening every 3 or 5 years if having a Pap test and a test for human papillomavirus (HPV).
Colorectal cancer	This is recommended starting at age 45 and can be done by performing a fecal occult blood test (FOBT) to detect blood in the stool or colonoscopy. If FOBT is positive, a colonoscopy will be recommended.
Cholesterol screening	Adults who have a family history of high cholesterol levels may need to be tested more regularly.
Dental examination	The American Dental Association recommends a dental exam and cleaning yearly. Dental health can affect a patient's overall health.
Lung cancer	Annual screening for lung cancer with low-dose computed tomography (LDCT) is recommended for adults age 50 to 80 years who have a 20-pack-year smoking history and currently smoke or have quit within the past 15 years.
Bone density	Screening is recommended for osteoporosis with bone measurement testing to prevent osteoporotic fractures in postmenopausal patients younger than 65 years at increased risk of osteoporosis, as determined by a formal clinical risk assessment tool.
Diabetes	Blood glucose tests are recommended every 3 years for adults, or sooner, depending on medical history.
Dilated eye examination	Patients who have an increased risk of eye disease should have a dilated eye exam. Risk factors include diabetes, African American race, age over 40 years, and family history of glaucoma.

10.5 Recommended One-Time Screenings

SCREENING	DESCRIPTION
Abdominal aortic aneurysm	Recommended one-time screening for *abdominal aortic aneurysm* (AAA) with ultrasonography in male patients aged 65 to 75 years who have ever smoked.
Hepatitis C	A person who has risk factors should be tested. Risk factors include being born between 1945 and 1965; history of blood transfusions or organ transplant before 1992; use of injected illegal drugs; and chronic liver disease, HIV, or AIDS.
Human immunodeficiency virus (HIV)	Clinicians should screen for HIV infection in adolescents and adults aged 15 to 65 years. Younger adolescents and older adults at increased risk of infection should also be screened.

10.6 Additional Screenings

SCREENING	DESCRIPTION
Alcohol use	Drinking in moderation means that female patients have no more than one drink a day and male patients have no more than two drinks per day. Drinking more than the recommended daily amount may lead to other health issues.
Nicotine or tobacco use	Various tools can be used. Typically, questions asked are related to current and past nicotine usage. The focus is on whether tobacco products are used, which kind, how much per day, history of use, and quitting behaviors.
Drug use	Tools focus on prescription medications used for nonmedical reasons and illegal substances. Medical assistants need to identify any history of or recent drug abuse. Common signs of substance use disorder include the following. • Poor hygiene • Change in eating habits or sleep patterns • Loss of interest in favorite things • Very energetic, talking fast, very sociable • Tired, sad, nervous, agitated, and bad moods • Missing school, work, or appointments • Spending money excessively • Slowed reaction time, paranoid thinking
Intimate partner violence	This screening covers domestic abuse for all genders. Intimate partner violence includes controlling behaviors, physical abuse, sexual abuse, and emotional or verbal abuse.
Older adult safety	This tool focuses on how safe an older person feels at home. This tool should screen for abuse and neglect.
Depression	Several tools are used for screening for depression. The screening tools ask a question related to moods, thoughts, and feelings.

abdominal aortic aneurysm. An enlarged area in the lower part of the aorta that supplies blood to the body.

CHAPTER 10: PATIENT CARE COORDINATION AND EDUCATION
Review Patient Records Prior to Visit

CHALLENGE

1. At which of the following ages is it recommended to begin regular colorectal cancer screenings?
   A. 30 years
   B. 35 years
   C. 40 years
   D. 45 years

   D is correct. The American Cancer Society recommends that screenings for colorectal cancer starting at age 45, usually with a stool test.

2. At which of the following ages is a cervical cancer screening recommended to start?
   A. 18 years
   B. 19 years
   C. 20 years
   D. 21 years

   D is correct. Cervical cancer screenings are recommended at age 21, with a Pap test every 3 years.

3. Which of the following are common signs of substance use disorder? (Select all that apply.)
   A. Normal reaction time
   B. Tired and sad
   C. Very energetic and talking fast
   D. Going to work on time

   B and C are correct. Feeling tired and sad, being very energetic, and talking fast are signs of a substance use disorder.

REVIEW PATIENT RECORDS PRIOR TO VISIT

The MA often has increased responsibilities in team-based care settings and may be responsible for previsit planning. Previsit planning can begin days before the appointment and include reviewing the patient's medical record to establish the following.

- Due dates of preventive testing (Pap smears, colonoscopies, mammograms)
- Due dates of immunizations (Check the CDC website for immunization schedules.)
- Due dates of patient care management items (HgbA1c, diabetic foot check, cholesterol testing)
- Expired or soon-to-be-expired prescriptions

Review the **preventive care** section of the patient's medical record to determine if any preventive and diagnostic testing, immunizations, or exams are due, such as diabetic foot checks. Also, review the medication section of the chart to see if the patient needs prescription refills. Electronic orders for diagnostic testing or prescriptions can be created in the order section of the patient's EHR. The provider will review the orders and either sign off on the orders or make revisions and discuss them with the patient.

Clinical Quality Measures
Responsibilities During the Visit

Part of the MA's routine consists of gathering specific information from the patient. This will facilitate a smooth patient visit with the provider and eliminate additional work that could delay the patient or the medical provider.

10.7 Take Note

Clinical quality measures are ways to identify treatments, processes, experiences, and outcomes. These can include patient engagement and safety, care coordination, use of health care resources, and preventive patient screening.

---

preventive care. Check-ups, patient counseling, and other screenings to prevent illnesses, disease, or other health-related issues.

Review Patient Records Prior to Visit

When conducting the patient interview, include the following.

- Discuss any changes in health status.
- Perform medication reconciliation, determining if any refills are needed.
- Confirm any allergies.
- Screen for any health conditions per facility protocols.
  - Fall risks
  - Mental health status
  - Various developmental screening tests
- Update health history.
- Educate the patient regarding preventive services needed based on recommended timelines.
- Discuss any needed or recommended immunizations.

Many electronic *clinical quality measures* are available to assist in measuring and tracking the quality of health care services.

Many health care providers are required to report clinical quality measures to measure health care quality for their patients.

Clinical quality measures can identify areas for quality improvement, differences in care, and outcomes and improve the coordination of care between providers.

While medical assistants are not authorized to give recommendations, they are often the liaison between the provider and the patient and help to reinforce instructions and ensure comprehension. They are patient educators, and patient education results in better adherence with treatment.

Document Preventive Maintenance and Screenings

An MA is responsible for documenting patient education and communications regarding preventive maintenance and screenings in the patient's medical record. The MA should indicate the topic that the provider requested for coaching, materials used, and general discussion points covered, along with questions and responses from the patient. Document all patient education in the patient record to indicate that the patient has been provided with and knows the educational material needed to successfully adhere to treatment plans.

CHALLENGE

1. Which of the following is an advantage of patient education?
   A. It allows patients to take a passive role in their medical care.
   B. It results in greater adherence to prescribed treatment programs.
   C. Anyone can educate the patient, even a friend.
   D. Information is easily found online by searching.

   B is correct. Patient education often results in better adherence to treatment programs.

2. What components does the medical assistant look for in the chart prior to the patient's visit?

   The medical assistant should identify the patient's medical history, medications, chronic problems, and any family issues that may impact health. The medical assistant should also review preventive care measures that may be due such as laboratory work and immunizations.

---

clinical quality measures. Ways to identify treatments, processes, experiences, and outcomes.

EDUCATION AND COMMUNITY RESOURCES

Research and Supply Information on Community Resources

Several community resources are available in local communities that provide services and education to patients. The MA will inform patients of local community resources and educational programs available to assist with preventive measures in their health and lifestyle choices. They can develop a community resource library by gathering local listings of agencies available when needed. The correct name, address, web address, phone number, contact person, and any additional instructions are important to include in the resource library.

Patient Education Related to Nutrition and Healthy Eating

Patient education can be used to promote good health habits by teaching patients the importance of healthy lifestyle choices such as the following.

- Nutrition
  - Encourage limiting fat intake and eating an adequate amount of fruits, vegetables, and fiber.
  - Heart-Healthy Diet from the American Heart Association (AHA) recommends limiting sugary drinks, sweets, fatty meats, and salty or highly processed foods. Eating foods lower in sodium and eating less than 2,300 mg of sodium a day can lower blood pressure.
  - Patients who have diabetes should monitor carbohydrate intake. Carbohydrates are broken down into glucose. Carbohydrates are measured in grams. Tracking carbs consumed in a day can give patients better control of their diabetes, but it is a learning process.
- Exercise
  - Weight can be affected by calories burned and consumed. Regular exercise can help patients maintain weight.
  - To lower blood pressure or cholesterol, 40 minutes of aerobic exercise of moderate to vigorous intensity three to four times a week is recommended.
- Get adequate rest (7 to 8 hours of sleep at night).
- Avoid tobacco and drug use.
- Limit alcohol consumption. Moderation is the key to alcohol consumption. Limitations include female patients having up to 1 drink and male patients having up to 2 drinks per day.
- Practice safe sex.
- Balance work and leisure activities.
- Adhere to medication regimens prescribed by the provider, including filling prescribed medications, taking them on time, understanding prescribing instructions, and being aware of drug interactions or contraindications.

Recommend these guidelines to patients of all ages. Adopting healthy habits can reduce risks for certain illnesses. Healthy habits can be adopted at any point in a patient's life to improve their overall health.

10.8 Community Resource Examples

- **Transportation and medical equipment:** Assist with transportation to and from medical appointments and obtaining needed medical equipment.
- **Adult day programs:** Offer daily activities for older adults.
- **Assistive living:** Housing for older adults or disabled individuals that provide nursing care, housekeeping, and preparing meals as needed. Patients must be able to partially care for themselves.
- **Long-term care:** Offer services for individuals who can no longer perform basic daily living activities independently.
- **Educational program and support groups:** Educate and support individuals with specific needs.
- **Low-cost medication programs:** Assist low-income individuals with obtaining needed medications.
- **Community health programs:** Provide programs to promote health and overall well-being in the community.

Resources for Clinical Services

Determine the needs of the medical office and formulate a list of the types of community resources that may be needed. Use the internet and phone directory to research the names, address, web addresses, and phone numbers of local resources such as state and federal agencies, home health care agencies, long-term nursing facilities, mental health agencies, and local charities. Locate local agencies such as food services, substance use disorder support groups, shelters for abused individuals, hospice care, and Women, Infants, and Children (WIC), as well as support groups for grief, weight management, and various diseases.

Contact each resource and request information such as business cards, pamphlets, and brochures. Compile a list of community resources with the proper name, address, phone number, email address, web address, and contact name. Include any information that may be helpful to the office. Update and add to the information often, at least every 6 months. Post the information in a location where it is readily available both in the office and on the practice's website. Navigate patients to community resources when necessary.

CHALLENGE

1. Which of the following guidelines should be incorporated when educating patients about healthy habits?
   A. High-fat and low-fiber diet
   B. Smoking no more than one pack a day
   C. Sporadic exercise
   D. 7 to 8 hours of sleep a night

   D is correct. Patient education to promote good health habits should include the importance of getting about 7 to 8 hours of sleep at night, a low-fat and high-fiber diet, exercising regularly, and refraining from tobacco use.

2. Which of the following is within the daily recommended sodium intake if a patient hopes to lower blood pressure?
   A. 2,600 mg
   B. 2,500 mg
   C. 2,400 mg
   D. 2,300 mg

   D is correct. Patients who have hypertension should consume less than 2,400 mg of sodium daily.

COORDINATE WITH PROVIDERS AND ORGANIZATIONS FOR CONTINUITY OF CARE

Assisting patients as they navigate through health care can be a complex responsibility. This can include identifying patients' financial, cultural, physical, and emotional barriers and needs to fulfill their medical care and treatment needs. Work closely with the health care team and patients to ensure barriers are eliminated and patients receive care promptly. Provide patients with resources for caregivers, adult day programs, and addiction and substance abuse support groups for patients and family members in need of support. If immunizations are required and finances are a barrier, a referral to the local board of health can be provided to assist in obtaining recommended immunizations needed to optimize health maintenance at an affordable cost. Address these areas with privacy and consider the patient's current situation. Patients should be respectfully addressed regarding their needs and how best to help meet them. This can be a sensitive area that must be addressed carefully. Ensure that the patient education and resources provided are documented in the patient's record.

Available Community Resources for Non-Clinical Services

Patients often need the assistance of non-health-related services within the community. Some of these can include the following.

- Food pantries
- Adult day programs
- Transportation assistance
- Fitness programs
- Financial and income support resources
- Employment programs
- Youth services
- Fuel assistance for heating bills
- Weatherization assistance programs

Many community resources are available in the local area that provide needed services to patients for various needs other than health-related. Address any assistance the patient needs, which expands their resource outlet and helps build a stronger individual and community.

Resources for Disabilities

Intellectual disabilities can provide restrictions such as caring for themselves, communicating, and social skills. These limitations can cause individuals to develop slower than their peers. Resources include the following.

- TASH: Advocates for human rights and inclusion for people who have significant disabilities and support needs.
- National Disability Rights Network
- Specialty-designed instruction programs
- American Association on Intellectual and Developmental Disabilities network
- The Arc: Develops programs, funding, and public policy assisting individuals with goals.

Research ahead of time to find local resources available for patients in the area.

CHALLENGE

1. When speaking with a patient to determine if any community resources are needed, which of the following actions should be taken?

   A. Handle it with privacy.
   B. Ask them how much money they have.
   C. Provide them with the list and ask them to call each one.
   D. Determine the best needs to meet.

   A is correct. Address these areas with privacy and consider the patient's current situation. Discuss with the patient and do not make assumptions.

FACILITATE PATIENT ADHERENCE

Setting Up Appointments Following The Encounter

When patients are finished with their encounter with the provider, the MA will often assist them in answering any questions and provide additional information as necessary. Provide education and information regarding follow-up appointments, adherence to medication treatments, and any referrals the patient has with outside resources.

Before the patient leaves, schedule follow-up appointments with the provider. Reminder cards, text message reminders, phone calls, or electronic reminder systems are great resources to help patients remember appointments. Also discuss medication education prior to leaving the office. This helps optimize patient outcomes and maintain patient adherence. The patient needs to know how and when to take their medications at home and their importance. If patients have difficulty remembering to take their medication, they can be provided a medication dosage box to separate medications. Cell phone apps or timers can be used to assist with remembering to take prescribed medications. Remind patients of the office policy related to prescription refill requests to ensure there is not a lapse in medication that results in missed dosages.

To ensure patient adherence, follow-up phone calls can be made to the patient to inquire about any questions they may have or to assist with any barriers they may have encountered with medications or other treatments.

Check in With the Patient or Family

The best method to promote adherence is communication. This can be achieved through telephone calls or e-mailing through a secure server, depending on patient preference. The health care organization must always maintain HIPAA compliance in all forms of communication. The patient's medical record must always be checked to identify who has been delegated as an authorized individual to receive private health information on the patient's behalf. It is the patient's right to restrict who receives any information and to sign a release to provide information to any person they designate.

Follow-up communication is critical to promoting adherence and clarity of short- and long-term goals. This follow-up allows for the patient's questions to be answered and alleviates anxiety or apprehension related to new medications or treatments. Answer any questions that the patient may have. The patient feels cared for, and the provider knows that the treatment plan is being followed.

Barriers to Care

Negative determinants of a patient's health can include several social factors, health services, individual behaviors, and genetic factors. The interaction of personal, social, economic, and environmental factors influences a person's health in some way. When speaking to patients regarding patient adherence, discuss any barriers the patient may have that would prevent them from following the provider's treatment plan.

10.9 Effects of Barriers to Care

BARRIER	POSSIBLE EFFECTS
Behavior	Decisions regarding diet, exercise, smoking cessation, avoiding illicit drug use
Biological or genetic	Sickle cell anemia, hemophilia, cystic fibrosis, heart disease, and cancer
Environment	Opportunities for employment and education, access to fresh foods, exposure to crime and violence, adequate transportation
Physical	Natural environment on health including weather/climate change, housing and neighborhoods, work sites, and recreational settings (parks, green space); exposure to toxic substances
Cultural	Role of the family and community: Who makes the health care decisions; who pays for the health care; beliefs of the illness; views on health, wellness, death, and dying; complementary therapies and alternative therapies; gender roles; relationships; beliefs related to foods, diet, illness, health, sexuality, fertility, and childbirth

Referral Forms and Processes

Primary care providers often refer patients to specialists for further diagnosing, testing, or treatment. After the encounter with the provider, the MA will be responsible for facilitating the referral process. Some health care organizations maintain a list of specialists to refer their patients to. Check with the specialist's office regarding accepting the patient's insurance before making the appointment. Give the patient the name and contact number of the specialist they are being referred to. In some cases, the MA will call the specialist's office to schedule the appointment for the patient upon check-out; other times, the patient may want to call and set up the appointment. Always follow up with patients to ensure they have an appointment.

CHALLENGE

1. Which of the following professionals orders referrals for patients to see specialists?
    A. Primary care provider
    B. Medical assistants
    C. Nurses
    D. Medical administrative secretary

    A is correct. The primary care providers usually create an order for referrals for patients to see specialists.

2. Which of the following barriers to health does exposure to crime and violence fall under?
    A. Behavior
    B. Biological
    C. Environment
    D. Physical

    C is correct. Environmental barriers include opportunities for employment and education, access to fresh foods, exposure to crime and violence, and adequate transportation.

PROVIDE EDUCATION TO PATIENTS ON COMMUNICABLE DISEASE PREVENTION

Preventive measures related to communicable diseases can be taught to patients to minimize exposure. Preventive measures are behaviors and actions that help protect patients' health, such as covering the mouth while coughing or sneezing and proper hand hygiene, including handwashing and using alcohol-based hand sanitizer.

Be aware of what communicable diseases need to be reported to the local agencies and the process of how and when to report those communicable diseases per the health care facility's protocol. This is important for identifying outbreaks and epidemics.

Prevention of Transmission of Communicable Diseases

Methods for preventing the transmission of communicable diseases include the following.

- Using proper handwashing techniques
- Cleaning and disinfecting frequently used surfaces
- Coughing and sneezing into the tissue or sleeve of shirt
- Avoiding sharing personal items
- Obtaining recommended vaccinations
- Staying away from others when sick
- Practicing safe sex

10.10 Take Note

Educate the patient on proper handwashing techniques and safe lifestyle practices, in addition to ways that help identify signs and symptoms of infection or diseases.

10.11 Communicable Diseases to Report

- Tuberculosis (TB)
- *Escherichia coli* (E. coli)
- Foodborne diseases
- Lyme disease
- Hepatitis B, C, D, and E
- Human immunodeficiency virus (HIV)
- Gonococcal infections
- COVID-19

CHALLENGE

1. The medical assistant can coach patients on disease prevention. Which of the following would be considered disease prevention coaching?
   A. Hygiene practices and information on recommended vaccines
   B. Preparations for a colonoscopy
   C. Self-management of diabetes
   D. Scheduling follow-up appointments

   A is correct. Hand hygiene and immunization education are related to preventive measures for disease.

kinesthetic learning. Learning by seeing the action and performing it.

TELEHEALTH TECHNOLOGIES

Telehealth is delivered and used in various ways, such as electronic submissions and live video calls. Electronic submissions allow providers and other allied health personnel to exchange patient health information, diagnostic results, and other important information related to a patient by sending and receiving data electronically. This has become an excellent way for primary health providers, specialists, and radiologists to communicate with patients, no matter their physical location.

Live video allows the provider and patient to communicate in real time through two-way interactions. There are several advantages to using live video, including transportation issues, financial restraints, or poor health.

Patient Education via Telehealth or Virtual Visit Systems and Processes

Technology allows providers to deliver health care and education, such as telehealth and virtual appointments. During these encounters, the patient and provider can speak to and sometimes see each other over an electronic device, such as a tablet, laptop, or cell phone. This can be a great way for providers to provide patient education without needing the patient to come in for an appointment. Telehealth has opened opportunities for rural areas to obtain the treatment they did not have access to.

An MA assisting with a telehealth appointment may be responsible for the following.

- Setting up the telehealth encounter and assisting with technical issues
- Documenting pertinent information in the patient's medical record
- Providing provider-approved patient education
- Scheduling follow-up and referral appointments
- Answering any questions within their scope of practice regarding the patient's treatment plan

Education Delivery Methods, Instructional Techniques, and Learning Styles

Learning is the process of gaining new knowledge or skills through instruction or experience. Patient education aims to put the information into the patient's long-term memory, but not everything will be picked up all at once. Understand the different learning styles and determine which is best for the patient.

Learning Styles

There are three main ways people attain new information. Ask patients their preferred learning methods.

- Auditory learning is achieved by hearing information. This can be accomplished by providing information verbally while the patient listens. An example is reading follow-up instructions to the patient while they listen to the MA.
- **Kinesthetic learning** involves movement or performing the task; it is physical. Learning this way involves seeing the action and performing it. A demonstration of the skill needed with a return demonstration or an anatomical model the patient can touch works best. A common example is demonstrating how to check blood sugar using a glucometer.
- Visual learning involves reading information and seeing diagrams or graphics.

Education Delivery Methods and Instructional Techniques

There are many ways to provide education to patients. Provide a quiet location for the teaching session, as distractions are detrimental to learning. Speak at an adequate pace, not too fast or slow, and make eye contact with the patient. Therapeutic communication allows the patient to be comfortable and engaged in the learning process. Provide written information for the patient to take home. Written information should be in lay terms, avoiding medical terminology, and at the appropriate reading and comprehension level for the patient.

CHALLENGE

1. Match the learning style with the example.

LEARNING STYLE	EXAMPLE
A. Kinesthetic learning	1. The MA reads the follow-up instructions to the patient.
B. Auditory learning	2. The patient demonstrates how to measure blood sugar.
C. Visual learning	3. The patient watches how to self-administer an insulin injection.

A: 2; B: 1; C: 3
Kinesthetic learning is having the patient demonstrate how to obtain blood sugar. Auditory learning is having the MA read the follow-up instructions. Visual learning is having the patient watch how to administer an insulin injection.

2. Which of the following forms of telehealth can be used or substituted for an in-person encounter?
   A. Remote patient monitoring
   B. Live video
   C. Store and forward telemedicine
   D. Transport TV

B is correct. Live video is substituted for an in-person encounter when limitations or the environment cannot provide the ability for face-to-face visits.

Understanding the patient's learning style helps identify the best methods of information delivery. Provide visual material for those who learn by seeing, including DVDs or approved online videos. For kinesthetic learning, provide demonstration materials so the patient can practice the skill. Active involvement allows the patient to have ownership of the skill they are learning. Demonstration with a return demonstration and repetition of the skill will aid in information retention and allow the patient to perfect the skill with positive feedback. Gaining a better understanding of the patient's preference and learning style can assist with knowing which type of patient education and coaching will be most beneficial.

Regardless of the learning style of the patient and the delivery method, it is important to ask for feedback. This is crucial to evaluate the effectiveness of the teaching session. Restating, repeating, and rephrasing the material is a method for evaluating the patient's understanding. Positive reinforcement helps lessen apprehension or resistance to learning information that is intimidating or overwhelming.

WRAP-UP

Providing patient education gives patients the skills, knowledge, support, and confidence to help manage their care. Individuals have different learning styles; knowing which is best for each patient when providing educational material is best. Identify learning styles and barriers that prevent the patient from adhering to their health care regimen. Be knowledgeable about community resources available to assist patients with strategies and obstacles to overcome barriers. Develop rapport with the patient and communicate effectively to allow them to properly convey important information regarding health plans and adherence. Providers can have telehealth encounters with patients using technology, which has many advantages.

CHAPTER 11
Administrative Assisting

OVERVIEW

This chapter includes administrative assisting tasks that the MA will be responsible for completing. There are several important administrative tasks that are essential to know and understand to be an effective team member. This chapter will address aspects of scheduling and determining the type, duration, and medical needs for the appointments. It also includes important factors that affect the *revenue cycle*, the use of electronic health records, and how *referrals* are completed using practice management software.

PATIENT APPOINTMENTS

Practice Management Systems and Software

Health care facilities typically use practice management systems and applications to assist with patient medical records, scheduling, registration, and billing. Practice management systems are most often integrated with an electronic health record (EHR) application.

The terms electronic medical records (EMR) and electronic health records are often used interchangeably, but there is a distinction.

Objectives

Upon completion of this chapter, you should be able to

- Schedule and monitor patient appointments using electronic and paper-based systems.
- Determine the type of appointment needed.
- Prioritize appointment needs based on urgency.
- Monitor patient flow sheets, superbill, or encounter forms.
- Verify insurance coverage/financial eligibility.
- Identify and check patients in/out.
- Confirm appropriate diagnostic and procedural codes.
- Obtain and verify prior authorizations and precertifications (for prescriptions, procedures, radiology).
- Prepare documentation and billing requests using current coding guidelines.
- Ensure that documentation complies with government and insurance requirements.
- Perform charge reconciliation (enter charges, post payments, make adjustments, process accounts receivable).
- Bill patients, insurers, and third-party payers for services performed.
- Resolve billing issues with insurers and third-party payers, including appeals and denials.
- Manage electronic and paper-based medical records.
- Process office mail and faxes to appropriate staff member.
- Facilitate/generate referrals to other health care providers and allied health care professionals.
- Make follow-up patient calls and appointment confirmations.
- Enter information into databases or spreadsheets (electronic medical record [EMR], electronic health record [EHR], Excel, billing chapters, scheduling systems).
- Participate in safety evaluations and report safety concerns.
- Maintain inventory of clinical and administrative supplies.
- Activate and facilitate use of patient portals.
- Provide technical instruction on the use of telehealth/virtual visits and troubleshoot issues.

revenue cycle. A series of administrative functions that are required to capture and collect payment for services provided by a health care organization.

referrals. An order from a provider for a patient to see a specialist or to obtain specific medical services.

Current Procedural Terminology (CPT®) is a registered trademark of the American Medical Association. CPT copyright 2023 American Medical Association. All rights reserved.

A *practice management system (PMS)* is the administrative side of the EHR. This type of system allows scheduling appointments, entering and tracking patient demographics, performing billing procedures, submitting insurance claims, processing payments, and other administrative duties.

- The electronic medical record (EMR) is a digital version of a patient's medical and health care information within a specific health care organization.

- The electronic health record (EHR) is a record of patient medical and health care information accessible to providers and other staff members with log-in credentials regardless of location, which contributes to more efficient patient workflow. This results in more accuracy and efficiency and a greater continuity of care for the patient. This integration allows for lab and diagnostic test orders to be entered and viewed by the patient and their providers in real time.

Paper Medical Records

Some health care providers still use paper-based filing systems (charts) for medical records. Paper charting can be cumbersome and only allows access of one user at a time, with no *real-time adjudication (RTA)* interoperability among health care providers. Additionally, searching for and locating charts can be time consuming. There are various storing and filing methods, but alphabetic filing (by the patient's last name) is the most common. Inside the chart, paper records are assembled in reverse chronological order, with the most recent medical services on the top.

Most organizations and medical providers have made the shift to electronic records for many reasons, including accuracy, efficiency, and requirements and incentives from the Department of Health and Human Services (HHS) and the *Centers for Medicare & Medicaid Services (CMS)*.

Storage of Medical Records

Electronic health records are typically stored using cloud storage; most back up in real time and are easily accessed and retrieved. Electronic records and backup data must be stored at a location off-site in case the original data source is lost or damaged.

For paper medical records, current records are stored on site, and archived records would be stored at a convenient off-site location to allow for retrieval as necessary. Archived records may need to be retrieved for the purpose of medical history, general patient care, or in the event of a legal matter, such as a subpoena.

The time required for medical record retention varies by state. However, they must be stored appropriately and in accordance with the minimum time required by each state. Regardless of the method of storage (electronic or paper), records must be maintained and well organized for effective health care delivery. Ensure that all federal and state privacy and confidentiality regulations are maintained relating to the medical records regardless of the methods used.

---

practice management system (PMS). Software used to electronically manage administrative functions, such as scheduling appointments, integrating patient documentation from electronic health records, coding, billing, and revenue cycle tasks such as running aging reports and managing the accounts receivable.

real-time adjudication (RTA). A tool that allows for a submission of the coded visit to the insurance company by participating providers for reimbursement decisions by third-party payers while the patient is present.

Centers for Medicare & Medicaid Services (CMS). A federal agency that oversees the Medicare program and assists states with Medicaid programs.

Schedule and Monitor Patient Appointments Using Electronic and Paper-Based Systems

Medical assistant (MA) responsibilities encompass many interactions with patients. This includes assisting with scheduling and cancelling and rescheduling appointments. The process of managing appointments can be done electronically and in a paper format. Electronic scheduling can be completed on a computer, kiosk, or tablet. Paper scheduling requires handwritten schedule information in a book or on a form. At times, the electronic method is replaced by the paper format when there is downtime due to power outages or technology issues. Patients can also have the ability and convenience to schedule their own appointment online using the health care organization's website or by logging in to their own patient portal.

Scheduling requires meeting the needs of the patient while managing the time of the provider. When scheduling and managing the time of the health care organization, allow for interruptions and urgent medical issues that can occur each day.

The schedule must also consider any times that need to be blocked out from the schedule *matrix*, such as hospital rounds, vacation days, regular days off, lunch hours, or conferences. Find and maintain the balance that works for the organization, providers, and patients.

Each health care organization also determines the method of appointment scheduling that is to be used.

11.1 Take Note

Effectively and accurately maintaining the schedule will positively contribute to the workflow and success of the organization, resulting in staff, patient, and provider satisfaction.

11.2 Schedule Methods

SCHEDULING METHOD	EXPLANATION
Specific time	A specific time gives each patient an individual time for their appointment.
Wave scheduling	This system schedules multiple patients in the same time period, perhaps the top of the hour or within the first 30 minutes, and then patients are seen based upon who arrives first. This gives more flexibility within each hour.
Double-booking	This system books two patients at the same time for their appointment and then provides medical services concurrently; it is beneficial if one has labs or tests that need to be done and the provider can alternate between their care.
Clustering	Patients are scheduled in groups with common medical needs (schedule all new patients on Tuesdays or all wellness exams on Fridays).

matrix. The designed time frame for appointments based on the method of appointment durations.

wave scheduling. Scheduling two or three patients during a designated hourly time period (last 30 min of the hour, patients seen in order of arrival).

double-booking. A type of scheduling in which two or more patients are scheduled within the same time slot.

clustering. Scheduling patients in groups with common medical needs.

Types of Office Visits and Associated Requirements

There are many reasons that a patient will seek medical services. This includes everything from acute urgencies to planned wellness visits. It also encompasses in-person visits as well as virtual visits (telehealth). Types of appointments include the following.

11.3 Types of Office Visits

TYPE OF APPOINTMENT	PURPOSE
New patient	Has not received services from the provider or same group (and same specialty) within 3 years — includes known complaint/condition
Established patient (could include follow-up, sick, or consultation)	Received services from the same provider or same group (and same specialty) within 3 years—includes known complaint/condition
Comprehensive	New or established patient for a specified complaint at highest coding level, multiple complaints, injuries, or worsening chronic conditions
Preventive care (complete physical exam, annual wellness exam, chronic care management)	Thorough review of body systems including preventive care and screenings
Urgent	Medically necessary within 24 hr
Other entities	Non-patient related (depositions, sales, representatives, staff meetings, training)

Determine the Type of Appointment Needed

Determining the type of appointment needed will help ensure the appropriate amount of time has been scheduled for the patient visit. Consider the medical resources needed to conduct the appointment. When a patient calls for an appointment, always ask the reason for the visit to determine the type and amount of time needed for the appointment.

Review the patient record to gather more information about the appointment. Is the patient coming in for chronic care management, a wellness exam, or a follow-up of a current condition? Once the reason for the visit is determined, ask the patient their preference of time and day for the appointment and then give them a few options of availability. Another consideration of scheduling is to ask if they prefer a virtual (telehealth) or an in-person visit.

Telehealth (virtual) visits can save patients time and money by avoiding travel time or transportation challenges. Determine their access to and comfort level with technology with telehealth visits. Telehealth encounters can be determined by the type of medical specialty, type of service required to treat the patient, provider preference, patient preference, or third-party payer guidelines allowed.

---

new patient. The initial patient appointment or the first encounter after a 3-year absence from the organization.

established patient. Patient who received same-provider services within the last 3 years.

Screening Methods to Identify Type of Appointment Needed

Screening refers to asking questions to determine the patient's signs and symptoms as well as the history of the current condition to prioritize the medical services. Screening is an especially important process to help determine the type of appointment that is needed. The health care organization will have established written policies and protocols for questions to ask when screening calls.

Questions can include patient name and contact information, reason for the visit, nature of the current condition, and other health care–related questions that relate to the nature of the current condition.

Screening procedures are also used to determine if there is a need to route the call, such as forwarding to the clinical staff or another department such as the billing department. The screening policies should clearly define what are considered urgent matters and how the calls should be handled. The policy can include a decision tree that has questions and directs the correct action to take depending upon the responses. The MA must use active listening for key words to determine what the next step will be, such as scheduling an appointment or giving the medical provider a detailed message requesting a return call.

Once the screening questions have been asked, verify the third-party payer (insurance) information and *eligibility*. Inform the patient of policies regarding patient financial responsibility requirements, such as *copayment* due at the time of services.

11.4 Take Note

It is best practice to also ask patients to come in at least 15 minutes earlier than the appointment to allow for time to fill out or update required paperwork.

Requirements Related to Duration of Visits

Many factors contribute to determining the amount of time needed for the appointment. The provider's habits and preferences can also contribute to the duration of the visit; they can take more or less time for different situations. The MA must consider the office processes and provider preferences as well as determining the type of appointment that is being scheduled. Schedules are often divided into 15-minute increments. Based on appointment need, the MA will block off the appropriate number of slots. Types of appointments and approximate time required are based on factors such as the type of provider and provider preference. Examples can include the following.

11.5 Requirements Related to Duration of Visits

TYPE OF APPOINTMENT	APPROXIMATE TIME REQUIRED
New patient	60 min
Established patient (could include follow-up, sick, or consultation)	15 min
Comprehensive	45 to 60 min
Preventive care (complete physical exam, annual wellness exam, chronic care management)	45 to 60 min
Urgent	20 min
Other entities	30 min

eligibility. Meeting the stipulated requirements to participate in the health care plan.

copayment. A set amount determined by the plan/payer that the patient pays for specified services, usually office visits and emergency department visits.

Prioritize Appointment Needs Based on Urgency

The MA is trained on asking the right questions to determine the appointment priority. A patient who calls in with a request for an urgent visit for minor injuries or acute conditions not requiring emergency care would be prioritized. This is not an appointment that would be scheduled for the next available time slot; instead, fit them in as soon as possible. The screening process (as established by the organization) will determine if the situation is an emergency (life-threatening) and should be referred to an emergency department or if it is urgent and could be accommodated by the office schedule.

This supports the need to ask the patient their name, phone number, and location at the beginning of the call.

The MA is not qualified or trained to diagnose or offer treatments for medical conditions. General guidance on recommendations for nonprescription treatments can be offered as patient education under the direction and policy of the organization.

11.6 Take Note

With emergency situations, the patient can be asked to call 911 or the MA can call 911 themselves to request personnel go to the patient's location, remaining on the phone with the patient until EMS personnel arrive.

CHALLENGE

1. Which of the following is a new patient?
   A. A patient who was seen in the office last November
   B. A patient who comes in for a recheck and brings their new insurance card in
   C. A patient who has not been seen since their annual visit last year
   D. A patient who has not been seen in the office for 4 years

   D is correct. New patients are those who have not been by the provider in 3 years or more and have not been seen by another provider of the same specialty within the same group.

2. Which of the following methods of scheduling categorizes patients into groups with similar medical needs?
   A. Specific time
   B. Double-booking
   C. Wave
   D. Cluster

   D is correct. Cluster scheduling is where patients are scheduled in groups with common medical needs.

3. Which of the following is a challenge of paper records?
   A. Minimal storage space is needed.
   B. Multiple users can access records concurrently.
   C. They are easy to search.
   D. They can be cumbersome.

   D is correct. Paper files can be cumbersome and take up a lot of space, only one user can access at a time, and they are challenging to search.

IDENTIFY AND CHECK PATIENTS IN/OUT

Patient check-in starts when the patient arrives for their appointment. It should be cordial and professional. The MA will verify the patient's identity, eligibility, and insurance information. Ask to see a photo identification, such as a valid state identification card or driver's license, to ensure that the name and birth date matches the information on the insurance card and patient medical record. The MA will ask the patient to verify their patient demographics and ask if anything has changed so information can be updated if needed. Claim denials often result from missing, incomplete, or inaccurate demographic information, and the check-in process is the time to ensure accuracy.

Patient registration forms will be checked to confirm they have been signed and uploaded to the patient account. The insurance card and valid state photo identification will be scanned into the system. Some health care facilities will take a picture of the patient to upload into the medical record. This helps to verify patient identity and decrease the possibility of identity fraud. Patients have the option to agree to or decline having a picture taken or photo ID scanned.

When verifying the patient insurance eligibility, the MA will also determine any copayments or patient financial responsibilities to be collected before medical services are rendered. It is far more efficient to collect the amounts due up front than after the appointment or once the patient has left. The patient should have been informed of amounts due at the time of service when the appointment was made.

Provide any assistance needed for patients when they are being escorted to the exam room. The patient should be asked if they need any accommodations or assistance; it should never be assumed.

The patient check-out process occurs after the medical encounter has been completed. It is essential to review the *after-visit summary (AVS)* and ask if the patient has any questions or concerns. Any follow-up needed should be noted and highlighted for the patient, including scheduling follow-up appointments or assisting with scheduling diagnostic tests or lab work. In the event of additional patient financial responsibility, such as *deductible* or *coinsurance* owed, it would be collected during check-out. The patient check-out should be just as cordial and professional as the greeting prior to the appointment.

Required Documentation for Patient Review and Signature

When patients come in to receive medical services, ensure that proper paperwork is reviewed, completed, and signed by the patient. The paperwork for new patients is more comprehensive than established patients, as they already have signed documents on file. This documentation can include patient demographics and medical history, the organization's *Notice of Privacy Practices (NPP)*, Patient's Bill of Rights, Assignment of Benefits, and any medical records release forms. These forms inform the patient of expectations and office policies and procedures and collect patient information for the medical record and billing purposes.

CHALLENGE

1. Which of the following can be used to verify a patient's identification?
   A. Driver's license
   B. Utility bill
   C. Social Security card
   D. Car registration

   A is correct. A photo identification, such as a driver's license, will verify identification of the patient. A utility bill, Social Security card, or car registration does not prove the identification of the patient.

---

after-visit summary (AVS). Information that includes follow-up appointments, provider orders, instructions, educational resources, and financial account information.

deductible. The amount that must be paid before benefits are paid by the insurance company.

coinsurance. The percentage of the allowed amount the patient will pay once the deductible is met.

Notice of Privacy Practices (NPP). Document that identifies how the provider will distribute and disclose a patient's protected health information.

MANAGE ELECTRONIC AND PAPER-BASED MEDICAL RECORDS

Sections of the Medical Record

The administrative section includes the following.

- Patient's demographic information (name, address, phone number, birthdate, sex (assigned at birth), insurance information, place of employment)
- Notice of Privacy Practices (NPP)
- Advance directive
- Consent forms
- Medical release forms
- Correspondence and messages
- Appointments and billing information

The clinical section includes the following.

- Health history
- Physical examinations
- Allergies
- Medication record
- Problem list
- Progress notes
- Laboratory data
- Diagnostic procedures (electrocardiograms, radiology reports, spirometry reports)
- Continuity of care (consultation reports, home health reports, hospital documents)

The patient medical record is a legal document, and when corrections are made to a paper record, it is done by adding a correcting entry or addendum or by drawing a line through data and adding new data—it should never be permanently deleted. Include the date and name of the person making the addendum. All information included in the medical record should be kept confidential and private and accessed only by those authorized. Compliance must always be maintained.

Monitor Patient Flow Sheets, Superbill, or Encounter Forms

11.7 Document Purposes

DOCUMENT	PURPOSE
Patient flow sheet	Records and tracks patient health data, such as vitals or lab results
Encounter form/Superbill	Records the diagnosis and procedures covered during the current visit
Encounter notes	Clinical notes that include history of present illness and current medications list
Laboratory report	Includes results from lab tests that were performed
Radiology reports	Includes results and interpretation from radiology services provided

The diagnosis and procedure code must link to support medical necessity, such as how a sore throat would support a strep test. The *encounter form* (which may also be referred to as the superbill) has a list of the diagnosis and procedure codes most commonly used by the practice. These codes are selected for a claim to be created to bill for the medical services. The encounter form is often created electronically, but in some cases it may also be a paper document. The encounter form can be updated and modified to meet the specific needs of the health care organization or specialty practice.

encounter form. A record of the diagnosis and procedures covered during the current visit; also known as superbill.

Chart Review

Charting is the process of documenting patient findings in their health records. This includes evaluations, determinations, treatments, and any follow-up needed. It supports continuity of care and incorporates any communications with other medical professionals as well as the patient. With electronic health records, the system automatically documents the person; date; and time when additions, modifications, or corrections are made. Paper records must have the physical writing of the person with their name, date, and time.

Electronic health records include interactive flow sheets that streamline continuity of care and assist with management of the patient's medical conditions. EHRs allow for effective communication within the medical organization and across other organizations that have integrated EHR systems to aid in the patient's care. Patient medical records are used to assist with providing effective medical care and billing a third-party payer, and they can even be used to support research efforts to improve overall health.

Ensure that the documentation process is efficiently and accurately reviewed before closing the record. A chart review is performed to make sure the encounter, prescriptions, follow-up, and communications are all completely and accurately documented.

11.8 Take Note

The diagnosis code(s) (ICD-10-CM) are the reason for the visit, such as tonsillitis or an annual exam. The procedure code(s) (CPT®) include what medical services were provided, such as an exam or laboratory work.

CHALLENGE

1. Which of the following is included on the encounter form (superbill)?
   A. Third-party payer
   B. Reason for the visit
   C. Employer
   D. Guarantor

   B is correct. The encounter form (superbill) includes the reason for the visit and what was done during the visit.

OBTAIN AND VERIFY PRIOR AUTHORIZATIONS AND PRECERTIFICATION

Utilization review is a process used by payers to inform providers about policy payments, benefits, and authorizations. Predetermination, *precertification*, *preauthorization*, and referrals are requested by providers based on the type of payor and the services required for the patient. Elective and costly procedures, therapies, diagnostic imaging, prescriptions, and laboratory tests can require utilization review before they are scheduled or provided. This includes services, such as a hip replacement surgery, or providing durable medical equipment, such as a walker.

Referral and Insurance Authorizations, Precertification Requirements

There are several insurance plans, and each works in its own way. Be familiar with requirements needed for optimum reimbursement.

The first part of the process is to verify eligibility. This will determine if the patient has health insurance coverage and will be able to receive the benefits during the proposed period. The second part is to verify if the patient's insurance covers the proposed service. Lastly, complete the insurance's requirements for obtaining authorization to provide the service to the patient.

precertification. A request to determine if a service is covered by the patient's policy and what the reimbursement would be.

preauthorization. Approval of insurance coverage and necessity of services prior to the patient receiving them.

CHAPTER 11: ADMINISTRATIVE ASSISTING
Facilitate/Generate Referrals

Preauthorization and precertification indicate the patient's health insurance carrier has verified that the service is covered or that the insurance carrier has reviewed the *medical necessity* for the service and has agreed that the procedure is medically necessary.

Preauthorization is typically required for certain medical procedures, therapies, diagnostic procedures, consultations with a specialist, non-emergency surgery, and hospitalizations. These requests are usually submitted electronically for faster response time. The provider's information; patient's demographic and insurance information; a description of the service requested; the patient's diagnosis, including ICD-10-CM code and the relevant *CPT codes/HCPCS codes* along with any additional information to justify the need for the service; and proposed time that the service will be performed will need to be detailed on these forms.

CHALLENGE

1. What is the difference between precertification and preauthorization?

   Precertification is a request to determine if a service is covered by the patient's policy. Preauthorization is sometimes required by the patient's insurance company to determine medical necessity for the proposed services.

Precertification can be obtained by verifying the patient's benefits and can be performed during the eligibility check. Precertification does not authorize the service or guarantee reimbursement because it does not determine medical necessity. Medical necessity must be established for the services to be approved.

FACILITATE/GENERATE REFERRALS

A patient can request their primary care provider to refer them to a specialty care provider to receive medical services. A referral may be required when a patient is seeking services outside the realm of the primary care provider. Referrals can be completed by a phone call, creation/sending via the EHR, or visiting the payer website or provider portal, or it could have a formal written process depending upon the policies of the third-party payer. The third-party payer can help to determine the route to take with a referral for a patient because proper reimbursement is contingent on their policies. Many third-party payers require the patient to schedule an appointment with their primary care provider to discuss the need for a referral. After the visit, the MA will assist with explaining the process and procedure for following up on the referral. They can also assist with making the appointment for the patient. For compliance purposes, referrals are considered part of the HIPAA exclusions for Treatment, Payments, and Operations (TPO), so a separate, signed release of medical information form is not required unless the organization has a policy stating otherwise.

---

medical necessity. Reasonable and appropriate services based on clinical standards per CMS and the OIG.

CPT codes. Current Procedural Terminology codes that identify medical services and procedures performed by a provider.

HCPCS codes. Healthcare Common Procedure Coding System codes that identify supplies and procedures not described by CPT codes.

Electronic Referrals

The health care organization can submit an electronic request to refer a patient to a specialty medical provider. This can be done using the electronic health record or practice management software. Many third-party payers have a specific electronic form that must be used by the medical provider to provide a referral to a patient. Some third-party payers have the form accessible on their website. Once again, documentation would be attached to support the medical necessity of the referral. A copy of the request and follow-up of the referral would be included in the patient health records.

The electronic referral must be completed on a secure site and can only be emailed or sent using a secure service where encryption is used to ensure that it cannot be downloaded or viewed by an unauthorized user.

CHALLENGE

1. Which of the following methods can be used to request a referral? (Select all that apply.)
   A. Electronic via EHR
   B. Phone call
   C. Website
   D. With a clearinghouse
   E. Through the employer

A, B, and C are correct. Referrals can be requested in writing, by phone, or on the third-party payer's website. They are not done through the employer or with a clearinghouse.

BILLING AND CODING

Verify Insurance Coverage/Financial Eligibility

Patient eligibility must be verified when an appointment is scheduled and on the date of service. Verifying patient eligibility is ensuring that the patient's policy is in effect and the third-party payer covers the medical services. When a patient receives services or calls to schedule an appointment, verify demographic detail and ask if there are any updates to the information. This includes name, address, phone, and insurance information. When the patient presents to receive medical services, verify a government-issued photo identification card and scan a copy of the insurance card into the system. Patient eligibility can be verified by either calling the insurance or using an eligibility application in the EHR or the payer's web-based verification service. This helps to determine the amount of patient financial responsibility so that it can be communicated with the patient and payment collected.

11.9 Explanation of Benefits

Bantam Health Care
PO Box 5566, Hartford, CT 06101

This is your Explanation of Health Care Benefits. This statment shows how we applied your coverage to claim(s) submitted to us. If you have a question, call the customer service number shown at the bottom of this page. This is **NOT** a bill.

Patient Name: **Kent, Martha**
Issue Date: 12/30/20XX

Bantam ID #: **453BBD77**

Date of Service	Patient Account Number Health Care Provider	Claim Number Type of Service	Amount Charged 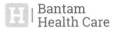	Network Savings	Amount Paid by Health Plan	Deductible	Copayment	Coinsurance 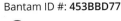	Amount Not Covered
12/13/23	11223-11223344 Physician Name	0000000000000 Offce Medical care	$100.00	$25.00	$55.00	$0.00	$20.00	$0.00	$0.00
		Office Laboratory	$36.00	$15.00	$21.00	$0.00	$0.00	$0.00	$0.00
		Office Laboratory	$30.00	$20.00	$10.00	$0.00	$0.00	$0.00	$0.00
		Claim Total:	$166.00	$60.00	$86.00	$0.00	$20.00	$0.00	$0.00

You are responsible for $20.00

Insurance Terminology

Some payers classify plans by tiers, which represent levels of coverage by the plan. Typically, the lower-level plans result in higher out-of-pocket expense to the patient. For example, the lowest-tier plan can have a lower monthly premium, but coverage could be 60% by the payer and 40% by the patient. Conversely, the highest-level plan can have a higher monthly premium, but the coverage could be 90% by the payer and 10% by the patient.

Patient financial responsibility can include copayment, coinsurance, and deductible.

Financial Eligibility, Sliding Scales, and Indigent Programs

The medical professional must be sensitive and considerate when collecting patient financial responsibility amounts. Some patients might not realize they will have to pay a portion when they have insurance, so be sure to explain the patient responsibility amounts to help them understand. Remember that people come in for medical services when they are not feeling well, and they may not want to discuss financial obligations when asked to pay their portion. Other patients can present with financial challenges, so be sure to communicate effectively about their options for payment. Offer a variety of payment options to meet the patient's needs. This can include cash, credit card, or payment plans.

11.10 Patient Financial Responsibility

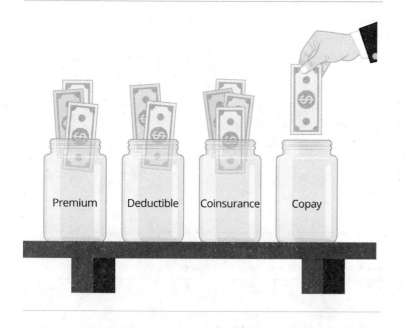

There are government programs to assist with financial responsibilities. The MA should be familiar with these programs to refer patients who can benefit by these services being offered. Assumptions should never be made, so communicate with the patient to determine how to best help them meet their needs. It is beneficial to know which programs provide public assistance. Some clinics can offer free health care services or payments for services based on a sliding scale of income.

Finances should not be the primary reason people do not seek medical services when needed, and assistance or guidance with programs or resources can help them gain access to medical services. This should be handled with sensitivity and respect for the patient and their medical needs. When the patient has insurance, follow the agreed-upon contractual obligations for the patient financial responsibility.

CHALLENGE

1. What methods can be used to verify patient eligibility?

   Patient eligibility can be verified by calling the insurance or using an eligibility application in the EHR or the payer's web-based verification service.

CONFIRM APPROPRIATE DIAGNOSTIC AND PROCEDURAL CODES

The medical provider will include diagnostic and procedural information in the documentation for the visit. Confirm the medical services provided and that the coding aligns with the documentation. The diagnosis and procedure codes play an important factor in keeping accurate patient medical records and are the basis for accurate reimbursement from the third-party payer. The provider determines the diagnosis code by evaluating and assessing the patient. This includes the condition in the patient's own words, the provider's observations, and results from any tests or related diagnostic services. The procedures include any treatment or services rendered from the provider. The MA must review the medical documentation to confirm that appropriate codes are being assigned and support medical necessity. The codes selected must be an accurate representation of the medical documentation.

11.11 Take Note

ICD-10-PCS codes are for hospital/inpatient only.

Diagnostic and Procedural Codes

Diagnosis codes (ICD-10-CM) are assigned according to the reason for the visit, meaning "Why did the patient seek medical services?" They are assigned for billing purposes with the third-party payer and are a part of the medical record for the patient. Diagnosis codes are three to seven alphanumeric characters long and begin with a letter. They describe the condition, cause, manifestation, location, severity, and type of injury or disease.

Procedural codes (CPT® and HCPCS) are assigned according to what medical services were provided relating to the diagnosis code. Procedure codes include medical procedures and services provided. They are assigned from the CPT, HCPCS, and ICD-10-PCS code sets.

11.12 Take Note

Physicians and other medical professionals use CPT to bill professional services. Procedure codes are five digits and can have a two-digit modifier to provide additional information.

11.13 Diagnostic and Procedural Codes

CODE SET	CODE IDENTIFIES	EXAMPLE
Current Procedural Terminology (CPT®)	Medical services	Office visit
	Procedures performed by the provider	Laboratory test
		Lesion removal
Healthcare Common Procedure Coding System (HCPCS)	Supplies	Medical supplies
	Procedures	Therapies
	Services not described by CPT	Transportation
International Classification of Diseases, 10th revision, Clinical Modification (ICD-10-CM)	Diseases	Hypertension
	Injuries	Falls, poisoning
	Medical conditions	Signs/symptoms
	Patient status affecting health care	Screenings
		Vaccinations
	Other reasons for health care encounters	Implanted medical devices or hardware

diagnosis codes. International Classification of Diseases, 10th revision, Clinical Modification (ICD-10-CM) codes based on the provider's diagnosis (why the patient is in need of medical services).

Prepare Documentation and Billing Requests Using Current Coding Guidelines

Documentation must be reviewed to ensure the correct information has been abstracted for code assignment and the codes selected by the medical provider are complete, correct, and sequenced appropriately. Follow current coding guidelines to ensure that accurate and efficient billing is performed when codes are confirmed and claims are submitted. The medical provider supplies the information needed to determine the best and specific codes to be used, and many times will select the codes. When any code does not match the documentation or is missing information, the medical provider would be queried for additional information. The sequencing of the codes is another aspect that must have attention to detail to ensure that the sequence is correct. Ensure that medical necessity is supported with the code selections.

CHALLENGE

1. Which of the following is an example of a diagnosis?
   A. Repair of wound
   B. Wheelchair
   C. Administer vaccination
   D. Laceration of abdominal wall

D is correct. Diagnosis describes the condition, cause, manifestation, location, severity, and type of injury or disease.

ENSURE DOCUMENTATION COMPLIES WITH REQUIREMENTS

The MA will be limited in terms of the documentation that they will provide in the health record. It is dependent upon their state's scope of practice requirements and the health care organization's policies. Generally, a MA can document items such as communication with the patient, recording vital signs and obtaining the chief complaint, history of present illness, and completing preauthorization requests based upon the medical provider's documentation for the encounter.

Many third-party payers have specific rules that apply to claims that are submitted to them, and it is important for the MA to stay current and informed. Third-party payers will send out annual updates as well as notices for changes prior to them being implemented. All rules and guidelines must be followed so that claims are accurate, timely, and efficiently recorded for the patient medical record and billing purposes. Governmental rules and guidelines must also be followed for documentation.

Government Regulations

Many governmental regulations are in place to ensure proper coding and documentation supports the medical services provided. Interoperability supports the importance of documentation and sharing patient information using common standards. This includes storage, interpretation, and exchanging of information. Sharing and exchange of patient health records reduces unnecessary services and tests and prevents duplication of services. Interoperability helps to ensure health care organizations and professionals have access to the patient health record to provide timely and appropriate care. The documentation must be accurate and in support of these goals. Patients have access to their own medical information, and it can be used for continuity of care. Proper documentation will also assist in proving that the appropriate standards of care were provided.

Effective documentation is also essential to receiving optimal reimbursement. Regulations such as the Medicare Access and CHIP Reauthorization Act of 2015 (MACRA) implemented changes in the reimbursement methods of payment for Part B providers. The details about the patient condition, care, and screenings provided are used to report quality metrics and qualifying conditions for risk-adjustment payment models. Quality metrics, risk adjustment, and value-based care require that the documentation is an accurate representation of the medical screenings and services provided. Programs and payment models like these can provide financial incentives to medical providers in support of quality of care being provided; it puts a concentration on quality, not quantity, of medical services. Medical providers are reimbursed based on achievement of the program goals. Preventive screening measures are included as proactive health care to improve patient outcomes and can reduce the need for future medical services and decrease the costs associated with future care. An example is medication reconciliation (a process of identifying the most accurate list of all medications the patient is taking compared to the medical record obtained from a patient, hospital, or other provider) to record and evaluate the medications a patient is taking, and an example of proactive measures is to provide smoking cessation education to a patient who wishes to quit smoking.

CMS Billing and Documentation Requirements

The Centers for Medicare & Medicaid Services (CMS) is a federal agency that oversees the Medicare program and assists states with the Medicaid programs. The CMS publishes documentation guidelines to ensure timely, accurate, and efficient documentation occurs. The publications are provider-type specific to give detailed information on documentation requirements. The publications include guidance with documentation errors that commonly occur and possible resolutions. An example is incomplete progress notes, orders, or procedures and how to address updating the documentation. The lack of proper documentation can have a detrimental effect on the overall patient care and also can result in denied or inaccurate reimbursements from the third-party payers.

Advanced Beneficiary Notice

The Advance Beneficiary Notice of Noncoverage (ABN) is a form used for fee-for-service (FFS) Medicare beneficiaries when the service may not be covered. The patient must be informed that it may not be covered and has the option to agree to be financially responsible for the payment. The ABN form is presented and signed before the services are provided. The ABN assigns the service as patient responsibility if Medicare denies the service. If an ABN is not signed prior to service and Medicare denies the claim, the patient is not responsible for the amount and the provider will not be paid. Medicare uses Healthcare Common Procedure Coding System (HCPCS) modifiers to convey the ABN status on the claim.

11.14 Common Insufficient Documentation Errors

- Incomplete progress notes
- Unauthenticated medical records (missing signatures and dates)
- No evidentiary radiographs to support medical necessity
- Insufficient documentation supporting conservative medical management was attempted
- Documentation that did not support certification of the plan of care for physical therapy
- Incorrect coding of Evaluation and Management (E/M) services to support medical necessity

CHALLENGE

1. Which of the following is a goal of interoperability?
   A. Increased reimbursements
   B. Exchange of information
   C. Maximized coding
   D. Decreased denials

B is correct. Interoperability supports the importance of documentation and sharing information using common standards. This includes storage, interpretation, and exchanging of information. Sharing and exchange of patient health records reduces unnecessary services and tests and prevents duplication of services. Interoperability helps to ensure health care organizations and professionals have access to the patient health record to provide timely and appropriate care.

PERFORM CHARGE RECONCILIATION

An important responsibility of the MA is patient account (charge) reconciliation when reimbursements are made. The EHR or practice management system will automatically apply payments from third-party payer claims and record the payment to the patient account, including contractual adjustments and any denied portion. The MA can also manually post charges, payments, and adjustments. All reimbursements received must be posted to the correct account, including third-party and patient payments. Reconciliation is the process of ensuring that the accounts are all balanced and accurate. The amounts must be accurate and recorded routinely to allow for updated balances to be reflected, indicating any patient financial responsibility. Patients receive statements indicating charges and amounts paid and their final financial obligation that is due.

Insurance Fundamentals

Revenue Cycle

The revenue cycle for a health care organization includes all finance-related aspects. The entire health care team has a direct impact on the potential revenue that will be earned and collected. The MA is involved in each step of the revenue cycle, from the first step of verifying patient eligibility to the final step of ensuring that the appropriate reimbursement has been received. Each component of the revenue cycle process is integral to ensuring the financial health of the health care organization.

11.15 Take Note

While the revenue cycle can vary by organization, the patient records, documentation, coding and billing, claim submission, payment posting, and follow-up are parts of an effective revenue cycle.

Effective communication positively contributes to healthy revenue cycle management, including communicating within the health care team, with patients, and with third-party payers.

11.16 Revenue Cycle

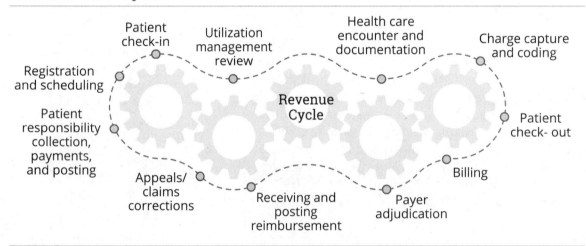

Incentive Models

Incentive models are part of the transition from strictly FFS (fee for service) to value-based programs. Incentive models include FFS reimbursement but have added incentives/disincentives based on provider performance of achieving certain quality and clinical measures and providing patient satisfaction. Areas of concentration include preventive care and screenings, minimizing risks such as preventing hospital readmissions, or other condition-specific measures that can improve the overall health care outcome of patients. Examples of incentive models include Pay for Performance (P4P), Accountable Care Organizations (ACO), and Patient -Centered Medical Home (PCMH).

Aging Reports, Collections Due, Adjustments, and Write-Offs

Accounts receivables (A/R) for a health care organization include any amount of money that is anticipated to be paid to it, including medical services billed. The MA will follow up to ensure that money that is due has been collected. An A/R *aging report* is used so that the older debts can be addressed first. This information can also be used to identify potential collections from delinquent accounts. The health care organization will also record adjustments when appropriate; an example is posting a contractual adjustment, which is the difference between the billed and allowed amounts for medical services or any write-off amounts.

Online Banking for Deposits and Electronic Transfers

Bank deposit slips will need to be generated for checks and cash received—for example, patient copayments. Many financial transactions will occur with banking online. Third-party payers often use electronic transfers when reimbursing for claims submitted electronically. EHR and practice management software will assist with keeping accurate records of the financial transactions. Performing financial transactions online and electronically is timelier and more efficient.

Auditing Methods, Processes, and Sign-Offs

Health record auditing is done to ensure that documentation is complete, correct, and signed by the provider and that the details support the codes (e.g., CPT, HCPCS, and ICD-10-CM) reported for reimbursement and quality purposes. Internal audits are done within the health care organization by the staff. Internal audits are often prospective audits, meaning they are performed prior to billing. This type of audit supports an organizations compliance policy by supporting coding and billing accuracy, aiding in the detection of potential fraud or abuse, and for documentation improvement opportunities. Prospective audits also support the revenue cycle by ensuring that all services rendered are correctly billed. Health records are chosen by type or at random and undergo a thorough review by the auditor. Any noted discrepancies in the record are resolved by the provider and then signed off. The documentation is then compared to the related billing claims, and any differences are corrected by the billing staff.

Retrospective reviews are done after the claims have been billed. These audits may be performed internally for statistical or quality purposes or externally by a third-party payer. Retrospective audits can be randomly chosen health records or targeted to specific data parameters.

A concurrent review is a type of audit performed at inpatient facilities. These audits are done during a patient's stay to ensure documentation completeness and efficacy of treatment.

CHALLENGE

1. Describe the purpose of reconciling a patient's financial records.

   Reconciliation is the process of ensuring that the accounts are all balanced and accurate. The amounts must be accurate and recorded to the correct patient account so that current balances are updated and the patient financial responsibilities are provided via a statement to collect the amount due.

aging report. A report that lists outstanding balances that have not been paid by either the patient or the insurance payer.

BILL PATIENTS, INSURERS, AND THIRD-PARTY PAYERS FOR SERVICES PERFORMED

Billing patients, insurers, and third-party payers for medical services rendered is an essential component to the revenue cycle. Utilizing the EHR and practice management software makes the process easier and more efficient. Practice management software allows for generating patient statements for their financial responsibility of the overall costs by generating to the patient portal or paper for mailing. The health care organization determines the timing of the billing and can use monthly billing or cycle billing. The size of the organization will help determine the frequency and method for billing. Smaller facilities can use monthly or bimonthly billing, and larger facilities would rely on cycle billing. Cycle billing is billing in segments throughout the month—for example, accounts with last name starting with A through F are billed in the first week of the month, G through M the second week, and so on.

Collecting patient financial responsibility must be done proactively to make it an easier and more successful process. Copayments and predetermined patient financial responsibilities should be collected at the time of service, and patients should be informed prior to arriving to the appointment. Offer patients different methods of payments, such as cash, check, or credit/debit card. Effectively communicate in a professional manner, which is considerate of the patient situation. Payment plans can be an option if the full payment cannot be paid at the time of service. Payments must be posted to the account when they are received to update the patient account.

Third-Party Payer Billing Requirements

The MA must follow third-party payer billing requirements to help ensure that proper reimbursement is received. The claims must be prepared following third-party guidelines before submitting them to the third-party payer or *clearinghouse*. These guidelines can include requirements such as timely filing, meaning that a clean claim must be submitted within a certain number of days from the date of service to be eligible for reimbursement. Some payers allow for up to one year from the date of service, but many have much shorter filing requirements. Another payer-specific example includes providing the date of injury on the worker's compensation claim for a patient who was injured or became ill as a result of performing their job.

A clearinghouse is an intermediary that is contracted by the provider to accept and process the claims for the third-party payers and assists with reducing claim errors. Clearinghouses can be private or public companies and serve as go-betweens between providers, billing groups, and payers for transmitting electronic claim information into specific forms required by the payers. Using a clearinghouse is beneficial for scrubbing claims prior to final submission and reducing the number of errors in claims and allows you the opportunity to correct before submission to the payer. Most claims will be submitted electronically. Claims are prepared using the practice management software that uses information captured directly from the patient encounter.

CHALLENGE

1. Which of the following is an example of cycle billing?
   A. Billing all patients on the 1st of the month
   B. Billing patients in segments
   C. Requiring full payment on the date of service
   D. Billing patients daily

   B is correct. Cycle billing is billing in segments throughout the month, for example accounts with the last name starting in A through F are billing in the first week of the month, G through M the second week, and so on.

clearinghouse. An organization that accepts the claims data from a health care provider, performs edits comparable to payer edits, and submits clean claims to the third-party payer.

RESOLVE BILLING ISSUES

Adjudicated claims can result in a denial or incorrect reimbursement, which requires follow-up to determine the reason for the denial or partial payment and the proper action to take. If a claim was denied because the service is not covered, verify the correct diagnosis and procedure codes were billed and supported medical necessity. Claims should be resubmitted after any needed corrections to the original claim have been made. If an incorrect reimbursement was received, verify the claim was processed correctly, submit a request to the payer to review it, and adjust the payment. Reimbursement errors could include issues related to in-network status or the failure to recognize a preauthorization number. If the claim is denied for patient eligibility, submit a copy of the patient eligibility verification performed and resubmit for reconsideration. If the claim is denied stating the service "does not meet medical necessity," it can be necessary to attach supporting documentation and submit with an appeal. When the denial cannot be determined or is unclear, the MA can contact the third-party payer for clarification and to determine any appropriate action needed.

CHALLENGE

1. When a claim pays with an incorrect reimbursement amount, which of the following actions should be taken?
   A. Bill the patient for the difference.
   B. Submit an appeal with documentation.
   C. Bill the insurance company for the difference.
   D. Write off the balance.

B is correct. If an incorrect reimbursement was received, verify the claim was processed correctly, such as in-network status or the preauthorization number was considered, and submit a request to the payer to review it and adjust the payment.

OTHER ADMINISTRATIVE DUTIES

Follow-Up Patient Calls and Appointment Confirmations

Most outgoing calls to patients are in response to appointment requests or confirmations, delivery of laboratory and imaging results, post-procedure follow-up calls, or returning patients' inquiry phone calls. Often, patients are anxious and eager to receive results from laboratory and diagnostic testing. Many patients now have instant access to their results via their patient portal (a personal account set up with their provider or a health care system linking to the components of their electronic health record). Health care providers notify patients of the findings within the patient portal, by phone, or by mail. The provider's organization may have a policy in place to contact the patients by phone for abnormal results or to instruct the patient to call the office to follow up after a specified time to get the results. This may be done to reduce the workflow of the staff while prioritizing contact with patients who require follow-up. The ordering provider must always review the results and provide direction related to conveying test results.

11.17 Take Note

Only leave the name of the practice if it does not reveal the purpose of the call.

Confirming and reminding patients of scheduled appointments can decrease *no-show* rates. Reminders can be done in a variety of ways, including automated calls or patient portal messages, appointment cards, email or text messages, or a combination of these. Inform patients of the practice's no-show and late-cancel policy.

It is helpful to plan ahead when returning patient phone calls.

no-show. When a patient has a scheduled appointment and does not show up or contact the medical office.

All patient communication and follow-up must be documented in the patient record. Always maintain confidentiality, not releasing unauthorized protected health information (PHI), and follow confidentiality guidelines when conducting conversations with patients over the telephone.

Tips when placing outgoing calls to patients include the following.

- Open the patient's medical record.
- Have all the information needed available prior to placing the call.
- Allow enough time and double-check the telephone number.
- The MA should identify themselves and confirm if this call time is convenient.
- Only provide information to the patient or authorized individuals who are identified on the patient's signed privacy agreement.

Tips when reaching a voicemail include the following.

- The MA should state only the name of the individual the message is intended for, date and time of the call, their name and the name of the practice, return call back number, and hours for returned calls.
- Follow any office policy and procedure guidelines regarding office privacy agreements signed by the patient.

CHALLENGE

1. Which of the following methods should be applied to phone call follow-ups?
   A. Triage the return calls.
   B. Make all return calls on Mondays.
   C. Wait to see if the patient calls again.
   D. Refer the patients to a different organization

A is correct. The MA will need to screen calls and determine the order of follow-up depending upon the reason for the call.

Process Office Mail and Faxes to Appropriate Staff Member

Receiving office mail and faxes is another responsibility that will need appropriate follow-up. All correspondence with vested members must be handled in a professional manner. When written correspondence is received by the health care organization, determine the appropriate person or department that will follow up. Scan a copy of the correspondence and the response in the patient's medical record, as the information is part of the legal record.

Written correspondence can be created using a template, which is a sample form that requires specific personalization dependent upon the reason for the contact. This includes appeal letters, interoffice memos, faxes, and emails. It must be HIPAA compliant, free from spelling errors, and grammatically correct. Written communication is a direct reflection of the health care organization.

CHALLENGE

1. Which of the following is an important part of written correspondence?
   A. Spell-check and proofread.
   B. Use colorful fonts.
   C. Send generic responses.
   D. Leave it in a pile on the front desk.

A is correct. Correspondence must be free from random errors and grammatically correct, must be personalized, HIPAA must be followed, and a copy must be placed in the patient records.

Enter Information Into Databases or Spreadsheets

Information must be entered accurately into the electronic health record. This data has an impact on the patient's overall health care and billing process. Diligence is necessary when entering information into any database or spreadsheet in the medical practice. The EHR and practice management software used by health care organizations includes important patient information in each section. This information is used to maintain health records, scheduling, billing, and any purpose that includes health data such as research. The databases used in the health care organization include code sets and fee schedules and must be regularly updated. This information can include a charge directory that has a list of billable items as well as the correct codes and amounts to be billed. This must be updated to reflect the correct, up-to-date amounts. Spreadsheets or data analysis applications can be used by the health care organization to compile data, sort, and retrieve information that can be used to create reports.

Data Entry and Data Fields

Electronic health records and PM systems use data entry fields in their applications. Each of the fields must include data that is correct for the intended purpose. Fields can include demographic information such as name, patient gender, address, and insurance information. The fields will be set specifically to accept information, such as a birthdate including numeric characters and insurance information accepting alphanumeric data. Some of the fields include drop-down menus that enable a person to select from a list of choices. Drop-down menus can help to increase the accuracy of data entered as they do not allow for typographical errors. Reports can also be generated using the data that is entered into the system, such as determining patients who are due for an annual wellness exam.

CHALLENGE

1. Describe the impact that data can have on the medical records.

Data has an impact on the patient's overall health care and billing process; it is a legal record. This information is used to maintain health records and for scheduling, billing, and any purpose that includes health data, such as research.

Maintain Inventory of Clinical and Administrative Supplies

Maintaining adequate supplies is essential. Keeping an office supplied may not seem like a complicated responsibility, but there is more to it than first appears. There are procedures for ordering supplies and making sure the practice has what is needed. The methods used, the companies that provide the supplies, and how supplies are delivered is called the supply chain. A supply chain consists of a relationship between a company and its suppliers to produce and distribute a specific product to buyers. There is a complex process of ordering, receiving, stocking, and organizing supplies as well as documenting and verifying correct amounts.

Supplies are generally ordered electronically through suppliers. The MA, if placing the order, will first review the *inventory supply log* of office supplies to make sure the number of supplies ordered is appropriate. The supplier's website will generally provide all supply information including item numbers, price, and description. Some offices may choose to have a supplier issue a printed catalog to have on hand.

inventory supply log. Form that tracks the amount of inventory the office has and can be used to predict anticipated amounts needed based on the history.

Supplies are sent different ways, so not all supplies require a signature. If a signature is required, a form will be sent by the supplier to ensure appropriate delivery of supplies. Once supplies arrive, the MA will check to make sure the supplies sent match what was ordered and in the correct amount. If any errors are noted with the supply delivered, notify either the practice manager or the supplier directly. Delivery orders need to be checked as soon as possible because they can contain supplies that must be refrigerated, such as vaccinations. The practice can have an electronic inventory system to log in and document the items received.

Stocking Supplies

Do not keep supplies stored in the shipping box because the box was transported outside and can bring germs or insects into the building. Remove supplies from the shipping boxes and place them in the storage room.

When stocking supplies, some of the supply boxes can be heavy. Make sure to use proper body mechanics when lifting and/or moving boxes.

A minimum number of supplies is usually determined by the type of office and the total patients seen each day. The threshold (also referred to as *par level*) is the minimum amount of inventory the office will have on the shelf before placing another order. It is always better to have adequate supplies on hand than to be without.

The health care team will determine the appropriate levels of supply to have in stock, referred to as the par level. Inventory of clinical and administrative supplies must be on hand to ensure items are there when they are needed. This includes keeping track of the current inventory and ordering when the levels are below the health care organization's par level. Administrative supplies can include paper, pencils, and other clerical supplies. Clinical supplies include items such as exam room table covers, bandages, and supplies for injections, blood draws, and other more detailed procedures performed. Always make sure there are enough supplies on hand, but also try to avoid waste by having a big surplus. Inventory should be verified on a routine basis, per policy. Document the item, the vendor, the cost, and how often the item may need to be ordered.

CHALLENGE

1. Which of the following describes the par level?
   A. Appropriate amount to have on hand
   B. Cost of the item
   C. The surplus amount to order
   D. Annual amount ordered

A is correct. The health care team will determine the appropriate levels to have in stock, referred to as the par level.

par level. Minimum amount of inventory an office will have on the shelf before placing another order.

Activate and Facilitate Use of Patient Portals

Patient portals play a big part in empowering the patients in managing their health care records and choices. The patient portal provides access to their records, including progress notes, lab results, radiology reports, immunizations, patient financial responsibility, and medications. The patient can contact the health care organization using the messaging feature of the patient portal as well as schedule appointments directly. Sometimes this is referred to as the "digital front door."

When a patient begins receiving medical services, they will be given a username and access code to log in to their patient portal. Only their information can be accessed using the code. The health care organization will also provide guidance with the log-in and maneuvering around the site.

> **CHALLENGE**
>
> 1. Which of the following is a use of the patient portal?
>   A. To review a family member's test results
>   B. To review their radiology report
>   C. To select an insurance plan
>   D. To submit a claim for reimbursement
>
> *B is correct. The patient portal gives patients a way to access their own records, including progress notes, lab results, radiology reports, immunizations, patient financial responsibility, and medications.*

Provide Technical Instruction on the Use of Telehealth/Virtual Visits and Troubleshoot Issues

Telehealth/virtual encounters are medical services provided using a secure phone or visual platform. The medical provider and the patient are in separate locations and have a synchronous conversation. The medical provider may be able to diagnosis by asking questions, observing symptoms, and reviewing objective data such as test results to diagnose and treat the condition. This can include conditions such as skin conditions, gastrointestinal system symptoms, aches and pains related to the musculoskeletal system, and headaches, to name a few. Based on the payer, medical nutrition therapy and many mental health services can also be done with telehealth services.

Telehealth visits can be completed using a computer, cell phone, or computer tablet. The MA will call the patient to ensure that they have access and have any documentation needed to complete the visit, such as a list of current medications. Telehealth visits have become popular as they minimize geographical barriers, save travel time, and give more flexibility in scheduling.

Telehealth/Virtual Visit Technologies, Barriers to Access

Technology can be a barrier for all vested members in being able to complete telehealth/virtual visits. Some patients might not have access to internet service or devices or may not be familiar or comfortable with telehealth technology. Telehealth visits can be done using a secure patient portal platform, and the MA can provide technical guidance and support to the patient to assist with logging in and verifying their settings are correct. If a patient has chosen to see the provider via telehealth, be prepared to explain and inform the patient of technology requirements for a telehealth visit and make sure they are prepared. In many cases, patients receiving a telehealth encounter also receive instructions on how to download a telehealth app, how to use the video tool, or where to log in for the visit via patient portal, text, or email instructions. The patient may need assistance with a microphone or camera to complete the visit. The MA can also help to troubleshoot any challenges that occur before or during the telehealth visit. Coaching and education can help to alleviate many of the technological barriers to telehealth visits.

> **CHALLENGE**
>
> 1. Which of the following is a barrier to telehealth/virtual visits?
>   A. Geographical locations
>   B. Travel time
>   C. Flexibility in scheduling
>   D. Familiarity with technology
>
> *D is correct. Some patients might not have access to internet service or may not be familiar or comfortable with telehealth technology.*

Participate in Safety Evaluations and Report Safety Concerns

The medical office must present a safe environment that minimizes risks for all. Potential hazards must be addressed before they become a risk to patients, medical providers, and other team members. Have a safety plan in place and routinely complete safety evaluations. All members of the health care team must be familiar with the plan and actions appropriate to address and prevent any concerns. The Occupational Safety and Health Administration (OSHA) is a federal agency that is responsible for inspecting, evaluating, and ensuring a safe work environment. There must be a process for reporting any safety concerns in the safety plan so that they can be addressed.

Inspection Logs, Schedules, Compliance Requirements, and Medical Equipment Servicers

All administrative and clinical equipment should have routine preventive checks to ensure safety and proper working condition. Examples of administrative equipment include printers, computers, copy machines, and fax machines. Examples of clinical equipment can include electrocardiographs, centrifuges, blood glucose monitors, and electronic blood pressure machines. Some clinical equipment will require calibration checks; know how and when to perform these. This is documented in equipment inspection logs, which also provide the timeline of recommended and required maintenance. There will be internal inspections as well as contacting the appropriate vendors to inspect when needed. These inspections will help to minimize risk of potential injury in the health care organization and ensure that the equipment is free from any malfunctions.

CHALLENGE

1. Which of the following documents can help to ensure that equipment is maintained?
   A. Safety plan
   B. Inspection log
   C. Superbill
   D. Safety evaluation

B is correct. Equipment inspection logs provide the timeline of recommended/required maintenance.

WRAP-UP

Administrative tasks can be a part of a MA's day-to-day responsibilities. Understand scheduling requirements and how to determine the type, duration, and medical needs when scheduling an appointment for a patient. Effective patient correspondence is an important aspect of quality patient care and a positive patient experience. Documentation is a critical element for billing, coding, and reimbursements. When claims are denied, the MA should know why and actions to take to correct denials. Maintaining supplies and inventory is an essential process in having an effectively run medical office.

CHAPTER 12
Communication and Customer Service

OVERVIEW

This chapter addresses effective *communication* and the positive impact it can have on the health care organization. Effective communication includes different types and styles of communication. Communication can occur in many different facets of the field, including telephone and written forms. The MA's responsibilities will include effectively communicating with patients and family members, members of the health care team, and third-party payers. Verbal and *nonverbal communication* and the impact it has on the communication process must be considered to ensure effective communication. Different adjustments or modifications may be needed to effectively communicate with a diverse population.

The chapter also addresses how to handle challenging situations and minimize the potential for them to escalate. Teamwork and effective communication positively contribute to the work environment and help to increase the positive workflow and patient health outcomes. *Professionalism* must be adhered to in all aspects of the health care environment. This includes appearance, communication, presence, and relationships. The MA must be an effective communicator who is both professional and respectful of the ultimate goal of assisting, providing a positive health care experience for patients.

Objectives

Upon completion of this chapter, you should be able to

- Recognize the diversity of patient cultures and backgrounds when providing care.
- Recognize stereotypes and biases and interact appropriately with patients, colleagues, and others.
- Modify verbal and nonverbal communication for diverse audiences.
- Modify verbal and nonverbal communications with patients and caregivers based on special considerations.
- Modify communications based on type of visit.
- Clarify and relay communications between patients and providers.
- Communicate on the telephone with patients and caregivers, providers, third-party payers using HIPAA guidelines.
- Prepare written/electronic communications/business correspondence.
- Handle challenging/difficult customer service occurrences.
- Utilize conflict management and complaint resolution to improve patient satisfaction.
- Engage in crucial conversations with patients and caregivers/health care surrogates, staff, and providers.
- Facilitate teamwork and team engagement.
- Demonstrate professionalism (for example, appropriate demeanor, clothing, language, tone).

communication. Sending and receiving information, thoughts, or feelings through verbal words, written words, or body language.

nonverbal communication. Communication that occurs through expressive behaviors and body language rather than oral or written words.

professionalism. The attitude, behavior, and work that represent a profession.

COMMUNICATION

Communication Cycle

Effective communication is a tool used in all aspects of the medical experience and includes all vested members (medical professionals, third-party payers, patients). The communication cycle integrates a sender, a receiver, and a message. The communication is effective when the message is sent and received with the intended purpose.

12.1 Cycle of Effective Communication

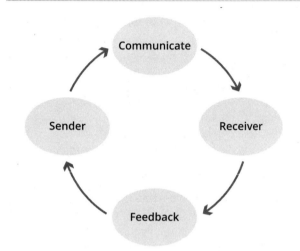

Therapeutic Communication

Therapeutic communication is used in health care and includes strong communication skills that help determine the implications of sending and receiving messages within a diverse patient audience.

Therapeutic communication creates the opportunity to build a positive rapport and relationship between the health care provider and the patient. It has a direct impact on the patient's comfort and well-being related to their health care experience and can encourage a more active participation in choices, preventive measures, and decision-making.

Active Listening Techniques

Active listening is an essential component of therapeutic communication. Active listening goes beyond hearing the words; it is being mindful of what is being said, how it is said, and the intended purpose. When a person is actively listening, their body language and signals show the sender that they are vested in the communication. This technique gives the opportunity for a more open and clear conversation. Characteristics of active listening include remaining nonjudgmental, positive body language, and allowing time to digest words and the intended message.

12.2 Take Note

Therapeutic communication techniques include displaying empathy, rephrasing, asking questions, remaining quiet and pausing to allow a message to be conveyed, and summarizing the received message.

---

therapeutic communication. Interaction between a patient and a medical professional focused on improving the physical and emotional well-being of the patient.

active listening. Engaging with the sender regarding the message and the intended interpretation (e.g., focus solely on the conversation, do not interrupt, confirm the message speaker has said, be respectful and professional).

Oral, Telephone, Email, and Text Communications

Communication types and styles will have a direct impact on the sending and receiving of the intended message. The communication style being used may depend upon the reason for the communication or the intended purpose and can be a blended combination of styles. The communication style being used by the sender may also determine the receiver's response or action.

Communication styles include the following.

- **Assertive.** This is the ideal communication style in health care. Assertive communication is a firm and direct style of communication. It includes proper eye contact and body language with a respectful volume of voice.
- **Passive.** This style is more submissive. Individuals that use this communication style will use a quiet, soft voice and may display hesitancy. Approach this style with a more assertive response.
- **Aggressive.** This style is abrasive in words and body language. Individuals that use this style tend to allow for minimal personal space and use loud and fast gestures. Communicating with someone using the aggressive style can feel intimidating. Respond calmly and never try to match a level of aggression.
- **Manipulative.** This style does not tend to be effective, as it is not a genuine communication—it can be very one-sided with ulterior motives. This style can feel patronizing.

Another factor in choosing a communication style includes whether the participants prefer visual, auditory, or kinesthetic communication. This can also contribute to the effectiveness of the communication process when adjusting to the preferred type of communication.

- Visual communicators use pictures and prefer seeing information in writing. Visual communicators tend to move their hands and use facial expressions. Body language can often say more about the message than the words being used.
- Auditory communicators use the skills of listening when comprehending the message.
- Kinesthetic communicators tend to focus on hands-on learning.

Recognizing communication styles allows you to tailor your response to be more effective for the person you are communicating with.

CHALLENGE

1. Which of the following communication styles is ideal for health care?
   A. Passive
   B. Aggressive
   C. Assertive
   D. Manipulative

   C is correct. The ideal communication style in health care would include assertive due to the direct and firm delivery.

2. Which of the following communication styles is patronizing?
   A. Passive
   B. Aggressive
   C. Assertive
   D. Manipulative

   D is correct. The manipulative style of communication can be very patronizing due to the one-sided delivery.

COMMUNICATION BETWEEN PATIENTS AND PROVIDERS

MAs can be integral in assisting with the communication between patients and providers. A good practice to use when relaying communication between the patient and the medical provider is paraphrasing what is being said to ensure it is correctly being received. It is also essential to clarify and ask questions when any uncertainty is present. Active listening helps to ensure that accurate and effective communication is occurring with the provider and then relayed to the patient.

12.3 Open-Ended vs. Closed-Ended

Open-ended questions ask for general information and can be used to start a conversation. This type of question can establish the conversation and create a comfort level of discussion. It can give the patient freedom to share what they feel is imperative regarding the topic.

- "How are you feeling today?"
- "Can you describe your symptoms?"
- "Can you explain the type of pain you are feeling?"

Closed-ended questions are seeking specific information and are more direct in nature. They can include brief answers such as yes or no to confirm information.

- "What is your current address?"
- "Are you feeling better today?"
- "Do you have a sore throat?"

Interviewing and Questioning Techniques

Ask clear and professional questions when interviewing a patient. Screening questions can be used to determine the medical needs when scheduling appointments and to determine the reason for an office visit. These questions can be asked in an open or closed form. To obtain more information from a patient, ask probing questions—open-ended questions that ask general information to start a conversation. For example, "Can you explain how this happened?"

Scope and Boundaries

When acquiring information from patients, it is important to remain within the professional boundaries and seek information relating to their health. Do not ask personal questions unless it directly pertains to a person's health. For example, it would be appropriate to ask a patient if they may be pregnant when a radiology order is being written. It would not be appropriate to ask a patient if they are suffering from depression when they came in for a suture removal.

Do not share personal information, personal experiences, peer experiences, or other patient experiences when talking with a patient. Maintaining appropriate boundaries and respecting privacy are essential components of communicating in the health care field.

Coaching and Feedback

Consider the patient and any considerations that should be put into place when effectively communicating with them. Ensure opportunities for the patient to give *feedback*.

- Consider the patient's ability to comprehend information. For example, the level of understanding approach of communicating information with a child compared to an older adult would be different.

- Practice empathy. When speaking with a patient who has received a new diagnosis of a disease that will require intensive medical treatments, be patient and keep the conversation around how the patient can be assisted. Patients can be in pain or have strong emotions; remember that a frustrated patient's words are not personal attacks.

- Provide positive reinforcement of behaviors and choices to encourage continued positive life choices that have a direct impact on the patient health.

feedback. Information relayed to the message sender regarding how the message was received and interpreted.

CHALLENGE

1. Which of the following is an open-ended question?
   A. Is the pain in your left knee?
   B. Who is your primary care provider?
   C. Did the injury occur on the job?
   D. How are your current symptoms impacting your life?

   D is correct. Open-ended questions ask for general information and can be used to start a conversation. Closed questions have a direct answer, such as yes or no.

2. What considerations ensure effective communication when speaking with a patient?

   Consider the patient's ability to comprehend the information. Show empathy for the patient's current situation. Be encouraging and patient.

CUSTOMER SERVICE

Audience Considerations

Customize the communication process to meet the needs of the intended receiver. Use active listening skills to help to ensure that effective communication is achieved.

- If a patient has hearing loss, speak clearly while facing the patient to ensure that they can read lips.

- Provide patients who have visual impairments larger print documents when needed.

- Ask patients if they have any questions or require any type of clarification.

- When communicating with a patient who has a cognitive impairment, use words and phrases at the appropriate level the patient can comprehend.

- Consider the age of the patient. An individual would communicate differently with a 5-year-old than a 65-year-old.

Nonverbal Communication

Nonverbal communication can be just as important as the words being spoken. Nonverbal communication is any type of communicating that does not use words. Nonverbal communication should be used to support a message being given and should not contradict the intended message. Body language is an example of nonverbal communication. Body language is the use of gestures and movements while communicating. It can include facial expressions, eye contact, gestures, and mannerisms. Ensure that the message and nonverbal communication match to add to the accurate understanding of the receiver. For example, when expressing empathy for a patient who has just received a terminal diagnosis, follow with a look of care instead of a smile.

12.4 Forms of Nonverbal Communication

- Eye contact
- Facial expressions
- Posture
- Haptics or touch
- Gestures
- Personal space

Another component of nonverbal communication is the concept of personal space and not crowding a person when talking with them. A person can shut down the communication process if they feel they are not at a safe distance, or their personal space is invaded. When a person is frustrated, is not understanding the situation, and has shut down, silence can be a powerful way to give the patient room to process and re-engage. Patience and active listening can assist with keeping the flow of communication.

A final area of nonverbal communication worthy of attention is therapeutic touch. A genuine comforting touch can help to calm a patient and show them that they matter and their medical needs are important. It can be a simple as a high-five or a gentle touch on the shoulder, when appropriate. Therapeutic touch can be encouraging and supportive for the patient. Make sure that the patient is receptive to therapeutic touch before offering it, as an unexpected touch could also be offensive or feel uncomfortable. In all cases, ask the patient for express consent prior to touching them.

Communication for Diverse Audiences

Patient and Families

The goal of all communication in health care is to positively contribute to the quality of patient care. The language used when communicating with a patient will be different than communicating with medical professionals. Medical professionals will use and understand more complex medical terms, while patients usually understand lay terms better. When speaking with the families of patients, be respectful of the patient's privacy. Confirm with the patient what information can be shared with their family. Ensure a release of information form has been completed and signed by the patient and has been documented in the patient's health record.

Medical Professionals

Communication with other medical professionals must be professional and respectful. A positive working relationship must be maintained by all members of the health care team. A good rapport built on trust and teamwork positively contributes toward ensuring great quality of care is provided to the patient by the health care team. An assertive communication style is effective in the health care field with medical professionals. Open communication will minimize the potential for miscommunications or misunderstandings. Nonverbal communication must also reflect a professional disposition and match the intended message being given by the words spoken.

Stereotypes and Biases

Stereotypes are generalized assumptions about a person or group of people. *Biases* are prejudice against a person or group of people. Both can enter the communication process and should be identified and eliminated to ensure effective communication with patients, families, and medical professionals. Addressing stereotypes and biases efficiently will help to contribute to the sending and receiving of the intended messages. A greater understanding of the diversity of people can help to decrease stereotypes and biases. Language, customs, culture, economic status, and age are all factors that contribute to the diversity encountered in health care. Always be respectful and professional.

---

biases. Beliefs that are not proven by facts about someone or a particular group of individuals.

Gender Identity and Expression

When addressing patients and other medical professionals, ask them their preferred name, preferred title, and what pronouns to use. Do not assume a person is married or single. Openly communicating with patients helps to build a rapport and relationship that will be conducive to creating a safe and comfortable atmosphere where they feel free to talk. When a health care service requires considerations based on sex characteristics (such as genitalia, uterus, prostate), refer to the patient's chart first. If clarification is still needed, it is appropriate to ask the patient.

Patient Characteristics Affecting Communication

Many factors that can affect communication must be considered. This includes potential barriers such as language, culture, or comprehension level. Proactively determine and address conditions or situational needs that apply. It is just as important to adjust accordingly as it is to identify any accommodations. As a rule, it is better to ask the patient how they would prefer to be assisted rather than making assumptions about their abilities and needs.

- Provide an interpreter for patients that have minimal understanding of the language being spoken. Family members can be considered if the patient has agreed to allow them to be informed of their medical information. In such circumstances, avoid using medical terminology and always convey messages using lay terms.

- Patients who have physical impairments can be assisted best by asking them how they would like to be assisted.

- When speaking with a child, use terms that they can understand based on their developmental level.

- Effective communication with a patient who has experienced hearing loss can be accomplished with appropriate language use, facing the patient, enunciating each word, and asking if they have any questions or concerns. When summarizing information for the patient, use a repetition of words from the explanation provided. Then, ask the patient to repeat the information back to assess their understanding of what was communicated.

Patient Cultures and Backgrounds

Be considerate of any cultural differences. A respectful disposition when reading nonverbal communication can increase the possibility of effectively communicating. Facial signs of confusion or grimacing in pain can help to understand the possible approach to take with assisting the patient. Do not make assumptions. Words and actions will vary with different types of cultural backgrounds. The health care services provided can also be dependent upon the patient's belief of medicine and treatments.

12.5 Take Note

Providing effective cultural, religious, psychosocial, and economic sensitivity to the needs of the patient is essential in health care and greatly increases the overall health care experience and outcome.

Cultural, Religious, Psychosocial, and Economic Considerations

The patient population is diverse. Patients will have different backgrounds, traditions, values, and beliefs. Knowledge and understanding of different cultures can help to prevent the possibility of stereotyping and offensive assumptions. However, be careful not to generalize about patient care based on your understanding. Generalizing is making a general assumption based on a small amount of information. An example of a generalization is assuming that a patient will not accept blood transfusions or organ donations based on their religion. Always verify with the patient in a professional and unassuming way their treatment preferences. Affiliation with a group does not always direct an individual's behaviors or choices, so all treatment options should be presented.

12.6 Psychosocial Health

Mental Health	Spiritual Health
Social Health	Emotional Health

Cultural differences can arise in the way that people believe conditions should be treated, whether it be holistically or with medications. In certain cultures, it can be seen as a sign of weakness to express the feeling of pain. A patient from such a culture may have difficulty communicating their needs with the health care team. Work with the patient and provider to identify where cultural differences may affect understanding and adjust your language as needed to ensure the medical team can meet the patient's needs.

A benefit of being culturally aware is providing psychosocial care. Psychosocial care is providing psychological, social, and spiritual care through therapeutic communication with cultural sensitivity. When provided effectively, it improves patients' overall health and quality of life. Examples of psychosocial care include motivational enhancement, relapse prevention, structured counseling, and psychotherapy.

A patient may also not seek medical services or minimize their signs and symptoms if they cannot afford treatment. To help ensure these patients can receive the right medical care, provide information about resources available to a person who has limited financial resources.

Regardless of the type of health care facility, it is important to take initiative to learn about the cultures represented in the health care practice.

CHALLENGE

1. Which of the following is an example of body language?
   A. Vocal pitch
   B. Empathy
   C. Shaking hands
   D. Enunciation of words

   C is correct. Body language is use of the body with gestures and movements while communicating.

2. What is the importance of the words matching the actions?

   Nonverbal communication should be used to support a message being given and should not contradict the intended message. Body language and nonverbal communication can be just as important as the words being spoken in avoiding miscommunication.

3. What is the importance of effectively communicating with the health care team?

   A good rapport built on trust and teamwork positively contributes toward ensuring great quality of care is provided to the patient by the health care team.

4. What should be done to minimize stereotypes of bias in communication?

   Gaining a greater understanding of the diversity of people helps to decrease stereotypes and biases and includes respect and professionalism in all communication with all people. Building a rapport and relationship with the patient will be conducive to creating a safe and comfortable atmosphere where they feel free to talk.

5. What is a benefit of psychosocial care?

   When provided effectively, it improves patients' overall health and quality of life.

TYPE OF VISIT CONSIDERATIONS

The type of visit will help to determine the best route to take when evaluating the communication process to use. Checking the audio and visual components of virtual visits is a must at the beginning of the visit. This will facilitate an easier visit, save time, and increase the opportunities for effective communication. Appearance, facial expressions, gestures, and eye contact are essential parts of the communication process for both in-person and virtual visits. For patients who have hearing or visual impairments using telehealth, it is important to use active listening skills to evaluate the patients' medical needs. In addition, some telehealth features offer a closed caption option that allows patients the opportunity to read live written captions of their visit, which allows for more effective communication.

Nonverbal Cues in Telehealth

Body language and nonverbal language are more noticeable during in-person visits. Virtual visits rely on the words spoken for effective communication. Because nonverbal communication is not as apparent with virtual visits, it can be challenging to assess for understanding. Therefore, appropriate and effective verbal communication is essential. Ask for questions or concerns and for information to be repeated back to assess comprehension. Demonstrate proper eye contact and display facial expressions that support the interest in the patient's medical needs and reason for their visit.

Telephone Communication

Privacy, security, and confidentiality must be followed using Health Insurance Portability and Accountability Act (HIPAA) guidelines when speaking with all vested members in the health care process (patients, caregivers, third-party payers) on the telephone. HIPAA will be covered in greater detail in another chapter.

Telephone Etiquette

When communicating using the telephone, it is important to be succinct because nonverbal communication and body language are more challenging to interpret. Avoiding medical jargon and complex medical terms will help to ensure the patient is able to communicate and understand what is being said. Ensure your vocal pitch and tone are not monotone or too loud. Clearly enunciate. It can be helpful to smile while on the phone, as it helps to present and convey a positive disposition. Active listening is important when using telephone skills. Give undivided attention to the person on the other end of the phone and be respectful and professional at all times.

12.7 Five Ps of Telephone Etiquette

- **Polite.** Use a soft tone.
- **Prepared.** Have all the relevant details (names, numbers, dates).
- **to the Point.** Don't beat around the bush.
- **Perceptive.** Don't waste people's time by talking on irrelevant topics.
- **cooPerative.** Provide the information needed. If you can't help, find someone who can or tell the caller you will call back with the information.

Written and Electronic Communication

Written communication can occur with emails, letters, faxes, and chat features and are included in the permanent legal records. Communicating using written words must adhere to the professional and respectful requirements for the MA. It must also follow HIPAA guidelines for privacy, security, and confidentiality. Written communications must be grammatically correct and free from errors, as they are representative of the MA and the health care facility.

telephone etiquette. Being respectful by using proper verbiage, tone, and manners when conveying information.

Email Etiquette

There are many advantages to using email, such as speed of receipt and simplicity of responding. Always send emails using a secure email software program. Check for spelling and grammar errors and do not include jargon or slang. Professionalism is a requirement of writing emails to patients, medical providers, or third-party payers. The message should be concise and to the point. The email must include a subject line, salutation, and proper closing with contact information. Proper etiquette includes using polite conversation and not writing using a conversational approach, such as that used when texting with a friend. Do not abbreviate words, as this could lead to misinterpretation and miscommunication. Documents such as reports or statements can be attached and should be referenced in the body of the email.

Business Letter Formats

Letters can be created for many purposes, and *templates* are often used for creating them. Templates are sample letters that provide the format, and the user adds the words where appropriate. Proofreading is important to ensure the letter is free from errors and is grammatically correct. Letters may be created to address a concern with a third-party payer, write a patient about their past-due balance, or request a consultation from another medical provider. Letters include the date, address, salutation, body, and complimentary closing and are done on letterhead for the health care organization. They are more formal in nature and usually mailed using the United States Postal Service (USPS) or another professional service. Certified mail can be used to ensure the letter has been received by the intended party in circumstances where it is imperative that the information is received. An example of this would be if a patient needs to be informed of concerning lab results and cannot be reached by phone or email or if a provider makes the decision to terminate a relationship with a patient.

Letter Styles
- **Full block format.** All lines are flush with the left margin.
- **Modified block format.** The address and body are left justified, and the rest start at the center of the document.
- **Modified block format with indented paragraphs.** The address is left justified and, the rest start at the center of the document with indented paragraphs.
- **Simplified format.** The information is left justified, and it does not include a salutation or complimentary closing.

Health care organizations tend to use the full block format. It is a formal document that must be created using time and care to ensure it is professional, as it represents the health care professionals. A proactive measure to ensure the accuracy is to have another medical professional review it before it is sent out.

---

template. A sample of written correspondence or email that is established with appropriate components that will be personalized to fit the need of the sender.

12.8 Example Letter

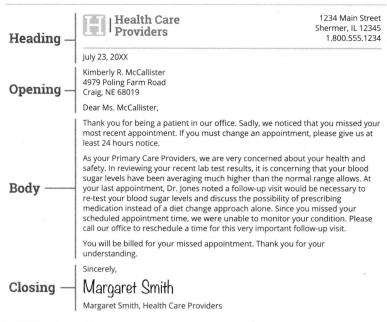

Heading — Health Care Providers · 1234 Main Street, Shermer, IL 12345 · 1.800.555.1234

Opening —
July 23, 20XX

Kimberly R. McCallister
4979 Poling Farm Road
Craig, NE 68019

Dear Ms. McCallister,

Body —
Thank you for being a patient in our office. Sadly, we noticed that you missed your most recent appointment. If you must change an appointment, please give us at least 24 hours notice.

As your Primary Care Providers, we are very concerned about your health and safety. In reviewing your recent lab test results, it is concerning that your blood sugar levels have been averaging much higher than the normal range allows. At your last appointment, Dr. Jones noted a follow-up visit would be necessary to re-test your blood sugar levels and discuss the possibility of prescribing medication instead of a diet change approach alone. Since you missed your scheduled appointment time, we were unable to monitor your condition. Please call our office to reschedule a time for this very important follow-up visit.

You will be billed for your missed appointment. Thank you for your understanding.

Closing —
Sincerely,

Margaret Smith

Margaret Smith, Health Care Providers

CHALLENGE

1. Which of the following is an important aspect of communication in the virtual setting?
   A. Personal space
   B. Therapeutic touch
   C. Word choice
   D. Proofreading

   C is correct. Virtual visits rely on the words spoken for effective communication. Because nonverbal communication is not as apparent during virtual visits, it can be challenging to assess for understanding. It is important to use words to ask for questions or concerns and to ask for information to be repeated back to assess comprehension.

2. Which of the following actions should be followed when on the phone with a patient?
   A. Multitasking for efficiency
   B. Smiling while talking
   C. Using a loud tone to ensure they hear
   D. Speaking fast to save time

   B is correct. It can be helpful to smile while on the phone, as it helps to present a positive disposition.

3. Which of the following is an example of email etiquette?
   A. Using humor
   B. Using informal language
   C. Abbreviating when possible
   D. Being concise

   D is correct. Etiquette must be followed when sending email. This includes having manners and using appropriate language.

CRUCIAL CONVERSATIONS

At times it is necessary to communicate in a challenging situation, and it is not always possible to say what the other person is hoping to hear. It may be a conversation with a patient that is frustrated and in pain and possibly not thinking as logically as they normally would. A conversation may occur with a patient that is financially struggling and is being asked to pay the balance of their account while other bills are compounding. A patient who received a terminal diagnosis may call with a question or concern about their treatment plan, and they may feel anxious and uncertain. Challenging conversations should be handled with extra care and compassion. These types of situations require patience, active listening skills, and collaboration with the patient. At times, emotions can run high, and empathy can go a long way in helping the patient gain understanding and acceptance. Speaking with caregivers or health care surrogates also is an integral part of assisting the patient with their medical needs. Always ensure that the patient has consented to their health information being released to the person prior to the conversation.

Speaking with other members of the health care team is another part of communication that occurs in the daily life of an MA. This communication must also be conducted in a professional and respectful manner. Show respect for the knowledge and authority of medical providers when communicating with them. It is essential to communicate openly and honestly. All members of the health care team should communicate with the common goal of quality patient medical care. Medical professionals do not need to be best friends; however, they must be always friendly and professional regardless of the situation.

Incident/Event/Unusual Occurrence Reports

"If it isn't documented, it didn't happen." This common phrase reflects the importance and necessity of documentation. All types of communication must be documented to ensure the event is on record. It must be detailed with the date, time, persons involved, and overview of the conversation including specific details. This practice protects the patient, as well as the health care professional.

Challenging Customer Service Occurrences

Handle challenging customer service occurrences with professionalism and respect. It may be challenging to communicate with a person who is upset or frustrated. It is important to maintain composure. It is never appropriate to match any negative energy in response to the challenging situation. Refrain from becoming defensive and remember the goal is to provide quality health care services. Building a good relationship based on trust and professionalism can help to enhance the patient-centered care experience. Another action that can help to minimize any defensive responses can be to use "I" statement instead of "You" statements. For example, "I understand that it is difficult making healthy eating decisions," instead of "It seems you have a hard time making healthy eating decisions."

When to De-Escalate Problem Situations

Communication experiences that can become challenging should be de-escalated as soon as possible to prevent them from becoming uncontrolled. Communications within the health care team must be professional and respectful. When conflict arises, it may be necessary to involve a supervisor for assistance with resolution. Open communication, allowing the patient to vent, and active listening skills can help to minimize the potential for conflict and will aide in effectively communicating. Professionalism and respect will help in minimizing any drama, gossip, or judgements.

When a conflict arises while communicating with patients, remember to be patient and listen to their concerns. The communication process must be free from distractions and interruptions. The patient should feel heard and that their concern will be considered. Set healthy boundaries in the discussion, both physical and psychological. The assertive communication style should include a tactful and courteous response. Use active listening and respect, and engage in appropriate communication by responding to appropriate verbal and nonverbal cues from the patient. If the situation escalates and attempts at resolution have not helped in controlling the situation, it may be beneficial to include a supervisor or another additional person to help in the de-escalation process.

Another proactive measure in trying to minimize potential challenging communication experiences and de-escalating a situation is to remove any potential barriers. Barriers can include language differences, lack of personal boundaries, cultural differences, judgements, and stereotypes.

Conflict Management and Complaint Resolution

Conflict management is managing a situation where differences occur and there appears to be no resolution that will be effective. Effective communication can help to minimize the possibility of conflicts. There must be a process in place to assist when situations escalate to a level where intervention is needed. Patients must have a resolution process that can be followed when they feel their concerns are not being heard and addressed. The goal is effective and respectful communication and that a win-win resolution can be achieved. Patient satisfaction surveys can be offered to see how happy patients are and what possible suggestions or concerns can be addressed.

Methods of conflict resolution can include allowing the other person to express concerns, practicing active listening, determining possible solutions or outcomes, and concluding that all vested members are satisfied. At times, it isn't about one side being right and the other side wrong; it can be respectfully coming to a conclusion that is satisfactory for all.

Understanding the underlying goals, rather than the specific asks, of each party can promote resolution. Many times, there are likely to be more similarities found when positive communication is pursued.

While effective communication can often lead to resolution, this is not always the case. Patients must be provided with a route to take when they are not satisfied with the outcome, such as having an unbiased person evaluate the situation and give potential options or solutions. The patient has the right to overall satisfaction when it relates to their health care experience.

12.9 Example

- A patient declines a blood pressure medication that the provider feels strongly about prescribing.
- On the surface, the preferences of the patient and provider are mutually exclusive: either taking the medication or not.
- After the MA discusses the situation with the patient and provider, it becomes clear that both agree that the patient's blood pressure should be lower and that it should be managed in a way that is safest for the patient. They disagree on the best way to accomplish their shared goals.
- Once there is a shared understanding and alignment, further conversation can include both parties sharing their individual views.
- To resolve this concern, the provider agrees to pause the conversation around the potential prescription for 6 weeks, while the patient agrees to meet with the MA for health coaching around diet and exercise to lower blood pressure and monitor their blood pressure every day.
- They agree to revisit the conversation in six weeks to discuss how impactful the diet and exercise have been. This also provides time for reviewing the risks and benefits of the medication if the provider still feels it is needed.

Cause-and-Effect Analysis

Cause and effect play a factor in the overall health care organization's ability to provide patient satisfaction. Being proactive in this measure can decrease customer complaints. Additionally, patient safety and ensuring a safe work environment for employees must be considered. Risk management is the process of ensuring a safe environment for all vested members. It evaluates and analyzes the environment and how to apply improvements to make it safer. An example is walking through the facility to ensure there are no loose cords or areas where a person could trip over items in the open areas. Identify any potential causes of incidents and the effects that could result and put a plan in place to minimize that potential.

CHALLENGE

1. What is the best approach for an MA when speaking with a patient who is upset?

   The MA must be patient, use active listening skills, and work with the patient throughout the communication process.

2. Which of the following actions should an MA take with a patient that is yelling at them?
   A. Talk louder.
   B. Interrupt them.
   C. Allow them to vent.
   D. Ask them to come back later.

   C is correct. It is important to never match any negative energy in response to the challenging situation. Refrain from becoming defensive and remember the ultimate goal is to provide quality health care services.

3. What can be done to assist patients who feel they are not being heard?

   There must be a process in place to assist when situations escalate to a level where intervention is needed. Patients must have a resolution process that can be followed when they feel their concerns are not being heard and addressed.

TEAMWORK

Facilitate Teamwork and Team Engagement

Effective teamwork and engagement are a must for any health care organization. They contribute to the flow of a positive environment, which helps ensure patient satisfaction. Each member of the health care team makes an impact on the overall health care experience for patients. Each member performs their own responsibilities, and the members work together to ensure that all tasks are completed. Gossip, negative tone and word use, and dramatic outbursts have no place in the work environment. While personal feelings related to workplace events and interactions are expected, health care professionals must not allow those feelings to hinder their professionalism or the way in which they provide patient care. Working together in a cooperative environment helps to engage each of the team members, which increases the patient satisfaction levels. Quality health care services are provided to patients by a team that works well together where each member is involved in the process.

CHALLENGE

1. Which of the following should be included in the work environment?
   A. Personal feelings
   B. Engagement
   C. Gossip
   D. Drama

   B is correct. Personal feelings, gossip, and drama have no place in the work environment.

PROFESSIONALISM

Demonstrate Professionalism

Professionalism is a must in a health care organization. It must be present in all aspects of the overall environment.

Professionalism encompasses the following.

- Behaviors
- Appearance
- Communication
  - Voice: tone, attitude, and word selection
  - Written
- Work ethic
- Relationships

All members of the health care team have their own roles and responsibilities that fit together to form a well-organized machine. All team members must be courteous, knowledgeable, and respectful in their presence and approach with the patient. The MA will be one of the first encounters that a patient has in the health care experience, and the first impression is important. Maintain a professional manner with a positive attitude of encouragement and support. These behaviors will help to build a relationship based on trust and respect.

Professional Presence

Displaying a professional presence is essential for an effective career. Other contributory factors in ensuring a professional environment include work ethic, positive and polite demeanor, willingness to assist, cooperation, and effective time management skills. Personal boundaries are essential within all relationships in the health care organization—personal relationships must be kept outside the work environment. Dress and appearance must be within the professional limits established within the field, and individual health care organizations will have policies and procedures to be followed relating to dress and appearance. When communicating, follow professional standards at all times regardless of the behavior of the other participants in the process.

CHALLENGE

1. How can an MA build a relationship with a patient based on trust and respect?

   Exhibit a professional manner with a positive attitude of encouragement and support. These behaviors will help to build a relationship based on trust and respect.

2. Which of the following is included in professionalism?
   A. Criticism
   B. A monotone voice
   C. Courtesy
   D. Casual dress

   C is correct. All team members must be courteous, knowledgeable, and respectful in their presence and approach.

WRAP-UP

The chapter included information that contributes to effectively communication between all vested members in the health care experience. It includes active listening, verbal and nonverbal communication, and knowing the appropriate words and language. The MA must effectively communicate with patients in an encouraging and supportive manner. Stereotypes and biases must be omitted or minimized from the communication process, as it will occur with a diverse population with diverse needs.

Conflict resolution and management may need to be used when put in a position of a challenge within the communication experiences. It is important to know how to de-escalate and also determine when a third member might need to be added to find a resolution. Using communication etiquette will also help to positively contribute to effective communication. A team that is professional, engaged, and effective communicators will ensure that the patients receive the best quality of care and are satisfied with their health care experience.

CHAPTER 13
Medical Law and Ethics

OVERVIEW

All health care providers and professionals have a primary responsibility to provide high-quality patient care and to prevent and manage diseases and conditions while respecting patient privacy, maintaining confidentiality, and communicating responsibly in fulfillment of this role. To ensure patient protection, health care professionals, including medical assistants, are bound by a variety of laws and regulations and by a wide range of legal and ethical responsibilities to their patients, their employers, and society.

This chapter will discuss the different laws and standards that help protect patients, their health information, and their health care. It is important to understand how to apply laws and regulations that guide the practice of patient care, including consent and who can give it and how to protect patient confidentiality and health information. Knowing how to apply ethics and values and how they are the foundation of many laws and regulations for patient care is essential when working in health care. A medical assistant should understand diversity and how biases may prevent some individuals from accessing health care and what role they have in improving that through cultural competency.

Objectives

Upon completion of this chapter, you should be able to

- Identify legal and regulatory requirements.
- Identify patient consent as needed.
- Identify professional codes of ethics.
- Describe and differentiate medical directives.
- Describe patient privacy and confidentiality, including medical records.
- Identify legal requirements regarding reportable violations or incidents.
- Identify personal or religious beliefs and values and provide unbiased care.

MEDICAL LAWS

Patient's Bill of Rights

An important aspect of patient care is understanding *medical law* and defining the rights and responsibilities of both the patient and health care provider. For patients, the American Hospital Association (AHA) created the original Patient's Bill of Rights in 1973, which provides guidelines and guarantees by federal law to ensure the protection and safety of patients. Although the Patient's Bill of Rights was originally intended for the hospital setting, most medical practices, hospitals, insurance companies, and even governments have adopted some form of the legislation.

13.1 Take Note

The primary purposes of the Patient's Bill of Rights are to help patients feel more confident in the health care system, to strengthen the relationship between patients and their health care provider by defining their rights and responsibilities and those of their health care provider, and to emphasize the role patients play in their health.

---

medical law. Laws that explain the rights and responsibilities of medical providers and patients.

The Patient's Bill of Rights outlines 15 guarantees for all patients seeking medical care in a health care organization and basic rights and responsibilities for effective patient care. Medical assistants must adhere to patient rights and uphold duties while administering and assisting with patient care. A summary of these guarantees is as follows.

13.2 The Patient's Bill of Rights

- The patient has the right to be treated fairly and respectfully.
- The patient has the right to get information they can understand about their diagnosis, treatment, and prognosis from their health care provider.
- The patient has the right to discuss and ask for information about specific procedures and treatments, their risks, and the time they will spend recovering. They also have the right to discuss other care options.
- The patient has the right to know the identities of all their health care providers, including students, residents, and other trainees.
- The patient has the right to know how much care may cost at the time of treatment and long term.
- The patient has the right to make decisions about their care before and during treatment and the right to refuse care. The hospital must inform the patient of the medical consequences of refusing treatment. The patient has the right to other treatments provided by the hospital and the right to transfer to another hospital.
- The patient has the right to have an advance directive, such as a living will or a power of attorney for health care. A hospital has the right to ask for their advance directive, put it in their file, and honor its intent.
- The patient has the right to privacy in medical exams, case discussions, consultations, and treatments.
- The patient has the right to expect that their communication and records are treated as confidential by the hospital, except as the law permits and requires in cases of suspected abuse or public health hazards. If the hospital releases their information to another medical facility, they have the right to expect the hospital to ask the medical facility to keep their records confidential.
- The patient has the right to review their medical records and to have them explained or interpreted, except when restricted by law.
- The patient has the right to expect that a hospital will respond reasonably to their requests for care and services or transfer them to another facility that has accepted a transfer request. They should also expect information and explanation about the risks, benefits, and alternatives to a transfer.
- The patient has the right to ask and to be informed of any business relationships between the hospital and educational institutions, other health care providers, or payers that may influence their care and treatment.
- The patient has the right to consent to or decline to participate in research studies and to have the studies fully explained before they give their consent. If they decide not to participate in research, they are still entitled to the most effective care that the hospital can provide.
- The patient has the right to expect reasonable continuity of care and to be informed of other care options when hospital care is no longer appropriate.
- The patient has the right to be informed of hospital policies and practices related to patient care, treatment, and responsibilities.
- The patient has the right to know whom they can contact to resolve disputes, grievances, and conflicts. And they have the right to know what the hospital will charge for services and their payment methods.

CHALLENGE

1. Which of the following is a goal of the Patient's Bill of Rights?
   A. Ensure that patients feel more ambivalent about their health care
   B. Ensure that health care providers make decisions for patients to ensure their best care
   C. Ensure the rights and responsibilities of both patients and health care providers and that patients play a role in their own health
   D. Ensure patients have access to necessary medications

   C is correct. The goals of the Patient's Bill of Rights are to help patients feel more confident in the health care system in the United States, to strengthen the relationship between patients and their health care provider, and to emphasize the role patients play in their health by ensuring patients understand their rights and responsibilities and those of their health care provider. It also outlines 15 guarantees for all patients seeking medical care in a health care organization.

2. According to the Patient's Bill of Rights, which of the following is a guarantee? (Select all that apply.)
   A. Patients have the right to refuse care.
   B. Patients have the right to privacy while in the hospital.
   C. Patients can be a participant in a research study without consent.
   D. Patients can request a transfer to another hospital.
   E. Patients will be provided information about the cost of treatment following discharge.

   A, B, and D are correct. The Patient's Bill of Rights gives patients the right to privacy as well as refusing care. The hospital must inform the patient of the medical consequences of refusing treatment. Patients have the right to other treatments provided by the hospital and the right to transfer to another hospital.

LAWS AND REGULATIONS

The health care field is a heavily regulated environment, given that people's lives and health are affected. There are several federal, state, and local regulatory agencies that establish rules and regulations for the health care industry to ensure compliance and to provide safe health care to every person who accesses the system.

Medical assistants should be familiar with laws that affect their profession. The most common laws and regulations that affect medical practices and patient care are shown in the table below.

13.3 Comply With Legal and Regulatory Requirements

LAW/REGULATION	DESCRIPTION
Patient Protection and Affordable Care Act	Commonly called the Affordable Care Act (ACA) or "Obamacare," named after former president Barack Obama, who signed it into law in 2010, this federal statute was a major step in health care reform by expanding access to more affordable, quality health insurance, increasing consumer insurance protection, emphasizing prevention and wellness, and curbing rising health care costs.
Health Insurance Portability and Accountability Act of 1996 (HIPAA)	HIPAA gives patients rights over their health information and sets rules and limits on who can look at and receive patients' private information. HIPAA applies to protected health information (PHI), whether electronic, written, or oral.
Health Information Technology for Economic and Clinical Health (HITECH) Act	The HITECH Act expands on HIPAA and includes provisions that allow for increased enforcement of the privacy and security of electronic transmission of patient information, such as prohibiting the sale of PHI, making business associates and vendors liable for compliance with HIPAA, and creating a penalty and violation system.

Health Insurance Portability and Accountability Act of 1996 (HIPAA). Federal law that required the creation of national standards to protect sensitive patient health information from being disclosed without the patient's consent or knowledge.

Health Information Technology for Economic and Clinical Health (HITECH) Act. Law that includes provisions that allow for increased enforcement of the privacy and security of electronic transmission of patient information, such as prohibiting the sale of PHI, making business associates and vendors liable for compliance with HIPAA, and creating a penalty and violation system.

13.3 Comply With Legal and Regulatory Requirements (continued)

LAW/REGULATION	DESCRIPTION
Occupational Safety and Health (OSH) Act	The OSH Act is overseen by the Occupational Safety and Health Administration (OSHA) and states that employers are accountable for providing a safe and healthful workplace for employees by setting and enforcing standards and by providing training, outreach, education, and assistance.
Controlled Substances Act (CSA)	CSA is a federal policy that regulates the manufacture and distribution of controlled substances. Controlled substances can include narcotics, depressants, and stimulants. The CSA classifies medications into five schedules, or classifications, based on the likelihood for abuse and if there are any medical benefits provided from the substance.
Emergency Medical Treatment and Active Labor Act (EMTALA)	The EMTALA of 1986 requires any hospital emergency department that receives payments from federal health care programs, such as Medicare and Medicaid, to provide an appropriate medical screening to any patient seeking treatment. This was enacted to eliminate "patient dumping," where a facility would transfer a patient based on a potentially high-cost diagnosis or refuse to treat a patient based on their ability to pay. This legislation requires the emergency department to determine whether a condition is emergent or not and to provide stabilizing treatment in the case of an emergency medical condition. It does not require that treatment be given for nonemergency conditions. Furthermore, outpatient clinics are not medically equipped to handle emergencies and therefore are not bound by the EMTALA.
Clinical Laboratory Improvement Act (CLIA)	The CLIA of 1988 is a group of laws that regulate all laboratory facilities for safety and handling of specimens. The objective of CLIA is to regulate accuracy and timeliness of testing regardless of where the test is performed. The Food and Drug Administration (FDA) is the federal agency that authorizes and implements the CLIA laws and determines the test complexity categories.
Title VII of Civil Rights Act of 1964	The Civil Rights Act prohibits an employer with 15 or more employees from discriminating on the basis of race, national origin, gender, or religion. The Civil Rights Act has also been amended several times to protect other groups. For example, the Pregnancy Discrimination Act of 1978 amended the Civil Rights Act and prohibited discrimination based on pregnancy and other related medical conditions. Sexual harassment is a form of sex discrimination that also violates the Civil Rights Act.
Americans with Disabilities Act of 1990 (ADA)	ADA forbids discrimination against any applicant or employee who could perform a job regardless of a disability. ADA also requires an employer to provide "reasonable accommodations" that are necessary to help the employee perform a job successfully unless these accommodations are unduly burdensome.

Controlled Substances Act (CSA). Statute that identifies all regulated substances into one of five schedules depending on potential for abuse.

Emergency Medical Treatment and Active Labor Act (EMTALA). Law that requires any hospital emergency department that receives payments from federal health care programs, such as Medicare and Medicaid, to provide an appropriate medical screening to any patient seeking treatment.

Clinical Laboratory Improvement Act (CLIA). A 1988 amendment that regulates federal standards that apply to all clinical laboratory testing performed on humans in the United States.

Title VII of Civil Rights Act of 1964. Law that prohibits an employer with 15 or more employees from discriminating on the basis of race, national origin, gender, or religion.

Americans with Disabilities Act of 1990 (ADA). Law that forbids discrimination based on disability.

13.3 Comply With Legal and Regulatory Requirements (continued)

LAW/REGULATION	DESCRIPTION
Heads of the European Radiological Protection Competent Authorities (HERCA)	Provides clarity on the regulator's approach to the roles of the undertaking and a range of professionals regarding the justification process.
Good Samaritan Acts	Allows bystanders to get involved in emergency situations without fear that they will be sued if their actions inadvertently contribute to a person's injury or death.
Genetic Information Nondiscrimination Act of 2008 (GINA)	Prohibits discrimination on the basis of genetic information with respect to health insurance and employment.
Patient Safety and Quality Improvement Act (PSQIA)	Framework for gathering and analyzing information regarding patient safety within the confines of protected health information laws.
Anti-Kick Back Statute (AKBS)	Criminal law that prohibits receiving benefits for referral or business involving federal health care programs.
No Surprise Act (NSA)	The No Surprise Act protects individuals from surprise billing if they have a group health plan or individual health insurance coverage. This includes banning surprise bills for emergency services from an out-of-network provider or facility without prior authorization.

CHALLENGE

1. Which of the following laws or regulations would include precautions and rules related to needlestick safety and injuries?
   A. CLIA
   B. EMTALA
   C. OSH Act
   D. HITECH Act

   C is correct. The Occupational Safety and Health (OSH) Act provides enforceable standards and regulations on safety and health in a workplace setting. This includes employers providing proper equipment and training on disposing of needles and precautions on needlestick injuries.

2. Which of the following laws classifies medications based on the likelihood for abuse and if there are any medical benefits provided from the substance?
   A. ADA
   B. CLIA
   C. CSA
   D. OSHA

   C is correct. The Controlled Substances Act (CSA) is a federal policy that regulates the manufacture and distribution of controlled substances. Controlled substances can include narcotics, depressants, and stimulants. The CSA classifies medications into five schedules, or classifications, based on the likelihood for abuse and if there are any medical benefits provided from the substance.

Heads of the European Radiological Protection Competent Authorities (HERCA). Association that provides clarity on the regulator's approach to the roles of the undertaking and a range of professionals regarding the justification process.

Good Samaritan Acts. Law that allows bystanders to get involved in emergency situations without fear that they will be sued if their actions inadvertently contribute to a person's injury or death.

Genetic Information Nondiscrimination Act of 2008 (GINA). Law that prohibits discrimination on the basis of genetic information with respect to health insurance and employment.

Patient Safety and Quality Improvement Act (PSQIA). Framework for gathering and analyzing information regarding patient safety within the confines of protected health information laws.

Anti-Kick Back Statute (AKBS). Criminal law that prohibits receiving benefits for referral or business involving federal health care programs.

No Surprise Act (NSA). Law that protects individuals from surprise billing if they have a group health plan or individual health insurance coverage.

PROTECT PATIENT PRIVACY AND CONFIDENTIALITY
Legal Requirements for Maintenance, Storage, and Disposal of Records

Sharing Information and Release of Information

The medical record contains sensitive information regarding patient history, current health status, and planned treatment. Training in proper documentation and maintenance of medical records and following federal and state laws and guidelines is essential to maintain patient privacy. There are many laws and regulations that guide how patient information and medical records should be managed.

The most important law regarding protection of medical records is HIPAA, which outlines patient privacy and confidentiality and how patient information is managed. HIPAA gives patients rights over their health care information. Patients have the right to receive a copy of their information, ensure the medical record is correct, and know who has had access to the record. Covered entities, such as health insurance companies, clearinghouses, and providers, must adhere to HIPAA. Employers are not considered covered entities because employee health records maintained by an employer are not used for HIPAA-covered transactions.

The HIPAA Security Rule requires implementing reasonable and suitable safeguards to protect protected health information and to prevent breaches of confidentiality.

HIPAA also requires providers to explain patient rights. The law requires patients to sign a form indicating they have received a privacy notice from a health care provider or hospital. HIPAA requires written consent when sharing health care information. HIPAA does not require a provider or health plan to share information with a patient's family or friends unless the person is legally identified as the patient's personal representatives.

13.4 Take Note

There are three safeguards set in place that medical facilities use to keep patient information private.

- Administrative safeguards are used to refer to the policies and procedures documented in writing that show how covered entities comply with HIPAA.
- Physical safeguards refer to the physical monitoring and access to PHI.
- Technical safeguards refer to the responsibility of the health care provider to monitor and safeguard patient information through all technology-related items.

Patient data ownership can be broken into the ownership of the data versus the medical records and the ability of patients to access their data. Medical records are legal documents generated by the health care provider or facility. Because it is a legal document and even though the information in the medical records pertains to the patient, the patient's original medical records must remain with the health care facility, and the health care provider is the owner of the medical records. However, based on HIPAA, the patient has a right to the information that is in the medical record. Thus, with few exceptions, patients have the right to inspect, review, and receive a copy of their medical records and billing records that are held by health plans and health care providers. In addition, only the patient and any of their authorized representatives, such as a family member with the patient's consent, have the right to access the patient's medical record. To summarize the concept, the medical provider or the facility owns the actual medical record, but the patient owns the information, or data, found within the record.

Patients may also request release of medical records or to receive copies of their medical records from the health care provider with a signed release form. This signed release form ensures that the confidentiality of the medical record is protected and can be shared only with an approved and authorized health care provider or entity. For example, if a patient transfers to another health care provider, the new health care provider may obtain the medical records only after the patient signs a release form.

CHAPTER 13: MEDICAL LAW AND ETHICS
Protect Patient Privacy and Confidentiality

Health care staff should always prioritize patient privacy. However, there are a few exceptions that would allow for the release of medical records without the patient's authorization or a signed release form from the patient. These exceptions include the following.

- Criminal acts: Evidence used in abuse cases, stabbings, gunshot wounds, or sexual assaults.

- Legally ordered: The court can order medical records to be submitted as evidence in court case through the process of a subpoena. When the court orders someone to appear in court (a summons) and bring records with them it is termed *subpoena duces tecum*.

- Communicable diseases: The Centers for Disease Control and Prevention or local health departments can require release of information in case of the possibility of diseases that potentially could cause a pandemic or sexually transmitted diseases, such as human immunodeficiency virus (HIV), syphilis, or tuberculosis.

- Mandated examinations: Ordered by employers' insurance companies for workers' compensation cases.

CHALLENGE

1. In which of the following situations would patients have to authorize the release of their medical records?
   A. The patient is relocating and needs to find a new health care provider.
   B. The patient is being investigated as a victim of elder abuse.
   C. The patient has tested positive for tuberculosis.
   D. The patient has filed for workers' compensation.

   A is correct. Patients must authorize release of medical records with a signed release form, including transferring to another health care provider. There are a few exceptions that would allow for the release of medical records without the patient's authorization or a signed release form from the patient. This includes criminal acts, cases of court orders or subpoenas, certain communicable diseases, and mandated examinations ordered by employers' insurance companies for workers' compensation.

2. According to HIPAA, which of the following owns the patient's medical record?
   A. The patient
   B. The health care provider
   C. The patient's insurance company
   D. The federal government

   B is correct. Patient data ownership can be broken into the ownership of the data and the ability of patients to access their data. Medical records are legal documents generated by the health care provider or facility. Because medical records are legal documents, patients' medical records must remain with the health care facility, and the health care provider is the owner of the medical records. However, the information that is in the medical record belongs to patients, allowing them the right to inspect, review, and receive a copy of their medical records and billing records that are held by health plans and health care providers.

3. The HIPAA Security Rule requires implementing reasonable and suitable safeguards for protected health information and to prevent breaches of confidentiality. Match the situation with the type of safeguard.

SAFEGUARD	SITUATION
1. Administrative safeguard	A. Keeping workstations with patient information out of high-traffic areas.
2. Physical safeguard	B. Data encryption system for patient information
3. Technical safeguard	C. Performing internal audits
	D. Implementing a "double lock system" (using a locked room and locked file cabinet)
	E. Appointing a security officer
	F. Installing firewalls in the facility's computer systems connected to the Internet.

   1: C, E; 2: A, D; 3: B, F. Administrative safeguards refer to the policies and procedures documented in writing that show how covered entities comply with HIPAA. Physical safeguards refer to the physical monitoring and access to PHI. Technical safeguards refer to the responsibility of the health care provider to monitor and safeguard patient information through all technology-related items and uses.

subpoena duces tecum. A requirement to bring requested documentation to the court of law when appearing for the summons.

INFORMED AND IMPLIED CONSENT

Consent is an act of reason, meaning the person giving consent must be of sufficient mental capacity and be in possession of all essential information to give valid consent. Consent must be free of force or fraud. There are many distinct types of consent. It is important for medical assistants and all health care professionals to be aware of them to protect themselves and their practice against cases of *malpractice* and *torts*, including assault and battery.

Implied Consent

This is inferred based on signs, actions, or conduct of the patient rather than oral communication. For example, an MA asks the patient if they can take their temperature, and the patient responds by opening their mouth and lifting their tongue. This concept also applies to emergent care for individuals who are unconscious or unable to speak. The law assumes *implied consent* to administer CPR and other lifesaving medical treatments to stabilize the patient.

> **13.5 Take Note**
>
> Consent is a critical aspect of patient autonomy, in protecting the legal rights of patients, and guides the ethical practice of health care.

Expressed Consent

This is given either by oral or written words. For example, when an MA is giving an injection, they ask the patient if they are ready to receive the injection, as well as which arm they prefer. The patient responds by agreeing to the injection and stating which arm they would like the injection to go into.

Informed Consent

This is a process that ensures the patient (or the guardian of the patient) knows, understands, and accepts the treatment that has been explained. For example, a patient is informed they must have a procedure performed, it has been explained to them, and they sign off on having the procedure performed.

In the health care setting, one of the most important types of consent is *informed consent*, which is a clear and voluntary indication of preference or choice, usually oral or written, and freely given in circumstances where the available options and their consequences have been made clear. Informed consent involves shared decision making between the patient and the health care provider. The health care provider must disclose appropriate information to a competent, adult patient so that the patient may make a voluntary choice to accept or refuse treatment. A competent adult must be oriented to time and place. They must be of clear mind and be able to understand all of the information given by the health care provider.

---

malpractice. Any treatment by a medical professional that does not follow the standards of care.

tort. "Wrong," or a harmful act committed by one individual to another.

implied consent. Consent granted when a patient assumes the position and allows the medical professional to perform it.

informed consent. An oral or written agreement of mutual communication that ensures the patient has been notified about their health care choices before making them.

The health care provider must detail all possible risks and potential prognoses for having a treatment or procedure performed and the available alternatives. Failure to obtain informed consent may lead to a case of medical **negligence** and malpractice. Unless it is an emergency, health care professionals should not proceed with any procedure without the consent of the patient.

Minors (those under the age of 18) cannot give consent except in these two situations. First, if the minor is seeking birth control, pregnancy care, sexually transmitted disease treatment, or substance abuse treatment, then they may do so without the consent of a parent. Second, if the minor has been declared by the courts as emancipated, then they are able to make medical, financial, and housing decisions for themselves without the approval of a parent or guardian. Emancipated minors win the approval of the courts by being enlisted in the military, being financially independent, living independently, or being married.

OBTAIN, REVIEW, AND COMPLY WITH MEDICAL DIRECTIVES

Advance Directives

CHALLENGE

1. While running in the park, an MA witnesses a man collapse. The man is unconscious and is not breathing, and the MA feels no pulse. The MA is trained in CPR and begins performing it on the man. Which of the following allows the MA to act in an emergency without the man's permission?
   A. Explicit consent
   B. Expressed consent
   C. Implied consent
   D. Informed consent

   C is correct. Consent is when a patient gives permission to a health care professional to provide care. However, in emergency situations when the patient is unable to provide it, the law allows for implied consent. The law assumes that an unconscious patient would consent to emergency care if the patient were conscious and able to consent.

2. Which of the following patients can give informed consent for a routine procedure? (Select all that apply.)
   A. Parents giving consent for the patient, who is a minor
   B. An adult who is under the influence of alcohol or narcotic drugs
   C. A minor who is employed
   D. A minor who is living independently
   E. A minor who is legally married

   A, D, and E are correct. Competent adults can give informed consent. Minors cannot give informed consent, except in the case they are married, emancipated, or living independently. Minors may also give consent, including the case of seeking birth control or care during pregnancy, treatment for sexually transmitted infections, or treatment for substance abuse.

It is important to be familiar with laws and different **advance directives** related to end-of-life issues. Advance or medical directives consist of a set of requests that patients put in writing for their health care provider, family, and other health care professionals to carry out in the case patients are incapacitated and are unable to speak for themselves. An advance directive allows patients to express values and desires related to end-of-life care. It will indicate what medical treatment patients wish to have if they are dying or permanently unconscious and identifies a health care agent for the patient who can help make decisions on the patient's behalf. The health care provider must obtain, review, and comply with these directives. The two main elements in an advance directive are a living will and durable power of attorney for health care.

---

negligence. When a patient does not receive adequate and appropriate care, which leads to suffering and harm.

advance directives. Written statements of a person's wishes regarding medical treatment, such as a living will.

Living Will

A living will is a legal document stating what procedures patients would want, which ones they would not want, and under what conditions these decisions would apply, such as the following.

- Analgesia (pain relief)
- Antibiotic and antiviral treatment
- IV hydration
- Artificial feeding
- Cardiopulmonary resuscitation (CPR)
- Ventilators
- Dialysis
- Organ donation
- *Do-not-resuscitate (DNR)* orders

Durable Power of Attorney

The *durable power of attorney (DPOA)* for health care is a legal document naming a health care agent or proxy to make medical decisions for patients when they are not able to do so, in the case they become incapacitated or unable to communicate. The agent will be able to decide as the patient would when treatment decisions need to be made. The agent communicates the same rights to request or refuse treatment that the patient would have if capable of making and communicating these decisions. A DPOA for health care enables patients to be more specific about their medical treatment than a living will. The agent may decide on a wide range of health care issues, including whether to admit or discharge the patient from a hospital or nursing home, what treatments may or may not be given, who can have access to the patient's medical records, and even how the patient's body is disposed of after death. For example, the agent may donate the patient's organs, order an autopsy, and even direct funeral arrangements. If the patient has specific requests, such as how to dispose of the patient's body after death, it must be in writing.

If an individual does not designate a health care agent or proxy and cannot make health care decisions, state law often appoints an individual who can make decisions on the individual's behalf, including the following.

- Court-appointed guardian or conservator
- Spouse or domestic partner
- Adult child
- Adult sibling
- Close friend
- Nearest living relative

Advance directives are legally valid throughout the United States as soon as the patient signs them in front of the required witnesses. Once the patient has completed a medical directive, a copy should be given to the family, hospital, and providers to review and have on file. The laws governing advance directives vary by state. Providers must fully evaluate the patient's condition before advance directives can be applied. Advance directives do not expire; they remain in effect until they are officially changed. The directive should be reviewed often and revised if necessary.

do-not-resuscitate (DNR). An order written in the hospital or on a legal form to communicate the wishes of a patient to not undergo CPR or advanced cardiac life support if the patient's heart stops or the patient stops breathing.

durable power of attorney (DPOA). A legal document naming a health care agent or proxy to make medical decisions for patients when they are not able to do so, in the case they become incapacitated or unable to communicate.

Do Not Resuscitate

Medical assistants should also be aware of several other forms that may be supplements to a patient's advanced care plan. As discussed earlier, a do-not-resuscitate order (DNR order) is a legal order written either in the hospital or on a legal form to communicate the wishes of a patient to not undergo CPR or advanced cardiac life support if the patient's heart stops or the patient stops breathing. A DNR order does not affect any treatment other than that which would require intubation or CPR. Patients who have a DNR order can continue to get chemotherapy, antibiotics, dialysis, or any other life-sustaining treatments.

POLST Form

Physician Orders for Life-Sustaining Treatment (POLST) is another type of advance directive, typically reserved for patients who may be near end of life. A physician fills out a life-sustaining treatment (POLST) form that contains a set of medical orders completed by the health care provider detailing the patient's end-of-life care. The POLST forms involves a shared decision-making process between the health care provider and patient with advanced or terminal illness and adheres to the patient's goal of care. An important aspect of the POLST form is the portability, meaning that the medical orders move with you as you move to other health care providers and practices.

CHALLENGE

1. Match the situation with the correct term.

TERM	SITUATION
A. POLST form	1. A legal directive that designates specific individuals to act on the patient's behalf
B. Living will	2. A legal order to not undergo CPR or advanced cardiac life support if the patient's heart stops or stops breathing
C. Durable power of attorney (DPOA)	3. A written document detailing the treatment preferences in the event a patient is unable to make medical decisions and identifying a health care proxy
D. DNR order	4. A written document that specifies what types of medical treatment are desired should the patient become incapacitated or permanently unconscious or cannot make decisions about emergency treatment.

A: 4; B: 3; C: 1; D: 2. There are many forms and decisions to make regarding end-of-life planning. This includes advance directives to detail one's treatment preferences and decision makers, living wills, durable power of attorney, do-not-resuscitate (DNR) order, and physician orders for life-sustaining treatment (POLST).

Physician Orders for Life-Sustaining Treatment (POLST). Type of advance directive, typically reserved for patients who may be near end of life.

LEGAL REQUIREMENTS REGARDING REPORTABLE VIOLATIONS OR INCIDENTS

Criminal and Civil Acts

To ensure patient protection, health care professionals are bound by a variety of laws and regulations and by a wide range of legal and ethical responsibilities to their patients, employers, and society. The MA should be familiar with the different types of laws and how to protect themselves and their employer against medical malpractice.

In general, there are two main categories of law: criminal and civil.

Criminal Law

This is concerned with violations against society based on the criminal statutes or codes. The remedies or punishments for violating state or federal criminal laws are monetary fines, imprisonment, and capital penalty (death). Violations of criminal laws are called crimes.

Misdemeanors

These are lesser crimes punishable usually by monetary fines established by the state but may also include imprisonment of 1 year or less.

Felonies

These are more serious crimes punishable by larger fines and/or imprisonment for more than 1 year, and in some states, the death penalty may be levied on a convicted felon for severe crimes, such as murder. In many states, a felony conviction for a health care professional may also include the revoking of a license to practice in their profession.

A health care professional may be prosecuted for a crime for practicing without a license, falsifying information in obtaining a license, or failing to provide life support for a patient. As discussed in the previous section, a health care provider failing to get informed consent from a patient may constitute a type of felony called battery, which is the actual nonconsensual physical contact on another person.

Civil Law

These laws protect the private rights of a person or a person's property. Civil laws include the areas of contracts, property, labor, privacy issues, and family law. A violation of civil law may lead to a civil lawsuit by the victim, which is a case brought to the courts to hold a party responsible for a wrongdoing. A wrongdoing or violation of civil law is called a tort. A tort is an action that wrongly causes harm to an individual but is not a crime.

Torts

There are two major classifications of torts: intentional and unintentional, which is classified as negligence.

Intentional Tort

This is a deliberate act that violates the rights of another. Examples of intentional torts include assault, battery, defamation of character, invasion of privacy, and administration of an injection without the consent of the patient.

Negligence

This is a common tort in the health care setting. Negligence does not require a specific intent to harm someone and is not a deliberate action but is the result of an individual or party failing to act in a reasonable way where a duty was owed.

Malpractice

Malpractice is an act of negligence and describes an improper or illegal professional activity or treatment, often used regarding a health care professional causing an injury to a patient. The negligence might be the result of errors in diagnosis, treatment, or postoperative care or a violation of patient confidentiality. Malpractice requires proof of a breach of a standard of care, and the breach must cause damage or harm. In general, the standard of care in a medical malpractice case is defined as the type and level of care an ordinary, prudent health care professional, with the same training and experience, would provide under similar circumstances. In other words, the critical question in a medical malpractice case is: "Would a similarly skilled health care professional have provided me with the same treatment under the same, or similar, circumstances?"

> **13.6 Take Note**
>
> There are four basic elements in negligence. They are known as the four Ds of Negligence.
>
> - Duty of Care: One party has a legal obligation to act in a certain manner toward the other.
> - Dereliction of Duty: Also called a breach, this is a failure to use reasonable care in fulfilling the duty.
> - Direct Cause: The failure in the duty leads to harm suffered by the injured person.
> - Damages: The harm or injury can be remedied by monetary compensation.

Penalties in civil law are almost exclusively monetary, which the court decides on for damages. The plaintiff or injured party may receive a monetary award for injuries sustained as a result of a particular incident, as well as compensation for medical expenses, lost wages, and the pain and suffering associated with the negligence.

Mandated Reporting

There are federal and state laws and statutes that mandate health care providers and professionals to report and document incidents of concern for a patient's safety and for the safety of the public at large. In the health care field, mandatory reporting duties refer mainly to the responsibility of health care professionals to report vital information and incidence to the appropriate agencies for the protection and welfare of the public, as well as specific vulnerable populations. Although these mandatory reporting guidelines may vary by state, prompt reporting of the following is mandatory.

- Births
- Deaths
- Certain communicable diseases, including specific sexually transmitted infections (STIs)
- Assaults or criminal acts
- Abuse, neglect, and exploitation—child, older adult, and intimate partner

According to the Centers for Disease Control and Prevention (CDC), there are more than 120 national notifiable diseases, or diseases required by law to be reported to government authorities. This includes tuberculosis, meningitis, acquired immunodeficiency syndrome (AIDS), and many sexually transmitted diseases. If a disease can be quickly transmitted to many individuals and may endanger the general population and may create an epidemic, it is the responsibility of health care providers and professionals to notify the proper authorities to prepare and, hopefully, prevent or limit the spread of that disease or illness. In fact, it is a legal and ethical mandate that these cases are reported to the local department of health, which may then be reported to the CDC. In addition, the information gained from reporting allows the local, state, and federal government to make informed decisions on laws and policies about specific activities, such as food handling, insect control, sexually transmitted infections, and disease tracking and immunization programs.

Although this may vary by state, in general, physicians; veterinarians; podiatrists; nurse practitioners, nurses, and nurse midwives; physician assistants; medical examiners and coroners; dentists; and administrators of health facilities and clinics, dispensaries, correctional facilities, or any other institution that diagnoses or treats a communicable disease are required to report communicable diseases to their local health department. Most local and state health departments have specific forms for reporting.

Abuse

Every state has mandatory reporting laws for abuse, specifically child abuse and elder abuse, and many states have requirements for reporting domestic violence. Abuse is defined as a misuse or maltreatment and may take many forms but includes the following types and actions.

- *Physical:* Pushing, hitting, shoving, punching, biting, choking, and physically trapping or impeding movement
- *Verbal/emotional:* Criticizing, degrading, swearing, blaming, and attacks that harm self-esteem
- *Psychological:* Isolation from family and friends, controlling actions and decisions, stalking, and invading privacy or space
- *Sexual:* Forcing or demanding sex, forcing unwanted sex with another person, forcing engagement into prostitution or pornography, and refusing to use safe sex practices
- *Economic:* Forbidding an individual from working, controlling access to money, and exploiting citizenship or lack of citizenship to work or to prevent from working

Statutes in each state provide more specific details describing the behaviors that are considered grounds for abuse or neglect and the penalties and proof needed to sustain the cases.

In the case of child or older adult abuse, there are several signs, such as the following.

- Previously filed reports of physical or sexual abuse of the child
- Documented abuse of other family members
- Different stories between parents and child on how an accident happened
- Stories of incidents and injuries that are suspicious
- Injuries blamed on other family members
- Repeated visits to the emergency department for injuries
- Discolorations/bruising on the buttocks, back, and abdomen
- Elbow, wrist, and shoulder dislocations
- Delays in the normal growth and development patterns
- Erratic school attendance
- Poor hygiene
- Malnutrition
- Obvious dental neglect
- Neglected well-baby procedures (e.g., immunizations)

Every state has statutes that require specific professionals and persons to report suspected abuse and neglect to appropriate agencies. They often include the following.

- Social workers
- Teachers, principals, and other school personnel
- Physicians, nurses, and other health care professionals
- Counselors, therapists, and other mental health professionals
- Childcare providers
- Medical examiners or coroners
- Law enforcement officers

Since each state varies in terms of what constitutes abuse and the reporting mechanism, the MA should familiarize themselves with the child protection statutes in the area in which they work as a medical assistant. The law requires reporting all cases of suspected, but not necessarily proven, abuse. Anyone who reports their suspicions in good faith is protected from lawsuits. Information elicited during a child abuse evaluation may potentially be used in a legal proceeding against the alleged perpetrator.

CHALLENGE

1. Many states have mandatory reporting laws. Which of the following professions are commonly considered "mandatory reporters" and mandated to report across every state? (Select all that apply.)
   A. Health care professionals
   B. Law enforcement officers
   C. Childcare providers
   D. Clergy members
   E. Social workers

   A, B, C, and E are correct. Depending on the relationship, attorneys and members of the clergy may be exempt from mandatory reporting due to privileged communications. This privilege of maintaining confidentiality may exist under many state laws.

2. During a pediatric visit, a medical assistant notices suspicious cuts and bruises on a child. The child's parent say that the child fell. Which of the following should the medical assistant do?
   A. Chart the injury in the patient's medical record.
   B. Notify the physician or health care provider.
   C. Immediately notify the police.
   D. Take no action, as the parent explained the child's injury.

   B is correct. It is imperative for the medical assistant to inform the physician or health care provider of the injury or any suspicion or signs of abuse.

ETHICS AND VALUES

Medical assistants are accountable to a health care provider or a hospital, but this does not exclude them from personal responsibility. Understanding the law, standards of practice, and ethical principles that govern them and their profession will help them make legal and sound decisions when confronted with an ethical situation or dilemma.

Ethics are the rules, standards, and moral principles that govern a person's behavior and on which the person bases decisions. Ethics are concerned with questions of how individuals in a society should act by defining right and wrong and appropriate conduct to serve the greater good. Ethics encompasses several different facets. One aspect of morals describes how "good or bad" or how "right or wrong" an action is. Similarly, values, or an individual's ethics, refer to one person's moral principles or what an individual believes is right or wrong. Values govern a person's decisions, with a goal of maintaining one's integrity or conscience. An individual's values may be influenced by concepts of honesty, fidelity, equality, compassion, responsibility, humility, and respect for life.

There are many types and fields in ethics, including personal, common, and professional. Personal ethics determines what an individual believes about morality and right and wrong. It includes one's personal values and moral qualities and is influenced by family, friends, culture, religion, education, and many other factors. Personal ethics has an impact on areas of life such as family, finances, and relationships and may change during one's life. An example of one's personal ethics may be for a person to believe in the death penalty but support a woman's right to an abortion.

Common ethics, also called group ethics, is a system of principles and rules of conduct accepted by a group based on ethnicity, political affiliation, or cultural identity. An example of common ethics is for a person who is religious to believe all abortion and the death penalty are bad and all life should be preserved.

Professional ethics is a type of ethics that aims to define, clarify, and criticize professional work and its typical values. Professional ethics sets the standards for practicing one's profession and can be learned only through education or training or on the job. It involves attributes such as commitment, competence, confidence, and contract. Professional ethics is often used to impose rules and standards on employees in an organization or members of a profession. Examples of professional ethics are in employee handbooks, codes of ethics, and the Hippocratic Oath taken by physicians.

A branch of ethics is medical ethics, which is the morals, moral principles, and moral judgments that health care professionals use to determine whether an action should be allowed based on "right and wrong." In addition to examining facts, medical ethics uses moral analysis to assess the obligations and responsibilities of health care professionals on various issues and challenges related to health care and medicine. It specifically addresses how to handle ethical issues arising from the care of patients and focuses on the health care professional's duty to the patient. The basic principles of medical ethics are the following.

13.7 Adhere to Professional Codes of Ethics

PRINCIPLE	DESCRIPTION
Autonomy	The capacity to think, decide, and act on one's own free will and initiative. The patient's decision-making process must be free of coercion or coaxing. Health care professionals should help patients come to their own decisions by providing full information.
Justice	The principle that ethics should be based on is what is consistent and fair to all involved. Patients in similar situations should have access to the same care. Health care professionals must consider four main areas when evaluating justice: fair distribution of scarce resources, competing needs, rights and obligations, and potential conflicts with established legislation.
Beneficence	This is the general moral principle of doing the "most good" or doing what is best for patients. This must consider the patients' pain, their physical and mental suffering, the risk of disability and death, and their quality of life. What is best for the patient may agree or disagree with the health care provider's clinical judgment.
Nonmaleficence	This is the principle of "do no harm" to the patient or to the fewest number of people in society. It is difficult for health care providers to always apply successfully the "do no harm" principle because, for example, most treatments involve some degree of risk or adverse effects.

CHALLENGE

1. Which of the following types of ethics includes basic principles of do no harm, justice, and autonomy?
   A. Common ethics
   B. Professional ethics
   C. Medical ethics
   D. Personal ethics

   C is correct. Medical ethics is the morals, moral principles, and moral judgments that health care professionals use to determine whether an action should be allowed based on "right and wrong." Basic principles of medical ethics are autonomy (free will), justice (do what is consistent and fair), beneficence (do what is best for patients), and nonmaleficence (do no harm).

2. Which of the following ethical principles is "do no harm"?
   A. Autonomy
   B. Justice
   C. Beneficence
   D. Nonmaleficence

   D is correct. Nonmaleficence is the principle of "do no harm" to the patient or to the fewest number of people in society.

3. Which of the following is an example of a moral value?
   A. A medical assistant interacting with patients and coworkers with integrity and empathy
   B. A medical office's employee handbook that details the organization's mission statement
   C. A medical assistant joining a professional organization that offers education, continuing education, and networking opportunities
   D. The Equal Employment Opportunity Commission's policy and practices on legal and fair hiring practices

   A is correct. Moral values are one's personal concept of right and wrong, formed through the influence of the family, culture, and society.

autonomy. The capacity to think, decide, and act on one's own free will and initiative.

justice. Fair distribution of benefit, risk, resources, and cost to ensure equal treatment.

beneficence. A moral obligation to act in the best interest of others.

nonmaleficence. A commitment not to cause harm.

IDENTIFY BELIEFS AND VALUES AND PROVIDE UNBIASED CARE

MAs will interact and provide care to a diverse patient population with different backgrounds, beliefs, values, experiences, and identities. This may include race, ethnicity, sex, age, religion, language, education, sexual orientation, and gender identity. Health care providers, professionals, and systems must create and deliver culturally competent patient care. Cultural competence is defined as the ability of providers and organizations to effectively deliver health care services that meet the needs of patients.

To build communities that are successful at improving conditions and resolving problems, MAs need to understand and appreciate many cultures, establish relationships with people from cultures other than their own, and build strong alliances with different cultural groups. This is particularly true in health care as they will need to successfully interact with patients, family members, and coworkers from many different cultures.

Although it is a broad concept, culture can be defined as the act of belonging to a designated group or community that shares common experiences that shape the way its members understand the world. Cultural practice and norms are often learned, shared, and passed on through generations. It may include groups that a person is born into, such as race, national origin, sex, class, or religion. Culture is a strong part of people's lives. It influences their views, their values, their humor, their hopes, their loyalties, and their fears. Culture helps guide thinking, decision making, and actions. Culture also affects interpersonal relationships, including marriages, communication patterns, and sexual habits.

A bias denotes a preference for a certain group, concept, or set of things. Biases may be held by an individual, group, or institution and can have negative or positive consequences. The two main types of biases are conscious bias (also known as explicit bias) and unconscious bias (also known as implicit bias). Most people understand that there is no place for this in the modern workplace. In fact, there are many laws and policies that exist to prevent prejudice based on race, age, sex, gender identity, physical abilities, religion, sexual orientation, and many other characteristics. Violations of these laws and policies may result in disciplinary action, termination of employment, and even criminal charges.

It is important to note that biases, conscious or unconscious, are not limited to ethnicity and race. Though racial bias and discrimination are well documented, biases may exist toward any social group. One's age, sex, gender identity, physical abilities, religion, sexual orientation, weight, and many other characteristics are subject to bias. Whether recognized or not, bias and prejudice can substantially undermine multicultural acceptance and inclusion in the health care setting. Confronting one's own biases and prejudice is a great first step toward building multicultural competence.

Cultural competence is an ongoing learning process. Health care professionals must continue to be aware of the influences that sociocultural factors have on patients and health care providers and professionals and the clinical relationship.

CHALLENGE

1. Which of the following is the act of belonging to a designated group or community that shares common experiences?
   A. Bias
   B. Ethnicity
   C. Culture
   D. Value

   C is correct. Culture is the act of belonging to a designated group or community that shares common experiences that shape the way its members understand the world. Cultural practice and norms are often learned, shared, and passed on through generations.

2. Management is hiring for a new medical assistant. After reviewing resumes and completing interviews, which of the following may be considered a bias in their hiring decision? (Select all that apply.)
   A. Hiring a candidate because they are from the same ethnicity
   B. Hiring a male candidate because they will not need to take parental leave
   C. Hiring a younger individual since they are not close to retirement
   D. Hiring a candidate that has a diploma over another candidate with no training

   A, B, and C are correct. A bias denotes a preference for a certain group, concept, or set of things and may include race, age, sex, gender identity, physical abilities, religion, and sexual orientation. Selecting a candidate based on education, training, and other qualities are legitimate reasons and not based on biases.

WRAP-UP

This chapter has provided an overview of laws that pertain to health care, standards, and guidelines that help to regulate the practice of patient care. All members of the health care profession must understand their responsibility to themselves, their employers, and their patients.

By understanding the different types of law and how they apply to the role as a medical assistant, MAs will be better able to provide better patient care and conduct themselves in a manner that is legal and compliant. In addition, they will be more capable of making sound decisions concerning their role in providing quality patient care and in protecting themselves and their employer from negligence and malpractice lawsuits.

IN PRACTICE
Patient Experience Coach

FOUNDATIONAL KNOWLEDGE AND BASIC SCIENCE

It's not uncommon for primary care providers to refer a patient to a specialist for the management of complex diseases.

However, some patients aren't always able to see the specialists they're referred to. This occurs for multiple reasons, including misunderstanding of the necessity to see a specialist, lack of clear coordination of care, cost, and scheduling concerns. When a referral is recommended, a detailed conversation between the medical assistant and the patient is vital. This increases the likelihood the patient will follow through with seeing the specialist.

Ask the patient if they understand the need for the referral and why it is being ordered. Then ask them about any concerns they might have. These questions help identify where to focus the conversation. As the patient explains their understanding, fill in any gaps or misinformation immediately.

For example, the patient might think they're being referred to an endocrinologist due to a problem with their blood. Explain that the referral is due to an abnormal result in their blood test, such as a high fasting glucose level. Supplement basic understanding with information about the risks of the condition, the benefits of treatment, and examples of the type of care to expect, including any diagnostic testing.

Convey a sense of urgency in relation to the importance of prioritizing the referral visit to improve the patient's current health condition and status. Whenever placing a referral, it's important to give the patient all necessary information for scheduling, including contact and location information for the specialist's office.

Then explain to the patient what will happen next. Should the patient call the specialist, or will the specialist's office reach out to the patient to schedule the initial appointment? Identify when the patient should contact your office if any issues should arise in order to avoid unnecessary delays in scheduling an appointment. Clear communication will improve the experience for the patient.

CHALLENGE

1. How can you help empower the patient to seek care from appropriate specialists to improve patient satisfaction within an organization?

Providing patients with the information and resources needed to seek care from specialists helps to motivate patients to take an active role in managing their medical care. Active patient involvement in decision making assists in positive patient satisfaction and outcomes.

MEDICAL TERMINOLOGY, ANATOMY, AND PHYSIOLOGY

Medical terminology is a new language that health care professionals learn over the course of their training and career. It's important to remember once this new language becomes familiar to you, it's not familiar to most patients.

When interacting with patients, make sure to translate the conversation accurately. Make sure you understand the information the patient is providing. Also, confirm that the patient understands the information you're giving them.

The best way to understand what the patient is telling you is to ask follow-up or clarifying questions. For example, if a patient tells you they've been feeling dizzy lately, clarify if they've been truly feeling dizzy and not lightheaded. These are different symptoms that could lead to a different diagnosis.

CHALLENGE

1. What are some strategies a medical assistant can use to discuss complex information with patients to ensure they have a positive experience?

   Identify and address any language barriers. Provide supplemental materials related to the information. Limit other distractors. Use patient-friendly terminology and simplify explanations. Make sure the patient has a full understanding of the information prior to leaving.

To seek clarification, you might say, I'm sorry to hear you're experiencing that. Would you say it feels like the room is spinning or like you might faint? The patient's response will give the provider a more accurate report of the patient's symptoms.

It's important to be consistent in the language you use. Avoid using technical medical terms, as they can confuse the patient. One example is using prescription versus medication. Often, they're used interchangeably. Be sure to only use one of these words during your interactions with a patient because they might assume there is a difference, leading to confusion. For this reason, language consistency is key to facilitating effective communication.

PATIENT INTAKE AND VITALS

Patients entering the medical office get their first impression of the visit from your professional demeanor and your initial interaction.

During the visit, you'll obtain the patient's vital signs. These readings provide a snapshot of the patient's current health status. You'll also perform height and weight measurements and review the pain scale and pain levels to understand pain the patient may be experiencing. Begin by explaining the process of obtaining vital signs, including how you'll take their temperature and measure their blood pressure, pulse, and respiration rates. When a patient knows what to expect, they feel more at ease.

Ask if the patient has any questions, and address any concerns that arise. Remember to always ask the patient for permission prior to making any physical contact. You'll need to obtain vital signs accurately, despite the various factors that can impact vital sign readings. For instance, when obtaining an oral temperature, make sure the patient hasn't smoked or had anything hot or cold to drink within the last 15 to 30 minutes, as this can alter the reading.

Additionally, a patient's pulse might be higher if they have high anxiety or if they were rushing to their appointment. The patient's physical position can also influence blood pressure readings. Before obtaining a reading, make sure the patient isn't crossing their legs or feet, as this may cause an inaccuracy. You might also obtain a high blood pressure reading when a patient either states they're nervous or appears uncomfortable. Document any factors that may contribute to an altered vital sign measurement in the patient's record.

You'll help the patient feel more confident about the encounter by following the precise steps for obtaining vital signs, clearly explaining procedures, and correcting factors that impact the measurement. This facilitates a better outcome for the patient while establishing a positive rapport.

CHALLENGE

1. How can the medical assistant help alleviate a patient's anxiety regarding having a vital sign measurement taken?

Recognize anxiety and talk to the patient about it. Listen and offer empathy. Help the patient relax. Suggest breathing techniques.

GENERAL PATIENT CARE: PART 1

It is important for the medical assistant to recognize signs and symptoms of an allergic reaction and respond immediately and appropriately.

Allergic reactions can range from mild to severe. Mild reactions may present as itchy skin, a rash, or mild swelling and irritation. However, severe allergic reactions can result in anaphylaxis or anaphylactic shock. These can be life threatening without immediate intervention.

It is important to recognize common signs and symptoms of an anaphylactic reaction. These include dyspnea, difficulty breathing and swallowing, weakness, sweating, and even convulsions. Anaphylactic reactions can occur within minutes after exposure to the allergen. As a medical assistant, you should be familiar with the location of medications and supplies you might need in emergencies.

If a patient demonstrates signs of anaphylaxis, immediately call for help from other health care team members and providers. Activate the emergency response system if a provider isn't on site or if directed to do so. If the patient stops breathing, you'll need to begin CPR immediately until the emergency response team arrives.

Epinephrine is the first line of treatment for a patient experiencing an anaphylactic reaction. You administer it using an auto-injector pen. Epinephrine can only be administered if a provider has given verbal or written orders. Time is of the essence in these situations. For quick administration, inject epinephrine through the patient's clothing. With auto injectors, hold the injector at the administration site for at least 10 seconds to allow the medication to fully inject into the patient.

Remember, always check the patient's drug and allergy status prior to administering any medication. Review the patient's medication and drug allergy status at the beginning of each visit. This prevents adverse reactions while placing priority on the patient's safety and wellness.

CHALLENGE

1. What are ways a medical assistant can be ready to respond to a patient experiencing an anaphylactic reaction in the medical office?

Complete periodic emergency supply checks. Practice responding to mock emergency situations in the office and identify ways to improve. Identify techniques to help with anxiety in emergency situations. Speak with other colleagues about the emergency action plan for a patient experiencing an anaphylactic reaction.

IN PRACTICE: PATIENT EXPERIENCE COACH
General Patient Care: Part 2

GENERAL PATIENT CARE: PART 2

As a medical assistant, it's important to be alert and ready to quickly respond to various situations that may arise, including potential threats or emergencies.

The first hour of an emergency is the most critical time because it correlates with the patient's prognosis and possibility of recovery. Medical assistance must be willing to jump into action while working within their scope of practice. The MA might need to bandage a wound for a patient who was injured at the medical office, perform CPR on a person having a heart attack, or properly position a person having a seizure to avoid injury.

CHALLENGE

1. The contact information for what organizations in the community is useful to have available for help with emergency situations?

Local emergency response team, poison control center, HAZMAT response team, state and local health departments, local hospitals, Red Cross, local disaster relief agencies

As a health care professional, people may look to you to help take control during an emergency. Think about how you can be an effective member of the health care team when responding to an emergency. Remain calm. Establish priorities to gain control of the situation.

Seek additional help. Never leave an emergency patient unattended. Use effective and clear communication while conveying accurate information to fellow health care team members, providers, and emergency response teams. Display knowledgeable skills, confidence, and empathy towards the situation. Remember, time is of the essence, and a patient's prognosis could depend on your actions.

INFECTION CONTROL AND SAFETY

Some think of illness or injury, and it may cause anxiety for others. However, the goal for people visiting a medical facility is to maintain or improve their health.

As a health care professional, it's your job to follow policies and procedures to keep infection control and patient safety top priorities. A clean and safe environment is welcoming to patients and encourages trust that their health and safety matter.

But what if a patient still has concerns? Don't brush off a patient's concern about infection control or hygiene practices. Engage them in policies before they have a chance to express concern. When appropriate, initiate infection control measures in front of patients. These include washing or sanitizing your hands, wiping off common surface areas, and providing alcohol-based sanitizer and face masks.

When a procedure requires full personal protective equipment, take the time to connect with the patient by introducing yourself prior to the procedure. Explain the PPE you are or will be wearing and why you'll be wearing it during the procedure. Ask them what you can do to help them feel more comfortable. This reduces anxiety or fear and helps the patient relax throughout the visit, allowing for a more pleasant office encounter.

CHALLENGE

1. What are some ways the medical assistant can assist with infection control?

Wash/sanitize your hands, sanitize surface areas, and wear appropriate PPE.

IN PRACTICE: PATIENT EXPERIENCE COACH
Point-of-Care Testing and Laboratory Procedures

POINT-OF-CARE TESTING AND LABORATORY PROCEDURES

As a medical assistant you'll perform a variety of these laboratory tests. These include blood glucose testing, urine pregnancy testing, and rapid strep screening.

Quality assurance involves a written set of policies and procedures. This helps guarantee that laboratories and clinics are running safely, efficiently, and correctly to produce reliable patient results. Quality control is a set of measures you perform to guarantee the reliability of test results through detecting and eliminating error. These measures allow for accuracy, reliability, and precision. Failure to perform quality control measures could result in various errors, including an incorrect diagnosis.

Imagine you receive a box of rapid strep testing kits that aren't functioning properly, and you're unaware there's something wrong. Without performing proper quality control measures, a patient could receive a false-negative diagnosis and not receive proper treatment for the strep throat. In addition to not receiving treatment in a timely manner, an incorrect diagnosis will cause the patient to return to the office or seek treatment at another facility.

How do you think the patient will feel about returning to the office to test again, knowing there was an error with their original screening? It's essential to perform quality control measures to maintain testing accuracy and integrity. Both quality assurance and quality control improve the patient experience and facilitate a sense of trust. Patient safety and quality care should always be of great importance.

CHALLENGE

1. What are some ways the medical assistant can assist with quality assurance in the laboratory?

   Proper collection and labeling of specimens, properly transport specimens, ensure instruments and equipment are maintained and calibrated, periodically check expiration dates on supplies, confirm patients have prepared properly for test, perform quality controls

PHLEBOTOMY

When people think about phlebotomy, they often associate the procedure with fear, discomfort, and anxiety. However, with the proper engagement, patients can experience minimal discomfort, and often have a pleasant experience.

As a health care worker, it's your job to prioritize the patient's safety. Use therapeutic communication to convey important information about the procedure and create a welcoming environment that is both safe and unintimidating. In addition, it's important to identify and address any uneasy feelings or emotions the patient may have regarding the procedure. For example, if the patient appears anxious, it's important to establish a rapport with them by detailing the steps of the procedure, answer any questions, and address any concerns they may have.

The MA can also provide tips on how the patient can relax during the procedure. Encourage them to practice deep breathing through each step, or have them focus on a specific point in the room while the procedure is taking place. Remain fluent and precise in your skill. Avoid shortcuts that could potentially lead to errors. And prepare your equipment and supplies with focus. These steps can help provide a professional image, make the patient feel at ease, and can reduce stress and anxiety related to the procedure.

CHALLENGE

1. What are some traits that can help a medical assistant have a positive patient experience when having a phlebotomy procedure?

   Patience, compassion, attention to detail, friendly, hand-eye coordination, ability to multitask, excellent social skills

EKG AND CARDIOVASCULAR TESTING

When people think about going to the doctor's office and having an EKG or other cardiac tests, there's often apprehension and worry. However, the medical assistant can make the experience more pleasant by enhancing patient communication and showing empathy.

As a medical assistant, it's important to establish a rapport with all patients to gain their trust and reduce any fears, validate their thoughts and feelings, and provide support and encouragement. Take time to explain the procedure. Answer any questions the patient may have. And explain what you're doing along the way. Avoid awkward periods of silence and engage in discussion before and after the exam to comfort and reassure the patient.

Prior to the procedure, take time to prepare the room by cleaning and sanitizing before bringing the patient in for testing. Stock gowns and sheets or blankets in the testing room so patients can have privacy and preserve their dignity during the exam. All these steps are important for patients to feel secure and less apprehensive during the testing procedure.

CHALLENGE

1. How can the medical assistant help alleviate a patient's anxiety when undergoing cardiac testing?

Display sensitivity; address patient questions and concerns; provide excellent communication and clear instructions; if possible, provide the patient with a timeline on when to expect results; offer reassurance

PATIENT CARE COORDINATION AND EDUCATION

Medical assistants educate the patient on their medications, procedures, and follow-up summaries. It's important for a medical assistant to have the knowledge and resources to educate a patient regarding their diagnosis and their treatment plan. This can encourage patient adherence. Medical assistants also provide community resource information to patients to assist with their personal needs.

A medical assistant can develop resources to distribute to patients within the medical office. This might include a printed brochure or handout identifying community resources and accompanying contact information. This establishes a rapport within the community and boosts confidence within your patients. Assisting patients to navigate their health care helps to improve the patient's investment in their own health and well-being. When there's effective communication and education among everyone on the health care team, patient adherence increases and optimizes outcomes.

CHALLENGE

1. What are examples of community resources that you can have available that could be beneficial to patients within the community?

Prescription drug discount programs, agencies serving individuals with disabilities, advocacy groups for victims, food distribution centers, emergency housing shelters, substance abuse programs, day programs for seniors, transportation services, community centers, short- and long-term care facilities

IN PRACTICE: PATIENT EXPERIENCE COACH
Administrative Assisting

ADMINISTRATIVE ASSISTING

Maintaining an effective daily patient schedule can increase your patients' experience and help the office run smoothly.

First, think about the characteristics of the provider and the organization. What time does the office start scheduling patients? Does the provider prefer a break time during the day? What is the office's appointment matrix? And what are the protocols for the various types of appointments?

Next, think about information you need from the caller when they request an appointment. How urgent is the request for the appointment? What type of appointment is the patient requesting? Is there a day or time during the week that's more convenient for the patient?

Once you obtain all the necessary information for scheduling the appointment, offer the patient available time slots for their preferred day and time. If you can't accommodate the patient's preferences, explain to the patient why, and let them know alternate appointment times that are available. Before ending the call, repeat the appointment back to the patient, speak clearly, and don't rush. Make sure you answer all of the patient's questions regarding their appointment. It's also good practice to contact the patient with a reminder prior to the appointment. This can help with fewer no shows. Obtaining necessary and accurate information from the patient is key to effective scheduling and maintaining an efficient workflow.

CHALLENGE

1. What are some qualities an individual needs to make an excellent medical office scheduler?

   Excellent communication skills; flexibility and understanding of the practice; positive and proactive attitude; compassion for patients; time management skills; problem-solving skills; excellent interview and triage techniques

COMMUNICATION AND CUSTOMER SERVICE

Have you ever encountered a lack of professionalism when obtaining health care services? Think about your experience. Were you eager to go back to the same facility or did you choose to go somewhere else, and even possibly change health care providers? Patients are choosing a health care provider to seek a service they are paying for. If they experience unprofessional behavior during their encounter, do you think they're likely to come back? Do you think they'll tell their friends and family about their experience?

It's important to remember health care is a business. And our patients are customers. Customer service is what we do to improve their experience while they receive care. Patients should have a sense of fulfillment or satisfaction when they receive services.

Medical assistants should demonstrate professional characteristics to deliver excellent customer service and represent the health care facility well. These characteristics include respect, kindness, empathy, compassion, honesty, and dependability. Remember, in addition to the characteristics discussed, maintaining a professional appearance also demonstrates you are a dedicated representative of your profession and also your organization.

CHALLENGE

1. What are some ways a MA can help to ensure that a patient is satisfied with their health care experience?

   A medical assistant can display a positive, professional attitude towards each patient. Provide excellent communication and listen to patient concerns. Engage with each patient respectfully. Inform patients about delays. Respect patient privacy. Develop rapport with patients. Provide a clean and safe environment. Ask patients to provide feedback.

MEDICAL LAW AND ETHICS

Today, we'll discuss cultural competence and providing patient care to a diverse range of patient population groups. It's important to identify cultural variations and unconscious biases that can limit communication and influence patient relationships.

For example, when asking transgender individuals to report the sex they were assigned at birth, this may not align with their gender: male, female, both, neither, or other. The transgender population risks social stigma, discrimination, and harassment, including when seeking and receiving medical services. Additionally, individuals from various cultural backgrounds perceive health and illness in different ways.

It's important to understand the differences that could be a barrier to providing the best care for patients who might have cultural backgrounds different from yours. As a critical and valued member of the health care team, it's your duty to provide the same care to all patients regardless of their values, beliefs, and behaviors, and this care may often need to be tailored according to the patient's social, cultural, and linguistic needs.

CHALLENGE

1. What are some ways you can make a transgender patient feel more comfortable during the patient visit?

   Some ideas include treating transgender individuals with respect, as you would for all patients. Politely ask the patient to state their name and pronouns. When asking for name and pronouns, ask what they "use" rather than what they "prefer." Refer to patients by the name and pronouns they state. Make a habit of requesting this from all patients to avoid singling out only those who present as gender-nonconforming. If a patient has changed their name, use their current name. Avoid offensive language and inappropriate questions. Educate yourself and your coworkers about transgender health care and issues.

IN PRACTICE
Case Studies

FOUNDATIONAL KNOWLEDGE AND BASIC SCIENCE

Case Study 1

A patient is prescribed amphetamine mixed salts (Adderall, a schedule II drug) for a new diagnosis of attention-deficit/hyperactivity disorder (ADHD). At the direction of the provider, the MA meets with the patient after the visit to review the process for refilling the medication.

Hello! My name is Sarah. The provider asked me to speak with you to make sure you understand how to pick up your new medication and what the refill process will look like. As you discussed with the provider, this medication has a lot of benefits when taken appropriately and as prescribed, but it can also be dangerous in terms of side effects and potential for abuse. Because of the risks, there are extra regulations on this medication that medical professionals and patients must follow. While these regulations can feel frustrating sometimes, following them helps ensure that patients like yourself can safely access the medications they need. Let's discuss how we can work together to ensure we follow regulations to treat ADHD safely.

Prescribing providers cannot include refills on this medication. At our clinic, the provider typically will send in three separate prescriptions after each visit with you. When you need another fill, you will call the pharmacy to request a fill each month by letting them know you have a prescription on hold or on file for the medication. You will need to come in for a checkup with the provider every 3 months to continue the prescription. These checkups ensure you are on the right dose, the medication is effectively treating your symptoms, and you are not experiencing any dangerous side effects.

You should never adjust your medication dose without speaking to the provider first. This is to ensure your safety with the medication and prevent any concerns with early refills. Our office cannot authorize early refills of this medication. Insurance and pharmacies also track this and would not allow an early refill due to regulations. If you have any concerns about your dose before you are due for your next visit, please call us.

IN PRACTICE: CASE STUDIES
Foundational Knowledge and Basic Science

Case Study 2

Ronald Turner, a 58-year-old male patient, was recently discharged from the hospital following a heart attack. When Mr. Turner comes into the clinic for his follow-up visit, the MA learns that prior to the heart attack, he had not seen a doctor in over 20 years. In addition to his newly diagnosed heart condition, Mr. Turner is overweight and has low exercise tolerance and kidney disease, which was diagnosed at the hospital.

Mr. Turner comes into his first visit stating that he wants to take control of his health. He was prescribed several new medications during his hospital stay. However, he is concerned about making sure he is on the right medications. Mr. Turner was told to see two specialists but could not remember which ones or why. He says he wants to be informed of everything that occurs with his health to be proactive and start living a healthier lifestyle. He does not know where to start but is motivated to do whatever needs to be done to prevent another heart attack and get things on the right track.

CHALLENGE

1. Based on the description above related to his hospital stay, which specialists would Mr. Turner have likely been referred to for follow-up care?

   He was most likely referred to a cardiologist for his heart condition and a nephrologist for his kidney disease.

2. What steps should the medical assistant take to help ensure Mr. Turner gets in to see the specialists in a timely manner?

   After verifying with the provider, explain to Mr. Turner what specialists he needs to see and why. Determine if the referrals have already been placed or need to be sent. Make sure Mr. Turner has all the information he needs to schedule, including clinic name, address, phone number, and instructions on how to get scheduled.

3. Which available tool would help provide streamlined communication and increased transparency to his health record?

   Signing Mr. Turner up for the patient portal will provide better transparency into the care being provided and could serve as a resource for direct communication between the patient and his care team.

Case Study 3

After completing the patient interview with Mr. Turner, including gathering his patient history and current health information, a medication list, and concerns, the provider performs their evaluation. After the exam, the provider asks the MA to see Mr. Turner and assist with patient education related to his new medications. The provider reports that Mr. Turner wants to be sure he understands what each medication is for, how he should take it, and what side effects might occur.

Additionally, the provider has given the patient information about changing his nutrition and health habits. The MA has been asked to review the nutritional guidelines with Mr. Turner and to schedule a follow-up appointment for the patient in 2 weeks. This appointment will evaluate how he is responding to his medications and answer any questions the patient might have related to his diet.

The MA returns to the exam room to discuss things with the patient.

CHALLENGE

1. What class of medications is Mr. Turner most likely prescribed to lower his blood pressure and why?

   Following his heart attack, Mr. Turner would likely be prescribed antihypertensives to control his blood pressure. High blood pressure is a risk factor for heart attacks.

2. How could the MA explain the mild side effects he may experience with the medications to help him understand that they are not worrisome?

   New medications can be scary, especially for a patient who has never taken them. Explain to Mr. Turner that side effects are common, sometimes expected, and overall harmless effects of medication. Explain that while the medication is still working as intended, all medications can also have unintended impacts. Review the common side effects of each of his medications with him, including signs to look for more concerning adverse reactions and any steps he can take to mitigate the side effects if possible

Case Study 4

Mr. Turner leaves his first appointment, expressing that he already feels more equipped to care for himself. He confirms his understanding of the next steps and schedules a follow-up appointment.

When Mr. Turner arrives back at the clinic a few weeks later, the MA is happy to see that his motivation to improve his health has not dissipated. He reports that he is feeling more comfortable with his medications and has noticed that some of the side effects of the medications he initially experienced have decreased. He states that he is ready to lose weight but has no idea where to start because all the information seems overwhelming. The MA validates his feelings of being overwhelmed and explains that he is right—small, steady changes are imperative to success with sustained change. The MA explains that diet and exercise are two main weight loss components. Because the goal is to start small and build on new habits, the MA asks where he would like to start. He replies that he wants to know which foods to eat and which foods he should avoid, noting that exercising intimidates him, and he is not yet ready to discuss it. The provider has asked the MA to provide this information to Mr. Turner.

Mr. Turner expresses that he is grateful for this information and sets a plan to check in with the MA and the provider about diet in 2 weeks using the patient portal.

CHALLENGE

1. What resource would be a good starting point in creating a nutritional plan with Mr. Turner?

   MyPlate would be an appropriate tool for developing an individualized nutritional plan for the patient.

2. Given his heart and kidney diseases, what specific recommendations should you inform Mr. Turner of?

   Counsel Mr. Turner on eating a low-sodium diet, which will help with both blood pressure and his heart, as well as protect his kidneys. Given his kidney disease, Mr. Turner should also focus on eating lean, healthy proteins and low-fat products.

3. What allied health professional can help Mr. Turner with weight loss by working with him to improve his strength and increase his mobility?

   A nutritionist, personal trainer, or dietitian

MEDICAL TERMINOLOGY, ANATOMY, AND PHYSIOLOGY

Case Study 1

Dionne is a medical assistant, primarily working in the front office of a cardiology clinic. She loves working with and helping patients. She prefers structure and is great at helping the office stay organized and on task but struggles to adapt to unexpected needs, including patient accommodations. Looking at the schedule, Dionne sees that a patient, Mr. Singh, is coming in this afternoon and needs to complete annual paperwork. Her previous experience with him is that he talks loudly, to the point of yelling, and that he becomes easily agitated with paperwork. Dionne decides to seek out support before he comes in. She approaches Vonetta, a nurse in the clinic who always seems to know what to do in challenging patient interactions.

Scene 1

Dionne: "Hi Vonetta, I need help. Mr. Singh is coming in today and I need him to complete paperwork, but that always seems to make him angry. I don't know what to do."

Vonetta: "Oh yeah, I know him and can understand your experiences with him. He's hard of hearing and has recently had some vision loss. When he's talking loudly, it's because of his own hearing loss. It's not anger. I think paperwork may be frustrating for him due to his vision problem."

Dionne: "Thank you so much for the information. That helps me understand him much better!"

Scene 2

Dionne: (speaking clearly in a friendly tone) "Hi, Mr. Singh! Welcome. Can I check you in over here? It's quieter, and it will be easier for us to talk."

Mr. Singh: "Hello. Sure, that's fine."

Dionne: (walks him over to a quiet, well-lit area) "We have paperwork we would like you to complete. I know it's hard to hear me in the busy lobby, so I thought this would be better."

(Hands over the paperwork printed in larger font.)

Mr. Singh: "Wow! This is so much better than that other junk you give me where the words are tiny. You better stick around because I might have questions."

Dionne: "I would be happy to assist you!"

CHALLENGE

1. Did Dionne take the right approach when Mr. Singh arrived to fill out paperwork?

Yes, Dionne and Mr. Singh were able to work together to complete the necessary paperwork. She also put a note in his medical record, directing others to have him come in early when paperwork would be required and to follow a similar process. From this experience, Dionne learned that patients who seem angry are often frustrated, and the team can plan ahead to make appropriate accommodations to improve their care experience.

Case Study 2

Diego is a medical assistant working in a primary care clinic. He is scheduled to draw blood on a patient, Ms. Aiko, to confirm a new diagnosis of diabetes. He speaks to the provider ahead of time and is informed that Ms. Aiko does not believe she has diabetes and finds it unnecessary to do any blood work. The doctor asks that Diego, an experienced MA who has specific training in diabetes management, try to give her some educational materials during her appointment, to prepare her for future conversations. Diego agrees.

Scene 1

Diego: Hi, Ms. Aiko. I am here to draw your blood today. Is there anything I can do today to make things easier?

Ms. Aiko: Absolutely nothing. This is a waste of time anyway. No one in my family has diabetes, and neither do I.

Diego: I can understand it must have been very surprising to hear you might have diabetes. This blood test will help us confirm one way or the other. If you don't mind me asking, what is your understanding of diabetes?

Ms. Aiko: It's a disease of people who eat nothing but candy and other desserts. I eat fairly healthy and go on walks sometimes. I don't have it.

Diego: I hear that living a healthy lifestyle is important to you, and it doesn't seem possible that someone who does so could end up with diabetes. While eating a lot of sugar and not exercising can be risk factors for diabetes, it can also occur in people who don't have as many risk factors. You should hear from our office within the next two days with the results. I would like to give you a handout on diabetes just in case the results are positive. I want you to know we will be here to help you through it.

Ms. Aiko: I don't have diabetes, but I'll take the handout if it makes you happy.

Scene 2

The blood work comes back indicating that Ms. Aiko has diabetes. The provider speaks to her about this and informs her of treatment steps, including diet management, exercise, and medication. Ms. Aiko expresses that she is not happy with the provider. Despite being upset, she agrees to schedule an in-office visit with Diego and the provider for further education and management discussions. Diego meets with her first, for an education and coaching session.

Ms. Aiko: Well, I guess you were right. Maybe I have diabetes right now, but we're going to fix this and get rid of it so tell me exactly what we need to do!

Diego: I'm sorry that you are going through this, and I know it is hard. I'm happy to hear you are motivated to lower your blood sugar and invest in your health in this way. I want to be sure that you understand diabetes can be well managed, sometimes just through diet and exercise.

Mrs. Aiko: We'll see about that. Just tell me what to do and I'll do it.

Diego: I appreciate your openness with me. A new diagnosis like this can be overwhelming. Learning to manage it will be a process, but we will work with you along the way. If it's okay with you, let's take small steps to start. I want you to know this is a safe place, and if you are feeling scared, angry, or overwhelmed, please let me know.

Conclusion

Medical assistants often work with people who are going through very challenging experiences. Whether feeling acutely sick, getting a new diagnosis, living through a medical crisis, or coming up on end of life, patients experience many emotions as they navigate the health care system and personal wellness. Supporting a patient while they are experiencing grief is a skill that must be developed.

CHALLENGE

1. How did Diego support Ms. Aiko's reaction to receiving the diabetes diagnosis?

Diego showed great professionalism and empathy for Ms. Aiko throughout these interactions. He understood and recognized that she was going through the stages of grief associated with the new diagnosis. He remained calm and gentle while still being direct about the facts of the situation. It is important to recognize what stage the patient is in and react accordingly, as Diego did, without taking the expressions of anger, fear, and sadness personally.

PATIENT INTAKE AND VITALS

Case Study 1

Aaniyah Jones, a 60-year-old female patient, comes into the clinic every Monday, Wednesday, and Friday at 12:30 p.m. for a blood pressure check. Ms. Jones's blood pressure has been intermittently high over the past 6 months. Dr. Lopez prescribed a new blood pressure medication 2 weeks ago, which seems to control the patient's blood pressure. However, today Ms. Jones looks upset and hurried. They tell the MA they need to be seen immediately because they need to get back to work as soon as possible. As the MA walks back to the examination room, Ms. Jones tells the medical assistant that the blood pressure medication the doctor prescribed has made them nauseated, and they have not taken it for the past 2 days.

The MA looks back into Ms. Jones' chart and notes that their blood pressure readings had averaged 134/86 mm Hg while taking the blood pressure medication. Their vitals today are 98.9° F, heart rate 88/min, respirations 22/min, and blood pressure 178/92 mm Hg.

Scene 1

Medical Assistant: "Ms. Jones, I noticed you seem upset today. Is everything okay?"

Ms. Jones: "No, I have been very stressed at work lately and am unsure how to decrease my anxiety. Now I cannot take my medication for my blood pressure, and I am scared something bad will happen."

Scene 2

Medical Assistant: "Yes, not taking your blood pressure medication is a concern, and anxiety can also contribute to higher blood pressure readings. Let me get this information to Dr. Lopez and see if he can help you with your medication to start to relieve some of that worry, and we can also have him talk with you about the anxiety. Would you like me to speak to the provider about finding resources to help decrease the anxiety and manage the stress level?"

Ms. Jones: "Thank you! I would appreciate any help I can get. I want to be able to take my medication and not have it make me sick."

Conclusion

The MA must provide empathy while identifying and documenting behaviors outside the norm. It is also important for the MA to identify factors that can contribute to abnormal vital sign readings.

CHALLENGE

1. Did the medical assistant take the right approach with Ms. Jones regarding their blood pressure reading?

    Yes. In this example, the MA identified that Ms. Jones is upset and expressed support around this while recognizing that this can contribute to their elevated blood pressure. The MA demonstrated the importance of reporting the abnormal measurement to the provider and reporting and requesting to help support a potential underlying cause (stress) at the provider's discretion.

Case Study 2

Annie Chang is 30 years old and overweight. Ms. Chang comes into the office for their annual checkup. She appears nervous and anxious and refuses to get on the scale when it comes time to measure her weight. Ms. Chang says she does not want anyone to know how much she weighs, not even the MA.

Scene 1

Medical Assistant: "Ms. Chang, you have the right to refuse to get weighed, and I will respect that. Everything we do in this office is confidential, and nothing is said to anyone. We are only here to help you. No one would ever judge you."

Ms. Chang: "I have gained a lot of weight over the last few years. I was involved in a lot of group fitness activities that were stopped or changed due to the pandemic. At first, I didn't like staying home all the time, but now the thought of being in group settings and leaving the house on a regular basis scares me. I'm ashamed that I've put on weight, making it harder to get out and start exercising again. I'm afraid that being weighed today will only make me feel worse."

Medical Assistant: "I'm sorry for what you have been going through. I appreciate you sharing that with me. You are not alone in this experience. As I said before, we are here to help you. We can hold off on weighing you for now. I will let the provider know what you shared and encourage you to speak further with her about it."

Scene 2

After Ms. Chang sees the provider.

Medical Assistant: "Hi, Ms. Chang. I understand you talked more with the provider about your concerns with your weight and the emotions you have been experiencing lately. I hope the conversation was helpful to you."

Ms. Chang: "It really was. Thank you for listening to me earlier rather than just pushing me to step on the scale. I now know that my weight gain is more likely a symptom of some mental health concerns I didn't realize I was experiencing. We're going to start me on medication to help with the root cause, and I have a goal of going on three 20-minute walks a week for the next month. I'm not sure if it will help me lose weight, but it sounds like a great step toward regaining control of my body, habits, and environment."

Medical Assistant: "That's great to hear! The provider mentioned that getting a baseline weight would still be helpful, so we can monitor it over time and watch for potential side effects from the new medication. Would you be okay with that?"

Ms. Chang: "That would be okay. I'm just still not sure I'm ready to know."

Medical Assistant: "I understand that. One option is for me to record it without telling you. That will allow us to monitor for change over time, and you have the right to call and ask for this information if you ever decide you want it. How does that sound?"

Ms. Chang: "That sounds great. Thank you."

IN PRACTICE: CASE STUDIES
General Patient Care: Part 1

Conclusion

All patients have the right to refuse treatment or measurements. Medical assistants need empathy and understanding of the patient's perspective on why they are refusing but always educate the patient on the importance of treatment, procedure, or medication. Medical assistants must always maintain professionalism and instill confidentiality in their patients.

CHALLENGE

1. In this situation, did the MA take the right approach with Ms. Chang in the beginning regarding their refusal to measure their body weight?

   Yes. The MA gathered beneficial information about Ms. Chang that related to their weight and affected other aspects of their health. Even if the MA suspected depression or anxiety based on Ms. Chang's report of their concerns, they remained professional and stayed within their scope of work by relying on the information to the provider rather than sharing their thoughts with Ms. Chang directly.

2. Was the MA's approach to taking Ms. Chang's weight in their final interaction appropriate?

   Yes. The MA continued to build trust with Ms. Chang by validating their positive feelings about the plan and listening for their true concerns regarding being weighed. (Ms. Chang was more concerned about knowing their weight than being weighed.) In the end, the MA reframes the weight as a measurement that contributes to the bigger medical picture rather than defining who Ms. Chang is.

GENERAL PATIENT CARE: PART 1

Case Study 1

Tracy is completing an externship as part of her medical assistant program. Her site is at a local clinic that serves a diverse patient population, including many older patients. Her externship preceptor is Mandy, who has been a certified medical assistant for over five years.

Scene 1

Mandy: "You've been doing great so far in your externship, Tracy. You've done an excellent job taking vital signs, rooming patients, instructing patients on urinalysis, and taking blood. Do you have any questions so far?"

Tracy: "Thank you! No questions so far. I'm looking forward to learning more."

Mandy: "Great. I think you're ready to learn how to administer an injection. You said you learned how to do this in your program and you also learned about patient safety, sterile procedures, and medication administration safety. Is that correct?"

Tracy: "That's correct. I did learn that and was able to practice on a practice injection arm."

Mandy: "Good. We have a few patients coming in today that need immunizations and insulin shots. You can watch me do them, and once you're comfortable, I'll observe you doing them."

Scene 2

Tracy: "Hi, Jada. Is Mandy here today?"

Jada: "Hi, Tracy. She's not. She had a family emergency and won't be in today. But I'll be taking over her medical assistant duties today. I know she's been supervising your externship, so just ask me any questions that you have today. Do you want to take Mrs. Wendon? She needs an injection of ampicillin."

Tracy: "Okay. I can give her the injection."

IN PRACTICE: CASE STUDIES
General Patient Care: Part 1

Scene 3

Tracy: "I think I made a mistake, Jada. I think I gave Mrs. Wendon the wrong medication."

Jada: "Okay. Let's look at the medication order. She was supposed to receive ampicillin. What did you give her?"

Tracy (holding a vial): "I gave her amitriptyline instead. I guess I misread the labels when I took it from the medication cabinet."

Jada immediately reported the medication error to the provider. Mrs. Wendon was monitored for any reactions, and an ambulance was called to transport her to the emergency room as a precaution.

Conclusion

It is important to identify and report any medication errors immediately. Failure to respond appropriately to critical errors could have fatal results.

Case Study 2

You are working as a medical assistant at a family medicine clinic. Your 2 p.m. appointment is with Jim Tocol, a 57-year-old male, who is here for his annual physical examination. Mr. Tocol generally feels well, although he's been having difficulty breathing. According to his medical records, he has a history of diabetes, hypertension, and emphysema. After the provider has completed Jim's physical examination, you are asked to administer an influenza vaccine to Jim.

Scene 1

MA: "Hello, I will be administering your influenza vaccination today. Can you provide me with your name and date of birth?"

Mr. Tocol: "Yes, it is Jim Tocol. My date of birth is 01/04/1966."

Scene 2

MA: "Okay, Mr. Tocol, we're all finished with your injection."

Mr. Tocol: "Oh, wow! That was my first time having a flu vaccine. That wasn't bad at all."

MA: "I need you to wait here for 20 minutes to make sure you do not have a reaction."

Mr. Tocol: "I'm having more difficulty breathing all of a sudden, and my throat feels numb. What's wrong with me?"

MA: "Mr. Tocol, I believe you may be having an allergic reaction. Do you have any allergies? I forgot to ask you earlier."

Mr. Tocol: "I only have a severe allergy to eggs."

Conclusion

The MA immediately administers an epinephrine, as directed by the provider, with an autoinjector to Mr. Tocol in the thigh.

CHALLENGE

1. Did Jada make the right decision reporting Tracy's medication error?

   Yes. Mrs. Wendon could have had an anaphylactic reaction to the medication she was administered. Jada took the right approach by reporting it immediately to the provider and monitoring Mrs. Wendon for possible reactions.

2. How could Tracy have avoided administering the wrong medication to Mrs. Wendon?

   Tracy should have completed the three medication label checks: first checking the label when obtaining the medication from its stored location, secondly, when drawing the medication up, and lastly, when returning the medication back to its stored location. Completing the three medication label checks can help avoid making this critical error.

CHALLENGE

1. Could Mr. Tocol's anaphylactic reaction been avoided? If so, how?

   Yes. The medical assistant failed to ask and update Mr. Tocol's allergy status. If the MA properly questioned Mr. Tocol about his allergies prior to administering the medication, they could have verified with the provider if it was okay to still administer the influenza vaccine to Mr. Tocol.

2. Did the medical assistant respond to Mr. Tocol's anaphylactic reaction appropriately?

   Yes. The MA administered epinephrine with an autoinjector and notified the provider for follow-up. Epinephrine is considered the first line of treatment for a patient experiencing anaphylactic shock and should be administered intramuscularly. It is also imperative that the MA call 911 immediately. The autoinjector is for emergency supportive care and does not replace the patient seeking advanced medical care afterward.

GENERAL PATIENT CARE: PART 2

Case Study 1

Alberto Gomez has been a patient at East End Family Clinic for more than 10 years. Thuy has been a medical assistant at the clinic for the last 2 years and knows Mr. Gomez well.

Before Thuy brings Mr. Gomez to the back office, he reviews Mr. Gomez's medical record. Mr. Gomez has a history of hypertension, diabetes, and hypertriglyceridemia. The patient is here for their quarterly check-up appointment.

Scene 1

Thuy: "Good morning, Mr. Gomez. How are you today?"

Mr. Gomez: "Hi, Thuy. I'm doing okay."

Thuy: "Well, it looks like you're here today for a check-up appointment."

Mr. Gomez: "Yes, but I'm not feeling so well the last few days and started having a little chest pain. Hopefully Dr. Vishal can figure out why."

Thuy: "I'm sorry to hear that. Let me get your height, weight, and vital signs, and we will get Dr. Vishal in to see you as soon as possible."

Scene 2

Thuy: (panicked) "Anne! Mr. Gomez just passed out. He was complaining about chest pains. I think he had a heart attack."

Anne (at the front desk): "Oh no! Is he okay? What should I do?"

Thuy: "Call 911 and then let Dr. Vishal know."

CHALLENGE

1. Did Thuy and Anne react appropriately to Mr. Gomez collapsing in the office? What could have been done differently?

Thuy and Anne both had fast responses to Mr. Gomez collapsing in the office by activating the emergency response team and beginning CPR. They remembered to remain calm in the emergency situation, which is one of the most important steps.

Scene 3

Thuy: (patting Mr. Gomez's chest) "Mr. Gomez, are you okay? Can you hear me?"

Anne: (out of breath) "Okay, I called 911 and have them on the phone. Dr. Vishal is coming with the defibrillator. What else should I do?"

Thuy: "I don't feel a pulse. I'm going to start CPR."

Conclusion

Thuy begins chest compressions and then gives Mr. Gomez rescue breaths. They check the pulse and then repeat until the defibrillator arrives or emergency services arrives. Remembering to remain calm in emergency situations is critical.

Case Study 2

You are working as a medical assistant in an internal medicine facility. Anna, a coworker, is in the break room with you preparing to have lunch.

Scene 1

MA: "Hi, Anna. Are you ready for lunch?"

Anna: "Yes, just cutting my apple now!"

Scene 2

Anna: Oh, no! The knife slipped, and I cut my finger open.

MA (noticing the steady flow of dark red blood): "Oh my goodness, that looks bad! Let me get the office manager right away! That's a lot of blood!"

Anna: "I don't know what to do. It won't stop bleeding!!!"

Conclusion

The MA and the office manager arrive back at the break room, where Anna continues to bleed onto the break room floor.

CHALLENGE

1. How could the MA have responded differently?

   Venous bleeding produces a steady flow of dark red blood. The MA could have covered the wound with a clean cloth or gauze, applying pressure on the wound, and had Anna elevate the hand before getting additional help.

INFECTION CONTROL AND SAFETY

Case Study 1

Steven Jones is a 53-year-old patient with a history of diabetes. He presents to the office to obtain his annual bloodwork. Upon reviewing the medical record, the medical assistant notes the bloodwork requested by the provider. The MA starts by washing their hands and getting all the equipment necessary for the procedure; blood draw begins with no issues or complications, and the necessary blood samples for the requested tests are obtained.

Scene 1

MA: "Mr. Jones, I'm filling the last vial of blood, and we then will be finished."

Mr. Jones: "Oh, good! It's starting to get uncomfortable."

MA: "OK, last vial is full. I'm going to remove the needle now."

Scene 2

Mr. Jones: "Ouch!!! That hurt. Sorry for jerking my arm."

MA: "Oh, no! I poked myself with the needle. Let me put it in the sharps container."

Mr. Jones: "Sorry about that. I'm not sure why I jerked my arm. Are you okay?"

Conclusion

The MA discards the contaminated needle into the sharps container and applies a bandage to Mr. Jones's venipuncture site before he leaves.

CHALLENGE

1. After the MA has cleaned the needlestick injury with soap and water, what would the next steps be for them to take?

   Immediately after washing the injured area, the next step is to find the supervisor to report the incident. An incident report must be filled out, and the employee must receive a medical evaluation.

2. What steps need to be taken related to screening the patient for HBV, hepatitis C, and HIV?

   Depending on the state regulation, consent may or may not be required from the individual to perform the screenings. If consent is required but not given, the employer must document the consent was not received from the patient. If the screening is done, OSHA requires that the employer be informed of the results of the patient's tests.

3. What steps could have been taken to help reduce the risk of a needlestick occurring?

   Find an area free from distractions, such as a specific room for blood draws, and/or use of retractable needles, which allows the device to be activated while still in the patient's arm and then removed.

IN PRACTICE: CASE STUDIES
Point-of-Care Testing and Laboratory Procedures

Case Study 2

You are working as a medical assistant when Julia Hernandez, a 32-year-old patient presenting with a cough, congestion, shortness of breath, and a sore throat, arrives to the office with a reception area that is full of patients waiting for well-visit appointments.

Scene 1

MA: "Hi, Ms. Hernandez. How are you?"

Ms. Hernandez: "I've had cough and shortness of breath, and I have had a fever of 102.0° F for the last 24 hours."

Scene 2

MA: "I'm sorry to hear that. Please have a seat and we will bring you back as soon as possible."

Ms. Hernandez: *cough* *cough* "OK. Thanks."

Conclusion

Ms. Hernandez waits in the crowded reception area for 20 minutes and is called back to the examination room by another MA. The MA notices some of the other patients in the reception area look concerned and uncomfortable being around Ms. Hernandez, as she is visibly ill and coughing.

CHALLENGE

1. What is the best way to handle this situation with Ms. Hernandez and the other patients in the waiting area?

   Provide a face mask to the patient if they are not already wearing one. Take the patient to a room where they can be away from all the well care patients to prevent others from being infected.

2. What patient education can be provided to Ms. Hernandez on how to prevent the transmission of disease?

   Provide instructions on how to properly cover a cough. Remind the patient that proper handwashing is routinely used to prevent the spread of infection. Proper handwashing should occur after coughing or sneezing, after use of the restroom, and before eating, to name a few. Advise a patient to carry alcohol-based sanitizer to use if handwashing is not available.

3. After Ms. Hernandez has received care and exited the examination room, how would the MA clean and disinfect the room?

   To help prevent the spread of infection, clean the room in the following steps: 1) Clean hands either by aseptic handwashing or use of an alcohol-based sanitizer. 2) Remove disposable paper covering over the examination table by tightly rolling it up to ensure contaminated side is on the inside. 3) Dispose of any paper gowns or disposable supplies used and then disinfect all work surfaces beginning with the examination table, sink, countertops, and any other surface the patient may have encountered.

POINT-OF-CARE TESTING AND LABORATORY PROCEDURES

Case Study 1

Austin, a 16-year-old patient, presents to the office. Austin's mother has brought him here today because he has been reported as being constantly thirsty and hungry. He also gets light-headed if he does not eat. The patient tells the medical assistant, "It seems like I always have to pee." The medical assistant takes the patient back to the examination room and obtains a set of vital signs for the provider. After examining the patient, the provider orders a urinalysis and blood glucose testing.

Scene 1

Medical Assistant: "Austin, we have to collect a clean catch urine. I will give you three cleansing towelettes. I need you to cleanse the area around one side of the tip of the penis and the urethral opening with a towelette. Repeat on the other side with a fresh towelette. Cleanse across the urethral opening with the last towelette. Open the specimen cup and place the lid with the top side down on a flat surface. Urinate in the toilet a little bit and then stop. Then, urinate into the cup, filling the specimen cup. Be careful not to touch the inside of the cup. Place the lid on the cup without touching the inside of the lid. When you are done, leave your specimen in the compartment in the restroom and come back to the exam room."

IN PRACTICE: CASE STUDIES
Point-of-Care Testing and Laboratory Procedures

Austin: "What are you testing for?"

Medical Assistant: "The provider wants to see if there is anything in your urine that should not be there that is causing your symptoms."

Austin: "OK, I understand. I'll go into the bathroom and try to get a sample."

Five minutes later, Austin returns to the exam room and tells the MA he left his urine sample in the bathroom.

Scene 2

Medical Assistant: "Now that we have collected your urine. I need to collect a blood glucose sample. It's a capillary stick, which means it will require me to take just a small drop of blood from your finger. I will put that drop of blood on this glucometer, which will give me a reading. Have you had anything to eat this morning?"

Austin: "I had a piece of toast this morning before I left about 2 hours ago."

Medical Assistant: "OK, is it all right if I use a finger on your left hand to get the sample?"

Austin: "Sure."

Medical Assistant: "OK, I am going to clean it and then obtain the sample. I will count 1-2-3, then poke."

Austin: "I hope it's okay."

Medical Assistant: "All complete! I'm going to relay the results to the provider, and they will be back in to go over the results."

Austin: "What were my results?"

Medical Assistant: "I cannot relay that information—the provider will need to review the results and will be in to discuss them."

The provider meets with Austin and his mother again, relaying that Austin's blood glucose was 195 mg/dL and that glucose was positive in the urine sample. Austin and his mother have agreed to return to the office the next day to have fasting bloodwork completed.

Conclusion

The medical assistant needs to be aware of abnormal labs so they can notify the provider to help diagnose patients and aid in further testing to confirm diagnoses.

CHALLENGE

1. Should the medical assistant have relayed the results to Austin?

    The medical assistant did the right thing by not relaying the results to the patient. MAs cannot release any lab results to patients without the provider reviewing and signing off on them first. Miscommunication of laboratory results can have a significant, negative effect on patients.

IN PRACTICE: CASE STUDIES
Point-of-Care Testing and Laboratory Procedures

Case Study 2

Austin's mom brings him back to the clinic the next day. The medical assistant determines that the patient has followed the pretesting fasting instructions. Austin is feeling shaky and light-headed. After the blood draw, the medical assistant notices he is trembling and seems very confused. They notify the provider and check Austin's blood sugar. His blood sugar is very low. The medical assistant administers instant glucose according to the provider's orders, and Austin quickly returns to a normal state. The provider suspects type 1 diabetes and schedules Austin for further testing at the hospital.

Scene 1

Medical Assistant: "Are you feeling better?"

Austin: "Yes, what happened?"

Medical Assistant: "Your blood sugar level dropped low. Your blood sugar was 50. Normal is 70 to 100 mg/dL, and your blood dropped significantly lower, which made you shaky and a bit confused. We gave you some instant glucose, or sugar, to bring it back up and make you feel better."

Scene 2

Medical Assistant: "The provider wants to schedule you for some further testing at the hospital. As he mentioned to you and your mom, he suspects you might have diabetes."

Austin: "Does that mean I will have to check my own blood every day?"

Medical Assistant: "Only the provider would be able to answer that. However, if you do, I can teach you how to collect your blood with a glucometer so you can monitor your blood glucose levels."

Austin: "Okay, thank you. That makes sense. I'm glad that I can do this on my own."

Conclusion

The medical assistant educated the patient on the need for further testing to confirm the diagnosis and also on provided preliminary education related to monitoring blood glucose levels at home.

CHALLENGE

1. What signs indicated to the medical assistant that Austin's blood glucose levels could be below normal?

    Austin appeared trembling, shaky, and confused. Austin also reported feeling light-headed during his visit. The medical assistant was able to recognize the patient's symptoms and notified the provider so an intervention could be done to reverse the effect of low blood sugar.

IN PRACTICE: CASE STUDIES
Phlebotomy

PHLEBOTOMY

Case Study 1

Aaron is a medical assistant in a primary care office. He is preparing to perform phlebotomy on a patient. The patient was diagnosed with high cholesterol and triglycerides 3 months ago. During their last visit, the patient was instructed to change their diet, increase exercise, and return to the office for a repeat lipid panel. The patient was asked to fast for 12 hours prior to coming to their appointment.

Scene 1

Aaron: "Hey, how are you? How's everything going? My name is Aaron, and I am the medical assistant who will be drawing your blood today for your lab work. It looks like your provider has ordered fasting labs. When was the last time you had anything to eat or drink?"

Patient: "I had some coffee and a biscuit for breakfast."

Scene 2

Aaron: "Fasting labs require that you have nothing to eat or drink except water for 12 hours prior to the blood work being performed. We will have to reschedule for another day."

Patient: "Why? I'm here now. I really do not have time to come back."

Aaron: "I am sorry, but we will have to reschedule. I would be happy to help get you to our schedulers so we can find a day that works for you."

Conclusion

Aaron escorts the patient out to the scheduler to reschedule the appointment, reminding the patient not to have anything to eat or drink except water 12 hours prior to the next appointment.

CHALLENGE

1. Did Aaron make the right decision by informing the patient they have to reschedule the blood work?

Yes. The presence of certain substances in the blood can be affected by fluid intake and food. For example, patients should fast prior to having a lipid panel. If the patient ate a meal prior to having blood drawn, the test values would likely detect fats from the food and the results would indicate elevated lipid levels, which could be an inaccurate overall result.

Case Study 2

Carrie is a medical assistant in a busy phlebotomy center. She is preparing equipment for a blood draw on her patient, Liam. Liam is getting routine lab work as part of an annual wellness examination.

Scene 1

Carrie: "Hi, Liam. My name is Carrie. It's a pleasure to meet you. I'll be drawing three tubes of blood today so we can perform the blood tests ordered by your provider. Do you have any questions for me?"

Liam: "No questions really, but I am incredibly nervous about this. Last time I had my blood drawn, I almost passed out. I'm scared of needles and the sight of blood."

Carrie: "Having your blood drawn can be intimidating, but I'll walk you through every step and we'll get through it together as quickly as possible! Is there anything I can do to make you more comfortable and relaxed?"

Liam: "I can't think of anything, but thank you for asking."

IN PRACTICE: CASE STUDIES
EKG and Cardiovascular Testing

Scene 2

Carrie: "I'd like to have you lie down on the table here. Would that be okay? Are you warm enough?"

Liam: "Okay, that sounds good, thanks."

Carrie: "I'm going to clean the area first, and then you'll feel a little pinch in your left arm near the crease by your elbow. I'm filling up the last blood tube now, and we're almost done!"

Liam: "Wow! I didn't feel that at all. Thanks for being kind and supportive."

Carrie: "That's it! All done. I'd like you to lie here for just a few minutes, and then I'll help you sit up and you'll be free to go."

Conclusion

Carrie stayed with Liam for a few minutes and continued to put him at ease by engaging in casual conversation. After ensuring Liam was okay to go, Carrie escorted him to the exit.

CHALLENGE

1. What qualities did Carrie exhibit during her interaction with Liam? What techniques did Carrie use to put Liam at ease and help them feel safe?

   Carrie introduced herself and approached Liam with a pleasant, warm demeanor. Carrie also explained the procedure steps to Liam and answered questions they had while displaying sensitivity to help put Liam at ease and feel safe.

EKG AND CARDIOVASCULAR TESTING

Case Study 1

Mr. Smith has been experiencing heart palpitations over the last month during exercise and while at rest. He just arrived in the clinic for a 12-lead EKG ordered by the provider to establish a baseline and possibly identify the cause of his palpitations.

Scene 1

Kim: "Good morning, Mr. Smith. I'm Kim, a medical assistant, and I will perform your EKG today. Have you ever had one before?"

Mr. Smith: "Nice to meet you, Kim. It has been about 10 years, but I remember it being pretty easy."

Kim: "It is a pretty simple procedure. Let's start by verifying your name and date of birth to make sure I've got the right guy."

Mr. Smith: "Michael Smith, 9/6/71."

Kim: "Perfect."

Scene 2

Kim: "Go ahead and lie down on the table. Please let me know if you are uncomfortable or have any difficulty breathing."

Mr. Smith: "Will do."

Kim: "I am going to place 10 electrodes on specific parts of your body and then connect wires to those electrodes that will allow the EKG machine to record electrical impulses from your heart. The report will print out for the provider to review and interpret. Do you have any questions so far?"

Mr. Smith: "Yeah. Will I feel this electrical current? And why are you only putting 10 electrodes on when the doc said I was supposed to get a 12-lead EKG?"

Kim: "Great questions! You will not feel any of the electrical impulses. This test allows us to amplify, capture, and record the heart's electrical activity that is already occurring. We measure 12 leads or recordings of your heart's activity from different angles. We only need 10 spots on the body to capture 12 different angles."

Mr. Smith: "Okay, great! Hook me up, then!"

Kim: "I am placing one electrode on each leg and one electrode on each arm, and then I have six that will go on your chest. I will touch your ribs and chest for some anatomical landmarks to place the electrodes in the correct spot."

Mr. Smith: "Do you ever get really hairy guys in here? How does that work?"

Kim: "Well, we have some surgical clippers in the drawer that I would use to clip some of the chest hair so the electrodes make a good connection."

Mr. Smith: "That makes sense!"

Conclusion

When preparing a patient for an EKG, explain the steps along the way to dispel any fears the patient may have. Patients may need help understanding how an EKG works and why the MA places electrodes in specific locations. They may not fully understand the language of the midaxillary line and fifth intercostal space, so it is helpful to explain the procedure in language the patient will understand. Give the patient the opportunity to ask questions to put the patient at ease and convey that the MA cares about their experience.

CHALLENGE

1. What patient instructions should Kim relay to Mr. Smith prior to performing the EKG?

Kim should instruct Mr. Smith to turn off all electronic devices, such as cell phones, and remove them from his pockets. Also, any jewelry should be removed. In addition, Mr. Smith should be instructed to lie still and not to talk or move during the EKG reading. These items could lead to artifacts on the EKG tracing.

Case Study 2

Mr. Smith has been prepped for the EKG, and the electrodes and leads are in place. Kim is preparing to perform the EKG and has covered Mr. Smith with a blanket for privacy.

Scene 1

Kim: "Okay, Mr. Smith, all your electrodes and leads are attached, and it looks like we have a good connection. We are ready to record the EKG. I will need you to lie still, breathe normally, and refrain from talking until I tell you we are done."

Mr. Smith: "Let's do this!"

Kim: "I am entering all your information into the EKG machine. I am now ready to press the button to start the test. Are you in a comfortable position?"

Mr. Smith: "I am."

Kim: "Okay, here we go!"

IN PRACTICE: CASE STUDIES
EKG and Cardiovascular Testing

Scene 2

(Kim presses the auto button and then the run button to start the EKG. She sees the correct standardization mark appear, and the tracing begins. Suddenly, she notices a wandering baseline artifact that moves away from the center of the page. She looks at Mr. Smith and notices the electrode on his left leg has shifted.)

Kim: "Mr. Smith, did you use any lotion or cream on your legs today?"

Mr. Smith: "I sure did. Every day after my shower."

Kim: "I am going to remove this electrode and use an alcohol prep to remove any residue and reattach the electrodes. Sometimes lotion can affect connectivity."

Mr. Smith: "Sorry about that. You told me not to use lotion, so I didn't use any on my chest. Who knew you were going to put those things on my legs?"

(Kim reattaches the electrodes and returns to the EKG machine)

Kim: "Okay, Mr. Smith, take two!"

Mr. Smith: "Ready!"

Kim: "Okay, this one was recorded correctly. Let me notify the provider that we are done, and then I will come and remove the leads and the electrodes."

Mr. Smith: "Wow. That was pretty simple. Thank you."

Conclusion

In addition to patient prep, it is necessary to check for artifact and electrode placement during the EKG. The electrodes or leads can sometimes shift and create issues, causing an inaccurate reading. It is imperative to catch this while the patient is still attached and present. It would be highly inconvenient to disconnect the patient and then prep and attach the electrodes and leads again because the EKG was not done properly.

CHALLENGE

1. How was Kim able to know to recheck the leads that were placed on Mr. Smith after starting the EKG?

   A wandering baseline results from movement associated with breathing or poor electrode connection. The baseline will wander away from the center of the paper, causing difficulty in tracing interpretation. Clean the skin before attaching the electrodes. Instructing the patient prior to their EKG appointment, to avoid using creams and lotions is helpful.

PATIENT CARE COORDINATION AND EDUCATION

Case Study 1

Ms. Bird came into the office today for a follow-up after being diagnosed with diabetes. The provider, Dr. Jones, examines Ms. Bird and notices that she has lost 7 pounds since her last visit, which was a month ago. Dr. Jones has identified that Ms. Bird does not have the resources to prepare meals at home to maintain her weight and blood sugar goals. Dr. Jones asks Sohni, the medical assistant, to obtain resources for Ms. Bird to get nutritional resources and make referrals to help her.

Scene 1

Sohni: "Hello, Ms. Bird. Dr. Jones has identified that you need some resources for nutrition at home to help maintain your weight and blood sugar goals relating to your diagnosis of diabetes."

Ms. Bird: "Yes, I don't have a grocery store nearby that I can get to, so I don't always have enough food at home to eat. I am not sure who can help me."

Scene 2

Sohni: "Don't worry. I will give you information to take with you, and we will set up what we can here before you leave. First, let's see if we can get the dietitian to talk to you while you are here. We can put in a referral for you to get food assistance services. I will give you all the related information, but we can send them the referral today. This service will bring you food so you have a meal prepared according to your diet and you don't have to prepare anything. Do you have the supplies to check your blood sugar at home?"

Ms. Bird: "Oh, that would be wonderful! That would help ease my mind and help me control my blood sugar and help me put some of my weight back on. You are a lifesaver! I have the supplies to check my blood sugar at home. Thanks for checking and asking."

Sohni: "You are very welcome, Ms. Bird. I am glad I could help and get that set up for you. If you need anything else, please don't hesitate to ask."

CHALLENGE

1. What key factors did the medical assistant identify and provide to assist Ms. Bird with her nutritional needs?

The MA identified the patient needed an outside resource, like seeing the dietitian, placing a referral for food assistance service, and determining if the patient required resources to check their blood sugar at home.

IN PRACTICE: CASE STUDIES
Patient Care Coordination and Education

Case Study 2

Mr. Hutchins is an established patient and is under care for herniated discs in his neck that occurred during a car accident approximately 6 months ago. He was in the clinic 2 weeks ago for a refill of muscle relaxants and pain pills. During that visit, he revealed that someone had stolen his medication and that he needed a refill. Dr. Gutierrez prescribed a 1-month supply with the understanding that this was a one-time occurrence and that Mr. Hutchinson was to be seen by a pain management specialist for further prescriptions.

Today, Mr. Hutchins is in visible pain and explains why he no longer has medications available for pain relief. He explains that he cannot be seen at the pain clinic until the end of next week and "just needs a 2-week refill." The medical assistant, Lin, suspects that Mr. Hutchins is misusing his medications. Lin informs Dr. Gutierrez, who, after speaking with Mr. Hutchinson, agrees with her concerns. Dr. Gutierrez would like Lin to act as a patient advocate for Mr. Hutchinson and provide him with a list of resources to obtain help and information on misusing medications.

Scene 1

Lin: "Mr. Hutchins, Dr. Gutierrez is concerned that you may be becoming dependent on muscle relaxants and pain medications. Dr. Gutierrez wanted the office to provide you with some resources for narcotic dependency clinics."

Mr. Hutchins: "You have got to be kidding me! How dare you accuse me of being an addict? I told you someone stole my medication, and now you think I am an addict and need help!"

CHALLENGE

1. What outside resources can the medical assistant provide to Mr. Hutchins to help with the misuse of prescribed medications?

   Educational resources can include misuse of prescription medications, preventive measures to prevent prescription abuse, prescription medication abuse support groups, and information on alternatives for pain management.

Scene 2

Lin: "No, Mr. Hutchins. I apologize for the misunderstanding. I was not accusing you or saying you are an addict, but we are concerned that you may be progressing to becoming dependent on those medications. You have called us within 2 weeks for refills for two reasons, and we want to ensure your health is the priority. I want to provide resources to help you wean off these medications and help you manage your pain."

Mr. Hutchins: "I see that you are trying to help. I have been taking more pain medications than I probably should have, and I may need some help managing my pain better. I appreciate that you're offering resources that will help me."

ADMINISTRATIVE ASSISTING

Case Study 1

The patient, Melinda Chao, has come in for their scheduled appointment at 1:00 p.m. for chronic care management. The MA is checking them in.

Scene 1

MA: "Hello, and welcome to ABC Clinic. Can I have your name, please?"

Melinda: "Hello, I am Melinda Chao for my 1:00 p.m. appointment."

MA: "Thank you. Can I see your insurance card and photo identification?"

Melinda presents the insurance card and photo identification. The MA verifies the patient's identity with what is in the EHR, using the insurance card and photo ID to confirm. Verifying patient's identity also prevents creation of a duplicate medical record.

Scene 2

MA: "Thank you. Have there been any changes to your address or insurance information?"

Melinda: "No, it is correct on the license."

MA: "Thank you. We have you checked in and we will call you when we are ready to take you to the exam room. Please have a seat."

Melinda: "Thank you."

Conclusion

Check-in is the process when the patient arrives for their appointment. It should be cordial and professional. The MA will verify patient eligibility, identification, and insurance information. They will ask to see a photo identification, such as a state identification card or driver's license, to ensure that the name matches the information on the insurance card and the information in the demographic section of the EHR.

CHALLENGE

1. What might be the repercussions if the MA did not verify Melinda's identification?

   Fraud or abuse can occur if Melinda is not the actual person who has the appointment and is listed on the insurance card. Fraud can have a large cost to consumers and insurance companies and reflects poorly on the practice.

2. Did the MA verify Melinda's identity using the correct form of identification?

   Yes. The MA verified Melinda's identity by requesting a photo identification to ensure the face matches the name.

IN PRACTICE: CASE STUDIES
Administrative Assisting

Case Study 2

A MA has answered the phone and is speaking with Jaquin Henderson, a patient who would like to schedule an appointment.

Scene 1

MA: "Jaquin, thank you for holding. What is the nature of the visit you are requesting?"

Jaquin: "I've had a headache for three days and nothing seems to help. My throat is sore, and I am very congested. I took medicine, and it hasn't helped."

CHALLENGE

1. Did the MA ask the correct screening questions to determine the urgency of the appointment?

    Yes. The MA obtained information from Jaquin that helped determine how urgent the request for the appointment was.

2. Which factors were used in screening the call with Jaquin? (Select all that apply.)
    A. Patient availability
    B. Insurance information
    C. Provider availability
    D. Past annual exam date of service
    E. Signs and symptoms
    F. History of current condition

    C, E, and F are correct. Screening is asking questions to determine the signs and symptoms as well as the history of the current situation to prioritize the medical services.

Scene 2

MA: "I am sorry you are not feeling well. Are you available this afternoon at 2:30?"

Jaquin: "Yes, I couldn't go to work for the last two days."

MA: "Is your address and insurance information the same as your last visit?"

Jaquin: "Yes, I came in last month for my annual wellness exam."

MA: "Thank you, and we will see you today at 2:30 p.m."

Conclusion

Screening is asking questions to determine the signs and symptoms as well as the history of the current situation to prioritize the medical services. It is done to screen the calls to determine which are urgent and which can be scheduled later when convenient. At times, the MA can ask questions to help the patient decide if medical attention is needed or if they will wait to see if it resolves on its own.

COMMUNICATION AND CUSTOMER SERVICE

Case Study 1

An MA is having a discussion with Ricola, a patient who received a statement that shows an additional balance of $238. Ricola is very upset.

Scene 1

MA: "Hello, how may I help you?"

Ricola: "I just got this bill for $238, and I don't have money for this."

MA (said in a calm voice): "Okay, I will gladly look at it with you."

Ricola: "I can't even pay my rent. How am I supposed to pay this, too?"

Scene 2

MA: "I understand your frustration. An additional bill can be stressful. Let's go ahead and look at the account to see what the charges are for."

Ricola: "I don't know why my insurance didn't cover it. I can't pay this."

MA: "Let's look at what the insurance covered, and we can even check out a payment plan so it isn't all due at once."

Ricola: "Okay, that could help."

Conclusion

It is essential for the MA to be able to remain calm, polite, and professional and not match the energy of the patient. It is professional to display empathy and helpfulness when listening and assisting with finding a resolution that works.

CHALLENGE

1. Did the MA handle this conversation appropriately with Ricola? Explain your answer.

   Yes, it may be challenging when communicating with a person who is upset or frustrated; however, it is important to maintain composure. Never match any negative energy in response to the challenging situation. Refrain from becoming defensive and remember the goal is to provide the patient with quality health care services.

2. Which of the following communication styles did the MA use when communicating with Ricola?
   A. Manipulative
   B. Aggressive
   C. Assertive
   D. Passive

   C is correct. The ideal communication style in health care would include assertive. Assertive includes being direct in addressing the issue, good eye contact and body language, and a respectful volume of voice.

3. What could the MA have done if the conversation had continued to escalate with Ricola and remaining calm didn't help?

   If it reaches a level that appears will not decrease and attempts have not helped in controlling the situation, it may be beneficial to include a supervisor or additional person to help in the de-escalation process.

IN PRACTICE: CASE STUDIES
Communication and Customer Service

Case Study 2

An MA is speaking with Chad, a patient who was just diagnosed with chlamydia.

Scene 1

MA: "Hello, Chad. We will be going over the visit summary. Please let me know if you have any questions or concerns at any point."

Chad: "Thank you. I appreciate it."

MA: "You are very welcome. Dr. Hernandez saw you today and has written a prescription. Would you like it sent to a pharmacy or have a paper copy?"

Chad: "Please send it to XYZ Pharmacy in Middletown."

MA: "I will gladly do that. Do you have any questions about your visit today?"

Scene 2

Chad: "Does the doctor see many patients with this diagnosis?"

MA: "We are not able to discuss other patients, but the medication will help with it. It is something that is commonly treated."

Chad: "Do you know anyone who has had it?"

MA: "I can tell you that it's a fairly common diagnosis. I am glad you came in so you could get a prescription. The pharmacist will answer any specific questions about the medication. Dr. Hernandez would like to see you for a follow-up appointment in 4 weeks. We can schedule that together at checkout. Can I help you with anything else today?"

Chad: "No, thank you."

MA: "You're welcome. We will head to checkout to schedule your next appointment. Please feel free to contact us with any questions or concerns if they arise."

Conclusion

It is important for the MA to refrain from sharing their own personal information when communicating with a patient. The MA should not share personal experiences, peer experiences, or the experiences of other patients when talking with a patient.

CHALLENGE

1. How can the MA help build a relationship with Chad based on trust and respect while still maintaining personal boundaries?

   The MA can use professional manner with a positive attitude of encouragement and support to Chad. These behaviors will help to build a relationship based on trust and respect. The MA can accomplish this without sharing any personal information or experiences.

2. Do you think the MA responded to Chad's question about knowing anyone else with the same diagnosis in the correct manner? Explain your answer.

   Yes. The MA responded appropriately. The MA refrained from sharing their own personal information when communicating with a patient. It is not appropriate to share personal experiences, peer experiences, or the experiences of other patients when talking with a patient, even if names aren't disclosed. HIPAA requirements state that personal patient information should not be shared without the patient's written consent.

MEDICAL LAW AND ETHICS

Case Study 1

Sandra is a medical assistant in a busy family medicine clinic. She works with several other medical assistants and Dr. Bonnai. It is a Friday, and the schedule is overbooked with patients. The clinic is already behind, with several patients in the waiting room. Sandra is seeing her sixth patient of the day, Thanh Vu. As she reviews his medical record, Sandra notes that he has been scheduled for a colonoscopy later in the week, and he will need instructions for preparing for the procedure.

Scene 1

Sandra: Good morning, Mr. Vu. How are you today?

Mr. Vu: I'm good, although my appointment was at 9:30, and it's almost 10:30 right now.

Sandra: I'm sorry about the long wait. We have a few patients that need a little bit more care. But we're glad you're here now, and we'll make sure to take care of you.

Mr. Vu: That's good to hear. I'm a little nervous because I was scheduled for a procedure by Dr. Bonnai, and I'm just not sure about it.

Sandra: I read that in your medical record, and Dr. Bonnai will certainly explain it to you. Then, afterward, I'll go over the preparation for the colonoscopy. Do you have any questions for me right now before I get the doctor?

Mr. Vu: No. That all sounds good so far.

Scene 2

Sandra: Hi, Mr. Vu. It's me again. May I come in?

Mr. Vu: Yes, of course.

Sandra: I heard you met with Dr. Bonnai and he talked to you about the colonoscopy. Do you have any questions about it right now before we go over a few things you'll need to prepare for it and for you to sign the consent form?

Mr. Vu: Prepare for it? I have no idea what the doctor was talking about! He mentioned something about being sedated and a scope going up me. Why am I even getting it? I don't have a history, and if it's just a recommended exam, do I really need to get it done? I'm just really uncomfortable about this whole thing.

Sandra: I'm sorry to hear that, Mr. Vu. Dr. Bonnai did schedule it, so I'm sure he feels it is important to your care. That being said, you have the final say on any medical procedure being recommended.

Mr. Vu: But do I really need it if I don't have any symptoms?

Sandra: That's a great question. I want to be sure you have all the information you need in considering this decision. Let me see if Dr. Bonnai is available to talk to you again.

IN PRACTICE: CASE STUDIES
Medical Law and Ethics

Scene 3

Sandra: Hi, Mr. Vu. May I come in again?

Mr. Vu: Yes, of course.

Sandra: I was hoping to get Dr. Bonnai for you, but he's with a patient, and it may be a while.

Mr. Vu: Oh, well. Let me go ahead and sign the consent form.

CHALLENGE

1. In this case, should Sandra have been okay with Mr. Vu signing the consent form? Why or why not?

Although it is the duty of Dr. Bonnai to provide information to the patient and to get informed consent prior to a procedure or treatment, it is Sandra's responsibility to prepare the consent forms and ask Mr. Vu if he has any questions and if everything that was explained was clearly understood. It seems the patient does not understand. Sandra should not allow Mr. Vu to sign, as he still had questions and does not understand the procedure or treatment and why the provider believes it to be necessary. Mr. Vu has not been fully informed and, thus, cannot legally give consent.

Case Study 2

Monique Williams has been a medical assistant in a pediatric clinic for the last 4 years. As a result, she has become familiar with many of the patients and their parents. Today, one of her patients is Allie Loflin, who is a 7-year-old girl. She is usually accompanied by her mom, Tracey.

Scene 1

Monique knocks on the door of the exam door and asks if she can enter. A man's voice says, "Come in."

She is surprised to see that Allie's dad, Ben, is here instead of her mom. Monique introduces herself and asks how everyone is doing.

Ben quickly says, "Fine."

Allie looks down and doesn't respond. Ben sternly says to Allie, "What do you say? She asked you a question."

"I'm fine," Allie says meekly. As she looks up, you notice a bruise on her face.

Monique proclaims, "Oh my, what happened here?"

Although she directed the question to Allie, Ben answers and says Allie was playing and ran into a branch, which happened a few days ago. But now they are here because he thinks she may have broken her arm.

Allie seems quieter than normal, and Monique is worried that something else is going on, such as child abuse.

Monique asks Allie how she injured her arm. Ben answers for her again and says she fell while riding her bike. Every time Monique tries to ask Allie a question, Ben answers. The reason for Allie's injuries does not seem to make sense.

Monique would like to get Allie by herself so she can ask questions privately. Monique asks Ben if she can recheck Allie's height and weight in another exam room.

He says no and that they are in a hurry and just wants to be seen by the doctor. Monique says she understands and that she will let the doctor know that they are ready to be seen

IN PRACTICE: CASE STUDIES
Medical Law and Ethics

Scene 2

Before Monique calls the doctor, she decides to review Allie's medical records.

As the medical assistant reviews Allie's medical record, she notices past incidents of injuries, such as burns and dislocations with questionable explanations from the parent. She compiles this information and reports it to the physician, Dr. Khan.

Dr. Khan examines Allie. When inquiring about her injuries, Dr. Kahn receives the same information and explanations from her father. Her father remains in the exam room and watches the physical examination very closely.

During the physical examination, Dr. Khan notes other bruises on Allie's body—some new and some old and healing. She suspects that Allie has fracture of the left arm and believes it to be consistent with child abuse.

CHALLENGE

1. Based on Dr. Khan's examination, what should be done next?

   The medical assistant or Dr. Khan should make an oral report to the local Child Protective Services and provide important information, such as the injuries reported, the history provided by the parent; and any past findings that may suggest a history of child abuse.

2. Are members of the health care team considered mandated reporters? What type of incidents are appropriate to report?

   Yes. There are federal and state laws and statutes that mandate health care providers and professionals to report and document incidents of concern for a patient's safety and for the safety of the public at large. In the health care field, mandatory reporting duties refer mainly to the responsibility of health care professionals to report vital information and incidents to the appropriate agencies for the protection and welfare of the public, as well as specific vulnerable populations.

IN PRACTICE
Quizzes

QUIZ 1: FOUNDATIONAL KNOWLEDGE AND BASIC SCIENCE

1. Which of the following statements describes a patient-centered medical home (PCMH)?

    A. It is an umbrella term for plans that provide health care in return for preset scheduled payments and coordinated care.

    B. It is a care delivery model supported by an interdisciplinary team and led by a primary care provider (PCP).

    C. It is nursing care and therapy delivered to a patient in their home following an acute event.

    D. It is an inpatient care facility for patients who are at the end of life.

2. Which of the following is an impact of patient portals?

    A. Increased wait times for results

    B. Increased demand on the care team

    C. Increased face-to-face visits

    D. Increased transparency

3. Which of the following is a component of the Quadruple Aim, which drives value-based care?

    A. Increased testing

    B. Increased revenue

    C. Improved patient outcomes

    D. Improved prevention screening

4. To which of the following allied health professionals should a medical assistant initiate a referral to for a provider who has ordered support to assist with improving a patient's range of motion?

    A. Radiology technician

    B. Occupational therapist

    C. Nurse practitioner

    D. Physical therapist

5. Which of the following responsibilities is appropriate for a medical assistant who works in an administrative capacity?

    A. Performing an EKG

    B. Preparing medications

    C. Obtaining vital signs

    D. Collecting copays

6. Which of the following medication classifications should be used for a patient who is experiencing seasonal allergies?

    A. Antihypertensives

    B. Antihistamines

    C. Diuretics

    D. Antipyretics

7. Which of the following schedules of controlled medications can be prescribed with up to a year's worth of refills, if authorized by the provider?

    A. Schedule II

    B. Schedule III

    C. Schedule IV

    D. Schedule V

IN PRACTICE: QUIZZES
Quiz 1: Foundational Knowledge and Basic Science

8. A patient who has chronic kidney disease is being directed to avoid ibuprofen due to the strain it puts on the kidneys. This is an example of which of the following?

   A. Side effect

   B. Adverse effect

   C. Contraindication

   D. Indication

9. Which of the following actions of pharmacokinetics is most impacted by age?

   A. Absorption

   B. Distribution

   C. Metabolism

   D. Excretion

10. Which of the following actions describes the medical assistant's role in confirming "the right medication," in terms of medication administration?

    A. Assessing the benefits and risks of a medication

    B. Stating the name of the medication, who ordered it, and the intended effect of the medication

    C. Informing the patient of the indication for the medication

    D. Evaluating the patient for effects

11. Albuterol (proventil HFA) is an example of which of the following medication classifications?

    A. Anticoagulant

    B. Bronchodilator

    C. Antiemetic

    D. Antipsychotic

12. A patient calls in with a question about one of their medications but does not remember the name of the medication and states, "It's a small, oval-shaped pink pill." The patient's medical record indicates they are currently taking 10 medications. Which of the following actions should the assistant take?

    A. Consult the Physicians' Desk Reference for clarification.

    B. Instruct the patient to seek help from a family member or the pharmacy.

    C. Ask the patient to bring the medication into the clinic to verify what it is.

    D. Type the patient's description into an online search engine to determine the answer.

13. Which of the following is an example of a simple carbohydrate?

    A. Honey

    B. Vegetables

    C. Pasta

    D. Beans

14. Which of the following is the first step a patient who has stage I chronic kidney disease should take to adapt their diet?

    A. Limit sodium.

    B. Decrease phosphorus intake.

    C. Control potassium intake.

    D. Avoid gluten products.

15. Which of the following supplements is also a naturally occurring hormone in the brain that is related to sleep?

    A. Gingko biloba

    B. Willow bark

    C. Melatonin

    D. Black cohosh

16. Which of the following is a warning sign for anorexia and should be reported to a provider immediately?

    A. Weight loss of at least 5%

    B. Increased frequency of menstrual periods

    C. Buying and consuming large amounts of food

    D. Excessive exercising

17. Which of the following routes of medication administration is a parenteral route?

    A. Subcutaneously

    B. Orally

    C. Topically

    D. Vaginally

18. Which of the following forms of medication are delivered orally?

    A. Foams

    B. Mist

    C. Lozenges

    D. Powders

19. A pediatrician prescribes a medication for a 5-year-old child, with the dosage listed as "X mg/kg/day, divided over 3 doses a day." Which of the following actions should the medical assistant take to determine how much medication the child should receive per dose?

    A. Measure and record the child's height.

    B. Convert the child's weight to kilograms.

    C. Multiply the daily dose by three.

    D. Ask the provider to clarify how much medication should be given in each dose.

20. How often should medication allergies be discussed with a patient?

    A. Annually

    B. At every visit

    C. Every 3 years

    D. Each phone call, portal message, or encounter with the patient

QUIZ 2: MEDICAL TERMINOLOGY, ANATOMY, AND PHYSIOLOGY

1. Which of the following abbreviations is used to indicate a heart attack?

    A. CVA

    B. BP

    C. PVD

    D. MI

2. According to The Joint Commission's "Do Not Use" list, which of the following should never be abbreviated?

    A. Disease names

    B. Body part names

    C. Medication names

    D. Test names

3. Which of the following does the root word dermat refer to?

    A. Sweat

    B. Skin

    C. Hair

    D. Nail

IN PRACTICE: QUIZZES
Quiz 2: Medical Terminology, Anatomy, and Physiology

4. Which of the following diseases is a patient referring to if they say "Lou Gehrig's disease"?

    A. Diabetes mellitus

    B. Multiple sclerosis

    C. Amyotrophic lateral sclerosis

    D. Transient ischemic attacks

5. Which of the following describes the position of the head to the chest when a person is in the anatomical position?

    A. Inferior

    B. Superior

    C. Anterior

    D. Dorsal

6. Which of the following is a common symptom of depression?

    A. Overwhelming worry

    B. Feelings of hopelessness

    C. Flashbacks

    D. Trouble following directions

7. Which of the following is an example of a physical stressor on the body?

    A. Pollution in the air

    B. Loss of a loved one

    C. Loss of job

    D. Medical bills

8. Which of the following is a helpful accommodation for a patient who has partial vision loss?

    A. Rubber coverings on floors

    B. Speaking louder

    C. Directing information through a family member

    D. Large print materials

9. Which of the following defense mechanisms is a patient engaging in if they state, "The lab must have mixed up the samples. I don't have diabetes"?

    A. Projection

    B. Identification

    C. Denial

    D. Regression

10. A patient is told their kidney disease has progressed to the point of dialysis. Which of the following stages of grief is the patient experiencing if they are beginning to explore dietary changes?

    A. Denial

    B. Anger

    C. Bargaining

    D. Depression

11. Which of the following mental health conditions tends to present as hyperactivity in young males?

    A. Anxiety

    B. Depression

    C. Posttraumatic stress disorder (PTSD)

    D. ADHD

12. In which of the following stages of development is the goal to achieve a balance between concern for the next generation and being self-absorbed?

    A. Generativity vs. stagnation

    B. Identity vs. role confusion

    C. Trust vs. mistrust

    D. Initiative vs. guilt

IN PRACTICE: QUIZZES

Quiz 2: Medical Terminology, Anatomy, and Physiology

13. Which of the following body cavities travels down the midline of the back?

    A. Thoracic cavity

    B. Spinal cavity

    C. Abdominal cavity

    D. Pelvic cavity

14. Which of the following is a bone of the lower extremities?

    A. Scapula

    B. Carpals

    C. Sacrum

    D. Metatarsals

15. Which of the following describes the body's systems and biological processes to maintain stability?

    A. Digestion

    B. Respiration

    C. Homeostasis

    D. Filtration

16. Which of the following is an autoimmune disorder leading to changes in the connective tissues of the body, especially the joints?

    A. Rheumatoid arthritis

    B. Gout

    C. Muscular dystrophy

    D. Myalgia

17. Which of the following is a symptom of shingles?

    A. Blistering rash

    B. Facial droop

    C. Decreased urine output

    D. Distorted vision

18. Which of the following can be diagnosed during a colonoscopy?

    A. Diverticulosis

    B. GERD

    C. Celiac disease

    D. Urinary tract infection (UTI)

19. For which of the following is a history of inflammatory bowel disease a risk factor?

    A. COPD

    B. Osteoporosis

    C. Chronic kidney disease

    D. Colorectal cancer

20. Which of the following describes an illness constantly present in a community?

    A. Outbreak

    B. Endemic

    C. Epidemic

    D. Pandemic

QUIZ 3: PATIENT INTAKE AND VITALS

1. A patient enters the office and lets a medical assistant know the handrail outside the office door is loose. Which of the following actions should the assistant take?

   A. Thank the patient and let the supervisor know immediately so it can be fixed.

   B. Thank the patient for the information and let the supervisor know when the assistant has time.

   C. Thank the patient for the information and write a note to let maintenance know at the end of the day so they can fix it.

   D. Thank the patient for the information and make no changes, since the patient may or may not be correct about the state of the handrail.

2. A patient who had a stroke has left-sided weakness and uses a cane to ambulate. Which of the following actions should the medical assistant take to ensure the patient's safety?

   A. Stay with the patient until the provider comes into the examination room.

   B. Set the patient's cane against the examination table so it does not obstruct the patient's path.

   C. Assist the patient onto the examination table.

   D. Wait until the provider is ready to call the patient into the examination room.

3. A patient states they have smoked a pack of cigarettes every day for the past 20 years. In which section of the patient's medical record should the medical assistant document this information?

   A. Family history

   B. Social history

   C. Past medical history

   D. Occupational history

4. A medical assistant enters a patient's examination room to administer a pneumococcal vaccination. Which of the following identifiers should the assistant use to verify the patient?

   A. Name and address

   B. Name and Social Security number

   C. Name and mother's maiden name

   D. Name and date of birth

5. Which of the following is found in the demographic section of a patient's medical record and needs verification at the beginning of each visit?

   A. Medications

   B. Address

   C. Medical record number

   D. Diagnosis codes

6. A patient states, "It burns when I urinate," when asked the reason for their visit. In which of the following sections of the patient's medical record should the medical assistant document this information?

   A. Review of systems

   B. Chief complaint

   C. Past medical history

   D. Social history

7. A 21-year-old patient arrives at the office and reports lower abdominal pain. During the patient interview process, the patient seems to have difficulty concentrating and appears to have a sense of panic. Which of the following should the medical assistant identify as a potential cause of their behavior?

   A. Depression

   B. Dementia

   C. Aggression

   D. Anxiety

IN PRACTICE: QUIZZES
Quiz 3: Patient Intake and Vitals

8. A patient states they work in construction and that their primary job is breaking up concrete with jack hammers. In which of the following sections of the patient's medical record should the medical assistant document this information?

   A. Medical history

   B. Chief complaint

   C. Occupational history

   D. Social history

9. A patient's blood pressure is 136/84 mm Hg. The medical assistant should identify that this blood pressure reading falls into which of the following categories?

   A. Normal

   B. Prehypertension

   C. Hypertension

   D. Hypertensive crisis

10. A stethoscope is typically placed over which of the following arteries when blood pressure is auscultated?

    A. Femoral

    B. Radial

    C. Brachial

    D. Carotid

11. A 64-year-old patient arrives at the office and reports frequent dizzy spells. After completing routine vital signs, which of the following actions should the medical assistant take next?

    A. Perform a pulse oximetry.

    B. Recheck body temperature.

    C. Perform orthostatic vital signs.

    D. Assess pain level.

12. A 7-year-old patient reports feeling "hot and sweaty." After taking the patient's oral temperature, a medical assistant documents a temperature that falls within the expected range for their age. Which of the following numbers should the assistant expect to see?

    A. 36° C (96.8° F)

    B. 37.6° C (99.7° F)

    C. 38.9° C (102° F)

    D. 37° C (98.6° F)

13. A 3-year-old child is being seen for ear pain. Which of the following should be used to obtain the child's temperature?

    A. Axillary

    B. Oral

    C. Tympanic

    D. Temporal artery

14. A medical assistant should identify that a patient who has a body mass index (BMI) greater than 30 falls into which of the following categories?

    A. Underweight

    B. Normal

    C. Overweight

    D. Obese

15. Which of the following methods should a medical assistant use to help patients feel comfortable about having their weight measured in the office?

    A. Reassure them that their weight is at a healthy level.

    B. Allow them to weigh themselves at home and bring the results into the office.

    C. Let them keep their shoes and outerwear on during the weighing process.

    D. Place the scale in a private area within the office.

IN PRACTICE: QUIZZES
Quiz 3: Patient Intake and Vitals

16. A medical assistant is obtaining a patient's vital signs. After measuring the heart rate, the MA documents 50/min. Which of the following terms best describes this?

    A. Hypotension

    B. Bradycardia

    C. Tachypnea

    D. Tachycardia

17. Which of the following vital signs for a 67-year-old patient is outside the expected reference range?

    A. Temperature 36.5° C (97.8° F), heart rate 106/min, respiratory rate 20/min, BP 116/74 mm Hg

    B. Temperature 37° C (98.6° F), heart rate 98/min, respiratory rate 14/min, BP 118/78 mm Hg

    C. Temperature 36.7° C (98.2° F), heart rate 98/min, respiratory rate 20/min, BP 114/76 mm Hg

    D. Temperature 37.0° C (98.6° F), heart rate 88/min, respiratory rate 18/min, BP 108/78 mm Hg

18. A 35-year-old established patient is in the office for an annual checkup. They report feeling great, and they appear to be in good physical condition. According to office policy, a medical assistant should check their blood pressure using the aneroid sphygmomanometer and temperature using an axillary thermometer. Their vital signs are BP 118/88 mm Hg, respiratory rate 16/min, temperature 39.1° C (102.4° F), heart rate 62/min. Given these vitals, which of the following steps should the assistant take next?

    A. Recheck the blood pressure using an electronic sphygmomanometer.

    B. Notify the provider of the patient's elevated temperature.

    C. Measure their temperature again with a different type of thermometer.

    D. Ask the patient if they have had anything hot or cold to drink within the last hour.

19. Which of the following manifestations should a medical assistant expect to see in a patient who has COPD?

    A. Orthopnea

    B. Weight gain

    C. Hypotension

    D. Bradycardia

20. Which of the following methods should a medical assistant use to obtain a weight measurement from a patient who uses a walker and has balance concerns?

    A. Use a scale with built-in handrails.

    B. Ask the patient to report their approximate weight.

    C. Place the patient's walker over the scale.

    D. Help the patient onto the scale and assure them they only need to stand for a few seconds.

QUIZ 4: GENERAL PATIENT CARE: PART 1

1. Which of the following supplies or equipment should be in each examination room?

    A. Sigmoidoscope

    B. EKG machine

    C. Biohazard waste container

    D. Examination table with stirrups

2. You work in a gastroenterology practice and need to prepare a patient for a colonoscopy. Which of the following positions should the patient be in?

    A. Prone

    B. Left lateral

    C. Semi-Fowler's

    D. Trendelenburg

3. In which of the following specialties would a medical assistant most likely perform a spirometry test in?

    A. Pulmonology

    B. Cardiology

    C. Gynecology

    D. Endocrinology

4. Which of the following is true of patient medication allergies?

    A. Medication allergies should be asked about and updated during each patient visit.

    B. Signs and symptoms of allergic reactions will occur within 2 min of exposure to the allergen.

    C. A patient without an allergic reaction to a medication will not have a reaction to it in the future.

    D. Most allergic reactions will result in anaphylaxis.

5. A medical assistant is preparing a prescription for a medical order. The patient is prescribed 20 mg of a medication once a day by mouth for 30 days. The dosage on hand is 10 mg tablets. Which of the following shows how many tablets the patient should take per day and how many the assistant should order?

    A. 2 tablets per day, 60 tablets

    B. 1 tablet per day, 60 tablets

    C. 2 tablets per day, 30 tablets

    D. 1 tablet per day, 30 tablets

6. A medical assistant has just opened a new multidose vial of insulin to administer to a patient. The manufacturer's expiration date is in 2 months and it is currently July 1st. Which of the following expiration dates should the assistant write on the vial?

    A. September 1

    B. July 29

    C. July 15

    D. January 1

7. When performing an eye instillation, which of the following instructions should the medical assistant give to the patient?

    A. The patient should look towards the ceiling with the affected eye open.

    B. The patient should look towards the ceiling with both eyes open.

    C. The patient should look towards the floor with both eyes open.

    D. The patient should look towards the floor with the affected eye open.

8. Which of the following categories will the patient's insurance information belong in the patient's health record?

    A. Correspondence data

    B. Clinical information

    C. Demographic data

    D. Social information

IN PRACTICE: QUIZZES
Quiz 4: General Patient Care: Part 1

9. A computerized provider order entry (CPOE) system allows more efficient medical entry and prescription-ordering electronically. Once a health care provider logs into the electronic health record (EHR), which of the following should be the provider's next step?

   A. Enter the prescription into the EHR.
   B. Send the order to the pharmacy.
   C. Select the patient from a patient list.
   D. Validate an order against the patient's medical record.

10. A patient is requesting a telehealth appointment with a provider. After a brief discussion with the patient, the medical assistant informs them that they are not eligible for a telehealth appointment. Which of the following could make the patient ineligible?

    A. The patient fell on vacation and suspects their leg is broken.
    B. The patient has a suspicious mole that needs to be inspected.
    C. The patient asks for a new prescription.
    D. The patient has depression and is seeking counseling.

11. When entering a patient's new prescription in the medical record, the medical assistant notices a message alerting them to a dosage error. Which of the following software options automatically checks for medication errors and interactions?

    A. Clinical decision support system (CDSS)
    B. Computerized provider order entry (CPOE) system
    C. Electronic health record (EHR) system
    D. Electronic medication administration record (eMAR)

12. A medical assistant is scheduling a patient's follow-up appointment and the patient is requesting a telehealth visit. Which of the following guidance should the assistant offer the patient?

    A. Tell the patient they must get their vital signs taken prior to the visit.
    B. Provide the patient a list of software and technical requirements for the appointment.
    C. Let the patient know that the appointment can be in a public place as lowered voices are used.
    D. Inform the patient that a public-facing video communication application, such as social media platforms are acceptable.

13. A medical assistant is discussing a controlled substance prescription for a new patient. The patient asks if it can be sent electronically to a specific pharmacy close to their house. Which of the following answers should the assistant give the patient?

    A. No. New prescriptions cannot be filled electronically.
    B. No. Medications that are controlled substances cannot be sent electronically.
    C. Yes, but a paper prescription is preferred.
    D. Yes, as long as the pharmacy is using approved and certified software.

14. A medical assistant is assisting a patient after a colonoscopy. Which of the following should the assistant inform the patient of in case the patient experiences pain or bleeding?

    A. Postprocedure discomfort and mild pain is common.
    B. The patient should notify the health care provider.
    C. Rest and inform the health care provider if it continues for more than 10 days.
    D. Do not notify the health care provider and go immediately to the emergency room.

15. An adult patient needs assistance onto the examination table. However, the medical assistant needs to prepare the supplies for administering an injection to the patient, of which the medication is in another room. Which of the following actions should the assistant take?

    A. Assist the patient down from the exam table until the medical assistant is able to assemble all the supplies.

    B. Schedule the injection for the patient's next appointment.

    C. Ask the patient's companion or another medical assistant to sit with the patient until the original assistant returns.

    D. Leave the patient in the room and quickly assemble the supplies needed.

16. A medical assistant observes a patient having an anaphylactic reaction. Which of the following steps should the assistant immediately take?

    A. Administer loratadine.

    B. Attach automated external defibrillator (AED) pads.

    C. Begin CPR.

    D. Notify the provider.

17. A medical assistant is administering a subcutaneous insulin injection to a patient. Which of the following is the angle of injection and type of tissue that the assistant should be targeting?

    A. 15°, dermis

    B. 45°, dermis

    C. 90°, muscle

    D. 45°, adipose

18. A patient needs an administration of an influenza vaccine during their medical visit. What needle size, angle, and site should the medical assistant select for an intramuscular (IM) injection?

    A. 25-gauge, 15° angle, anterior forearm

    B. 27-gauge, 45° angle, abdominal region

    C. 20-gauge, 90° angle, deltoid muscle

    D. 18-gauge, 5° angle, abdominal region

19. Which of the following is true of electronic prescribing of prescriptions?

    A. An electronic prescription may only be transmitted electronically.

    B. Since the patient is directly delivering the prescription, written prescriptions are faster than electronic prescriptions.

    C. Electronic prescriptions can reduce the risk of the prescription being tampered with.

    D. Electronic prescriptions may result in more calls to the health care provider.

20. When storing or organizing vials of vaccines, which of the following actions should the medical assistant take?

    A. If additional room is required, vaccines may be temporarily stored in the same refrigerator as the staff's items.

    B. Vaccines should be stored in the freezer between -50° C and -15° C (-58° F and 5° F).

    C. Use the vial with the latest expiration date to ensure the highest quality of a vaccine is being administered.

    D. Check the expiration date of all vials being stored or organized.

QUIZ 5: GENERAL PATIENT CARE: PART 2

1. Which of the following areas are considered sterile?

    A. The area below the Mayo stand

    B. The drape on the Mayo stand that is 12 inches or more away from the body

    C. The 1-inch edge of the inside of a sterile instrument packet

    D. The outermost wrapper of a sterile instrument packet

2. Which of the following is the proper technique for removing surgical staples?

    A. Use the scissors and forceps included in the kit.

    B. Begin with the first staple and remove each in a row until all have been removed.

    C. Place the lower tip of the sterile staple remover under the staple and squeeze the handle together until they are completely closed.

    D. Once the remover is under the staple, squeeze the handles and, at the same time, lift slowly but with moderate pressure.

3. Which of the following is the priority action for a major burn, such as a fourth-degree burn?

    A. Call 911.

    B. Apply a lotion, such as aloe vera.

    C. Place the burn under cool running water.

    D. Apply a bandage.

4. A medical assistant observes a patient in the waiting room placing their hands around their throat and collapsing. Which of the following is most likely the cause?

    A. Hypoglycemia

    B. Seizure

    C. Obstructed airway

    D. Syncope

5. Which of the following phases of wound healing occurs at approximately day 10?

    A. Proliferative

    B. Inflammatory

    C. Maturation

    D. Dehiscence

6. Which of the following procedures provide a better view of cervical cells to send to pathology?

    A. Endoscopy

    B. Colposcopy

    C. Cryosurgery

    D. Incision and drainage

7. Which of the following kinds of wound complication causes only the edges of the wound to separate?

    A. Dehiscence

    B. Evisceration

    C. Hemorrhaging

    D. Infection

8. A provider asks a medical assistant to start filling out the prior authorizations form for a power wheelchair for a patient. Which of the following is the purpose of submitting a prior authorization?

    A. To request an item be categorized as durable medical equipment, prosthetics, orthotics, and supplies (DMEPOS)

    B. To request approval for an item to be included on the CMS's Master List

    C. To request approval from the insurance company for coverage of an item before a claim is submitted

    D. To request approval for a provider to be an approved prescriber of DMEPOS

IN PRACTICE: QUIZZES
Quiz 5: General Patient Care: Part 2

9. Which of the following conditions would be an indication for the use of an automated external defibrillator (AED)?

   A. Cardiac arrest

   B. Hypovolemic shock

   C. Seizure

   D. Syncope

10. Which of the following is the ratio of compressions to breaths when performing CPR on an adult?

    A. 30 chest compressions: 1 breath

    B. 30 chest compressions: 2 breaths

    C. 15 chest compressions: 1 breath

    D. 15 chest compressions: 2 breaths

11. Which of the following should the medical assistant identify when assigned to check the emergency kit or crash cart?

    A. The automated external defibrillator (AED) is checked after every use.

    B. The emergency kit is in the same, accessible area.

    C. Expired medications are in the front to be used first.

    D. Pediatric doses on all medications should be marked with permanent marker.

12. An incision and drainage (I&D) procedure would be indicated for which of the following conditions?

    A. A tender mass or pustule under the dermal tissue

    B. Cervical dysplasia

    C. Suspicious mole on the face

    D. Soft tissue tumor on the breast

13. In which of the following medical emergency situations does a patient exhibit pale and clammy skin, rapid pulse and respirations, and the patient appearing weak and becomes unresponsive with dilated pupils?

    A. Hypoglycemia

    B. Hypothermia

    C. Syncope

    D. Shock

14. Which of the following steps should the medical assistant take to ensure an instrument packet is sterile?

    A. Check to make sure only one instrument is in each packet.

    B. Check to make sure the instrument packet has autoclave tape around it with white markings on it.

    C. Check to make sure the inside of the wrapper is sterile by placing a piece of autoclave tape on it.

    D. Check for the autoclave indicator strip and expiration date.

15. A 14-year-old patient has a laceration on their face from playing field hockey. Which of the following should be the recommended type of suture?

    A. Absorbable, size 4-0

    B. Absorbable, size 6-0

    C. Nonabsorbable, size 4-0

    D. Nonabsorbable, size 6-0

16. A medical assistant is examining a patient's wound, which appears red and swollen with yellowish drainage. Which of the following wound complications would be suspected?

    A. Dehiscence

    B. Evisceration

    C. Hemorrhaging

    D. Infection

IN PRACTICE: QUIZZES
Quiz 5: General Patient Care: Part 2

17. Prior to notifying the provider, which of the following steps should you take for a patient who has a deep cut on their arm?

    A. Apply a tourniquet.

    B. Determine if the bleeding is arterial or venous, which determines what action must be taken.

    C. Provide the patient with sterile gauze and instruct the patient to apply pressure and elevate the arm.

    D. Use either a suture or surgical staples to close the wound and prevent further bleeding.

18. Which of the following is an appropriate treatment for a patient who has a sprained ankle?

    A. Place a cool, wet cloth on the ankle to ease the pain.

    B. Apply ice, elevate, and wear a compression bandage on their ankle.

    C. Refer them to an orthopedic surgeon to have their ankle repositioned.

    D. Apply a sterile bandage around the ankle to prevent swelling.

19. A patient collapses in front of a medical assistant and is unresponsive. A co-worker is calling 911 and alerting the provider. Which of the following steps is the medical assistant responsible for taking first?

    A. Run with the co-worker to notify the provider.

    B. Begin chest compressions.

    C. Apply automated external defibrillator (AED) pads.

    D. Check the patient's pulse and breathing.

20. A provider requests additional forceps during a surgical procedure. Which of the following steps should the medical assistant take?

    A. Grab another instrument packet containing forceps. Open the packet and hand the forceps to the provider.

    B. Grab another instrument packet containing forceps and place the packet on the Mayo stand.

    C. Without touching the drape on the Mayo stand, open the sterile package and drop the forceps into the sterile field.

    D. Without touching the outer wrapper, open the sterile package and hand the provider the forceps to ensure they do not touch the sterile field.

QUIZ 6: INFECTION CONTROL AND SAFETY

1. Which of the following is a virus?

    A. *Escherichia coli* (E. coli)

    B. Histoplasmosis

    C. Pinworms

    D. Varicella

2. Which of the following can be further classified as protozoa, helminths, and ectoparasite?

    A. Parasites

    B. Bacteria

    C. Viruses

    D. Fungi

3. Which of the following is a direct mode of transmission?

    A. Contact with an infected person

    B. Contact with a contaminated examination table

    C. Contact with a tick

    D. Contact with a pen

4. A health care worker is not feeling well and has a fever. In which of the following scenarios can the health care worker resume caring for patients?

    A. After being fever-free for 48 hr with the help of fever-reducing medications

    B. After being fever-free for 24 hr with the help of fever-reducing medications

    C. After being fever-free for 48 hr without the help of fever-reducing medications

    D. After being fever-free for 24 hr without the help of fever-reducing medications

5. According to the CDC, which of the following is the first step a medical assistant should take after exposure to blood?

    A. Report it to their supervisor.

    B. Receive a medical evaluation.

    C. Receive health counseling.

    D. Wash the area with soap and water.

6. A medical assistant is performing aseptic handwashing. How long should the assistant rub their hands vigorously with soap?

    A. 5 to 10 seconds

    B. 10 to 15 seconds

    C. 15 to 20 seconds

    D. 2 to 3 min

7. How often are health care facilities required to train their staff on guidelines for exposure to bloodborne pathogens?

    A. Biannually

    B. Annually

    C. Every 2 years

    D. The health care facility can determine when they want to train their staff

8. What is the minimum temperature that must be reached to ensure the sterility of autoclaved items?

    A. 93.3° C (200° F)

    B. 107.2° C (225° F)

    C. 135° C (275° F)

    D. 121.1° C (250° F)

IN PRACTICE: QUIZZES
Quiz 6: Infection Control and Safety

9. According to CDC guidelines, when can sterilized packages be used?

    A. If the package is intact and has no tears but does show a watermark

    B. If the package has a small tear patched with tape

    C. If the package was stored near a sink on an open shelf

    D. If the package has been stored in a cool, dry area and does not show watermarks

10. When using chemical sterilization, how long do instruments need to be submerged to be considered sterilized?

    A. 6 hr

    B. 10 hr

    C. 8 hr

    D. 24 hr

11. How long should unwrapped items be sterilized in an autoclave?

    A. 10 min

    B. 15 min

    C. 20 min

    D. 40 min

12. Which of the following is the goal of surgical asepsis?

    A. To reduce the number of micro-organisms

    B. To eliminate pathogenic micro-organisms

    C. To try to reduce the risk of contamination

    D. To prohibit the growth of micro-organisms

13. In which of the following scenarios should a medical assistant use medical aseptic techniques?

    A. Washing hands prior to and after each patient encounter

    B. Assisting in the removal of a cyst

    C. Assisting with placing sutures on a cut leg

    D. Cleaning a deep wound on the forearm

14. Which of the following items should a medical assistant dispose of in a biohazard waste bag?

    A. Gauze that fell on the ground

    B. A used needle

    C. Gauze contaminated with blood

    D. A used mask

15. Gloves should be worn during which of the following medical office tasks?

    A. Cleaning the front office table

    B. Performing a blood pressure reading for a patient

    C. Handling anything contaminated with blood

    D. Handling unused suture scissors

16. How often should the exposure control plan be updated if there are no changes?

    A. Monthly

    B. Quarterly

    C. Annually

    D. Every 5 years

17. In a health care setting, which of the following is the minimum amount of alcohol content that can be used in an alcohol-based sanitizer?

    A. 40%

    B. 55%

    C. 60%

    D. 90%

18. OSHA regulations require employers to make which of the following vaccines available at no cost to health care workers?

    A. Hepatitis A

    B. Hepatitis B

    C. Varicella

    D. Measles, mumps, and rubella (MMR)

19. Which of the following is a common symptom of contracting an infectious disease?

    A. Numbness and tingling

    B. Headache

    C. Blurry vision

    D. Difficulty breathing

20. Which of the following precautions should a medical assistant consider when a person is coughing or sneezing?

    A. Droplet precautions

    B. Airborne precautions

    C. Contact precautions

    D. Transmission-based precautions

QUIZ 7: POINT-OF-CARE TESTING AND LABORATORY PROCEDURES

1. Which of the following can cause a false positive when obtaining a specimen for fecal occult blood testing?

    A. Collecting the sample from the first bowel movement of the day

    B. Consuming vitamin C and iron supplements

    C. Consuming a high-fiber diet

    D. Discontinuing prescription medications

2. Which of the following is considered proper technique to avoid contamination during collection of a urine sample?

    A. Do not urinate directly into the urine container.

    B. Avoid touching the inside of the container or the lid.

    C. Add a preservative to the midstream container.

    D. Ask the patient to wear gloves during collection into the container.

3. Which of the following should be included when labeling a patient's specimen?

    A. Insurance company

    B. Diagnosis

    C. Address

    D. Collector's initials

4. Which specimen collection performs tests for substances that are sporadically released into the urine?

    A. 24-hour urine

    B. Clean catch

    C. Random

    D. First void

IN PRACTICE: QUIZZES
Quiz 7: Point-of-Care Testing and Laboratory Procedures

5. Which of the following is a normal range for a hemoglobin A1C?

   A. Less than 12.0%

   B. Less than 5.7%

   C. Less than 7.0%

   D. Less than 8.0%

6. Which of the following is the normal range for a total cholesterol?

   A. 40 to 150 mg/dL

   B. 70 to 100 mg/dL

   C. 130 to 200 mg/dL

   D. 150 to 220 mg/dL

7. Which of the following identifiers should be used to verify the patient before obtaining a specimen for laboratory collection?

   A. Name and date of birth

   B. Address and patient identification number

   C. Diagnosis and insurance information

   D. Patient's name and insurance information

8. Which of the following is required to be included on a urine specimen label prior to sending it to the laboratory?

   A. Insurance carrier

   B. Medication patient is taking

   C. Time the urine was collected

   D. Diagnosis of the patient

9. Which of the following is required when obtaining and transporting a drug screening?

   A. Chain of command

   B. Chain of custody

   C. Medical insurance card

   D. Authorization forms from an employer

10. In which of the following phases of quality assurance are instruments maintained and calibrated?

    A. Preanalytical phase

    B. Analytical phase

    C. Midanalytical phase

    D. Postanalytical phase

11. Ishihara color plates are used to screen for what sensory disorder?

    A. Distance vision

    B. Near vision

    C. Vision acuity

    D. Color deficiency

12. Which of the following describes how an abnormal tympanogram appears on a graph when completed?

    A. A continuous up and down line

    B. A declining line

    C. A peak line

    D. A flat line

13. When performing a scratch test for allergen testing, which of the following is the amount of time that must pass before checking for a wheal formation?

    A. 5 min

    B. 10 min

    C. 15 min

    D. 25 min

14. How many days prior to skin testing should the patient discontinue antihistamines?

    A. 30 days

    B. 15 days

    C. 3 days

    D. 7 days

IN PRACTICE: QUIZZES
Quiz 7: Point-of-Care Testing and Laboratory Procedures

15. Which of the following is the number of successful and measured breathing maneuvers that a patient must complete during spirometry testing?

    A. Three
    B. Two
    C. Four
    D. One

16. Which of the following is the best instruction to give a patient on how to perform a peak flow test?

    A. "Take the deepest breath possible. Seal your lips around the mouthpiece. Blow out as hard and as fast as you can."
    B. "Take the deepest breath possible. Seal your lips around the mouthpiece. Inhale as much air as you can."
    C. "Blow all your air out of your lungs as much as possible. Seal your lips around the mouthpiece. Inhale as hard and as fast as you can."
    D. "Take the deepest breath possible. Seal your lips around the mouthpiece. Blow out in short, small puffs."

17. Which of the following could cause a specimen to be rejected from the lab?

    A. A fasting lab was drawn on a patient who ate breakfast.
    B. A handwritten lab requisition was sent with the specimen.
    C. The urine specimen was left at room temperature in a urine collection cup for 4 hr.
    D. The name on the specimen label does not match the lab requisition.

18. Which of the following is an error that would affect the test results in the preanalytical phase (before the specimen is sent to the lab) of quality assurance?

    A. Equipment malfunction
    B. Excessive turnaround time
    C. Failure to report
    D. Order entry error

19. An adult who has normal hearing should be able to hear tones at which of the following decibels?

    A. 15 decibels
    B. 20 decibels
    C. 25 decibels
    D. 10 decibels

20. Which of the following is the amount of time it takes to process a result for a urine pregnancy test?

    A. 3 min
    B. 1 min
    C. Immediately
    D. 5 min

QUIZ 8: PHLEBOTOMY

1. Which of the following questions should a medical assistant ask a patient prior to obtaining a blood specimen for a lipid panel?

   A. "Do you smoke cigarettes?"

   B. "When was the last time you had anything to eat or drink?"

   C. "Do you have any medical allergies?"

   D. "Have you taken acetaminophen within the last 12 hours?"

2. Which of the following steps should a medical assistant take if they are unsure which tube to use when obtaining a blood specimen?

   A. Draw one tube of each color to ensure one of them is the appropriate tube.

   B. Ask another medical assistant.

   C. Draw one extra red-top tube.

   D. Consult the laboratory reference manual.

3. How many times should an EDTA tube be inverted?

   A. 2 to 4 times

   B. 4 to 6 times

   C. 6 to 8 times

   D. 8 to 10 times

4. In which of the following places should a medical assistant first attempt to locate a vein?

   A. Antecubital space

   B. Foot

   C. Wrist

   D. Back of the hand

5. Which of the following is the preferred alcohol concentration for disinfecting the skin prior to a phlebotomy test?

   A. 70%

   B. 40%

   C. 90%

   D. 100%

6. Which of the following color tubes should be drawn first?

   A. Green

   B. Red

   C. Gray and red marbled

   D. Lavender

7. Which of the following is the appropriate needle size when using a butterfly system?

   A. 20-gauge, ⅝-inch

   B. 20-gauge, ½-inch

   C. 22-gauge, ¼-inch

   D. 22-gauge, ½-inch

8. Which of the following is a postanalytical consideration in phlebotomy?

   A. Improper data entry

   B. Insufficient quantity for testing

   C. Mislabeling of specimen tubes

   D. Error in patient identification

9. Which of the following is the minimum amount of time a medical assistant should instruct a patient to leave their bandage in place following a phlebotomy or capillary puncture?

   A. 5 min

   B. 15 min

   C. 10 min

   D. 20 min

IN PRACTICE: QUIZZES
Quiz 8: Phlebotomy

10. Which of the following is a characteristic of collecting timed specimens?
    A. They require specific preparation of the skin.
    B. They monitor therapeutic medication levels.
    C. They must be collected in the morning.
    D. They must be obtained from the basilic vein.

11. How long should serum specimens be allowed to clot prior to centrifugation?
    A. 30 min
    B. 2 hr
    C. 5 min
    D. 15 min

12. Which of the following information should be included on a laboratory requisition form?
    A. Provider's tax identification number
    B. Patient's height
    C. Patient's weight
    D. Diagnosis code

13. How should critical laboratory values be handled when they are received at the office?
    A. Call the patient and ask them to schedule an appointment.
    B. Enter the values in the patient's chart.
    C. Report the critical values to the provider right away and document that the provider was notified.
    D. Ask the nurse to check the report.

14. How should light-sensitive samples be prepared for transport?
    A. They should be wrapped in foil.
    B. They should be placed in gauze.
    C. They should be positioned in an ice bath.
    D. They should be rolled in a biohazard bag.

15. A clinic has just received laboratory results for a patient indicating an error with the sample. Which of the following actions should the medical assistant take first?
    A. Schedule a follow-up appointment with the patient.
    B. Input the results in the patient's medical record.
    C. Forward the results and alert the ordering provider.
    D. Call the patient to inform them a mistake was made in the laboratory.

16. Which of the following additives is found in light blue blood tubes?
    A. Serum separator gel
    B. Clot activator
    C. Sodium citrate
    D. Lithium heparin

17. Which of the following often requires chain of custody documentation?
    A. Blood cultures
    B. Drug screenings
    C. Chemistry studies
    D. Plasma determinations

18. A medical assistant is preparing to centrifuge a blood sample when they notice the centrifuge is 3 months overdue for calibration. Which of the following actions should the assistant take?

    A. Attempt to calibrate the device themselves.

    B. Run the sample.

    C. Notify the laboratory supervisor and use another device.

    D. Remove the service label and use the centrifuge.

19. A medical assistant is performing a phlebotomy draw on a patient who reports feeling lightheaded and restless. Which of the following actions should the assistant take?

    A. Ask the patient to take some deep breaths.

    B. Finish the procedure as quickly as possible.

    C. Stop the procedure and alert the provider.

    D. Have the patient squeeze the assistant's hand for comfort.

20. While preparing the phlebotomy equipment for a blood draw, the medical assistant notices the patient appears very anxious. Which of the following questions should the assistant ask the patient to ensure the patient's safety?

    A. "Would you like some water?"

    B. "Can you sit still for the procedure?"

    C. "Why are you so anxious?"

    D. "Have you ever fainted during a phlebotomy test?"

QUIZ 9: EKG AND CARDIOVASCULAR TESTING

1. Which of the following positions is best for performing an EKG?

    A. Prone

    B. Supine

    C. Fowler's

    D. Left lateral

2. Which of the following actions should be taken for a patient experiencing a somatic tremor artifact on their electrocardiogram due to uncontrolled muscle movements?

    A. Tie the patient's arms to the exam table while conducting the test.

    B. Ask for assistance to hold the patient's arms still while conducting the procedure.

    C. Clean the skin and securely tape down the electrodes on the extremities.

    D. Have the patient lay their hands palms down under their buttocks to reduce the muscle movements.

3. Which of the following places should the electrode for lead V2 be placed?

    A. The right leg

    B. The left arm

    C. The left side of the sternum, fourth intercostal space

    D. The left side of the chest, fifth intercostal space, midaxillary line

4. Which of the following places should the black limb lead be placed?

    A. The right leg

    B. The right arm

    C. The left leg

    D. The left arm

IN PRACTICE: QUIZZES
Quiz 9: EKG and Cardiovascular Testing

5. Which of the following actions can cause a wandering baseline artifact?

    A. A disconnected or broken lead wire

    B. A patient with lotion or cream on their skin

    C. The patient shaking due to anxiety

    D. Poor grounding of the machine

6. Which of the following artifacts is a result of patient movement with breathing?

    A. 60-cycle interference

    B. Interrupted baseline

    C. Wandering baseline

    D. Somatic tremor

7. A medical assistant notices frequent, regular spikes on the EKG tracing. Which of the following actions should the assistant take?

    A. Reattach the faulty electrode.

    B. Have the patient hold their breath for 10 seconds.

    C. Turn off nearby electrical equipment.

    D. Offer the patient a warm blanket.

8. Which of the following demonstrates how somatic tremors can differentiate from 60-cycle interference?

    A. Somatic tremors produce an interrupted baseline.

    B. Somatic tremors produce irregular spikes.

    C. 60-cycle interference produces a wandering baseline.

    D. 60-cycle interference produces an irregular QRS rhythm.

9. Which of the following statements made by a medical assistant demonstrates an understanding of patient privacy?

    A. "Please remove all clothing from the waist up and you can get dressed after the EKG is done."

    B. "I'll cover your abdomen with a blanket as soon as I'm done placing the EKG electrodes."

    C. "I can turn the heat up if you're cold as you'll need to remain unclothed for the duration of the EKG test."

    D. "You can leave all your clothes on and I'll try to work around them to obtain the EKG."

10. Which of the following is the correct number of electrodes needed to record a 12-lead EKG?

    A. 12

    B. 10

    C. 5

    D. 6

11. Which of the following serves as a conductor of impulses during an EKG?

    A. Electrocardiograph

    B. Lead wires

    C. Electrolyte gel

    D. EKG paper

12. While preparing to record an EKG, you notice there's a break in the baseline and the screen displays flat lines across all leads. Which of the following do you suspect?

    A. The patient is in asystole.

    B. An electrical interference has occurred.

    C. There is a disconnected lead wire.

    D. The patient is in ventricular fibrillation.

IN PRACTICE: QUIZZES
Quiz 9: EKG and Cardiovascular Testing

13. Which of the following is the duration of a standard calibration box?

    A. 4 seconds

    B. 2 seconds

    C. 0.04 seconds

    D. 0.2 seconds

14. Which of the following is the height of a standard calibration box?

    A. 20 mm

    B. 0.5 mm

    C. 15 mm

    D. 10 mm

15. A medical assistant is preparing to record an EKG on a patient who has a history of pulmonary disease. The patient reports shortness of breath after lying on the exam table. Which of the following actions should the medical assistant take?

    A. Elevate the head of the bed to 45° (semi-Fowler's position).

    B. Tell the patient to hold their breath.

    C. Administer oxygen to the patient.

    D. Record the EKG with the patient standing.

16. While assisting with a cardiac stress test, the medical assistant observes the patient's blood pressure reading is 204/108. Which of the following actions should the assistant take?

    A. Stop the procedure and notify the provider immediately.

    B. Finish performing the stress test and notify the provider.

    C. Decrease the treadmill speed and check the electrodes.

    D. Administer aspirin to the patient and stop the test.

17. Which of the following differentiates sinus tachycardia from ventricular tachycardia?

    A. Sinus tachycardia has narrow QRS complexes.

    B. Ventricular tachycardia has narrow QRS complexes.

    C. Sinus tachycardia doesn't have P waves.

    D. Ventricular tachycardia has P waves.

18. Which of the following dysrhythmias results in continuous fibrillatory waves between the QRS complexes?

    A. Atrial fibrillation

    B. Ventricular fibrillation

    C. Sinus rhythm

    D. Sinus arrest

19. Which of the following waves represents atrial depolarization?

    A. U wave

    B. Q wave

    C. T wave

    D. P wave

20. Which of the following places should the electrode for lead V4 be placed?

    A. The left leg

    B. Right arm

    C. The left side of the sternum, fifth intercostal space, midclavicular line

    D. The left side of the chest, fifth intercostal space, midaxillary line

QUIZ 10: PATIENT CARE COORDINATION AND EDUCATION

1. Which of the following screenings would be recommended for a 65-year-old male who has a history of smoking?

   A. Colonoscopy

   B. Prediabetic testing

   C. Hepatitis C

   D. Abdominal aortic aneurysm

2. Which of the following is the purpose of evaluating the patient after an educational session?

   A. To determine if the material was correct

   B. To determine if the patient has a learning deficit

   C. To determine if the patient understood the information or skill

   D. To demonstrate correct evaluation techniques to the provider

3. Which of the following is the advised timeframe for patients aged 40 years and older to have mammogram screenings?

   A. Every 3 years

   B. Biannually

   C. Annually

   D. Every 5 years

4. Which of the following is the best resource to refer to a caretaker of an adult patient who can no longer care for themselves?

   A. Local hospitals

   B. Assisted living facilities

   C. Adult day programs

   D. Long-term care facilities

5. Which of the following is the best way to assist a patient with finding resources for their specific needs?

   A. Schedule a visit with a social worker.

   B. Refer the patient to internet searches.

   C. Provide the patient with a screening questionnaire to return to the office.

   D. Maintain a list of local community resources.

6. Which of the following is the best method to instruct a patient on remembering to take their medication each day?

   A. Warn the patient they may not get better if they can't remember to take their medication.

   B. Ask the patient to write their medication schedule on their calendar.

   C. Send a daily text to remind the patient to take their medications.

   D. Utilize medication boxes that are arranged for the week.

7. Which of the following is the main goal of a patient-centered medical home (PCMH)?

   A. Increase the needs of health care services

   B. Positively contribute to the revenue cycle

   C. Improve patient outcomes and reduce costs

   D. Decrease travel and time for the patient

8. Which of the following is the main reason for patient deficiencies during a transition of care?

   A. Insufficient financial resources

   B. Lack of communication

   C. Lack of family support

   D. Insufficient staffing

IN PRACTICE: QUIZZES
Quiz 10: Patient Care Coordination and Education

9. Listening to a medical assistant explain ways to decrease dietary intake of sodium is considered which of the following learning styles?

    A. Kinesthetic learning

    B. Auditory learning

    C. Visual learning

    D. Tactile learning

10. Which of the following preventive measures can a medical assistant use to educate a patient regarding communicable diseases?

    A. Covering a cough

    B. Sneezing into the air

    C. Washing hands only if soiled

    D. Avoid touching hand sanitizer bottles

11. Which of the following is a social determinant that can prevent a patient from meeting their needs?

    A. Adequate transportation

    B. Smoking

    C. Sickle cell anemia

    D. Weather or climate change

12. Which of the following can be a barrier when providing patient education?

    A. Visual impairment

    B. Color deficiency

    C. College-level education

    D. Self-employment

13. Regarding prescription medications, which of the following steps must be completed prior to a patient leaving the medical office?

    A. Verifying insurance coverage

    B. Verifying the patient's pharmacy hours

    C. Inquire about the patient's employment status

    D. Provide medication education

14. Which of the following might be a result of ineffective communication between medical providers during transition of care?

    A. Decreased medical costs

    B. Rehospitalization

    C. Greater availability of medical resources

    D. Optimal health care services

15. The physician has spoken with the patient regarding the health benefits of quitting smoking. The patient agrees to seek help. Which of the following actions should the medical assistant take?

    A. Ask the provider for a written referral.

    B. Share with the patient that a previous patient had success with a smoking-cessation gum.

    C. Provide the patient with several names and numbers to contact for smoking cessation support.

    D. Ask the patient to contact their insurance provider for a referral for smoking cessation.

16. When reviewing a 48-year-old female's medical record prior to their annual wellness exam, the medical assistant sees they have not completed any preventive care screenings. Which of the following should be discussed with the patient during their appointment?

    A. Mammogram

    B. Prostate exam

    C. Chest x-ray

    D. Electrocardiogram

17. Which of the following forms of telehealth is a substitute for in-person visits?

    A. Store and forward telemedicine

    B. Live video

    C. Remote patient monitoring (RPM)

    D. Mobile health (mHealth)

18. Which of the following is a cultural factor that can affect a patient's adherence with treatment?

    A. Beliefs related to food and diet

    B. Beliefs related to education

    C. Beliefs related to traditions

    D. Beliefs related to values

19. Which of the following immunizations should be given regularly during a lifetime?

    A. Influenza vaccine

    B. Hepatitis B vaccine

    C. Hepatitis A vaccine

    D. Varicella vaccine

20. Which of the following timelines is suggested for individuals to screen for colorectal cancer?

    A. Starting at age 40 years old

    B. Starting at age 45 years old

    C. Starting at age 40 only with family history

    D. Starting at age 45 only with family history

QUIZ 11: ADMINISTRATIVE ASSISTING

1. Which of the following types of patient visits is more resource intensive?

    A. Sports physical

    B. Established patient

    C. Follow-up

    D. New patient

2. Which of the following has an impact on determining the duration of an appointment?

    A. Third-party payer requirements

    B. Provider preferences

    C. Patient availability

    D. Reimbursement methods

3. Which of the following questions should be asked during the screening process to determine the type of appointment needed?

    A. What is the reason for the visit?

    B. Who is your employer?

    C. What medications are you currently taking?

    D. What is your previous address?

4. Which of the following applications should be used to create an encounter form?

    A. Excel

    B. Word

    C. Inventory software

    D. Practice management software

IN PRACTICE: QUIZZES
Quiz 11: Administrative Assisting

5. A medical assistant is checking out a patient following their appointment. Which of the following actions should the medical assistant take?

    A. Request to see the patient's photo identification.

    B. Ask the patient what medications they are currently taking.

    C. Review the after-visit summary with the patient.

    D. Evaluate the patient's past, family, and social history.

6. Which of the following codes are determined by reviewing the reason for a patient's visit?

    A. Procedure codes (CPT)

    B. ICD-10-PCS

    C. HCPCS codes

    D. Diagnosis codes (ICD-10-CM)

7. Which of the following services can require case management and preauthorization from a third-party payer?

    A. Elective and costly medical services

    B. Preventive medical services

    C. Annual wellness exam

    D. Follow-up care for a burn

8. Using coding guidelines, which of the following should be supported with code selections when preparing a billing request?

    A. Predetermination findings

    B. Verification of insurance coverage

    C. Explanation of benefits

    D. Medical necessity

9. Which of the following describes the purpose of interoperability?

    A. Reimbursement methodologies

    B. Supports the importance of documentation

    C. Audits and reviews

    D. Credentialing

10. Which of the following is a function of performing charge reconciliations?

    A. Verifying patient eligibility

    B. Continuity of care

    C. Posting the amounts in the patient's account

    D. Obtaining preauthorization

11. Which of the following services does a clearinghouse provide?

    A. Billing patients for their financial responsibility

    B. Claims adjudication for the third-party payer

    C. Processing payroll for the health care organization

    D. Safety inspections and evaluating procedures

12. Which of the following actions should a medical assistant take for a claim that was denied for lack of medical necessity?

    A. Bill the patient.

    B. Resubmit the claim.

    C. Submit an appeal.

    D. Write off the amount.

13. A patient has a fee-for-service Medicare plan. Which of the following forms should be used for the patient when a service might not be considered medically necessary?

    A. Patient's Bill of Rights

    B. Notice of Privacy Practices

    C. Advance directives

    D. Advance Beneficiary Notice of Noncoverage

14. Which of the following is a benefit of a medical assistant calling to remind a patient of an upcoming visit?

    A. Increased reimbursement

    B. Decreased claim denials

    C. Decreased no-show rates

    D. Less patient financial responsibility

15. Which of the following is a benefit of using drop-down menus when entering patient information into the medical records?

    A. Less information needed

    B. Greater accuracy

    C. More specificity

    D. More consistency

16. Which of the following is a purpose of an equipment inspection log?

    A. To keep track of depreciation value

    B. To monitor who uses the equipment

    C. To document a timeline of scheduled maintenance

    D. To determine sales on equipment

17. Which of the following does the health care facility provide a patient with to log into their patient portal?

    A. A username and access code

    B. An email address

    C. A fee schedule

    D. A referral

18. Which of the following actions should a medical assistant take if a patient is having trouble logging into a telehealth visit?

    A. Ask the patient to contact tech support at their local computer store.

    B. Assist the patient with logging in and verify their settings are correct.

    C. Ask them to reschedule when a family member is there to assist.

    D. Request an interpreter to assist.

19. Which of the following reports is used to show health care service charge amounts that are outstanding to the organization?

    A. A/R aging report

    B. A/P aging report

    C. Remittance advice

    D. Bank deposit statement

20. In which of the following categories does a medical assistant record a cash payment of $20 that a patient pays towards their appointment at the time of services?

    A. Copayment

    B. Coinsurance

    C. Deductible

    D. Write-off

QUIZ 12: COMMUNICATION AND CUSTOMER SERVICE

1. A medical assistant is speaking with a patient who is being treated for kidney disease. One of the possible treatments is a kidney transplant, and the patient is refusing that option. Which of the following actions should the assistant take?

    A. Remind the patient they could die without a kidney transplant.

    B. Respect the patient's wishes and answer any questions or concerns.

    C. Inform the patient that they will help them get approval from the insurance company, so the procedure is covered.

    D. Ask the patient to have their family members contact the health care organization.

2. A medical assistant is speaking with an older adult patient regarding how to increase their appetite. Which of the following considerations should the assistant make when speaking with the patient?

    A. Speak in a loud voice.

    B. Provide the patient with large print documents.

    C. Speak clearly and maintain proper eye contact.

    D. Use complex medical terms that clearly define the diagnosis.

3. A medical assistant is speaking with a medical provider about correspondence that will be written for a patient. Which of the following factors applies to the communication process between the assistant and provider?

    A. Complex medical terms may be used.

    B. Lay terms will be used.

    C. Passive communication style is used.

    D. Aggressive communication style is used.

4. A medical assistant should recognize that which of the following characteristics describe a kinesthetic communicator?

    A. They tend to communicate using visual aids.

    B. They tend to communicate using auditory resources.

    C. They are one-sided communicators with ulterior motives.

    D. They tend to communicate by using their hands.

5. Which of the following is a true statement regarding patients who utilize virtual visits?

    A. Nonverbal cues are eliminated.

    B. Body language is not a factor.

    C. Personal space is essential.

    D. They rely more on the words being said.

6. A medical assistant is assisting with preparing a patient for their appointment by asking questions. Which of the following is a closed-ended question?

    A. "Who is your employer?"

    B. "What is your past medical history?"

    C. "What are your health concerns today?"

    D. "What questions or concerns do you have?"

7. Which of the following actions should a medical assistant take when communicating with patients on the phone?

    A. Use a monotone voice.

    B. Enunciate words.

    C. Speak loudly so they can hear.

    D. Use appropriate body language.

IN PRACTICE: QUIZZES
Quiz 12: Communication and Customer Service

8. Which of the following should a medical assistant recognize as the purpose of using a template?

    A. Templates alleviate the need to proofread.

    B. Templates guide the writer in using the proper format.

    C. Templates replace the need for etiquette.

    D. Templates are more informal than other letters.

9. A medical assistant is having a discussion with a patient who arrived late for their appointment and is upset that they are being requested to reschedule it. Which of the following actions should the assistant take to try to de-escalate the situation?

    A. Allow the patient to vent the reason for the tardiness.

    B. Inform the patient that they can go to a different provider who is available now.

    C. Remind the patient that they were late and that the provider has other patients to see.

    D. Ask the patient to sit and wait to see if they can be fit into the schedule.

10. A medical assistant is speaking with a patient who is unhappy with the medical services they received. The patient feels that their needs were not met and demands that the medical provider see them again. The schedule is full and it is not possible to fit the patient in today. Which of the following actions should the assistant take?

    A. Inform the patient they will have to schedule a new appointment on a different day.

    B. Give the patient a list of local providers they can choose to see.

    C. Tell the patient that their insurance will not likely cover a new appointment, so they will have to pay out-of-pocket costs.

    D. Inform a supervisor of the situation and ask them to assist.

11. The daughter of an adult patient has called to discuss the treatment plan for their parent. Which of the following actions should the medical assistant take?

    A. Inform the patient's daughter that the medical provider will contact them with the information.

    B. Answer the questions being asked.

    C. Confirm the patient's daughter is listed on the signed release of information form.

    D. Send the patient's daughter a copy of the patient's treatment plan via email.

12. Which of the following actions positively contributes to teamwork and engagement of the team members?

    A. Performing individual responsibilities and overall tasks

    B. Working through drama that is brought into the work environment

    C. Encouraging dating and personal relationships

    D. Creating a gossip board to share feelings

13. Which of the following characteristics demonstrates a professional attitude as a medical assistant?

    A. Healthy eating

    B. Good work ethic

    C. Physical fitness

    D. Accurate personal budgeting

14. A medical assistant is speaking with a patient who came in for management of diabetes. The assistant is giving the patient information about a diabetic diet. Which of the following is the goal of the therapeutic communication in this situation?

    A. To manipulate the conversation

    B. To demand changes

    C. To control the conversation

    D. To encourage and support

IN PRACTICE: QUIZZES
Quiz 12: Communication and Customer Service

15. A medical assistant is assisting to prepare for an upcoming virtual visit for chronic pain management. Which of the following is an important proactive measure to perform in preparation of the visit?

    A. Send the patient an after visit summary.

    B. Check that audio and visual components are working properly.

    C. Complete an encounter form prior to the visit.

    D. Schedule a follow-up visit.

16. Which of the following is a component of active listening skills?

    A. Paraphrasing what is being said

    B. Asking the patient to wait to ask questions until the information has been presented

    C. Responding to emails during the conversation

    D. Correcting the patient mid-sentence

17. Which of the following vocal traits should be used when speaking with patients over the telephone?

    A. Speak sternly using a lower tone.

    B. Speak warmly using a louder tone.

    C. Speak using a warm and natural tone.

    D. Speak slowly using monotone.

18. Which of the following actions assists with increasing patient satisfaction?

    A. Ask the medical provider to determine patient satisfaction levels.

    B. Include a satisfaction survey in the new patient packets to be completed before the appointment.

    C. Have the patient complete patient satisfaction surveys after their appointment.

    D. Include the patient satisfaction survey during the resolution process for conflict management.

19. A medical assistant is working to de-escalate a conversation with a patient who is upset about receiving a statement of their account with a balance due. The patient then begins to calm down and asks questions that indicate a better understanding. Which of the following actions should the assistant take following the conversation?

    A. Schedule an appointment to go over the patient's financial responsibility.

    B. Ask the patient to contact their insurance company to verify the amounts.

    C. Document the conversation in the patient medical record.

    D. Perform a courtesy write-off for the amount due.

20. Which of the following is included in risk management for a health care organization?

    A. Decreasing the number of staff

    B. Reducing spending in the budget

    C. Controlling inventory levels

    D. Ensuring a safe environment

QUIZ 13: MEDICAL LAW AND ETHICS

1. Which of the following protects patients' health information and sets rules and limits on who can view and receive the information?

   A. Affordable Care Act (ACA)

   B. Health Insurance Portability and Accountability Act (HIPAA)

   C. Health Information Technology for Economic and Clinical Health (HITECH) Act

   D. Protected health information (PHI)

2. Which of the following holds employers accountable for providing a safe workplace?

   A. CLIA

   B. OSH Act

   C. Emergency Medical Treatment and Active Labor Act (EMTALA)

   D. Controlled Substances Act (CSA)

3. A medical assistant is performing a strep test for an adult patient. As the assistant approaches the patient with a swab, the patient opens their mouth. Which of the following types of consent is the patient demonstrating?

   A. Express consent

   B. Guardian consent

   C. Implied consent

   D. Informed consent

4. Which of the following individuals can give informed consent to participate in a clinical trial?

   A. A 75-year-old who is in the advanced stage of dementia

   B. A 17-year-old adolescent who is employed and lives with their parents

   C. A 32-year-old who is in a coma

   D. A 16-year-old who has enlisted in the military

5. Which of the following prohibits the sale of a patient's protected health information (PHI)?

   A. Civil Rights Act

   B. Patient's Bill of Rights

   C. Affordable Care Act (ACA)

   D. Health Information Technology for Economic and Clinical Health (HITECH) Act

6. Which of the following allows patients to be informed of specific procedures and treatment options they have available?

   A. Civil Rights Act

   B. Health Insurance Portability and Accountability Act (HIPAA)

   C. Affordable Care Act (ACA)

   D. Patient's Bill of Rights

7. A patient has a terminal illness and wants to appoint a family member to make decisions for them when they are unable to. Which of the following forms should be completed?

   A. Medical orders for life-sustaining treatment (MOLST)

   B. Do-not-resuscitate (DNR) order

   C. Durable power of attorney for health care (DPAHC)

   D. Living will

8. Which of the following forms is specifically used to indicate that a patient does not want to receive CPR if their heart stops or they stop breathing?

   A. Do-not-resuscitate (DNR) order

   B. Advance directives

   C. Durable power of attorney for health care (DPAHC)

   D. Living will

IN PRACTICE: QUIZZES
Quiz 13: Medical Law and Ethics

9. Which of the following parties does ownership of a patient's medical record usually remain with?

    A. Courts

    B. Third-party payer

    C. Patient

    D. Health care provider

10. In which of the following situations does a patient have to authorize release of their medical record?

    A. The patient is being charged with assault, and there is a court order.

    B. The patient's family physician refers them to a specialist for additional care.

    C. The patient has injured themselves on the job and is applying for workers' compensation.

    D. The patient was in contact with a person who was diagnosed with tuberculosis.

11. A medical assistant receives a call from a patient's child, who is also a patient at the clinic and often accompanies the patient during their medical appointments. They ask the assistant to tell them what medication the patient is on. Which of the following is an appropriate response?

    A. Release the patient's information because their child is also a patient at the clinic.

    B. Release the patient's information because the child accompanying the patient at appointments constitutes implied consent.

    C. Release the patient's information after the patient authorizes it or confirms that their child is their personal representative.

    D. Release the patient's information but only what medication the patient is taking.

12. According to HIPAA, which of the following is not a covered entity?

    A. Employers

    B. Clearinghouses

    C. Health insurance plans

    D. Health care providers

13. Which of the following is mandatory for a health care provider to report?

    A. A 35-year-old patient who tested positive for strep throat

    B. A 10-year-old patient who has a history of fractures and bruises in different stages of healing

    C. A 68-year-old patient who reports they are unable to pay their bills because their Social Security payments are low

    D. A 6-month-old patient whose parents refuse to allow immunizations for them

14. Which of the following actions should a health care provider take if a child is brought in with a fractured arm and bruises, does not speak, and appears scared and possibly undernourished?

    A. Schedule a follow-up appointment to monitor for future injuries.

    B. Investigate the child's injury to prevent a wrongful report and potential lawsuit.

    C. Contact the police or Child Protective Services.

    D. Refer the child to a pediatrician for further follow-up.

IN PRACTICE: QUIZZES
Quiz 13: Medical Law and Ethics

15. A medical assistant should identify that a clinic is violating which of the following laws by failing to provide personal protective equipment (PPE) to its employees?

    A. Clinical Laboratory Improvement Amendments (CLIA)

    B. Occupational Safety and Health (OSH) Act

    C. Emergency Medical Treatment and Active Labor Act (EMTALA)

    D. Controlled Substances Act (CSA)

16. A medical assistant should identify that which of the following regulates blood and urine testing?

    A. Clinical Laboratory Improvement Amendments (CLIA)

    B. Emergency Medical Treatment and Active Labor Act (EMTALA)

    C. Controlled Substances Act (CSA)

    D. Occupational Safety and Health (OSH) Act

17. Which of the following basic elements of negligence protects a provider if they fail to provide care in an after-hours emergency involving someone in the community who is not an established patient?

    A. Duty of care

    B. Dereliction of duty

    C. Direct cause

    D. Damages

18. Which of the following individuals cannot serve as a health care proxy with a durable power of attorney in all states?

    A. A patient's spouse or domestic partner

    B. A patient's adult child

    C. A patient's health care provider

    D. A patient's court-appointed guardian

19. Which of the following can a patient still receive if they have a do-not-resuscitate (DNR) order on file?

    A. Antibiotics, chemotherapy, and dialysis

    B. Antibiotics, CPR, and chemotherapy

    C. Chemotherapy, CPR, and dialysis

    D. Chemotherapy, dialysis, and intubation

20. A medical assistant should identify that which of the following is an example of negligence?

    A. A patient is upset at their provider and posts on social media that the provider has lost their medical license.

    B. A medical assistant becomes frustrated with a patient who has dementia, yells that they are going to hit the patient, and raises their hand.

    C. A medical assistant forcibly pulls a patient out of the exam room because the patient refuses to leave.

    D. A medical assistant forgets to take a patient's blood glucose, and the patient leaves and is later hospitalized for diabetic ketoacidosis.

QUIZ ANSWERS

Quiz 1: Foundational Knowledge and Basic Science

1. **A.** Managed care is an umbrella term for plans that provide health care in return for preset scheduled payments and coordinated care.

   B. Correct. PCMH is a care delivery model in which a PCP coordinates treatment to make sure patients receive the required care when and where they need it and in a way they can understand.

   C. Home health refers to specific types of care, typically physical therapy, occupational therapy, and nursing, being provided in the home to those who are unable to leave their home easily.

   D. Hospice is a service for end-of-life care, and can be delivered to the patient either at their home or as inpatient care at a hospice facility.

2. **A.** Patient portals have decreased wait times for results, because they allow patients to see results directly online.

   B. Patient portals have been shown to reduce the demand on the care team, because they reduce the need for phone calls, which can be time consuming.

   C. Patient portals have not been shown to increase face-to-face visits.

   D. Correct. Patient portals provide increased transparency, because they allow patients direct access to their health information, including test results and imaging. Patient portals also enhance patient engagement by enabling patients to access their electronic medical records.

3. **A.** Increasing testing is not a component of the Quadruple Aim. The components of the Quadruple Aim should result in decreased testing, focused only on testing that truly provides value.

   B. Lower costs are a component of the Quadruple Aim.

   C. Correct. The Quadruple Aim is made up of improved patient outcomes, decreased cost of care, improved patient satisfaction, and health care worker wellness.

   D. While prevention screenings are an important aspect of value-based care, this is not one of the four components of the Quadruple Aim.

4. **A.** Radiology technicians use various types of imaging equipment to assist the provider in diagnosing and treating certain diseases.

   B. Occupational therapists assist patients who have developed conditions that restrict them developmentally, emotionally, mentally, or physically.

   C. Nurse practitioners provide basic patient care services, including diagnosing and prescribing medications for common illnesses.

   D. Correct. The assistant should initiate a referral to a physical therapist. Physical therapists assist patients with building strength and increasing range of motion.

5. **A.** Performing an EKG is a clinical responsibility that is not appropriate for a medical assistant who specializes in administrative responsibilities.

   B. Preparing medications is a clinical responsibility that is not appropriate for a medical assistant who specializes in administrative responsibilities.

   C. Obtaining vital signs is a clinical responsibility that is not appropriate for a medical assistant who specializes in administrative responsibilities.

   D. Correct. Collecting copays is an administrative responsibility that is assigned to administrative medical assistants.

6. **A.** Antihypertensives are medications used to lower blood pressure.

   B. Correct. Antihistamines are medications that are used to relieve allergy symptoms, including seasonal allergies.

   C. Diuretics are medications used to remove excess fluid.

   D. Antipyretics are medications used to reduce fever.

7. **A.** Schedule II medications are the most tightly controlled of controlled medications. Refills are not included for Schedule II medications.

   B. Schedule III medications can be prescribed with up to 5 refills to be filled within 6 months.

   C. Schedule IV medications can be prescribed with up to 5 refills to be filled within 6 months.

   D. Correct. Schedule V medications are the least controlled of the controlled medications. Providers can authorize up to a year's worth of refills for these medications.

8. **A.** Side effects are known, expected, and relatively harmless yet undesirable actions on the body from medications and are not a reason for the patient to avoid the medication.

    B. An adverse effect is an unintended, harmful action of the medication, such as an allergic reaction, and prevents further use of the medications. In this case, it is the disease process of kidney disease that makes the medication unsafe for the patient, not an action of the medication itself.

    C. Correct. A contraindication is a symptom or condition that makes a particular treatment or medication inadvisable or even dangerous. In this case, the patient's kidneys cannot safely filter the medication due to their decreased function.

    D. Indications are the problems or symptoms the medication is recommended for. In this case, ibuprofen may be indicated for pain relief, but an alternative medication should be recommended in its place due to the contraindication of ibuprofen in the setting of kidney disease.

9. **A.** The primary factors that impact speed of absorption include route of medication administration, formulation of medication, how dissolvable the medication is in fat, and surface area of the body part where absorption is occurring. Absorption is not significantly impacted by age.

    B. Distribution is not impacted significantly by age. Factors to consider with medications and distribution are if the medication would be stopped by the blood-brain barrier and if the medication can cross the placental barrier in patients who are pregnant.

    C. Correct. Metabolism refers to the body's ability to break down a medication. Several factors impact speed of metabolism, with age being one of the primary factors. Infants and older adults have slower metabolisms and, therefore, medication dosages must be altered for these groups.

    D. Excretion is the body's removal of medication metabolites from the body. Age does not play a significant role in excretion.

10. **A.** While medical assistants can be authorized to administer a medication, it is not within their scope of practice to determine if a medication is appropriate for a patient based on the benefits and risks associated with the medication.

    B. Correct. The role of the medical assistant in medication administration as it relates to "the right medication" is to provide the patient with the name of the medication, the name of the provider who prescribed it, and the intended effect of the medication.

    C. While informing the patient of the indication for the medication is a responsibility of the medical assistant, this relates to the concept of "the right reason," rather than "the right medication."

    D. While evaluating the patient for effects and reactions to the medication may be a responsibility of the medical assistant, this relates to the concept of "the right evaluation," rather than "the right medication."

11. **A.** Albuterol is not an example of an anticoagulant. Anticoagulants delay blood clotting.

    B. Correct. Albuterol is a bronchodilator used to relax airway muscles.

    C. Albuterol is not an example of an antiemetic. Antiemetics reduce nausea and vomiting.

    D. Albuterol is not an example of an antipsychotic. Antipsychotics control psychotic symptoms.

IN PRACTICE: QUIZZES
Quiz Answers:

12. **A. Correct.** The assistant should consult the Physicians' Desk Reference to identify the medication because it has a product identification guide with color photographs of medications.

    B. Medication confusion and errors can be extremely dangerous. Redirecting this patient could risk the patient opting to not pursue an answer, which could result in the patient taking their medication incorrectly.

    C. Asking the patient to bring the medication into the clinic could delay resolution to the question and is also not necessary. So long as the patient can give a detailed report of what the medication looks like, there are better solutions.

    D. While the internet could be a useful resource in this situation, searching online could lead to false or inaccurate information. If a webpage is being used for information regarding patient care, it must be a site approved by the medical assistant's employer.

13. **A. Correct.** Honey is an example of a simple carbohydrate, or a simple sugar.

    B. Vegetables are sources of complex carbohydrates.

    C. Pasta is a source of complex carbohydrates.

    D. Beans are a source of complex carbohydrates.

14. **A. Correct.** High blood pressure is one of the primary contributing factors of worsened kidney function. Therefore, a patient who has chronic kidney disease should limit their sodium intake to less than 2,300 mg per day.

    B. Decreasing phosphorus intake is indicated for patients who are in Stage IV and V of chronic kidney disease, because worsened kidney function leads to higher levels of phosphorus in the blood.

    C. Controlling potassium intake is indicated for patients who are in Stage IV and V of chronic kidney disease, because worsened kidney function leads to increased potassium levels in the blood stream.

    D. Those who have celiac disease should avoid gluten. Gluten is not a cause for concern with chronic kidney disease.

15. **A.** Gingko biloba is a supplement that improves memory and mental function by increasing blood flow to the brain.

    B. Willow bark is a supplement that supports pain relief.

    C. Correct. Melatonin is a naturally occurring hormone in the brain that is related to sleep. It is also a supplement that can be taken to help with sleep regulation.

    D. Black cohosh is a supplement that relieves symptoms associated with menopause.

16. **A.** Weight loss of at least 15% is a potential warning sign for anorexia.

    B. Amenorrhea, or lack of a menstrual period, is a potential warning sign for anorexia.

    C. Buying and consuming large amounts of food is a warning sign of bulimia, not anorexia.

    D. Correct. Excessive exercising is a warning sign of anorexia and should be reported to a provider immediately.

17. **A. Correct.** Subcutaneously is a parenteral route of medication administration.

    B. Orally is an enteral or nonparenteral route of medication administration.

    C. Topically is a nonparenteral route of medication administration.

    D. Vaginally is a nonparenteral route of medication administration.

18. **A.** Foams are delivered vaginally.

    B. Mists are delivered nasally or via inhalation.

    C. Correct. Lozenges are delivered orally.

    D. Powders are delivered topically.

19. **A.** Dosage calculations for children are based on weight, not height.

B. Correct. The assistant should convert the child's weight in pounds to kilograms to determine how much medication the child should receive per dose.

C. The assistant should divide the daily dose by three, not multiply the daily dose by three, as part of the equation to determine how much medication the child should receive per dose.

D. Calculating medication doses is within the scope of practice of a medical assistant. The information already provided by the provider is adequate for the medical assistant to calculate from there.

20. **A.** While annual visits are a good time to review a comprehensive list of medication allergies, relying only on this is not safe practice.

B. Correct. Allergies can change, and medical record information can be incorrect. Therefore, it is best practice to review medication allergies at every patient visit and any time a medication is prescribed.

C. Reviewing medication allergies every 3 years is not safe and can lead to outdated and incorrect information.

D. While medication allergies should be reviewed at every visit, as well as any time a medication is prescribed, it is not necessary to discuss medication allergies during every phone call or non-visit interaction with a patient.

Quiz 2: Medical Terminology, Anatomy, and Physiology

1. **A.** CVA is the abbreviation for cerebrovascular accident, or stroke.

B. BP is the abbreviation for blood pressure.

C. PVD is the abbreviation for peripheral vascular disease.

D. Correct. MI is the abbreviation for myocardial infarction, which is the clinical term for heart attack.

2. **A.** Some common diseases do have accepted standard abbreviations, such as DM for diabetes mellitus.

B. Some body parts do have accepted standard abbreviations, such as "abd" for abdomen.

C. Correct. To avoid medication errors, the full name of any medication should always be used.

D. Some test names do have accepted standard abbreviations, such as "CBC" for complete blood count.

3. **A.** The root word hidr refers to sweat.

B. Correct. The root word dermat refers to skin.

C. The root word trich refers to hair.

D. The root word onych refers to a fingernail or toenail.

4. **A.** Diabetes mellitus is commonly referred to as "diabetes" or "DM."

B. Multiple sclerosis is commonly abbreviated as "MS."

C. Correct. Amyotrophic lateral sclerosis (ALS) is commonly known as Lou Gehrig's disease. Lou Gehrig was a famous baseball player who had the disease and made it more well-known.

D. Transient ischemic attacks are commonly abbreviated as "TIA" or referred to as "mini strokes."

IN PRACTICE: QUIZZES
Quiz Answers: Quiz 2: Medical Terminology, Anatomy, and Physiology

5. **A.** Inferior would indicate the head is below the chest, which is not accurate of the anatomical position.

    B. Correct. The head is superior to the chest, meaning it is above or closer to the top of the body than the chest.

    C. Anterior refers to the front or belly side of the body. The head is not in front of the chest.

    D. Dorsal refers to the back of the body. The head is not behind or closer to the back of the body than the chest.

6. **A.** Overwhelming worry is more common with anxiety than depression.

    B. Correct. Those experiencing depression can experience extreme sadness, fatigue and lethargy, hopelessness, pain, digestive issues, an extreme lack of motivation, even with activities and hobbies that were previously enjoyable, and thoughts of suicide.

    C. Flashbacks are a common symptom of posttraumatic stress disorder (PTSD).

    D. Trouble following directions is a common symptom of ADHD.

7. **A. Correct.** Pollution in the air is a physical stressor on the body, as poor air quality directly impacts the body's ability to maintain a state of wellness and can cause many different diseases.

    B. Loss of a loved one is an environmental stressor as it puts a strain on the person experiencing it but not directly through physical means.

    C. Loss of a job is a socioeconomic stressor.

    D. Medical bills are socioeconomic stressors.

8. **A.** Rubber coverings on floors can be helpful for wheels on a wheelchair but are not related to supporting patients who have vision loss.

    B. Speaking louder might be helpful for patients who have hearing loss but is not helpful for those who have vision loss.

    C. So long as the patient is willing and able (with accommodations), information about their health and health care should always be directed to them first.

    D. Correct. For patients experiencing some level of visual impairment, but not total vision loss, large print materials can be helpful in supporting the patient's understanding and engagement with the topic at hand.

9. **A.** Projection is the transference of a person's unpleasant ideas and emotions onto someone or something else.

    B. Identification is the attribution of characteristics of someone else to oneself or the imitation of another.

    C. Correct. Denial is the avoidance of unpleasant or anxiety-provoking situations or ideas by rejecting or ignoring them.

    D. Regression is a reversion to an earlier, more childlike, developmental behavior.

10. **A.** In the denial stage, patients do not believe the information they are being told and are not looking for solutions because there is not a belief the problem exists.

    B. In the anger stage, patients feel upset and hostile. They are not looking for solutions.

    C. Correct. In the bargaining stage, patients might start looking for alternative solutions, such as lifestyle changes, even if it is too late for those changes to be effective.

    D. In the depression stage, patients might feel sad and hopeless. They understand alternative solutions are not going to be effective.

11. **A.** Anxiety symptoms include uncontrolled levels of stress, fast heart rate, sweating, and being consumed by worry.

    B. Depression typically presents as extreme sadness, fatigue, hopelessness, pain, issues with digestion, extreme lack of motivation, or thoughts of suicide.

    C. PTSD symptoms include flashbacks, negative thoughts, hopelessness, changes in reactions, trouble with concentration and sleep, self-destructive behaviors, and avoidance.

    D. Correct. ADHD can present differently in young males and females. Males tend to be more hyperactive while females tend to be more quietly inattentive.

12. **A. Correct.** In the generativity vs. stagnation stage, adults continue raising children and some become grandparents. They want to help mold future generations, so they often involve themselves in teaching, coaching, writing, and social activism. Achieving the tasks of this stage results in professional and personal achievements and active participation in serving the community and society. Nonachievement occurs when development ceases, which leads to self-preoccupation without the capacity to give and share with others. This is the psychosocial crisis for middle adults (35 to 65 years).

    B. The goal of this stage is for someone to know who they are as a person and how they fit into the world around them. This is the psychosocial crisis for adolescents (12 to 20 years).

    C. In this stage, the goal is to develop trust with the primary caregiver. This is the psychosocial crisis for infants (birth to 18 months).

    D. The goal of this stage is to try new activities and take on new responsibilities. This is the psychosocial crisis for preschoolers (3 to 6 years).

13. **A.** The thoracic cavity is found within the chest.

    B. Correct. The spinal cavity is a continuation of the cranial cavity as it travels down the midline of the back.

    C. The abdominal cavity is found within the abdomen.

    D. The pelvic cavity is inferior to the abdominal cavity.

14. **A.** The scapula is a bone of the upper extremities.

    B. The carpals are bones of the upper extremities.

    C. The sacrum is a bone of the axial skeleton.

    D. Correct. Metatarsals are found in the foot, making them bones of the lower extremities.

15. **A.** Digestion is the breakdown of foods and ingested substances by the body.

    B. Respiration is the process of moving air in and out of the lungs.

    C. Correct. Homeostasis is achieved when the body's systems and biological processes maintain stability.

    D. Filtration is the process of removing waste products from the blood.

16. **A. Correct.** Rheumatoid arthritis is an autoimmune disorder leading to changes in the connective tissues of the body, especially the joints.

    B. Gout is an excessive accumulation of uric acid in a joint.

    C. Muscular dystrophy is an inherited or spontaneous gene mutation in one of the genes involved in protecting muscle fibers from damage.

    D. Myalgia is a general term for muscle pain.

17. **A. Correct.** Shingles causes a rash with blisters, which follows the path of the affected nerve.

    B. Facial droop is a symptom of a cerebrovascular accident but is not associated with shingles.

    C. Decreased urine output is a common symptom of acute renal failure but is not associated with shingles.

    D. Distorted vision can be a symptom of a concussion but is not associated with shingles.

18. **A. Correct.** Diverticulosis is pouchlike herniations through the muscular wall of the colon caused by high pressure inside the colon pressing against weak areas of the colon wall. It is typically discovered during a colonoscopy.

    B. GERD is an acid reflux disease that can be diagnosed via an upper endoscopy.

    C. Celiac disease is a condition affecting the small intestine and can be diagnosed via an upper endoscopy which often includes a biopsy.

    D. A UTI is a urinary tract infection, which can be diagnosed through urine tests.

IN PRACTICE: QUIZZES
Quiz Answers: Quiz 3: Patient Intake and Vitals

19. **A.** Smoking is a risk factor for COPD.

    B. Age is a risk factor for osteoporosis.

    C. High blood pressure is a risk factor for chronic kidney disease.

    D. Correct. Eating a high-fat diet, family history of colorectal cancer, and a history of inflammatory bowel disease are all risk factors for colorectal cancer.

20. **A.** An outbreak is a generalized term for a sudden rise in cases of a disease.

    B. Correct. An endemic is an illness that is constantly present within a community.

    C. An epidemic is when a disease spreads rapidly to a large number of people.

    D. A pandemic is a world-wide outbreak of a disease.

Quiz 3: Patient Intake and Vitals

1. **A. Correct.** The supervisor should be notified immediately. The assistant is responsible for ensuring the patient area is comfortable and free of potential causes of harm.

    B. Patient safety is always a priority and should be addressed immediately.

    C. Patient safety is a priority and needs to be addressed immediately.

    D. It is not up to the assistant to determine the validity of a patient's reasoning or perception. The issue needs to be addressed immediately, because it could be a potential hazard.

2. **A.** This may not be feasible with the time management required within the office.

    B. The patient's cane should be always be kept near them.

    C. Correct. The assistant should help the patient onto the examination table to make sure they are safe and secure.

    D. Patients should not have to wait until the provider is ready to be called into an examination room.

3. **A.** The family history section includes the patient's immediate family members' history of diseases.

    B. Correct. The assistant should document this information in the social history section of the patient's medical record. This section includes diet, exercise, tobacco use, and substance use.

    C. The past medical history section includes past illnesses, diseases, or surgeries the patient has had.

    D. The occupational history section includes occupational hazards in the patient's life.

4. **A.** The patient's address is not an acceptable patient identifier.

    B. While the patient's Social Security number can verify the patient, many facilities do not have access to that information.

    C. A mother's maiden name is not an acceptable patient identifier.

    D. Correct. The patient's name and date of birth are the two standard identifiers used to verify a patient.

5. **A.** Medications are not listed in the demographic section.

    B. Correct. The patient's address is found in the demographic section and should be verified at the beginning of each visit to ensure it is still accurate.

    C. A medical record number is specific to an organization and used as a patient identifier within the medical facility, not with a patient directly.

    D. Diagnosis codes describe an individual disease or medical condition.

6. **A.** Review of systems is a component of the physical exam completed by the provider.

    B. Correct. This is the reason the patient is being seen and is usually in the patient's words. Therefore, the assistant should document the patient's statement in this section of the patient's medical record.

    C. Past medical history relates to past illnesses, surgeries, and childhood illnesses.

    D. Social history relates to diet, exercise, tobacco use, and substance use.

7. **A.** The patient is not displaying symptoms of sadness, fatigue, or lack of energy.

   B. Patients experiencing dementia are usually older adults and they typically do not experience a sense of panic.

   C. The patient is not displaying any violent behavior towards themselves or others.

   D. Correct. Signs of anxiety include difficulty focusing, a sense of panic, and irritability. Anxiety can be a response to fear or feeling anxious when visiting any type of health care facility.

8. **A.** Medical history relates to past illnesses, childhood disease, and surgeries.

   B. The chief complaint is usually in the patient's own words and is the reason for the visit.

   C. Correct. Occupational history relates to exposures in a patient's place of work that could be hazardous to their health, such as hazardous machinery.

   D. Social history relates to diet, tobacco, alcohol, and substance use.

9. **A.** Normal blood pressure is less than 120/80 mm Hg.

   B. Correct. Prehypertension is a systolic pressure of 120 to 139 mm Hg and a diastolic pressure of 80 to 89 mm Hg.

   C. Hypertension is greater than 140/90 mm Hg.

   D. A hypertensive crisis is greater than 180/110 mm Hg.

10. **A.** The femoral artery is used to determine circulation in the lower extremities.

    B. The radial artery is used with the palpatory method when the blood pressure cannot be auscultated.

    C. Correct. Blood pressure readings are most commonly auscultated over the brachial artery in the antecubital space.

    D. The carotid artery is commonly used in emergency situations to obtain a pulse.

11. **A.** Used for respiratory conditions, the pulse oximeter measures the level of oxygen saturation in the blood.

    B. Body temperature does not need to be rechecked due to complaints of dizziness.

    C. Correct. The assistant should obtain orthostatic vital signs to determine if there is a change in blood pressure or pulse since the patient is reporting dizziness.

    D. Pain is subjective and requires additional questions to determine location, onset, duration, and characteristics of the pain.

12. **A.** This temperature is within the expected reference range for older adult patients who are 70 years and older.

    B. This temperature is within the expected reference range for a 1-year-old child.

    C. This temperature is outside the expected reference range and should be reported to the provider immediately.

    D. Correct. This temperature is within the expected reference range for those who are 6 years and older.

13. **A.** This site is considered the least accurate and is not recommended to use on a 3-year-old child.

    B. It can be difficult to get a 3-year-old child to hold a thermometer under their tongue. They may not understand or comprehend the directions at this age.

    C. This site should not be used since the patient is complaining of ear pain. It is best to avoid inserting a thermometer in the ear.

    D. Correct. A temporal artery thermometer is not invasive and provides a fast and accurate reading since the artery is so close to the surface.

14. **A.** A BMI less than 18.5 is considered underweight.

    B. A BMI of 18.5 to 24.9 is considered normal.

    C. A BMI of 25 to 29.9 is considered overweight.

    D. Correct. A BMI greater than 30 is considered obese.

IN PRACTICE: QUIZZES
Quiz Answers: Quiz 3: Patient Intake and Vitals

15. **A.** This is not always correct.

    B. The weight at the time of the office visit is the weight that should be recorded in the patient's record.

    C. Shoes and outerwear need to be removed to obtain an accurate weight.

    D. Correct. Privacy is a significant factor when weighing a patient, and placing the scale in a private area typically helps them feel more comfortable.

16. **A.** Hypotension refers to having low blood pressure.

    B. Correct. Bradycardia best describes this pulse rate. Bradycardia refers to a slow heart rate. "Brady" means slow and "cardia" means heart.

    C. Tachypnea refers to respirations over 20/min.

    D. Tachycardia refers to a heart rate above 100/min.

17. **A. Correct.** The heart rate is elevated. An expected heart rate for this patient is 60 to 100/min.

    B. These vital signs are all within the expected reference ranges for this patient.

    C. These vital signs are all within the expected reference ranges for this patient.

    D. These vital signs are all within the expected reference ranges for this patient.

18. **A.** The blood pressure is within the expected reference range, so the assistant does not need to recheck it.

    B. The assistant should avoid reporting anything to the provider that might be a false reading.

    C. Correct. If a temperature reading using an axillary thermometer is higher than 37.2° C (99° F) and does not appear to match the patient's general condition, the assistant should repeat the temperature measurement using a different method.

    D. This doesn't correlate with an axillary temperature. This would only affect an oral temperature reading.

19. **A. Correct.** Orthopnea is difficulty breathing in a recumbent position and is relieved by sitting or standing. It often occurs in patients who have COPD because they need to sit up to breath or use multiple pillows to allow them to breathe as they sleep.

    B. Weight loss is often seen in patients who have COPD.

    C. Hypertension is often seen in patients who have COPD.

    D. Tachycardia is often seen in patients who have COPD.

20. **A. Correct.** Using a scale with built-in handrails is the safest and best option for a patient who has balance concerns.

    B. Only weights measured in the clinic, or otherwise directly approved by provider, should be entered into the patient's medical record. Asking the patient to estimate their weight could lead to inaccurate and unsafe medical decision making.

    C. While this is an appropriate method of obtaining weight from a patient who has balance concerns, there is a better, safer option for the assistant to use.

    D. This method could put the patient at risk for a fall and assumes they are able to stand alone safely, even for a few seconds.

Quiz 4: General Patient Care: Part 1

1. **A.** A sigmoidoscope is used in a specialized procedure and may need a dedicated room for the procedure.

   B. An EKG machine may not be needed for every patient and may have a dedicated room for performing EKGs.

   C. Correct. Every examination room should contain a biohazard waste container for safe disposal of contaminated material.

   D. Many medical offices will have a dedicated room where they perform pelvic exams which would require an examination table with stirrups.

2. **A.** The prone position requires the patient to lie face down, flat on their stomach. Although this would allow access to the back, it would not allow for a rectal exam or view.

   B. Correct. The left lateral position requires the patient to be placed on their left side with their right leg sharply bent upward and their left leg slightly bent. This position is used for rectal exams, such as a colonoscopy.

   C. The semi-Fowler's position is a modified full-Fowler's position with the head of the table at a 45° angle instead of a 90° angle. This position would not allow access for a rectal exam.

   D. The Trendelenburg position is often used in surgical and critical care procedures and is not normally used in a medical office except in cases of shock or hypotension.

3. **A. Correct.** A spirometer is used to monitor a patient's lung function and is common in a pulmonology specialty.

   B. Cardiology specializes in heart diseases and disorders.

   C. Gynecology specializes in health related to the vagina, uterus, fallopian tubes, and ovaries.

   D. Endocrinology specializes in the diseases of the endocrine system.

4. **A. Correct.** A patient's medication allergy history should be updated during every patient visit.

   B. Signs and symptoms of an allergic reaction can occur within 20 min to 2 hr after exposure.

   C. Although a patient might not have had an allergic reaction to a medication or allergen in the past, it is always possible to develop a reaction later.

   D. Most allergic reactions are common and present with mild symptoms, not anaphylaxis.

5. **A. Correct.** If the daily dosage is 20 mg and the tablets come as 10 mg, the patient will need to take 2 tablets per day. For a course of 30 days, 60 tablets should be ordered.

   B. This medication order would allow enough tablets for 30 days; however, taking 1 tablet per day would be less than what is prescribed.

   C. This medical order would only allow for a 15-day course of the medication.

   D. This medication order would be less than what was prescribed daily.

6. **A.** Multidose vials are good for 28 days after opening unless the manufacturer's expiration occurs sooner than 28 days.

   B. Correct. Multidose vials are good for 28 days after opening unless the manufacturer's expiration occurs sooner than 28 days. July 29 is 28 days after the opening of the vial.

   C. Multidose vials are good for 28 days, not 15 days, after opening unless the manufacturer's expiration occurs sooner than 28 days.

   D. Multidose vials are good for 28 days after opening unless the manufacturer's expiration occurs sooner than 28 days.

7. **A.** The patient should be instructed to look towards the ceiling with both eyes open.

   B. Correct. To perform an eye instillation, the patient should be instructed to look towards the ceiling with both eyes open.

   C. The patient should be instructed to look towards the ceiling with both eyes open.

   D. The patient should be instructed to look towards the ceiling with both eyes open.

IN PRACTICE: QUIZZES
Quiz Answers: Quiz 4: General Patient Care: Part 1

8. **A.** Correspondence data is any correspondence with the patient regarding legal or insurance matters.

    B. Clinical information includes all the data that has been recorded about the patient's health.

    C. Correct. Demographic data includes name, address, birthdate, sex, Social Security number, phone number, and insurance information.

    D. Social information pertains to the patient's living environment, occupation and lifestyle choices.

9. **A.** The third step in the process is entering the prescription into the EMR.

    B. The fifth step in the process involves the system sending the order to the pharmacy.

    C. Correct. The second step in the process is selecting the patient from a patient list in the system.

    D. The fourth step in the process is validating the order against the patient's medical history, health insurance plan, and other information within the system.

10. **A. Correct.** To rule out a fracture, the patient needs to have an x-ray, and based on the results, may need a cast or immobilizing device. This would be an inappropriate situation for a telehealth appointment.

    B. A dermatology visit can be conducted via telehealth since the physician is able to view the mole on video.

    C. A provider would be able to renew or write a new prescription for the patient via telehealth.

    D. Mental health counseling may be conducted via telehealth.

11. **A. Correct.** A CDSS can automatically check for medication interactions and allergies, and for errors in medication dosage and frequency.

    B. A CPOE is an electronic process that allows a health care provider to enter medical orders electronically into a system instead of using more traditional order methods.

    C. An EHR system is a digital version of a patient's paper chart.

    D. An eMAR is a digital report of the medications administered to a patient at a facility by a health care provider or professional.

12. **A.** Depending on the patient's diagnosis and the reason for the visit, the patient may be able to self-report their vital sign measurements.

    B. Correct. The patient should receive instructions and information on technology requirements for any telehealth services, which should include how to sign on and how to use the microphone, camera, and text chat.

    C. The patient should find a private room where no other people may be present in the room with the patient.

    D. Public-facing video communication applications such as social media platforms should not be used in the provision of telehealth due to privacy risks.

13. **A.** Prescription refills and new prescriptions may be sent electronically as long as the software being used to transmit the prescription is approved.

    B. The Drug Enforcement Agency's (DEA) rule on Electronic Prescriptions for Controlled Substances (EPCS) allows health care providers the option of writing prescriptions for controlled substances electronically.

    C. Many states are requiring health care providers to use electronic prescriptions for both controlled and noncontrolled substances instead of paper prescriptions.

    D. Correct. The pharmacy must use software that has been approved through a third-party audit and certified to attest the software is DEA EPCS-compliant.

14. **A.** Although discomfort or mild pain may occur after a procedure, the patient should notify the health care provider of any issues.

    B. Correct. The patient should notify the health care provider of any issues after a procedure, especially pain or bleeding.

    C. The patient should notify the health care provider of any issues after a procedure and should not wait several days before notifying the provider.

    D. The patient should go to the emergency room in case of a life-threatening situation. However, if the provider is immediately available, the patient should first try to contact the provider for advice to determine if an emergency does exist.

15. **A.** Having the patient move on and off the examination table may increase the risk of the patient falling.

    B. A procedure should not be rescheduled without the approval or authorization of the health care provider.

    C. Correct. If the medical assistant is unable to remain in the room, a family member or another assistant should be asked to sit with the patient. The patient should not be unattended as they could be at risk for a fall.

    D. The patient should not be unattended as they could be at risk for a fall.

16. **A.** Loratadine is a medication used for allergies, but not the first choice for an anaphylactic reaction.

    B. AED pads are attached when a patient is not breathing and does not have a pulse.

    C. CPR should be administered only in cases where the patient loses consciousness and stops breathing.

    D. Correct. The health care provider should be notified to give an order to administer epinephrine to the patient.

17. **A.** A 15° angle into the layer of skin between the epidermis and dermis would be appropriate for an intradermal injection, not for insulin.

    B. Although the angle of injection for a subcutaneous injection is 45°, the sites of subcutaneous injections are the upper outer arm, abdominal region, and the upper thigh, not the dermis.

    C. An intramuscular injection, not a subcutaneous injection, is administered in the muscle at a 90° angle.

    D. Correct. A subcutaneous insulin injection should be administered at a 45° angle into adipose tissue.

18. **A.** An intradermal injection is given with a 25-gauge needle at a 15° angle in the anterior forearm. This would not be appropriate for an influenza vaccine.

    B. A subcutaneous injection can be administered with a 27-gauge needle at a 45° angle in the abdominal region. This would not be appropriate for an influenza vaccine.

    C. Correct. An IM injection such as an influenza vaccine is usually administered in the deltoid muscle. The needle sizes range from an 18- to 25-gauge needle depending on the size of the patient's arm. The angle of injection for an IM injection is 90°.

    D. A 5° angle of injection is used for intradermal injections and an 18-gauge needle should be used for IM injections. This would not be appropriate for an influenza vaccine.

19. **A.** Along with computer-generated paper prescriptions and written prescriptions, electronic prescriptions can also be faxed.

    B. Being able to transmit an electronic prescription provides increased efficiency since the pharmacy can more quickly receive it and begin filling the prescription.

    C. Correct. Electronic prescribing (e-prescribing) can reduce opportunities for tampering and diversion of controlled substances.

    D. Pharmacies can pose routine questions via the e-prescribing system rather than through a phone call to the health care provider. This results in increased efficiency and fewer pharmacy calls to the provider.

20. **A.** Medications kept for patient administration must not be stored in the same refrigerator as office staff food or other items.

    B. Vaccines may be stored at room temperature in the refrigerator, or in the freezer.

    C. Medications must be rotated according to their expiration dates. The supply of vaccines should be rotated to use the ones with the shortest or soonest expiration date first.

    D. Correct. Expiration dates on medications and all supplies for injection should be routinely checked.

Quiz 5: General Patient Care: Part 2

1. **A.** The Mayo stand should be above the waist, with the area below the waist being unsterile.

   B. Correct. The Mayo stand should be at least 12 inches away from someone's body to maintain sterility.

   C. The 1-inch edge of the inside of the sterile instrument packet wrapper is considered nonsterile.

   D. The inside area of the wrapper is sterile. The outermost side of the wrapper is unsterile.

2. **A.** To remove staples, use the staple removal device.

   B. The proper technique would be to begin with the second staple of the wound and remove every other one until all have been removed.

   C. Correct. To use the sterile staple remover, place the lower tip under the staple and squeeze the handle together until completely closed. This will bend the staple in the middle and pull the edges of the staple out of the skin.

   D. Do not lift the staple remover when squeezing the handles.

3. **A. Correct.** When treating a major burn, emergency care is needed. Call 911 or seek immediate care for major burns.

   B. Immediately applying a lotion would only be appropriate for a minor burn.

   C. Immediately putting the burn under cool water would only be appropriate for minor burns.

   D. Apply a bandage only in the case of a burn blister breaking.

4. **A.** Initial symptoms of hypoglycemia are irritability, moodiness or change in behavior, hunger, sweating, and rapid heart rate.

   B. A person having a seizure might experience falling and shaking.

   C. Correct. A patient who is choking usually places their hands at their throat.

   D. Syncope is fainting, or a brief loss of consciousness. When experiencing syncope, a patient may collapse. However, they would not place their hands around their throat prior to collapsing.

5. **A. Correct.** The proliferative phase is between 3 and 21 days, with fibrin threads extending across the wound that starts pulling the edges together.

   B. The inflammatory phase usually occurs at day 3 and is accompanied by pain, swelling, and loss of function.

   C. The maturation phase is between 21 days and 2 years, with tissue cells strengthening and tightening. In addition, a scar forms.

   D. Dehiscence is a wound complication where the edges are separated.

6. **A.** An endoscopy provides views inside hollow organs and body cavities such as the larynx, bladder, or colon.

   B. Correct. A colposcopy is used to examine the inside of the vagina and cervix. This is performed after an abnormal Pap smear. A biopsy should be taken of the cervical tissue to send to a pathology lab to determine if it is cancerous.

   C. Cryosurgery is the destruction of tissue using cold liquid.

   D. Incision and drainage (I&D) procedures are used to relieve abscesses.

7. **A. Correct.** Dehiscence is a wound complication where the wound edges separate.

   B. Evisceration is a wound complication where the wound edges separate and the abdominal organs protrude.

   C. Hemorrhaging is a wound complication where the wound is bleeding.

   D. Infection is a wound complication where the wound shows sign of inflammation, swelling, and purulent drainage.

8. **A.** The Centers for Medicare & Medicaid Services (CMS) establishes which items are considered DMEPOS.

   B. The CMS establishes a list of DMEPOS items called the Master List.

   C. Correct. Prior authorization is a process where a request for approval of coverage is submitted for an item before a claim is submitted for payment.

   D. Any licensed and approved provider may prescribe DMEPOS.

IN PRACTICE: QUIZZES
Quiz Answers: Quiz 5: General Patient Care: Part 2

9. **A. Correct.** Cardiac arrest occurs when the heart suddenly and unexpectedly stops pumping. This condition is appropriate for the use of an AED.

   B. Treatment for hypovolemic shock includes IV blood and fluid replacement depending on the source of the loss.

   C. Seizures are uncontrolled muscle activity. Steps should be taken to prevent injury to the patient.

   D. Syncope is fainting, or temporary loss of consciousness. Treatment includes ammonia capsules to arouse the patient.

10. **A.** Two breaths should be given for every 30 compressions.

    B. Correct. Thirty chest compressions followed by two rescue breaths is standard recommended practice for CPR on an adult patient.

    C. Thirty compressions should be given for every two breaths for adult CPR.

    D. Fifteen chest compressions followed by two rescue breaths is standard recommended practice for CPR on a child or infant when there are two rescuers.

11. **A.** The AED should be regularly checked, usually monthly, and not just after use on a patient.

    B. Correct. The emergency kit should be in a location easily accessible to the examination rooms and all staff members should know where it is located.

    C. Expired medications should be promptly removed and replaced.

    D. Medication labels should not be written on to avoid misidentification.

12. **A. Correct.** An I&D procedure is commonly used to release pus from an abscess.

    B. Cervical dysplasia is the presence of abnormal cells in the cervix. An I&D procedure would not be appropriate for this condition.

    C. A biopsy would be needed to remove the mole for pathology to rule out skin cancer.

    D. A biopsy would be the needed to remove or take a sample of tissue for pathology to rule out breast cancer.

13. **A.** Hypoglycemia is low blood sugar and may lead to shock if not treated.

    B. Hypothermia is an abnormal lowering of body temperature, usually resulting from immersion in cold water or being stranded in subzero weather. Signs and symptoms include shivering, numbness, confusion, paleness, and eventual loss of consciousness.

    C. Although syncope is loss of consciousness, the patient presents with additional early symptoms.

    D. Correct. The patient most likely is going into shock and displays the early and late stages of the signs and symptoms.

14. **A.** A packet may contain a single instrument or multiple instruments.

    B. All sterile instrument packets must have autoclave tape on them and the tape must indicate that it has been properly sterilized. This indication is with black markings.

    C. Autoclave tape is placed on the outside of the instrument packet before the item is autoclaved.

    D. Correct. All instrument packets must show indication of being autoclaved using an indicator strip or autoclave tape that has darkened lines and have an expiration date to be considered sterile.

15. **A.** Absorbable sutures are used to attach tissues beneath the skin. The appropriate size for the face and neck are 5-0 and 6-0.

    B. Absorbable sutures are used to attach tissues beneath the skin. Nonabsorbable sutures are used on skin surfaces where they can be easily removed after an incision heals.

    C. Sizes 5-0 and 6-0 would be more appropriate to minimize scarring.

    D. Correct. Nonabsorbable sutures are used on skin surfaces where they can be easily removed after an incision heals. Sizes 5-0 and 6-0 are used for tissue on the face and neck to minimize scarring.

16. **A.** Dehiscence is the separation of wound edges.

B. Evisceration is the separation of wound edges and protrusion of abdominal organs.

C. Hemorrhaging is bleeding that does not always present with a pustular discharge.

D. Correct. Infection is a common complication in wounds and presents with inflammation, swelling, and purulent or pus-like drainage.

17. **A.** In some cases, a tourniquet will need to be applied if the bleeding continues. However, the provider should be notified and then they should advise whether a tourniquet should be used.

B. Regardless of the types of bleeding, the bleeding must first be addressed.

C. Correct. One of the first steps with a deep cut is to control the bleeding by applying pressure to the wound and elevating it.

D. A wound must first be cleaned before the wound is closed in order to prevent infection. This should only be performed by the provider.

18. **A.** This would be done for a minor burn, not a sprain.

B. Correct. For a patient who has a sprain, applying ice and a compression bandage to reduce any swelling would be appropriate.

C. A dislocation of a bone would require repositioning of the bone.

D. Although a bandage should be applied to prevent swelling, the bandage does not need to be sterile since there is no open wound. Ice should also be applied to the ankle.

19. **A.** The medical assistant should stay with the patient while the co-worker calls 911 and notifies the provider.

B. The medical assistant should check the patient's pulse before beginning CPR.

C. An AED would be used if the patient is not breathing or does not have a pulse, both of which must be checked first.

D. Correct. After calling 911, the medical assistant should check the patient's pulse and breathing before performing CPR or using an AED.

20. **A.** Sterile procedures must be used when opening any sterile instrument packet. The instrument should be gently placed in the sterile field and not handed to the provider.

B. Sterile procedures must be used when opening any sterile instrument packet. Placing a packet on the Mayo stand would make the sterile field now unsterile.

C. Correct. The sterile forceps should be dropped into the sterile field without touching the drape on the Mayo stand.

D. The sterile forceps should be gently dropped into the sterile field and not handed to the provider.

Quiz 6: Infection Control and Safety

1. **A.** E. coli is a common bacterium.

   B. Histoplasmosis is a fungus that causes a lung infection and is passed on by certain bird and bat droppings.

   C. Pinworms are a parasite.

   D. Correct. Varicella, or chickenpox, is a common virus.

2. **A. Correct.** Parasites can be further classified as protozoa, helminths, or ectoparasite.

   B. Bacteria cannot be further classified as protozoa, helminths, or ectoparasites. Their shape further classifies them.

   C. Viruses cannot be further classified as protozoa, helminths, or ectoparasite. The type of disease they cause further classifies them.

   D. Fungi cannot be further classified as protozoa, helminths, ectoparasite. How they reproduce further classifies them.

3. **A. Correct.** Contact with an infected person is a direct mode of transmission, which occurs when there is contact with an infected person or body fluid carrying the pathogen.

   B. Contact with a contaminated examination table is an indirect mode of transmission, which provides an immediate step between the portal of exit and the portal of entry.

   C. Contact with a tick is an indirect mode of transmission, which provides an immediate step between the portal of exit and the portal of entry.

   D. Contact with a pen is an indirect mode of transmission, which provides an immediate step between the portal of exit and the portal of entry.

4. **A.** A health care worker should be fever-free for at least 24 hr without the help of fever-reducing medications.

   B. A health care worker should be fever-free for at least 24 hr without the help of fever-reducing medications.

   C. A health care worker only needs to be fever-free for 24 hr without the help of fever-reducing medications.

   D. Correct. A health care worker should be fever-free for at least 24 hr without the help of fever-reducing medications.

5. **A.** Following exposure to blood, the assistant should first wash the area with soap and water.

   B. Following exposure to blood, the assistant should first wash the area with soap and water.

   C. Following exposure to blood, the assistant should first wash the area with soap and water.

   D. Correct. Following exposure to blood, the assistant should first wash the area with soap and water. Next, the assistant should report the incident to the supervisor. After that, the assistant must receive a medical evaluation. And lastly, the employee should receive health counseling.

6. **A.** According to the CDC, it is advised to rub hands together for 15 to 20 seconds. Too short of a time will not allow for the debris to lift from the skin and remove microbes. Too long of a time is not necessary and can dry out skin.

   B. According to the CDC, it is advised to rub hands together for 15 to 20 seconds.

   C. Correct. According to the CDC, it is advised to rub hands together for 15 to 20 seconds.

   D. According to the CDC, it is advised to rub hands together for 15 to 20 seconds.

7. **A.** Although it is okay to do training twice per year, it is only required to train staff annually.

   B. Correct. Facilities are required to train staff annually and upon being hired.

   C. It is a requirement to train staff at least once per year.

   D. OSHA regulates how often a facility should complete this training. Facilities can complete the training more frequently, but it needs to be completed at least annually to stay in adherence.

8. **A.** This is not a high enough temperature to ensure the sterility of autoclaved items.

   B. This is not a high enough temperature to ensure the sterility of autoclaved items.

   C. This temperature exceeds the minimum temperature that must be reached to ensure the sterility of autoclaved items. Increasing the heat to this temperature can damage the instruments.

   D. Correct. This is the minimum temperature that must be reached to ensure the sterility of autoclaved items. To kill all organisms, the autoclave must reach and stay at 121.1° C (250° F) throughout the autoclave process.

IN PRACTICE: QUIZZES
Quiz Answers: Quiz 6: Infection Control and Safety

9. **A.** Items that have been sterilized that have a wrapping intact but show a watermark cannot be used due to possible contamination.

   B. Any sterilized package that has a tear in it must be repackaged and go through the sterilization process again.

   C. Packaged autoclave instruments should be stored in a dry, covered area.

   D. Correct. Packages should be stored in a cool, dry, covered area and should not show signs of watermarks.

10. **A.** It is required for instruments to be submerged in the chemical bath for 8 hr with a closed lid to be considered sterilized.

    B. Submerging the instruments for 10 hours may cause damage.

    C. Correct. It is required for instruments to be submerged in the chemical bath for 8 hr with a closed lid to be considered sterilized.

    D. Submerging the instruments for 24 hr can cause significant damage.

11. **A.** Any time less than 20 min will not allow for proper sterilization of equipment.

    B. Any time less than 20 min will not allow for proper sterilization of equipment.

    C. Correct. Unwrapped items should be sterilized in an autoclave at 121.1° C (250° F) for 20 min to ensure all instruments are properly sterilized.

    D. Any time that exceeds 20 min might cause damage to the instruments.

12. **A.** The goal of medical asepsis is to reduce the number of micro-organisms.

    B. Correct. The goal of surgical asepsis it to eliminate pathogenic micro-organisms.

    C. Surgical asepsis must be used during invasive procedures and removes all micro-organisms.

    D. The goal of medical asepsis is to prohibit the growth of micro-organisms.

13. **A. Correct.** Washing hands is a medical aseptic technique and should be completed several times a day. It is done to help reduce the number of micro-organisms and help prohibit their growth.

    B. Surgical asepsis should be used any time a health care worker is doing an invasive procedure, or there is penetration of the patient's skin.

    C. Surgical asepsis should be used any time a health care worker is doing an invasive procedure, or there is penetration of the patient's skin.

    D. Surgical asepsis should be used any time a health care worker is doing an invasive procedure, or there is penetration of the patient's skin.

14. **A.** Gauze that is free from any biohazard contamination, such as blood, can go directly into a trash can.

    B. A used needle must be placed in a biohazard sharps container.

    C. Correct. Gauze that is contaminated with blood should be disposed of in a biohazard waste bag.

    D. A used mask that does not have any visible biohazard contaminations can be placed in the regular trash.

15. **A.** It is not necessary to wear gloves when cleaning the front office table. This would be considered low or no potential for the spread of infection since no blood or body fluids are present.

    B. It is not necessary to wear gloves when performing a blood pressure reading for a patient. This would be considered low, or no, potential for the spread of infection since no blood or body fluids are present.

    C. Correct. A health care worker must wear gloves when handling anything contaminated with blood or body fluids.

    D. It is unnecessary to wear gloves when handling instruments that have not been in contact with patients or do not have blood or body fluids on them.

16. **A.** Updating the exposure control plan monthly is not necessary if there are no changes.

    B. Updating the exposure control plan quarterly is not necessary if there are no changes.

    C. Correct. The exposure control plan needs to be updated annually, and whenever procedures that require exposure to potentially contaminated materials are added or changed.

    D. The exposure control plan needs to be updated annually, and whenever procedures that require exposure to potentially contaminated materials are added or changed.

17. **A.** Having less than the required percentage may not clean the area effectively.

    B. Having less than the required percentage may not clean the area effectively.

    C. Correct. Alcohol-based hand sanitizer must be at a minimum of 60% in a health care setting.

    D. Although 90% is an appropriate amount in an alcohol-based sanitizer, the minimum amount is 60%.

18. **A.** OSHA requires employers to make hepatitis B vaccines accessible to health care workers at no cost.

    B. Correct. OSHA requires employers to make hepatitis B vaccines accessible to health care workers at no cost.

    C. OSHA requires employers to make hepatitis B vaccines accessible to health care workers at no cost.

    D. OSHA requires employers to make hepatitis B vaccines accessible to health care workers at no cost.

19. **A.** Numbness and tingling are not common symptoms of contracting an infectious disease.

    B. Correct. Fever, headache, cough, runny nose, and malaise, or feeling tired, are common symptoms of contracting an infectious disease.

    C. Blurry vision is not a common symptom of contracting an infectious disease.

    D. Difficulty breathing is not a common symptom of contracting an infectious disease.

20. **A. Correct.** Droplet precautions should be taken when there is a risk of transmission through contact of secretions, such as coughing or sneezing.

    B. Airborne precautions should be taken when there is a risk of transmission through infectious agents floating in the air, exposing everyone in the area.

    C. Contact precautions should be taken when there is a risk of transmission through direct and indirect touching.

    D. Transmission-based precautions is a general term and is broken down into contact, droplet, and airborne precautions.

Quiz 7: Point-of-Care Testing and Laboratory Procedures

1. **A.** This may be the only stool the patient may have for the day and this will not create a false positive

    B. Correct. Vitamin C and iron supplements need to be avoided 3 days prior to collection because they can cause a false positive for fecal occult blood.

    C. Fiber will not alter the results. Fiber is used to help stimulate stools.

    D. Regular medications should not be stopped.

2. **A.** The urine needs to go into the container for collection and testing.

    B. Correct. The inside of the container should not be touched, it is sterile and should remain so.

    C. No preservatives need to be added, and doing so would alter the results.

    D. Gloves will still contaminate the specimen cup if touched inside.

3. **A.** This is included on the requisition.

    B. This is included on the requisition.

    C. This is included on the requisition.

    D. Correct. The person who collects the specimen should include their initials on the specimen.

IN PRACTICE: QUIZZES

Quiz Answers: Quiz 7: Point-of-Care Testing and Laboratory Procedures

4. **A. Correct.** This type of collection is important for the quantitative analysis of components such as protein when analyzing kidney function. This collection of urine can analyze substances that are sporadically released into the urine over a 24-hour period.

   B. A clean-catch specimen is used when the provider suspects a urinary tract infection and will not provide quantitative results.

   C. A random specimen will not provide quantitative results.

   D. A first voided specimen will have higher concentration but will not provide quantitative results.

5. **A.** Blood hemoglobin A1C below 5.7% is considered normal, and 12.0% would indicate diabetes.

   B. Correct. HbA1C should be less than 5.7% to have diabetes under control.

   C. This number is too elevated. Normal range should be below 5.7%.

   D. An A1C of 8.0% is indicative of uncontrolled diabetes. The normal range should be below 5.7%.

6. **A.** 40 to 150 mg/dL is the normal range for triglycerides.

   B. 70 to 100 mg/dL is the normal range for a fasting glucose.

   C. Correct. A normal range for a total cholesterol is 130 to 200 mg/dL.

   D. 150 to 220 mg/dL is a high total cholesterol.

7. **A. Correct.** Name and birthdate are used in all procedures to verify the patient. The patient should be asked their name and birthdate, and these should be compared to the requisition to verify the patient.

   B. An address and patient identification number are not used to verify the patient.

   C. Diagnosis and insurance information do not verify a patient.

   D. The patient's name and insurance do not verify the correct patient.

8. **A.** The insurance carrier's information can be on the requisition but not on the specimen.

   B. A patient's medication information is not proper identification for a specimen label.

   C. Correct. The time the specimen was collected should be documented on the specimen label. Specimen containers should be labeled with patient's name and date of birth, date and time of collection, and the initials of the person collecting it.

   D. A patient's diagnosis is noted on the laboratory requisition form but does not need to be identified on the specimen label.

9. **A.** A chain of command is not required. The specimen is a legal specimen that needs to be handled in a chain of custody to prevent any possibility of tampering with before the test is conducted.

   B. Correct. The specimen is a legal specimen that needs to be handled in a chain of custody to prevent any possibility of tampering with before the test is conducted.

   C. Medical cards are sometimes needed if applicable for billing. However, they are not required for the transportation of the drug screening.

   D. Authorization forms from employers are requested for drug screening but are not required in the transportation of a drug screening.

10. **A.** Although the preanalytical phase is included in quality assurance, instruments are maintained and calibrated in the analytic phase.

    B. Correct. Instruments are maintained and calibrated in the analytic phase along with several other processes.

    C. There is not a midanalytical phase in quality assurance. Machines are calibrated and checked in the analytic phase.

    D. Although the postanalytical phase is included in quality assurance, instruments are maintained and calibrated in the analytic phase.

11. **A.** Distance vision is tested by the Snellen chart.

    B. Near vision is tested by using the Jaeger chart to measure the patient's ability to read items at a close distance.

    C. Vision acuity is tested with an eye chart.

    D. Correct. Ishihara color plates test for color deficiency. Testing for color blindness can alert a patient to be aware of difficulty distinguishing between red and green as well as between blue and yellow. The most common type of color deficiency is a red-green deficiency. Screening is done by testing the patient on 11 color plates within an Ishihara book.

12. **A.** Results will not produce a continuous up and down line.

    B. Results will not produce a declining line.

    C. A normal tympanogram produces a peak on the graph, whereas an abnormal tympanogram will produce a flat line.

    D. Correct. A normal tympanogram produces a peak on the graph, whereas an abnormal tympanogram will produce a flat line.

13. **A.** A wheal should occur within the first 15 min. Waiting only 5 min is not long enough for a "reaction" time and may produce a false-negative result.

    B. 10 minutes is too short of a time to allow for a wheal to form.

    C. Correct. A diluted allergen is applied to a scratch or prick on the surface of the skin. If a wheal occurs in the first 15 min, the allergist can identify the substance as a possible allergen and consider intradermal testing.

    D. 25 min is too long to wait because a reaction should have already been noted at 15 min.

14. **A.** Discontinuing antihistamines 30 days prior to skin testing is not necessary.

    B. Discontinuing antihistamines 15 days prior to skin testing is not necessary.

    C. Correct. Discontinuing antihistamines 3 days prior to skin testing allows the body to rid itself of antihistamines and allows the proper skin testing process to take place.

    D. Discontinuing antihistamines for 7 days prior to skin testing is not necessary.

15. **A. Correct.** Three tests are done to do a comparison with the predicted values in order to detect pulmonary disease.

    B. A patient must complete three maneuvers to have a good comparison.

    C. A patient only needs to complete three maneuvers to compare.

    D. One maneuver does not provide enough data to evaluate lung function.

16. **A. Correct.** The peak flow test is to measure how well air is expelled from the lungs.

    B. The patient should not suck air in, as they are being tested on their ability to blow air out.

    C. The patient should fill their lungs with air and blow it out as fast as they can.

    D. The patient is being measured on the force of their exhale, so they should blow out fast and hard.

17. **A.** The lab will process the specimen, but the results will not be accurate since the patient was not fasting as directed from the provider.

    B. Handwritten or electronic lab requisitions are acceptable for specimen processing.

    C. The lab will process the specimen, but results will not be accurate considering urine should be kept in refrigeration if not processed within 1 hr.

    D. Correct. Misidentification will cause the lab to reject a specimen because they are unable to verify the correct patient with the specimen.

18. **A.** This is an error that occurs in the analytical phase or during the laboratory processing phase.

    B. This is postanalytical, so this error would occur after the specimen was run.

    C. This is postanalytical, so this would occur after the specimen has been run which impacts the test results.

    D. Correct. An order entry error is an error that could have occurred prior to the collection of the specimen and could affect the test results.

IN PRACTICE: QUIZZES
Quiz Answers: Quiz 8: Phlebotomy

19. **A.** Children who have normal hearing are able to hear tones at 15 decibels. An adult who has normal hearing should be able to hear tones at 25 decibels.

    B. 20 is not the normal decibels for adults to hear tones.

    C. Correct. Adults with normal hearing are able to hear tones at 25 decibels.

    D. Adults with normal hearing should be able to hear tones at 25 decibels, and a child should be able to hear at 15 decibels.

20. **A. Correct.** QuickVue pregnancy test kits require a 3 min reaction time for accurate results.

    B. 1 min is not long enough for the amount of hCG in the urine to react with the test cassette.

    C. For accurate results, the medical assistant must wait a full 3 min, which allows proper absorption of the hCG in the urine to react with the test cassette.

    D. Rapid streptococcus testing requires 5 min to process.

Quiz 8: Phlebotomy

1. **A.** Cigarette smoking will not affect a lipid panel test.

   B. Correct. It is important to ask about the timing of the patient's last meal to ensure they fasted prior to a lipid panel blood draw.

   C. The presence of medical allergies will not alter the lipid panel test.

   D. Taking acetaminophen will not affect the lipid panel results.

2. **A.** The assistant should only draw the necessary tubes, and ensure the tubes drawn coincide with the tests requested.

   B. While another medical assistant might know the answer, it is best practice to look it up in the reference manual.

   C. The assistant should only draw the appropriate amount of blood for the requested tube and avoid drawing any extra tubes of blood.

   D. Correct. The assistant should always check the laboratory manual to determine which tube to use for a particular test.

3. **A.** EDTA tubes should be inverted more than 2 to 4 times.

   B. EDTA tubes should be inverted more than 4 to 6 times.

   C. EDTA tubes should be inverted more than 6 to 8 times.

   D. Correct. EDTA tubes should be inverted 8 to 10 times.

4. **A. Correct.** The assistant should first attempt to locate a vein in the antecubital space because the antecubital space contains the largest peripheral veins.

   B. The assistant should not first attempt to locate a vein in the foot.

   C. The assistant should not first attempt to locate a vein in the wrist.

   D. The assistant should not first attempt to locate a vein on the back of the hand.

5. **A. Correct.** A 70% alcohol concentration is the preferred alcohol concentration.

   B. A 40% alcohol concentration is not sufficient to disinfect the skin.

   C. A 90% alcohol concentration is too strong.

   D. A 100% alcohol concentration is too strong.

6. **A.** The green-top tube should not be drawn first.

   B. Correct. The red-top tube should be drawn first.

   C. The gray and red marbled-top tubes should not be drawn first.

   D. The lavender-top tube should not be drawn first.

7. **A.** A 20-gauge needle is too large of a lumen to use with a butterfly system.

   B. A 20-gauge needle is too large of a lumen to use with a butterfly system.

   C. A needle length of ¼ inch is too small to use with a butterfly system.

   D. Correct. Butterfly needles typically have a 21- to 23-gauge with a needle length of ½ to ¾ inch.

IN PRACTICE: QUIZZES
Quiz Answers: Quiz 8: Phlebotomy

8. **A. Correct.** Improper data entry is a postanalytical consideration because it is an error that occurs after the specimen has been processed.

   B. Insufficient quantity for testing is a preanalytical consideration because it is an error that occurs during the venipuncture procedures.

   C. Mislabeling of specimen tubes is a preanalytical consideration because it is an error that occurs immediately after performing the venipuncture procedures.

   D. Error in patient identification is a preanalytical consideration because it is an error that occurs prior to performing the venipuncture procedures.

9. **A.** The assistant should instruct the patient to leave the bandaging in place for a minimum of 15 min.

   B. Correct. The assistant should instruct the patient to leave the bandaging in place for a minimum of 15 min.

   C. The assistant should instruct the patient to leave the bandaging in place for a minimum of 15 min.

   D. The assistant should instruct the patient to leave the bandaging in place for a minimum of 15 min.

10. **A.** Blood cultures, not timed specimens, require specific preparation of the skin.

    B. Correct. Timed specimens are crucial for therapeutic medication-level monitoring to confirm the patient's medication dosage and adherence.

    C. Timed specimens are not required to be collected in the morning.

    D. Timed specimens are not required to be obtained from the basilic vein.

11. **A. Correct.** Serum specimens should be allowed to clot for 30 min prior to centrifugation.

    B. Serum specimens should be allowed to clot for 30 min prior to centrifugation. Two hours is too long because it will cause leaching of substance changes.

    C. Serum specimens should be allowed to clot for 30 min prior to centrifugation.

    D. Serum specimens should be allowed to clot for 30 min prior to centrifugation.

12. **A.** The provider's tax identification number does not need to be included on the laboratory requisition form.

    B. The patient's height does not need to be included on the laboratory requisition form.

    C. The patient's weight does not need to be included on the laboratory requisition form.

    D. Correct. The diagnosis code that correlates with the tests being ordered (ICD-10) needs to be included on the laboratory requisition form.

13. **A.** The ordering provider should be notified of the critical laboratory values.

    B. The ordering provider should be notified of the critical laboratory values.

    C. Correct. When critical laboratory values are received at the office, the ordering provider should be notified and it should be documented that the provider was notified.

    D. The ordering provider, not the nurse, should be notified of the critical laboratory values.

14. **A. Correct.** Light-sensitive samples should be wrapped in foil to shield them from light.

    B. Gauze would not protect light-sensitive samples from light.

    C. Some samples require deep cooling, but light-sensitive samples require shielding from light. An ice bath would not protect light-sensitive samples from light.

    D. A biohazard bag would not protect light-sensitive samples from light.

15. **A.** The ordering provider must review the results prior to scheduling a follow-up appointment.

    B. The ordering provider must review the results prior to including them in the patient's medical record.

    C. Correct. All results must be forwarded to the ordering provider first.

    D. The provider should be notified first. The provider must then reorder the test for the patient prior to requesting them to return to the office.

IN PRACTICE: QUIZZES
Quiz Answers: Quiz 8: Phlebotomy

16. A. Serum separator gel is found in tiger-top tubes.

    B. Clot activator is found in red-top tubes.

    C. **Correct.** Sodium citrate is found in light blue blood tubes.

    D. Lithium heparin is found in green-top tubes.

17. A. Blood cultures do not require chain of custody documentation.

    B. **Correct.** Blood alcohol levels and drug screenings often require chain of custody documentation.

    C. Chemistry studies do not often require chain of custody documentation.

    D. Plasma determinations do not often require chain of custody documentation.

18. A. Only trained technicians should calibrate medical devices.

    B. Best practice is to place the device out of service until it is calibrated.

    C. **Correct.** The assistant should notify the laboratory supervisor or office manager of the overdue status and remove the device from service.

    D. The service label on medical devices should not be removed or altered.

19. A. The assistant should not ask the patient to take some deep breaths.

    B. The assistant should not finish the procedure as quickly as possible.

    C. **Correct.** The assistant should stop the procedure and alert the provider immediately.

    D. The assistant should stop the procedure, notify the provider, and ensure the patient's safety.

20. A. This question will not help to ensure the patient's safety during the phlebotomy test.

    B. If the assistant is truly concerned about a patient's ability to keep their arm stable during the procedure, they should work with the patient to understand the underlying concerns, rather than asking a question that might make the patient feel more uncomfortable.

    C. This question will not help to ensure the patient's safety during the phlebotomy test.

    D. **Correct.** Asking about prior fainting episodes allows the assistant to take measures to ensure their safety, such as having the patient lie down for the blood draw.

Quiz 9: EKG and Cardiovascular Testing

1. **A.** The patient is in a prone position when they are lying on their stomach. This is not a suitable position for performing an EKG.

   B. Correct. A supine position occurs when a patient is lying on their back. This is the best position for performing an EKG.

   C. Fowler's position is when the patient is sitting up at a 90° angle. This is not a suitable position for performing an EKG.

   D. The left lateral position is when the patient is lying on their side with one leg folded. This position is best used for a colonoscopy.

2. **A.** A patient's arms should not be tied to the exam table during a procedure.

   B. A patient should not be held down while conducting a procedure.

   C. Cleaning the skin and taping down the electrodes will not decrease the somatic tremor artifact.

   D. Correct. If patients have conditions that lead to uncontrolled muscle movement, have them lay their hands with the palms down under their buttocks to reduce somatic interference.

3. **A.** This is the location for the green limb lead electrode.

   B. This is the location for the black limb lead electrode.

   C. Correct. The electrode for lead V2 is placed on the left side of the sternum, fourth intercostal space.

   D. This is the location for the V6 lead electrode.

4. **A.** The green limb lead goes on the right leg.

   B. The white limb lead goes on the right arm.

   C. The red limb lead goes on the left leg.

   D. Correct. The black limb lead goes on the left arm.

5. **A.** An interrupted baseline is obvious when there is a break in the tracing. It is usually related to a disconnected or broken lead wire.

   B. Correct. A patient with lotion or cream on the skin is correct. Cleaning the skin prior to attaching the electrodes and instructing the patient to avoid using creams and lotions will assist in reducing a wandering baseline.

   C. Somatic tremors are characterized by irregular spikes throughout the tracing and are related to muscle movement.

   D. AC interference, or 60-cycle interference, is characterized by regular spikes in the EKG tracing. It is related to poor grounding or external electricity interfering with the tracing. Nearby electrical equipment, such as lights, computers, and other items plugged into wall sockets, can result in AC interference.

6. **A.** 60-cycle interference is due to nearby electrical equipment.

   B. Interrupted baselines are breaks in the EKG tracing and are not associated with breathing.

   C. Correct. Movement with patient breathing is the most common cause of wandering baseline.

   D. A somatic tremor is a result of involuntary muscle movement, typically of the arms and legs.

7. **A.** This technique could be used to address an interrupted baseline.

   B. This is not a recommended technique.

   C. Correct. Frequent regular spikes are seen with 60-cycle interference caused by nearby electrical equipment.

   D. This technique could be used to address somatic tremors.

8. **A.** Somatic tremors do not interrupt the baseline.

   B. Correct. Somatic tremors are caused by involuntary muscle movement and produce irregular spikes and artifacts. 60-cycle interference is characterized by regular spikes in the EKG tracing.

   C. 60-cycle interference does not affect the baseline.

   D. 60-cycle interference does not alter the regularity of the rhythm.

IN PRACTICE: QUIZZES
Quiz Answers: Quiz 9: EKG and Cardiovascular Testing

9. **A.** Patients should not be exposed during the entire EKG to protect privacy.

   B. Correct. The patient should remove clothing above the waist so the chest electrodes can be placed in the correct location. The patient should be covered as soon as the leads are attached.

   C. Patients should not be exposed during the entire EKG to protect privacy.

   D. Patients must remove clothes above the waist so the chest electrodes can be placed in the correct locations.

10. **A.** Typically, 10 electrodes are needed to record a 12-lead EKG.

    B. Correct. Typically, 10 electrodes are needed to record a 12-lead EKG.

    C. Typically, 10 electrodes are needed to record a 12-lead EKG.

    D. Typically, 10 electrodes are needed to record a 12-lead EKG.

11. **A.** An electrocardiograph is a machine that captures the data.

    B. The lead wires provide the data for the tracing.

    C. Correct. Each electrode is impregnated with an electrolyte gel that serves as a conductor of impulses. If the electrode doesn't come with an electrolyte gel already in it, a gel can be applied before applying the electrode to the patient.

    D. EKG paper is used to provide a visual of the electrical impulses from the heart.

12. **A.** Asystole takes time to display a perfectly flat line across all leads.

    B. An electrical interference would result in additional waves.

    C. Correct. The most common cause of an interrupted baseline is a detached lead wire.

    D. Ventricular fibrillation produces waves on the EKG.

13. **A.** The duration of a standard calibration box is 0.2 seconds.

    B. The duration of a standard calibration box is 0.2 seconds.

    C. The duration of a standard calibration box is 0.2 seconds.

    D. Correct. The duration of a standard calibration box is 0.2 seconds.

14. **A.** The standard calibration box is 10 mm tall.

    B. The standard calibration box is 10 mm tall.

    C. The standard calibration box is 10 mm tall.

    D. Correct. The standard calibration box is 10 mm tall.

15. **A. Correct.** Elevating the head of the bed will take pressure off the diaphragm and ease breathing.

    B. Patients should not hold their breath for the exam.

    C. Although the patient may benefit from supplemental oxygen, it must be ordered by the provider and there is another action that would benefit the patient immediately.

    D. The EKG should be recorded with the patient lying on their back or in a semi-Fowler's position.

16. **A. Correct.** The assistant should immediately notify the provider of the elevated blood pressure reading.

    B. The stress test should not be continued with such an elevated blood pressure.

    C. The stress test should be stopped immediately.

    D. The medical assistant should not administer medication without a provider's order.

17. **A. Correct.** Sinus tachycardia has narrow QRS complexes. Ventricular tachycardia has wide QRS complexes.

    B. Ventricular tachycardia has wide QRS complexes, whereas sinus tachycardia has narrow QRS complexes.

    C. Sinus tachycardia is a dysrhythmia where the heart rate is greater than 100/min and there is one P wave preceding each QRS complex.

    D. Sinus tachycardia has narrow QRS complexes, whereas ventricular tachycardia has wide QRS complexes.

18. **A. Correct.** Atrial fibrillation is characterized by an irregular rhythm, absence of P waves, and narrow QRS complexes.

    B. Ventricular fibrillation has no discernable waves.

    C. Sinus rhythm is very regular and has P waves.

    D. Sinus arrest has P waves and is only irregular when the P waves are absent.

19. **A.** The U wave represents late ventricular repolarization.

    B. The Q wave represents early ventricular depolarization.

    C. The T wave represents ventricular repolarization.

    D. Correct. The P wave represents atrial depolarization.

20. **A.** This is the location for the red limb lead electrode.

    B. This is the location for the white limb lead electrode.

    C. Correct. The electrode for lead V4 is placed on the left side of the sternum, fifth intercostal space at the midclavicular line.

    D. This is the location for the V6 lead electrode.

Quiz 10: Patient Care Coordination and Education

1. **A.** Colonoscopies are a recommended screening for colorectal cancer in adults aged 45 to 75.

    B. Prediabetic testing is a recommended screening for prediabetes mellitus and type 2 diabetes mellitus in adults aged 35 to 70 who are overweight or obese.

    C. Hepatitis C is passed from an infected person through blood. A person with risk factors should be tested. These risk factors include a history of injection of illegal drugs, an organ transplant before 1992, or someone who was born between 1945 and 1965.

    D. Correct. Males between the ages of 65 and 75 who have smoked at some point in their lives are more susceptible to an abdominal aortic aneurysm and should receive this screening.

2. **A.** It is essential to evaluate the patient on the information presented to ensure the patient has retained and understands the information to successfully adhere to treatment plans.

    B. The purpose of evaluating the patient after an educational session is to ensure the patient understood the educational information provided, not to determine if the patient has a learning deficit. The medical assistant cannot determine if a patient has a learning deficit.

    C. Correct. The information presented should be verified for accuracy before it is presented to the patient. It is essential to evaluate the patient on the information presented to ensure the patient has retained and understands the information to successfully adhere to treatment plans.

    D. It is important to correctly evaluate patients after an educational session. However, it is not to demonstrate correct evaluation procedures to the provider.

IN PRACTICE: QUIZZES
Quiz Answers: Quiz 10: Patient Care Coordination and Education

3. **A.** Patients are recommended to have annual mammograms beginning at age 40 and older.

   B. Patients are recommended to have annual mammograms beginning at age 40 and older.

   C. Correct. Patients are recommended to have annual mammograms beginning at age 40 and older.

   D. Patients are recommended to have annual mammograms beginning at age 40 and older.

4. **A.** Hospitalization is for acute onset of medical conditions and not for long-term living conditions.

   B. Assisted living facilities are for patients who are able to perform some of their own care.

   C. Adult day programs are for adults who are still able to take care of their basic needs during the day.

   D. Correct. Long-term care facilities are for treating patients who have conditions that require medical care ranging from mild care to acute care.

5. **A.** It is not necessary to schedule a social worker visit with the patient.

   B. The internet isn't a referral source, and using the internet to find resources might overwhelm the patient.

   C. The patient should not be provided with a questionnaire to return to the office.

   D. Correct. A medical assistant should maintain a list of community resources that can help further assist the patient.

6. **A.** Warning or scaring a patient that they may not get better if they can't remember to take their medication is not a way the medical assistant can help the patient remember to take their medications.

   B. Medication boxes can often be arranged to provide a week's worth of a patient's medications and are labeled for morning, afternoon, and evening doses, as necessary, to ensure the patient takes the correct medications at the correct time.

   C. Sending daily texts to a patient is time-consuming and not feasible.

   D. Correct. Many patients do not refer to their calendar daily, or at the right time, for their medication doses.

7. **A.** The goal of a PCMH does not affect the need for health care services.

   B. The goal of a PCMH does not contribute to the revenue cycle.

   C. Correct. The goal of a PCMH is to have a centralized setting that facilitates partnerships between the patient, the provider, and the patient's family (when appropriate).

   D. The goal of a PCMH does not impact the travel or time for the patient.

8. **A.** Lack of communication between providers regarding patient histories, medication therapies, and overall patient needs are the main reasons for increased risk of rehospitalization, adverse clinical events, increased spending, and poor care quality.

   B. Correct. Transitions are areas that fall short when it comes to providing quality care. Lack of communication between providers regarding patient histories, medication therapies, and overall patient needs are the main reasons for increased risk of rehospitalization, adverse clinical events, increased spending, and poor care quality.

   C. Lack of communication between providers regarding patient histories, medication therapies, and overall patient needs are the main reasons for increased risk of rehospitalization, adverse clinical events, increased spending, and poor care quality.

   D. Lack of communication between providers regarding patient histories, medication therapies, and overall patient needs are the main reasons for increased risk of rehospitalization, adverse clinical events, increased spending, and poor care quality.

9. **A.** Kinesthetic learning is a hands-on learning approach.

   B. Correct. Auditory learning is achieved by hearing the information.

   C. Visual learning is achieved by seeing the materials.

   D. Tactile learning is achieved by touching and demonstrating.

10. **A. Correct.** Preventive measures include healthy behaviors such as covering a cough or sneeze, handwashing or utilizing hand sanitizer after coughing, sneezing, using the restroom, or touching objects, and receiving immunizations and screenings.

    B. Preventive measures include healthy behaviors such as covering a cough or sneeze.

    C. Preventive measures include healthy behaviors such as handwashing or utilizing hand sanitizer after coughing, sneezing, using the restroom, or touching objects.

    D. Preventive measures include healthy behaviors such as handwashing or utilizing hand sanitizer after coughing, sneezing, using the restroom, or touching objects.

11. **A. Correct.** Accessibility to transportation is a social determinant that can prevent a patient from meeting their needs.

    B. Smoking is considered a behavioral determinant.

    C. Sickle cell anemia is considered a genetic determinant that can prevent a patient from meeting their needs.

    D. Weather and climate changes are physical determinants that can impact the needs of patients.

12. **A. Correct.** A visual impairment can be a barrier to learning.

    B. Color blindness should not be a barrier to learning.

    C. Having a college-level education should not be a barrier to learning.

    D. A patient being self-employed should not be a barrier to learning.

13. **A.** Verifying insurance coverage is important prior to the patient having an encounter with the provider. However, it is not a necessary step to complete regarding prescription medications.

    B. The patient will be responsible for verifying their preferred pharmacy's hours when filling a prescription medication.

    C. The patient's employment status is needed for their demographic section of their health record. However, it is not needed in regard to prescription medications.

    D. Correct. Medication education is an important step for the medical assistant to complete with the patient prior to the patient leaving the office as it enables patient adherence and optimizes patient outcomes.

14. **A.** Ineffective communication would result in increased long-term medical costs.

    B. Correct. Ineffective communication between medical providers might result in rehospitalization.

    C. Ineffective communication would not provide greater availability of medical resources.

    D. Ineffective communication would decrease the quality of care the patient receives.

15. **A.** This type of referral is not required to be in formal writing.

    B. Information about other patients should not be shared. It is important to refer the patient to a person who can assist them with quitting.

    C. Correct. A medical assistant can refer the patient to this resource without a written referral from the provider.

    D. This referral does not require contact with the insurance provider. The patient should be given contact information for the appropriate resource.

16. **A. Correct.** Female patients need to start annual mammograms at 45 years of age.

    B. Prostate exams are only for male patients.

    C. Chest x-rays are diagnostic measures, not preventive care screenings.

    D. Electrocardiograms monitor heart rhythms and are usually performed to diagnose a heart disorder or to document the patient's rhythm at an annual appointment. Electrocardiograms are not completed as a preventive care measure.

17. **A.** Store and forward telemedicine is transmission of medical data to a provider or medical specialist for assessment. It is not a substitute for in-person visits.

    B. Correct. Live video is substituted when patients cannot physically make it to the provider's office, or a situation restricts the patient from going to the provider's office.

    C. RPM is the collection of personal and medical data from a patient at one location via electronic communication technologies. It is not a substitute for in-person visits.

    D. mHealth includes health care, public health practice, and patient education supported by mobile communication devices, such as cell phones, tablet computers, and laptops. It is not a substitute for in-person visits.

18. **A. Correct.** These factors related to different cultures' belief in food and diet can impact adherence with treatment.

    B. Cultural beliefs related to education should not affect the patent's adherence with their medical treatment.

    C. Cultural beliefs related to traditions should not affect the patient's adherence with their medical treatment.

    D. Cultural beliefs related to values should not affect the patient's adherence with their medical treatment.

19. **A. Correct.** It is advised that individuals receive an influenza vaccination annually.

    B. This vaccine is only recommended for health care workers or those who are exposed to blood and bodily fluids.

    C. This is not a required vaccine unless traveling to developing nations.

    D. Many people over the age of 65 have already had the chickenpox, so the varicella vaccine is not required to be given regularly.

20. **A.** The recommended age to start screening for colorectal cancer is 45 years old.

    B. Correct. The recommended age to start screening for colorectal cancer is 45 years old.

    C. The recommended age to start screening for colorectal cancer is 45 years old, even with a family history.

    D. The recommended age to start screening for colorectal cancer is 45 years old, even without a family history.

Quiz 11: Administrative Assisting

1. **A.** Sports physicals are not as resource intensive as new patient visits.

    B. Established patient visits are not as resource intensive as new patient visits.

    C. Follow-up patient visits are not as resource intensive as new patient visits.

    D. Correct. New patient visits are more resource intensive. They involve getting to know the history and current medical condition of the patient.

2. **A.** Third-party payer requirements do not have an impact on determining the duration of an appointment.

    B. Correct. The provider's habits and preferences can have an impact on determining the duration of an appointment.

    C. Patient availability does not have an impact on determining the duration of an appointment.

    D. Reimbursement methods do not have an impact on determining the duration of an appointment.

3. **A. Correct.** Screening questions should include the patient's name, telephone number, and reason for the visit.

    B. Asking the patient about their employer is not necessary during the screening process.

    C. Asking the patient what medications they are currently taking is not necessary during the screening process.

    D. Asking the patient for their previous address is not necessary during the screening process.

4. **A.** Excel is spreadsheet software, it does not include encounter forms.

    B. Word is word processing software, it does not include documentation of the encounter form.

    C. Inventory software is used to record equipment and supplies it does not include encounter forms.

    D. Correct. Practice management software includes the patient medical record where the encounter form resides.

5. A. Requesting to see the patient's photo identification should be completed during the check-in process.

   B. Asking the patient what medications they are currently taking is part of the examination.

   C. **Correct.** The assistant should review the after-visit summary with the patient following their appointment.

   D. Evaluating the patient's past, family, and social history is part of the examination.

6. A. Procedure codes include any treatment or services rendered by the provider.

   B. ICD-10-PCS codes are for hospital, or inpatient, only.

   C. HCPCS codes are used for administration of medication and durable medical equipment and other services not reflected in CPT codes.

   D. **Correct.** Diagnosis codes are determined by reviewing the reason for a patient's visit.

7. A. **Correct.** Elective and costly medical services can require preauthorization before they are provided.

   B. Preventive medical services do not require preauthorization.

   C. An annual wellness exam does not require preauthorization.

   D. Follow-up care for a burn does not require preauthorization.

8. A. Predetermination is finding out the payer's allowed amount for a specified service. This process should be accomplished quickly on a payer's portal or website and does not relate to information on the billing request.

   B. Verification of insurance coverage should be confirmed prior to preparing the billing request and does not accompany information when preparing the billing request.

   C. Explanation of benefits informs the patient of what the insurance has covered for their service and the remaining balance the patient owes.

   D. **Correct.** Medical necessity should be supported with code selections.

9. A. Reimbursement methodologies determine how health care services are reimbursed.

   B. **Correct.** Interoperability helps to ensure that health care organizations and professionals have all the important information needed regarding patient care.

   C. Audits and reviews should be used to verify that information is accurate.

   D. Credentialing is licensing and certifications for medical professionals.

10. A. Patient eligibility should be verified when scheduling appointments and receiving services. It is not related to charge reconciliations.

    B. Continuity of care ensures the patient has the care they need by the people qualified on a continual basis. It is not related to charge reconciliations.

    C. **Correct.** Reconciliation is the process of ensuring that the accounts are all balanced and accurate. The amounts should be entered accurately into the correct patient account.

    D. Preauthorization is for elective and expensive medical services. It is not related to charge reconciliations.

11. A. The billing department is responsible for notifying patients of their financial responsibility.

    B. **Correct.** A clearinghouse is an intermediary that has contracted to accept and process the claims for the third-party payer. They also assist with reducing claim errors.

    C. Payroll should be done by human resources or outsourced to a human resources firm.

    D. OSHA should perform safety inspections and evaluate procedures.

12. A. The patient should not be billed.

    B. Resubmitting the claim will cause a denial for duplicate services, an adjustment should be submitted instead.

    C. **Correct.** The assistant should verify the diagnosis and procedure codes, attach supporting documentation, and submit an appeal for a claim that was denied for lack of medical necessity.

    D. The balance should not be written off.

IN PRACTICE: QUIZZES
Quiz Answers: Quiz 11: Administrative Assisting

13. **A.** The Patient's Bill of Rights informs the patient of their health care rights to receive quality care.

    B. A Notice of Privacy Practices informs the patient of the expectations of the health care facility.

    C. Advance directives allow medical decisions to be made by a specified person in the event the patient is unable to communicate them.

    D. Correct. The Advance Beneficiary Notice of Noncoverage (ABN) is a form used for Medicare beneficiaries when the service may not be covered by a fee-for-service Medicare plan.

14. **A.** Reimbursement rates are not impacted by reminder calls to patients about upcoming appointments.

    B. Claim denials are not impacted by reminder calls to patients about upcoming appointments.

    C. Correct. Confirming and reminding patients of scheduled appointments can decrease no-show rates.

    D. Patient financial responsibility is not impacted by reminder calls to patients about upcoming appointments.

15. **A.** Drop-down menus do not require less information.

    B. Correct. Drop-down menus can help to increase the accuracy of data entered as they do not allow for typographical errors.

    C. Specificity is decreased with drop-down menus because choices can be limited.

    D. Drop down menus do not impact the consistency of data.

16. **A.** Inspection logs do not keep track of depreciation value.

    B. Inspection logs do not monitor the users.

    C. Correct. Medical equipment inspection logs document a timeline of scheduled maintenance.

    D. Inspection logs keep track of preventive checks and scheduled maintenance. It does not determine sales on equipment.

17. **A. Correct.** When a patient begins receiving medical services at a health care facility, they will be given a username and access code to log into their patient portal.

    B. The facility provides the patient with a username and access code, not an email address.

    C. The facility provides the patient with a username and access code, not a fee schedule.

    D. A referral is when a primary care provider refers a patient to a different medical provider. It is not provided to a patient to log into their patient portal.

18. **A.** The assistant should provide technical guidance and support to the patient to assist with logging in and ensuring the settings are correct.

    B. Correct. The assistant should assist the patient with logging in an verify their settings are correct.

    C. The assistant should not ask the patient to reschedule when a family member is there to assist.

    D. Interpreters are for language and communication barriers, not technology issues. Therefore, the assistant should not request an interpreter to assist.

19. **A. Correct.** Accounts receivable (A/R) aging reports for a health care facility include any amount of money that is anticipated to be paid to them. An A/R aging report should be printed so that the older debts can be addressed first.

    B. Accounts paid (A/P) aging reports show money that will be paid out by the health care facility, not money owed to them.

    C. A remittance advice shows the results from claim adjudications.

    D. A bank deposit statement shows the financial transactions from the health care facility with the bank.

20. **A. Correct.** Copayment is a predetermined set amount that is due at the time of services.

B. Coinsurance is a shared financial amount that has a percentage due by the patient and a percentage due by the third-party payer after the deductible has been met.

C. The deductible is the annual amount that is paid by the patient before the third-party payer's financial responsibility is paid.

D. A write-off is an amount that the health care facility deems to be noncollectible.

Quiz 12: Communication and Customer Service

1. **A.** It is important to respect the patient's wishes and not try to convince them.

   B. Correct. The assistant should respect the patient's wishes.

   C. An aggressive communication style will not help and could make the patient feel forced to adhere.

   D. It is important to respect the patient's wishes and not be aggressive.

2. **A.** Assumptions should not be made about the patient or their hearing.

   B. Assumptions should not be made about the patient if their medical record does not state the patient has a visual impairment.

   C. Correct. The assistant should speak clearly while maintaining good eye contact.

   D. It is important to not use jargon but instead use language that can be understood by the patient.

3. **A. Correct.** Communication between medical professionals can include more complex medical terms.

   B. Lay terms are used with patients as they do not tend to have the training for medical terms.

   C. It is important to respect the provider's time by summarizing concisely and to the point about what needs to be written in the correspondence.

   D. If an aggressive communication style is used with the provider, it may come across as being disrespectful towards a team member, as well as not showing respect for the knowledge and authority the provider holds.

4. **A.** Visual communicators tend to communicate more by what they see.

   B. Auditory communicators tend to communicate more by what they hear.

   C. Manipulative communicators can be very one-sided with ulterior motives.

   D. Correct. Kinesthetic communicators focus on body language and the messages that it conveys.

5. **A.** Nonverbal cues are part of the communication process with virtual visits. However, in-person visits at the office provide an environment where it is much easier to assess nonverbal cues for understanding.

   B. Body language does apply. However, it is less prevalent than with in-person visits.

   C. Personal space is not a factor in virtual visits.

   D. Correct. Virtual visits rely on the words spoken for effective communication.

6. **A. Correct.** This is a direct question with one answer, so it is closed-ended.

   B. This is an open-ended question.

   C. This is an open-ended question.

   D. This is an open-ended question.

7. **A.** Vocal pitch and tone should be appropriate for speaking with patients, ensuring it is not monotone with a loud tone.

   B. Correct. It is important to speak clearly and enunciate words while communicating via telephone.

   C. Unless the patient has an impairment, speaking loudly usually indicates an aggressive communication style approach, which is not appropriate or necessary.

   D. Body language is not present on the phone. However, nonverbal cues can be used, such as allowing time for the patient to digest words of the intended message.

IN PRACTICE: QUIZZES
Quiz Answers: Quiz 12: Communication and Customer Service

8. **A.** Templates assist with format, but they do not spellcheck or proofread.

    B. Correct. Templates are sample letters that provide the proper format. Words can be added to templates when it is appropriate to do so.

    C. Templates assist with format, but they do not replace etiquette.

    D. Templates assist with a formal format by providing a consistent structure of communication as it serves as a legal record in a patient's chart.

9. **A. Correct.** Allowing the patient to vent can help to de-escalate the situation.

    B. Changing providers is not in the best interest of the patient since they would have to establish a new relationship during a stressful situation.

    C. Reminding the patient that they were late would likely escalate the situation to a higher level and make the patient feel they are not important.

    D. Asking the patient to wait would likely escalate the situation to a higher level of anxiety as they wait to see if they will get worked into the schedule. They may also be concerned about seeing a provider with whom they have no established relationship.

10. **A.** This will likely escalate the situation by uprooting the patient's schedule.

    B. This will likely escalate the situation by making the patient feel no longer welcome with their current established provider.

    C. This will likely escalate the situation and upset the patient by asking them to pay for another appointment when they feel the provider was at fault for not providing quality care.

    D. Correct. It is important to know when to ask for assistance when a situation escalates.

11. **A.** The assistant must ensure the proper documentation has been signed by the patient to release information.

    B. The assistant must ensure the proper documentation has been signed by the patient to release information.

    C. Correct. The assistant must ensure the proper documentation has been signed by the patient to release information.

    D. The assistant must ensure the proper documentation has been signed by the patient to release information.

12. **A. Correct.** Teamwork is achieved when each member performs their own responsibilities and works together to ensure that all tasks are completed.

    B. Personal feelings, gossip, and drama have no place in the work environment.

    C. Personal relationships should not impact the work environment.

    D. All team members must be courteous, respectful, and maintain a positive attitude towards one another which encourages harmony among staff.

13. **A.** Healthy eating does not impact professionalism.

    B. Correct. A good work ethic demonstrates professionalism.

    C. Physical fitness does not impact professionalism.

    D. Accurate personal budgeting does not impact professionalism.

14. **A.** Therapeutic communication is not used to manipulate.

    B. Therapeutic communication is not used to demand changes.

    C. Therapeutic communication is not used to control the conversation.

    D. Correct. Therapeutic communication can encourage a more active participation in choices, preventive measures, and decision-making.

15. **A.** After visit summaries are not proactive measures. A summary of the visit is given at the end of the appointment once documentation is complete.

    B. Correct. Checking the audio and visual components of virtual visits is a must at the beginning of the visit to increase the opportunities for effective communication.

    C. Encounter forms are completed both during the visit and prior, and thus not a proactive measure.

    D. Follow-up visits are scheduled after a virtual visit is finished, and thus not a proactive measure.

16. **A. Correct.** Active listening includes paraphrasing what is being said to ensure it is correctly being received.

    B. Active listening is hearing and comprehending the words, not discouraging the patient from asking questions.

    C. Active listening entails giving undivided attention to the person speaking.

    D. Active listening skills do not include interruptions.

17. **A.** Vocal pitch and tone should be appropriate for speaking with patients.

    B. Vocal pitch and tone should be appropriate for speaking with patients.

    C. Correct. Vocal pitch and tone should be appropriate for speaking with patients, ensuring it is not monotone or too loud. Words must be enunciated and clearly spoken. It can be helpful to smile while on the phone.

    D. Vocal pitch and tone should be appropriate for speaking with patients.

18. **A.** Patient satisfaction surveys can determine satisfaction levels. This is not within the scope of practice for the medical provider.

    B. Patient satisfaction levels should be asked for after receiving medical services, not on the patient's first day in the office.

    C. Correct. Patient satisfaction surveys can be offered to see how satisfied patients are with their care and if they have any possible suggestions or concerns that can also be addressed.

    D. It would not be accurate to have patients complete patient satisfaction surveys during the resolution process for conflict management.

19. **A.** An appointment is not needed to go over the patient's financial responsibility.

    B. The patient does not need to contact their insurance company as they can review the explanation of benefits to see patient financial responsibility.

    C. Correct. All types of communication must be documented to ensure the event is on record.

    D. Patient financial responsibility is due and should not be written off.

20. **A.** Risk management does not apply to staffing levels.

    B. Risk management does not apply to budgeting.

    C. Risk management does not apply to inventory.

    D. Correct. Risk management is the process of ensuring a safe environment for all vested members.

Quiz 13: Medical Law and Ethics

1. **A.** The ACA is a federal statute that allows access to affordable and quality health care and increases consumer insurance protection.

   B. Correct. HIPAA gives patients rights over their health information and sets rules and limits on who can view and receive their private information.

   C. The HITECH Act expands on HIPAA by including provisions that have prohibited the sale of PHI, made business associates and vendors liable for adherence with HIPAA, and created a penalty and violation system.

   D. PHI is protected health information, such as demographic information, medical history, and test results.

2. **A.** The Clinical Laboratory Improvement Amendments (CLIA) are a group of laws that regulate all laboratory facilities for the safety and handling of specimens.

   B. Correct. The Occupational Safety and Health (OSH) Act states that employers are accountable for providing a safe and healthful workplace.

   C. EMTALA requires emergency departments to provide stabilizing treatment for emergency medical conditions.

   D. The CSA is a federal policy that regulates the manufacture and distribution of controlled substances, such as narcotics, depressants, and stimulants.

3. **A.** Express consent means that an individual expresses a preference or choice, often verbally or in writing.

   B. The patient does not need a guardian to grant permission to do the procedure because they are an adult.

   C. Correct. Implied consent is not expressly granted by a patient, but rather inferred from their actions and the facts and circumstances of the situation.

   D. Informed consent is a clear and voluntary indication of preference or choice, usually verbally or in writing. This consent is only given by the patient after information is given either verbally or in writing.

4. **A.** A person who is in the advanced stage of dementia would not have the capacity to understand and make decisions regarding their health care.

   B. Minors do not have the legal rights of an adult and are unable to give consent.

   C. A patient who is in a coma cannot speak for themselves and therefore cannot give informed consent. A health care proxy would need to speak for the patient in this case.

   D. Correct. Minors are considered emancipated if they enlist in the military and can then give informed consent.

5. **A.** The Civil Rights Act prohibits an employer with 15 or more employees from discriminating based on race, national origin, gender, and religion.

   B. The Patient's Bill of Rights helps patients feel more confident in the health care system and strengthens the relationship between patients and their health care provider.

   C. ACA is a federal statute that expands access to more affordable, quality health insurance and increases consumer insurance protection.

   D. Correct. The HITECH Act expands on HIPAA by including provisions that have prohibited the sale of PHI, made business associates and vendors liable for adherence with HIPAA, and created a penalty and violation system.

6. **A.** The Civil Rights Act prohibits an employer with 15 or more employees from discriminating based on race, national origin, gender, and religion.

   B. HIPAA gives patients rights over their health information and sets rules and limits on who can view and receive their private information.

   C. The ACA is a federal statute that expands access to more affordable, quality health insurance and increases consumer insurance protection.

   D. Correct. The Patient's Bill of Rights guarantees patients the right to ask for information regarding procedures and treatments available to them.

7. **A.** A MOLST form is a set of medical orders completed by the health care provider detailing the patient's end-of-life care.

   B. A DNR order is a directive that prevents health care providers from performing CPR on a patient.

   C. Correct. A DPAHC is a legal document naming a health care agent or proxy to make medical decisions for patients if they become incapacitated or unable to communicate.

   D. A living will is a legal document stating which procedures a patient would and would not want, and under what conditions they would want them provided, if they cannot communicate their wishes themselves.

8. **A. Correct.** A DNR order is a legal document indicating that a patient does not want life-saving measures if their heart stops.

   B. Advance directives are legal documents consisting of a patient's requests for their health care provider, family, and other health care professionals to carry out if the patient becomes incapacitated or unable to speak for themselves.

   C. A DPAHC is a legal document naming a health care agent or proxy to make medical decisions for a patient if they become incapacitated or unable to communicate.

   D. A living will is a legal document stating which procedures a patient would and would not want, and under what conditions they would want them provided, if they become unable to communicate their wishes.

9. **A.** Because medical records are legal documents, a patient's medical record could be released by a court order or subpoena in a court case without the patient's authorization. However, courts do not own the medical records.

   B. Patients must authorize the release of information to third-party payers. Otherwise, they do not have access to patients' medical records or information.

   C. Because the information and data in a medical record belongs to the patient, patients have the right to inspect, review, and receive a copy of their medical and billing records that are held by health plans and health care providers. However, the patient is not considered the owner of their medical record.

   D. Correct. Although the information in the medical record pertains to the patient, the health care provider is the owner of the medical records. Therefore, the patient's original medical records must remain with the health care facility.

10. **A.** A patient's medical record could be released without authorization by a court order or subpoena and used as evidence in a criminal case.

   B. Correct. The patient must sign a release of information form if being seen by another health care provider.

   C. A patient's medical record could be released without authorization for mandated examinations, such as ordered by the employer's insurance company for a workers' compensation claim.

   D. A patient's medical record could be released without authorization if the patient has been exposed to a communicable disease, such as tuberculosis, syphilis, or HIV.

IN PRACTICE: QUIZZES
Quiz Answers: Quiz 13: Medical Law and Ethics

11. **A.** Being a patient at the same clinic as their parent does not constitute authorization for release of information to the child.

    B. A health care provider is allowed to give information to family members if they are present during the medical visit or a hospital stay. However, the patient would still have to complete a release of information form to authorize their child to receive the information.

    C. Correct. A health care provider cannot share a patient's information with family or friends, unless they are the patient's personal representative or the patient authorizes with written consent.

    D. Regardless of limiting the amount of information provided, the patient would still have to complete a release of information form to authorize their child to receive this information.

12. **A. Correct.** Employers, including those in health care, are not covered entities under HIPAA.

    B. According to HIPAA, health care clearinghouses are defined as covered entities.

    C. According to HIPAA, health insurance plans are defined as covered entities.

    D. According to HIPAA, health care providers are defined as covered entities.

13. **A.** Mandatory reporting is required for specific communicable diseases, but strep throat is not included in this.

    B. Correct. This patient shows signs of child abuse, specifically physical abuse, which is a mandatory reporting requirement.

    C. A patient being unable to afford medical care is concerning but not a reason to report for concern of abuse, unless there is reason to believe that someone is stealing their money.

    D. Although there are a series of recommended immunizations for infants at that age, refusal of immunizations is not a mandatory reporting requirement.

14. **A.** Delayed reporting may further endanger the child's safety and the parent may not return for the follow-up appointment.

    B. The law requires health care providers to report all cases of suspected, but not necessarily proven, abuse. Anyone who reports their suspicions in good faith are protected from lawsuits.

    C. Correct. A health care provider who suspects abuse must report it to Child Protective Services or other appropriate authorities.

    D. Delayed reporting may further endanger the child's safety and the parent may not return for the follow-up appointment.

15. **A.** CLIA is a group of laws that regulate all laboratory facilities for the safety and handling of specimens.

    B. Correct. The OSH Act states that employers are accountable for providing a safe and healthful workplace.

    C. EMTALA requires emergency departments to provide stabilizing treatment for emergency medical conditions.

    D. The CSA is a federal policy that regulates the manufacture and distribution of controlled substances, such as narcotics, depressants, and stimulants.

16. **A. Correct.** CLIA is a group of laws that regulate all laboratory facilities for the safety and handling of specimens and monitor the accuracy and timeliness of testing.

    B. EMTALA requires emergency departments to provide stabilizing treatment for emergency medical conditions.

    C. The CSA is a federal policy that regulates the manufacture and distribution of controlled substances, such as narcotics, depressants, and stimulants.

    D. The OSH Act states that employers are accountable for providing a safe and healthful workplace.

17. **A. Correct.** Duty of care is a provider's responsibility after agreeing to treat or provide medical services to a patient who requests treatment. If a relationship has not been established between the provider and patient, then no duty exists.

    B. Dereliction of duty, also called a breach, is a failure to use reasonable care in fulfilling the duty.

    C. Direct cause is the failure in the duty, leading to harm suffered by the injured person.

    D. Damages is the harm or injury that resulted from the action and can be remedied by monetary compensation.

18. **A.** A spouse or domestic partner may serve as a patient's health care proxy.

    B. A patient's adult child may serve as their health care proxy.

    C. Correct. Some states do not allow a health care provider or an employee of a facility to be a patient's health care proxy.

    D. State law may appoint a court-appointed guardian or conservator as a patient's health care proxy if they have not designated one.

19. **A. Correct.** Patients who have a DNR order can continue to get chemotherapy, antibiotics, dialysis, or any other life-sustaining treatments.

    B. Patients who have a DNR order can continue to get chemotherapy and antibiotics, but not CPR.

    C. Patients who have a DNR order can continue to get chemotherapy and dialysis, but not CPR.

    D. Patients who have a DNR order can continue to get chemotherapy and dialysis, but not intubation.

20. **A.** This is a case of defamation of character, which is a type of intentional tort.

    B. This is a case of assault, which is a type of intentional tort.

    C. This is a case of battery, which is a type of intentional tort.

    D. Correct. The medical assistant failed to act reasonably where a duty was owed, which was to take and monitor the patient's blood glucose. This is negligence because there was no intent to harm the patient, and it was not a deliberate action.

APPENDIX
Glossary

#

20/20 vision. The ability to see at 20 feet what the average person sees at 20 feet.

A

abdominal aortic aneurysm. An enlarged area in the lower part of the aorta that supplies blood to the body.

accountable care organizations (ACOs). Group of medical professionals associated with a defined patient population that are accountable for the quality and cost of care delivered to those patients.

active listening. Engaging with the sender regarding the message and the intended interpretation (e.g., focus solely on the conversation, do not interrupt, confirm the message speaker has said, be respectful and professional).

Advance Beneficiary Notice of Noncoverage (ABN). A form used for fee-for-service (FFS) Medicare beneficiaries when the service may not be covered.

advance directives. Written statements of a person's wishes regarding medical treatment, such as a living will.

adverse reactions. Unwanted or undesired effects that are possibly related to taking a medication, usually secondary to the main effect of the medication.

after-visit summary (AVS). Information that includes follow-up appointments, provider orders, instructions, educational resources, and financial account information.

aging reports. A report that lists outstanding balances that have not been paid by either the patient or the insurance payer.

alimentary canal. The passage in which food passes through the body from the mouth to anus.

aliquot. A whole portion of something must be divided up into equal parts.

allergic. A condition of sensitivity in which the immune system reacts abnormally to a foreign substance.

Americans with Disabilities Act of 1990 (ADA). Law that forbids discrimination based on disability.

ampule. Sealed glass capsule containing a liquid.

analytes. A substance or chemical that is being identified and measured.

anaphylactic shock. A systemic allergic reaction that can be life-threatening without immediate medical intervention.

anatomical position. Standard frame of reference in which the body is standing up, face forward, arms at the sides, palms forward, and toes pointed forward.

antecubital. The inner or front surface of the forearm at the elbow.

anthropometric. Related to measurement and proportion of the body.

Anti-Kick Back Statute (AKBS). Criminal law that prohibits receiving benefits for referral or business involving federal health care programs.

antibody. Protein the body creates in response to antigens.

antigen. Foreign substance within the body.

artifact. Alteration or interference on the EKG that is not related to cardiac electrical activity; appears as distorted lines or waves.

atrial flutter. A single area within the atrial tissue firing at a rate faster than the rate the ventricles are responding to.

audit log. A trail of entries made in the electronic record.

auscultation. Listening with a stethoscope.

automated external defibrillator (AED). Device that provides electrical shock to restore a normal heartbeat.

autonomy. The capacity to think, decide, and act on one's own free will and initiative.

APPENDIX: GLOSSARY

B

beneficence. A moral obligation to act in the best interest of others.

bevel. Area around the surface of the needle point.

biases. Beliefs that are not proven by facts about someone or a particular group of individuals.

biohazard waste. Materials that present a potential or actual risk to the health of humans, animals, or the environment.

biopsy. The surgical removal of tissue for later microscopic examination.

body mass index (BMI). An individual's weight divided by the square of their height, used to determine weight status.

bradycardia. Heart rate less than 60/min.

C

capillary puncture. The method of acquiring blood from a fingertip or heel.

capitation. A managed care method of monthly payments to the provider based on the number of enrolled patients, regardless of how many encounters a patient may have during the month.

cardiopulmonary resuscitation (CPR). Lifesaving technique that consists of chest compressions combined with artificial ventilation.

Centers for Disease Control and Prevention (CDC). National public health agency that protects the public's health.

Centers for Medicare & Medicaid Services (CMS). A federal agency that oversees the Medicare program and assists states with Medicaid programs.

certification. Verification by an outside agency that an employer is following established guidelines and standards of care and providing the highest quality of care for their patients.

chief complaint. Primary reason for the office visit.

cholesterol. A waxy, fatlike substance made by the liver.

clearinghouse. An organization that accepts the claims data from a health care provider, performs edits comparable to payer edits, and submits clean claims to the third-party payer.

Clinical Laboratory Improvement Amendments (CLIA). A 1988 amendment that regulates federal standards that apply to all clinical laboratory testing performed on humans in the United States.

clinical laboratory testing. Testing used in conjunction with health history and physical examination to provide essential data for the diagnosis and management of a patient's condition.

clinical quality measures. Ways to identify treatments, processes, experiences, and outcomes.

clotted blood. Blood obtained when drawn in a tube that does not contain an anticoagulant.

clustering. Scheduling patients in groups with common medical needs.

coinsurance. The percentage of the allowed amount the patient will pay once the deductible is met.

colposcopy. Examination of the vagina and cervix performed using a colposcope, which is a specialized type of endoscope.

communicable disease. Illness caused by an infectious agent that occurs through direct or indirect contact.

communication. Sending and receiving information, thoughts, or feelings through verbal words, written words, or body language.

comprehensive care. Care designed for the patient's physical and mental health needs using a team-based approach.

computerized provider order entry (CPOE). Process in which providers enter and send treatment instructions, including medications, laboratory, and radiology orders, via a computer application rather than paper, fax, or phone.

Controlled Substances Act. Statute that identifies all regulated substances into one of five schedules depending on potential for abuse.

copayment. A set amount determined by the plan/payer that the patient pays for specified services, usually office visits and emergency department visits.

CPT codes. Current Procedural Terminology codes that identify medical services and procedures performed by a provider.

crash cart. Portable cart stocked with emergency supplies; emergency kit.

critical values. Laboratory results at such variance to the normal value range that a potential life-threatening, pathophysiologic state is occurring. Action must be taken as soon as possible.

cytology. Microscope examination of cells to identify a diagnosis.

D

deductible. The amount that must be paid before benefits are paid by the insurance.

defense mechanism. Coping strategies individuals use to protect themselves from negative emotions such as guilt, anxiety, fear, and shame.

dehiscence. Partial or total separation of a wound's edges.

diagnosis codes. International Classification of Diseases, 10th revision, Clinical Modification (ICD-10-CM) codes based on the provider's diagnosis (why they are in need of medical services).

diastolic. Measurement of force while the heart is relaxing; bottom number on a blood pressure reading.

disinfection. Process of killing disease-producing micro-organisms but not spores.

do-not-resuscitate (DNR). An order written in the hospital or on a legal form to communicate the wishes of a patient to not undergo CPR or advanced cardiac life support if the patient's heart stops or the patient stops breathing.

double-booking. A type of scheduling in which two or more patients are scheduled within the same time slot.

durable medical equipment. Medical devices and supplies that can be used repeatedly outside of a hospital.

durable power of attorney (DPOA). a legal document naming a health care agent or proxy to make medical decisions for patients when they are not able to do so, in the case they become incapacitated or unable to communicate.

E

electrocardiogram (EKG). A cardiac test that records electrical activity of the heart, provides information about heart rate and rhythm, and can show evidence of a previous heart attack.

electronic medical record (EMR). Record in a medical practice or clinic to document the patient's demographic information, care, progress, and treatment.

eligibility. Meeting the stipulated requirements to participate in the health care plan.

emergency medical services (EMS). System that provides urgent pre-hospital treatment and care.

Emergency Medical Treatment and Active Labor Act (EMTALA). Law that requires any hospital emergency department that receives payments from federal health care programs, such as Medicare and Medicaid, to provide an appropriate medical screening to any patient seeking treatment.

emergency. Unforeseen circumstance that requires immediate attention.

encounter form. A record of the diagnosis and procedures covered during the current visit; also known as superbill.

endoscopy. Procedure that uses an endoscope to view a hollow organ or body cavity, such as the larynx, bladder, colon, sigmoid colon, stomach, abdomen, and some joints.

engineering controls. Devices used to isolate or remove the bloodborne pathogen hazard from the workplace.

environmental stressor. Situation that causes enough stress to become an obstacle to achieve goals or have positive experiences.

epidemic. Occurs when a disease spreads rapidly to a large number of people

Erik Erikson. Psychologist who developed the concepts of stages of life based on a person's age.

erythema. Superficial reddening of the skin.

established patient. Patient who received same-provider services within the last 3 years.

ethics. Set of principles that differentiate between right and wrong.

evisceration. Separation of wound edges and protrusion of abdominal organs.

F

fasting. The absence of eating food and sometimes drinking.

fecal occult blood test (FOBT). A lab test used to check stool samples for hidden (occult) blood.

fee for service. System used by private insurance companies and non-for-profits in which insurance carriers determine the allowed charge either by a fee schedule or through service benefits that define covered services but not necessarily the exact payments.

feedback. Information relayed to the message sender regarding how the message was received and interpreted.

first aid. Immediate care given to the victim of injury or sudden illness to sustain life and prevent death.

Food and Drug Administration. Organization responsible for protecting the public health by ensuring safety, efficacy, and security of human medications.

G

Genetic Information Nondiscrimination Act of 2008 (GINA). Law that prohibits discrimination on the basis of genetic information with respect to health insurance and employment.

glucose tolerance test (OGTT). Test process that evaluates glucose levels over time to assess for diabetes by measuring the body's response to sugar.

Good Samaritan Acts. Law that allows bystanders to get involved in emergency situations without feat that they will be sued if their actions inadvertently contribute to a person's injury or death.

H

HCPCS codes. Healthcare Common Procedure Coding System codes that identify supplies and procedures not described by CPT codes.

Heads of the European Radiological Protection Competent Authorities (HERCA). Association that provides clarity on the regulator's approach to the roles of the undertaking and a range of professionals regarding the justification process.

Health Information Technology for Economic and Clinical Health (HITECH) Act. Law that includes provisions that allow for increased enforcement of the privacy and security of electronic transmission of patient information, such as prohibiting the sale of PHI, making business associates and vendors liable for compliance with HIPAA, and creating a penalty and violation system.

Health Insurance Portability and Accountability Act (HIPAA). Federal law that required the creation of national standards to protect sensitive patient health information from being disclosed without the patient's consent or knowledge.

health maintenance organization (HMO). A medical insurance group that provides coverage of health care services for a period of time and a fixed annual fee.

Helicobacter pylori. Type of bacteria that infects the digestive tract.

hematocrit (Hct). Volume percentage of red blood cells in blood.

hematology. Study of cause, prognosis, treatment, and prevention of diseases related to blood.

hemoconcentration. An increase of formed elements of the blood and a decrease of fluid content.

hemoglobin (Hgb). Iron-containing oxygen-transport in red blood cells that is responsible for carrying oxygen from the respiratory organs to the rest of the body.

hemoglobin A1C. Identifies blood glucose levels over approximately 3-month period.

hemorrhage. Escape of blood from a ruptured blood vessel.

Holter monitor. A portable device for cardiac monitoring that is worn for at least 24 hours.

homeostasis. State in which the body's systems and biological processes maintain stability.

hormones. Chemicals used by the body to increase or decrease activity of the hormone's specific target cells.

human chorionic gonadotropin (hCG). Hormone secreted by the placenta during pregnancy.

I

implied consent. Consent granted when a patient assumes the position and allows the medical professional to perform it.

incision and drainage (I&D). Lancing a fluid or pressure build up under the skin to allow it to drain and relieve pressure.

informed consent. An oral or written agreement of mutual communication that ensures the patient has been notified about their health care choices before making them.

inventory supply log. Form that tracks the amount of inventory the office has and can be used to predict anticipated amounts needed based on the history.

Ishihara test. Vision test to assess for color deficiency.

J

justice. Fair distribution of benefit, risk, resources, and cost to ensure equal treatment.

K

kinesthetic learning. Learning by seeing the action and performing it.

laboratory directory. A catalog of information regarding laboratory tests with up-to-date test menus, testing information, specimen collection requirements, storage, preservation, and transportation guidelines.

L

lancet. A small blade with sharp point.

lumen. Open space in the needle.

M

malpractice. Any treatment by a medical professional that does not follow the standards of care.

managed care plans. System used by private and public insurance plans that controls health care cost and improve preventive care for its patients by having contracts with providers and medical organizations. The three types of managed care plans are health maintenance organization (HMO), preferred provider organization (PPO) or point-of-care (POS) service.

matrix. The designed timeframe for appointments based on the method of appointment durations.

medical asepsis. Clean technique that includes frequent hand hygiene, proper use of gloves, cleaning and sterilizing medical equipment, and sanitizing surfaces.

medical law. Laws that explain the rights and responsibilities of medical providers and patients.

medical necessity. Reasonable and appropriate services based on clinical standards per CMS and the OIG.

medication reconciliation. Comparing the patient's list of medications to the medical record as a safety measure to reduce the risk of improperly prescribing an incorrect or contraindicated prescription, including medication interactions and adverse reactions.

micro-collection device. Small plastic tube designed to collect capillary blood.

micro-organism. A microscopic organism that cannot be seen by the naked eye.

microbiology. Study of all living organisms that are too small to be visible by the naked eye.

mononucleosis. Contagious virus that is spread through saliva, also known as mono, most commonly caused by the Epstein-Barr virus.

myocardial infarction. The flow of blood that brings oxygen to the heart muscle suddenly becomes blocked. If not restored quickly, the heart muscle will begin to die and cardiac arrest can occur.

N

Needle Safety and Prevention Act. Law signed in November 2000 that requires safety measures in workplaces where there is an occupational exposure to blood or other potentially infectious materials.

negligence. When a patient does not receive adequate and appropriate care, which leads to suffering and harm.

new patient. The initial patient appointment or the first encounter after a 3-year absence from the organization.

No Surprise Act (NSA). Law that protects individuals from surprise billing if they have a group health plan or individual health insurance coverage.

no-show. When a patient has a scheduled appointment and does not show up and or contact the medical office.

nonmaleficence. A commitment not to cause harm.

nonparenteral. Given by mouth, delivered to the gastrointestinal tract.

nonpathogenic. Harmless and does not cause disease.

nonverbal communication. Communication that occurs through expressive behaviors and body language rather than oral or written words.

normal flora. Micro-organisms that live on or within the body without causing disease.

Notice of Privacy Practices (NPP). Document that identifies how the provider will distribute and disclose a patient's protected health information.

nuclear medicine. Type of diagnostic imaging that involves administration of radioactive isotopes that collect in areas of high metabolic activity.

nutrition. The field of study focused on food and the substances in food that help people grow, recover from illnesses, and stay healthy.

O

objective. Information that can be observed or measured.

Occupational Safety and Health Administration (OSHA). Agency that creates regulations that employers must follow for employees to remain safe while working.

ophthalmic. Relating to the eye and its diseases.

ophthalmoscope. Instrument used to examine the interior of the eye.

orthostatic hypotension. A significant drop in blood pressure during positional changes, particularly when the patient is moving from lying down to sitting or from sitting to standing; also known as postural hypotension.

otic. Relating to the ear.

otoscope. An instrument used for visual examination of the eardrum and ear canal, typically having a light for visibility.

P

par level or threshold. Minimum amount of inventory an office will have on the shelf before placing another order.

parenteral. Administered or occurring in the body bypassing the gastrointestinal tract.

pathogenic. Causes disease.

Patient Safety and Quality Improvement Act (PSQIA). Framework for gathering and analyzing information regarding patient safety within the confinements of protected health information laws.

patient-centered medical home (PCMH). A partnership between a patient and their care team in which total health is the focus and not just a single condition. A health care team consists of a provider (physician, nurse practitioner, physician assistant), CMAA, CCMA, nurses, and pharmacist.

peak flow meter. Device that measures the amount of air exhaled upon forceful exhalation.

personal protective equipment. Gear worn when there is a chance of coming in contact with blood or body fluids. In the health care setting, this includes gloves, gowns/aprons, shoe covers, lab coats, masks and respirators, protective eyewear, and face shields.

Physician Orders for Life-Sustaining Treatment (POLST). Type of advance directive, typically reserved for patients who may be near end of life.

Physicians' Desk Reference (PDR). Reference book that provides a guide to prescription medication information.

plasma. The liquid portion of the blood; mainly made of water; contains proteins, electrolytes, gases, some nutrients, and waste products; and required to recover from injury, distribute nutrients, and remove waste from the body.

point of service (POS). A type of managed care health insurance plan that is based on lower medical costs in exchange for more limited choice.

practice management system (PMS). Software used to electronically manage administrative functions, such as scheduling appointments, integrating patient documentation from electronic health records, coding, billing, and revenue cycle tasks such as running aging reports and managing the accounts receivable.

preauthorization. Approval of insurance coverage and necessity of services prior to the patient receiving them.

precertification. A request to determine if a service is covered by the patient's policy and what the reimbursement would be.

preferred provider organization (PPO). A network of physicians, other health care practitioners, and hospitals that have joined together to contract with insurance companies, employers, or other organizations to provide health care to subscribers for a discounted fee.

prefix. Word component that appears at the beginning of a word to change the meaning of the rest of the word.

premature atrial contractions (PAC). A premature contraction that results when the atria are triggered to contract earlier than they should.

premature ventricular contractions (PVC). Premature contractions in the ventricles.

preventive care. Check-ups, patient counseling, and other screenings to prevent illnesses, disease, or other health-related issues.

professionalism. The attitude, behavior, and work that represent a profession.

pulmonary function test. Test to assess lung functioning, which will help assist in the detection and evaluation of pulmonary disease.

pyrexia. Fever greater than 100.4° F.

Q

qualitative. Identifying or measuring by the quality of something rather than its quantity.

quality assurance (QA). Maintenance of a desired level of quality related to a service or piece of equipment.

quality control (QC). Steps performed to ensure the reliability of test results through detecting and eliminating error.

quantitative. Related to measuring the amount of something.

R

real-time adjudication (RTA). A tool that allows for a submission of the coded visit to the insurance company by participating providers for reimbursement decisions by third-party payers while the patient is present.

referral. An order from a provider for a patient to see a specialist or to obtain specific medical services.

respiration. One complete inhalation and exhalation.

respondent superior. "Let the master answer" doctrine of law that holds the employer vicariously liable for acts of an employee.

revenue cycle. A series of administrative functions that are required to capture and collect payment for services provided by a health care organization.

S

Safety Data Sheets. Sheets that provide information on the hazards and actions necessary when working with specific chemicals.

sanitization. The cleaning process that reduces the number of micro-organisms to a safe level.

scope of practice. A specific set of standards that a medical professional may perform within the limits of the medical license, registration, and/or certification.

seizure. Uncontrolled muscle activity that can be caused by high body temperature, head injuries, drugs, and epilepsy.

serum. Liquid portion of the blood obtained after a serum sample tube has clotted and has been centrifuged.

side effects. A secondary reaction to the one intended.

sinus rhythm. Rhythm that originates from the sinus (SA) node and describes the characteristic rhythm of the human heart.

sprain. A stretched or torn ligament.

standard precautions. Guidelines recommended by the Centers for Disease Control and Prevention (CDC) to ensure the safety and welfare of health care workers and the public.

sterile technique. A group of strategies used to reduce exposure to micro-organisms and keep the patient as safe as possible.

sterilization. The complete destruction of all micro-organisms through specific means.

strain. A stretched or torn muscle or tendon.

stress testing. Monitoring the heart during exercise on a treadmill or stationary bike to evaluate how the heart responds to stress.

subjective. Information gathered from what a patient communicates.

subpoena duces tecum. A requirement to bring requested documentation to the court of law when appearing for the summons.

suffixes. Word components that appear at the end of the word to change the meaning of the rest of the word.

surgical asepsis. Techniques to eliminate pathogenic and other potentially harmful microbes related to invasive procedures.

syncope. Fainting; a brief episode of unconsciousness.

systolic. Measurement of force while the heart is contracting; top number on a blood pressure reading.

T

tachycardia. Heart rate greater than 100/min.

telehealth. The virtual delivery of health care services remotely.

telephone etiquette. Being respectful using proper verbiage, tone, and manners when conveying information.

templates. A sample of written correspondence or email that is established with appropriate components that will be personalized to fit the need of the sender.

The Joint Commission (TJC). Accrediting body that focuses on quality improvement and patient safety, certifying health care organizations and programs in the U.S. including hospitals and health care organizations that provide ambulatory and office-based surgery, behavioral health, home health care, laboratory, and nursing care center services.

therapeutic communication. Interaction between a patient and a medical professional focused on improving the physical and emotional well-being of the patient.

therapeutic effects. The helpful effect that the provider is hoping will help the patient to feel better.

Title VII of Civil Rights Act of 1964. Law that prohibits an employer with 15 or more employees from discriminating on the basis of race, national origin, gender, or religion.

tort. "Wrong," or a harmful act committed by one individual to another.

U

universal precautions. Precautions that apply when it is possible to come into contact with human blood, tissue, body fluids or secretions, regardless of patient infection status.

V

value-based plan. Insurance coverage that changes the amount of reimbursement based on health outcomes of patients and the quality of the service they received.

ventricular fibrillation (V-fib). A type of abnormal heart rhythm in which ventricles twitch or quiver, not pumping blood to the rest of the body.

ventricular tachycardia (V-tach). A regular, fast rhythm characterized by large, irregular, wide QRS complexes on the EKG.

vital signs. Metrics (temperature, pulse, respiration, blood pressure) used to evaluate a patient's overall health status.

volume. Amount of blood being pumped through the heart; represented by strength of contractions and is documented in pulse as strong or "bounding" and weak or "thready."

W

wave scheduling. Scheduling two or three patients during a designated hourly time period (last 30 min of the hour, patient seen in order of arrival).

whole blood. Blood obtained when drawn in a tube that contains an anticoagulant.

word root. Core component of words that describe the basic meaning.

workplace controls. Practices in the workplace that reduce the chances of exposure by changing or mandating the way a task is performed.

World Health Organization (WHO). Agency that promotes health, and monitors and coordinates activities concerning health-related issues.

APPENDIX
References

Agency for Healthcare Research and Quality. (n.d.). *Acronyms and abbreviations.* https://www.ahrq.gov/research/findings/final-reports/iomracereport/reldataapa.html

Blesi, M. (2022). *Medical assisting: Administrative & clinical competencies.* (9th ed.). Cengage Learning.

Bonewit-West, K., and Hunt, S. A. (2020). *Today's medical assistant: Clinical and administrative procedures.* (4th ed.). Elsevier.

Booth, K., Whicker, L., and Wyman, T. (2020). *Medical assisting: Administrative and clinical procedures.* (7th ed.). McGraw Hill.

Centers for Disease Control and Prevention. (2002). *Hand hygiene in health care settings-core* [Slides]. https://www.cdc.gov/HandHygiene/download/hand_hygiene_core.pdf

Centers for Disease Control and Prevention. (2012, May 18). *Principles of epidemiology.* https://www.cdc.gov/csels/dsepd/ss1978/lesson1/section11.html

Centers for Disease Control and Prevention. (2019, May 24). *Disinfection & sterilization guidelines.* https://www.cdc.gov/infectioncontrol/guidelines/disinfection/index.html

Centers for Disease Control and Prevention. (2020, January 30). *Hand hygiene guidance.* https://www.cdc.gov/handhygiene/providers/guideline.html

Centers for Disease Control and Prevention. (2021, March 11). *Diabetes meal planning.* https://www.cdc.gov/diabetes/managing/eat-well/meal-plan-method.html

Centers for Disease Control and Prevention. (2022, April 14). *ACIP contraindications guidelines for immunization.* https://www.cdc.gov/vaccines/hcp/acip-recs/general-recs/contraindications.html

Garza, D., and Becan-McBride, K. (2018). *Phlebotomy handbook: Blood specimen collection from basic to advanced.* (10th ed.). Pearson.

Hewlett, A.L., Hohenberger, H., Murphy, C.N., Helget, L., Hausmann, H., Lyden, E., Fey, P.D., and Hicks, R. (2018). Evaluation of the bacterial burden of gel nails, standard nail polish, and natural nails on the hands of health care workers. *American Journal of Infection Control, 46*(12):1356–1359.

Judson, K., and Harrison, C. (2020). *Law & ethics for health professions.* (9th ed.) McGraw Hill.

Niedzwiecki, B., Pepper, J., and Weaver, P. (2020). *Kinn's the administrative medical assistant: An applied learning approach.* (14th ed.). Elsevier.

Occupational Safety and Health Administration. (2011, January). *OSHA FactSheet: OSHA's bloodborne pathogen standard* [Dataset]. https://www.osha.gov/sites/default/files/publications/bbfact01.pdf

Smith, T. M. (2020, January 10). What is value-based care? These are the key elements. *American Medical Association.* https://www.ama-assn.org/practice-management/payment-delivery-models/what-value-based-care-these-are-key-elements

APPENDIX: REFERENCES

The Joint Commission. (2016, April 11.) *When a repeat test value is still critical but is showing improvement, does it still need to be considered a "critical result" and reported in that time frame?* https://www.jointcommission.org/standards/standard-faqs/laboratory/national-patient-safety-goals-npsg/000001556/

Townsend Little, K. (2018). *Fundamental concepts and skills for the patient care technician.* Elsevier.

U.S. Department of Health and Human Services. (n.d.). Definition & facts for celiac disease. *National Institute of Diabetes and Digestive and Kidney Diseases.* https://www.niddk.nih.gov/health-information/digestive-diseases/celiac-disease/definition-facts

U.S. Department of Health and Human Services. (n.d.). Eating right for chronic kidney disease. *National Institute of Diabetes and Digestive and Kidney Diseases.* https://www.niddk.nih.gov/health-information/kidney-disease/chronic-kidney-disease-ckd/eating-nutrition

U.S. Department of Health and Human Services. (n.d.). Reduce the number of days people are exposed to unhealthy air - EH 01. *Healthy People 2030.* https://health.gov/healthypeople/objectives-and-data/browse-objectives/environmental-health/reduce-number-days-people-are-exposed-unhealthy-air-eh-01

U.S. Department of Health and Human Services. (n.d.). Social determinants of health. *Healthy People 2030.* https://health.gov/healthypeople/priority-areas/social-determinants-health

APPENDIX
Index

A

Abbreviations, 82–85
Abdominal aortic aneurysm (AAA), 284
Abdominal cavity, 52
ABN (Advance Beneficiary Notice of Noncoverage), 309
Abrasions, 189, 193
Absorption, 29, 36, 62, 153, 156–157, 180, 194
Abuse, 348–349
Acceptance stage of grief, 106
Accommodations, 100–101, 138–139
Accountable care organizations (ACOs), 277, 278, 280, 311
Accounts receivables (A/R), 311
AC interference, 265
Acronyms, 83–85
Active immunity, 58
Active listening, 299, 320, 322–324, 327, 329–331
Acupuncture, 14
Acute renal failure, 72
Acute respiratory distress (ARDS), 74
ADA (Americans with Disabilities Act of 1990), 100, 139, 338
ADHD (attention-deficit/hyperactivity disorder), 98
Adhesives for skin, 180, 181
Administrative assisting, 295–318. *See also* Appointments; *Revenue cycle*
    data entry tasks, 315
    follow-up patient calls, 313, 314
    inventory management, 315–316
    mail and fax processing, 314
    medical records management, 302–303
    patient check-in and check-out, 301
    patient portal activation, 317
    preauthorizations and precertifications, 303–304
    referrals, facilitation of, 304–305
    safety evaluations, 318, 332
    telehealth instruction, 317
Advance Beneficiary Notice of Noncoverage (ABN), 309
Advance directives, 105, 343–345
Advanced practice nurses (APNs), 279
Adverse reactions
    to electrocardiograms, 272
    to medications, 12, 18–20, 111–112, 158
    to phlebotomy procedures, 242
AEDs (automated external defibrillators), 194–197
Afferent neurons, 64
After-visit summaries (AVSs), 301
Aggressive communication style, 321
Aging reports, 311
AHA (American Heart Association), 287
AIDS. *See HIV/AIDS*
Airborne precautions, 204
Airway obstructions, 184, 186
AKBS (Anti-Kick Back Statute), 339
Alcohol use. *See also Substance use disorder*
    celiac disease and, 45
    eating disorders and, 46, 47
    patient education on, 282, 287
    testing for, 113, 230, 255, 284
Alimentary canal, 61
Aliquot, 256
Allergic reactions, 18, 19, 22, 111–112, 149–150, 158
Allergists, 12, 236
Allergy testing, 236

Allied health professionals, 5
Alzheimer's disease, 75
Ambulatory care. *See Outpatient care*
American Heart Association (AHA), 287
Americans with Disabilities Act of 1990 (ADA), 100, 139, 338
Ampules, 152, 159
Analgesics, 15, 17
Analytes, 224, 227
Anaphylaxis/anaphylactic shock, 19, 111, 149–150, 188
Anatomical position, defined, 94
Anatomy and physiology, 50–67
    cardiovascular system, 59–60, 63, 71, 87
    cavity sections, 52
    cell structure and functions, 50–51
    endocrine system, 64, 67, 76–77, 87
    gastrointestinal system, 61–62, 73, 88
    homeostasis and organ system interactions, 67
    immune and lymphatic systems, 57–58
    integumentary system, 53–54, 67–68, 87
    muscular system, 57, 70, 88
    nervous system, 63–64, 67, 75, 117
    planes of body, 52
    quadrants and regions, 52–53
    reproductive systems, 65–66, 78–79, 89
    respiratory system, 63, 74, 87
    skeletal system, 54–56, 69, 88
    urinary system, 60, 72, 89
Ancillary services, 14
Androgens, 65
Anemia, 71
Anesthesiologists, 12
Anger stage of grief, 106

Angiography, 80
Anorexia nervosa, 46, 127
Antacids, 15, 31, 147
Antecubital space, 115, 155, 248–249
Anthropometric measurements, 125–128
Anti-anxiety agents, 16
Antibiotics, 15, 20, 86, 155, 183
Antibodies, 58, 223
Anticholinergics, 15
Anticipatory grief, 105
Anticoagulants, 15, 20, 246
Anticonvulsants, 15
Antidepressants, 15, 19–20
Antidiarrheals, 15, 17
Antiemetics, 15
Antifungals, 15
Antigens, 58, 224, 226
Antihistamines, 15, 19, 236
Antihypertensives, 15
Anti-inflammatories, 15, 186
Anti-Kick Back Statute (AKBS), 339
Antilipemics, 15
Antimigraine agents, 15
Anti-osteoporosis agents, 15
Antipsychotics, 16
Antipyretics, 16
Antitussives, 16, 17
Anti-ulcer agents, 15
Antivirals, 16
Anus, 62
Anxiety
  anti-anxiety agents, 16
  blood pressure and, 115, 129
  defense mechanisms and, 102
  eating disorders and, 47
  electrocardiograms and, 265, 266
  phlebotomy and, 242
  screening for, 113
  signs and symptoms, 98, 113
  telehealth visits for, 173
  white-coat syndrome and, 99, 113

Anxiolytics, 16
Apathy, 103
Apical pulse, 118, 147
APNs (advanced practice nurses), 279
Appendicitis, 73
Appendicular skeleton, 54, 56
Appointments. *See also* Scheduling appointments
  confirmation of, 313
  duration of visits, 299
  follow-up, 137, 182–183, 190, 193, 258, 290
  medical records review prior to, 285
  no-shows, 313
  practice management systems and, 295–296
  reminders for, 313
  telehealth visits, 9, 293, 298
  types of visits, 298–299
  urgency of, 300
A/R (accounts receivables), 311
ARDS (acute respiratory distress), 74
Arrhythmias, 149, 263–264
Arterial bleeding, 190
Arteries and arterioles, 59, 60, 118
Arthritis, 69
Artifacts, 265, 267, 270–272
Artificially acquired immunity, 58
Artificial nails, 209
Aseptic techniques, 151, 175–177, 199, 207–208
Assertive communication style, 321, 324, 330
Assistive devices, 100, 101
Assistive living, 287
Asthma, 74, 238
Asystole fibrillation, 264
Atherosclerosis, 71
Atrial fibrillation, 263, 264
Atrial flutter, 263
Atria of heart, 59–60, 262–264
Atrioventricular (AV) node, 59, 60
Attention-deficit/hyperactivity disorder (ADHD), 98

Audiometry, 235, 236
Auditing methods, 311
Auditory communication, 321
Auditory learning, 293
Auscultation, 114, 115, 118, 120
Autoclaves, 176, 214
Automated external defibrillators (AEDs), 194–197
Autonomic nervous system, 64
Autonomy, as ethical principle, 351
Autonomy vs. shame and doubt stage, 96
AV (atrioventricular) node, 59, 60
AVSs (after-visit summaries), 301
Axial skeleton, 54, 56
Axillary temperature, 122
Axons, 63

B

Bacteria
  antibiotics and, 86
  artificial nails and, 209
  disease associated with, 199, 200
  expired medications and, 31
  microbiological study of, 222
  sebaceous glands and, 53
  in urine specimens, 230, 233
  white blood cells and, 246
Bandaging, 155, 157, 189–193, 253
Bargaining stage of grief, 106
Barriers to care, 2, 291
Basal cell skin cancer, 68
B-cells, 58
Beneficence, as ethical principle, 351
Benign prostatic hyperplasia (BPH), 79
Bevel of needles, 153, 245, 251
Biases, 324, 335, 352. *See also* Stereotypes
Bicuspid (mitral) valve, 59, 60
Billing, 305–309, 312–313

Binge eating disorder, 47
Biohazardous materials
  bags for transport of, 230, 257–258
  OSHA protocols for, 215, 217
  personal protective equipment and, 215–217
  symbol used for, 216–217
  waste from, 132–133, 152, 182, 190, 203, 215–217, 231
Biopsies, 134, 178
Birth control. See Contraceptives
Black cohosh, 41
Bladder. See Gallbladder; Urinary bladder
Bleach solutions, 211
Blind patients, 101
Blood banks, 222
Bloodborne pathogens, 203–205, 215, 241
Blood components, 246
Blood glucose, 173, 224–225, 283
Blood pressure
  allergic reactions and, 19
  antihypertensives, 15
  auscultatory method, 114, 115
  errors and troubleshooting, 115
  factors affecting, 115, 129
  hypertension, 71, 115, 116, 174
  hypotension, 117, 149
  medications and changes in, 20
  palpatory method, 115
  ranges by age, 116, 119, 128
  screening for, 283
  white-coat syndrome and, 99
Blood pressure cuffs (sphygmomanometers), 114–116, 132
Blood specimens. See also Phlebotomy
  errors involving, 255
  gloves for handling of, 203, 217
  for point-of-care testing, 224–226
  processing and handling, 254–257
  storage requirements, 219
  transporting, 257–258
  types of samples, 246

Body language, 320–321, 323, 327
Body mass index (BMI), 126, 127
Body surface area (BSA), 24
Body temperature
  factors affecting, 122, 129
  first aid for alterations in, 188
  heat exhaustion and heat stroke, 185
  hypothermia and, 185
  implied consent for taking, 342
  infectious agents and, 201
  measurement of, 122, 132, 141
  ranges by age, 123, 128
  regulation of, 34, 53, 54
  seizures and, 188
Bone density screening, 283
Bone marrow, 55, 58
Bones, 54–56, 187
Bounding pulse, 118
BPH (benign prostatic hyperplasia), 79
Brachial pulse, 118
Bradycardia, 93, 263
Bradypnea, 120
Brain, 63, 64
Brand name medications, 146
Breast cancer, 283
Breathing, 63, 64, 120–121
Bronchitis, 74
Bronchodilators, 16, 237
BSA (body surface area), 24
Buccal route of administration, 143
Bulbourethral (Cowper's) glands, 65
Bulimia nervosa, 46, 127
Bundle of His, 59, 60, 262
Burns, 34, 175, 184, 188, 192–193
Business letter formats, 328–329
Butterfly needle system, 245, 248

C

Calibration
  documentation of, 318
  of EKG devices, 274
  of laboratory equipment, 233, 234, 257
  for quality control, 219
  of syringes, 153, 157, 160
Cancer, 68, 73, 167, 283
Candidiasis, 78
Cannabis, 17
Capillaries, 59, 60
Capillary bleeding, 190
Capillary punctures, 224, 225, 251–253
Capitation models, 11
Carbohydrates, 35, 37, 38, 42, 287
Cardiac arrest, 160, 184, 194–196, 274
Cardiac cycle, 60, 114, 261, 262
Cardiac monitoring, 266, 274–275
Cardiac muscle, 57, 60
Cardiology and cardiologists, 12, 134, 262, 279
Cardiopulmonary resuscitation (CPR)
  allergic reactions and, 150
  anaphylactic shock and, 188
  asystole and, 264
  for burn victims, 193
  cardiac arrest and, 196
  certification for, 184, 197
  defined, 175
  do-not-resuscitate orders and, 345
  implied consent for, 342
Cardiovascular system, 59–60, 63, 71, 87
Care coordination, 277–291
  in ACOs, 277, 278, 280
  as clinical quality measure, 285–286
  communication and, 277, 281, 282
  with community agencies, 282
  for continuity of care, 282, 288–289
  medical providers and, 279–280
  in patient-centered medical homes, 8, 277, 278, 280

APPENDIX: INDEX

patients and family members
in, 281
of preventive care, 279, 282–286
referrals and, 9, 12, 291
support staff and, 281
for transitional care, 282
Carotid artery, 118
Cartilage, 54, 55
Catheterized urine collection, 228
Cause-and-effect analysis, 332
Cavities of body, 52
CBC (complete blood count), 232
CDSSs (clinical decision support systems), 171
Celiac disease, 45, 73
Cells, structure and function of, 50–51
Cellulitis, 67
Centers for Disease Control and Prevention (CDC)
on bloodborne pathogens, 205
on communicable diseases, 204, 341
on community resources, 282
on diabetes management, 42
disease monitoring by, 81
growth charts from, 125
hand hygiene recommendations, 209
on intramuscular injections, 158
post-exposure guidelines, 218, 219
reporting diseases to, 170, 348
on standard precautions, 203
on sterilization protocols, 215
on unsafe injection practices, 151
on vaccine schedules, 285
Centers for Medicare & Medicaid Services (CMS), 170, 198, 296, 309
Central nervous system (CNS), 64
Central nervous system stimulants, 16
Centrifuges, 224, 230, 246, 256
Centrioles, 50, 51
Cerebral concussions, 75

Cerebrovascular accidents (strokes), 75, 264
Certification
for AED use, 197
for CPR, 184, 197
for EPCS software, 166
for medical assistants, 2, 3, 6–7
precertification, 303–304
Cervical cancer, 283
Chain of custody, 230–231, 255
Chain of infection, 201, 208
Charge reconciliation, 310–311
Charting, 296, 303
CHF (congestive heart failure), 71
Chicken pox (varicella), 199
Chief complaints, 111, 128, 193
Children. *See Pediatric patients*
Chiropractic medicine, 14
Chlorine, 212
Choking, 110, 175, 186, 188
Cholesterol, 33, 35, 38, 222, 225, 232, 283, 287
Chronic kidney disease (CKD), 43–44
Chronic obstructive pulmonary disease (COPD), 74, 238, 272
Chronic renal failure, 72
Cigarettes. *See Tobacco use*
Cilia, 50, 63
Civil law, 346–347
Civil Rights Act of 1964, 338
Clean-catch midstream urine specimens, 228, 233
Cleaning. *See also Disinfection; Sterilization*
burn areas, 192
equipment, 132
examination rooms, 133
injection sites, 157
sanitization, 211
vial stoppers, 152
wounds, 181, 182, 189, 190, 193
Clearinghouses, 312, 340

Clinical and Laboratory Standards Institute, 253
Clinical decision support systems (CDSSs), 171
Clinical Laboratory Improvement Amendments of 1998 (CLIA), 221, 223, 226, 232, 338
Clinical laboratory testing, 221, 222
Clinical quality measures, 285–286
Clitoris, 66
Closed-ended questions, 322
Closed fractures, 187
Clotted blood samples, 246, 254
Cluster scheduling, 297
CMS (Centers for Medicare & Medicaid Services), 170, 198, 296, 309
CNS (central nervous system), 64
Coaching, 42, 97, 237, 286, 294, 317, 331
Codes and coding, 244, 303, 304, 307–308, 313
Coinsurance, 301, 306
Colon (large intestine), 61, 62
Colonoscopy, 136
Colorectal cancer, 73, 283
Color vision testing, 235
Colposcopy, 178, 179
Combining vowels, 87, 90
Comminuted fractures, 187
Common ethics, 350
Communicable diseases. *See also Infection control; specific diseases*
CDC guidelines for, 204
immunity against, 58
occupational exposure to, 205
prevention strategies, 292
release of information on, 341
reporting requirements, 170, 292, 348
signs and symptoms of, 202
telehealth visits and, 9
transmission of, 133, 199–200

APPENDIX: INDEX

Communication, 319–334
    active listening and, 299, 320, 322–324, 327, 329–331
    care coordination and, 277, 281, 282
    in challenging situations, 329–332
    in CPOE systems, 171
    cultural considerations, 325–326, 352
    customer service and, 323–326, 330
    cycle of, 320
    documentation of, 330
    in e-prescribing, 165
    families and, 262, 281, 324
    interpreters for, 101, 325
    medical professionals and, 324
    nonverbal, 242, 319, 323–325, 327
    older adults and, 138, 323
    patient adherence and, 290
    in patient-centered medical homes, 278
    pediatric patients and, 139, 242, 325
    persons with disabilities and, 100, 101
    privacy issues and, 322, 324, 327
    professionalism in, 319, 326–330, 332–333
    questioning techniques, 322
    in revenue cycle management, 310
    scope and boundaries of, 322
    specialty pharmacies and, 167
    stereotypes and biases in, 324, 330
    styles of, 320–321, 324, 330
    teamwork and, 324, 332
    telehealth and, 327
    telephone, 313, 314, 327
    terminally ill patients and, 102
    therapeutic, 100, 294, 320, 326
    written, 314, 327–329
Community resources, 282, 287–289
Compensation (defense mechanism), 103
Complaint resolution, 331
Complementary therapies, 14
Complete blood count (CBC), 232
Complex carbohydrates, 35

Compound fractures, 187
Compounding medications, 167, 168
Comprehensive care, 12, 278
Computed tomography (CT), 80
Computer-based monitoring, 273
Computerized provider order entry (CPOE), 171–172
Concussions, 75
Confidentiality. *See* Privacy issues
Conflict management, 331
Congestive heart failure (CHF), 71
Conjunctivitis (pinkeye), 200
Connective tissue, 54
Conscious bias, 352
Consent
    expressed, 324, 342
    implied, 342
    informed, 136, 342–343, 346
    for medication administration, 146
    for sharing health information, 340
    for specimen collection, 230–231
Contact precautions, 204
Continuing education, 3, 6
Continuity of care, 169, 282, 288–289, 296, 303, 308
Contraceptives, 16, 20, 343
Contraindications for medications, 18–20, 166
Contrast material, in diagnostic imaging, 80
Controlled substances, 17–18, 161–163, 166–167
Controlled Substances Act of 1970 (CSA), 17, 338
Conversion (defense mechanism), 103
Conversion (mathematical), 21, 24–25, 123, 126, 145
Coordination of care. *See* Care coordination
Copayments, 299, 301, 306, 311, 312

COPD (chronic obstructive pulmonary disease), 74, 238, 272
Coping strategies, 47, 98, 102–104
Coronal (frontal) plane, 52
COVID-19 pandemic, 7, 81, 173, 292
Cowper's (bulbourethral) glands, 65
CPOE (computerized provider order entry), 171–172
CPR. *See* Cardiopulmonary resuscitation
CPT (Current Procedural Terminology), 303, 304, 307
Cranial cavity, 52
Crash carts, 194–195
Criminal law, 346
Critical values, 232, 259
Cryosurgery, 178, 179
Cryptorchidism, 79
CSA (Controlled Substances Act of 1970), 17, 338
CT (computed tomography), 80
Cultural competence, 325–326, 352
Cushing syndrome, 76
Customer service, 323–326, 330
Cytology, 222
Cytoplasm, 50, 63
Cytoskeleton, 51

D

Day programs, 287–289
DEA (Drug Enforcement Administration), 161, 166, 167
Deaf patients, 101
Death and dying. *See* End-of-life care
Debridement of wounds, 134
Decongestants, 16
Deductibles, 301, 306
Deep full-thickness burns, 192
Deep-thickness burns, 192
De-escalation process, 330

APPENDIX: INDEX

Defense mechanisms, 102–104

Dehiscence, 191

Dendrites, 63

Denial (defense mechanism), 103

Denial (stage of grief), 106

Dentistry and dentists, 146, 278, 280, 283

Depression
  antidepressants, 15, 19–20
  eating disorders and, 46, 47
  nonachievement and, 97
  in older adults, 105
  screening for, 113, 284
  signs and symptoms, 98, 113
  as stage of grief, 106
  telehealth visits for, 173

Dermatitis, 67

Dermatology and dermatologists, 12, 134, 173, 279

Dermis layer of skin, 53, 54

Desired over have method, 23

Developmental delays, 101

Diabetes. *See also* Insulin
  dietary needs for, 42, 287
  obesity and, 47
  orthostatic hypotension and, 117
  screening for, 224, 283
  telehealth visits for, 173, 174
  type 1, 76
  type 2, 47, 76
  weight management and, 127

Diagnosis codes, 307, 313. *See also* ICD-10

Diagnostic imaging, 14, 80

Dialysis, 127, 197, 344, 345

Diastolic pressure, 114, 116, 119

Diet and nutrition, 33–47
  carbohydrates, 35, 37, 38, 42, 287
  for celiac disease, 45
  counseling on, 173
  for diabetes, 42, 287
  eating disorders, 46–47, 126, 127
  essential nutrients, 33
  fasting, 136, 233, 242
  fats, 35, 37, 38, 62, 242, 287
  food sources of nutrients, 37
  for kidney disease, 43–44
  label requirements, 38
  minerals, 14, 36–38, 54
  MyPlate guidelines for, 33, 42
  nonessential nutrients, 33
  patient education on, 46, 280, 287
  proteins, 34, 37, 38, 42, 43
  supplements, 14, 20, 39–41
  vitamins, 14, 35–40, 54
  water, 34, 37, 42

Dietary supplements, 14

Dietitians, 280

Digestion, 33, 35, 61–64

Digital thermometers, 122

Dilated eye examinations, 31, 283

Directional terminology, 95

Disabilities, 100–101, 138, 139, 289

Discrimination. *See* Biases; Stereotypes

Diseases, 67–81. *See also* Communicable diseases; Infection control; Pathogens; specific diseases
  cardiovascular system, 71
  diagnostic measures, 80
  endemic, 81
  endocrine system, 76–77
  epidemics, 81, 348
  gastrointestinal system, 73
  integumentary system, 67–68
  muscular system, 70
  nervous system, 75, 117
  pandemics, 81
  prevention measures, 81
  reproductive system, 78–79
  respiratory system, 74
  skeletal system, 69
  terminal, 8, 102, 105, 345
  urinary system, 72

Disinfection, 133, 151, 163, 176, 204, 207, 211–214

Dislocations, 187, 193

Displacement, 103

Dissociation, 103

Distribution of medications, 29

Diuretics, 15, 16, 47

Diversity, 325–326, 352

Diverticulosis, 73

DME (durable medical equipment), 197–198, 303

DNR (do-not-resuscitate) orders, 344, 345

Doctors. *See* Physicians

Doctors of osteopathy (DOs), 4, 6, 279

Documentation. *See also* Health records; Medical records
  of allergic reactions, 149, 150
  of calibration, 318
  of communication, 330
  for durable medical equipment, 198
  of employee medical training, 205, 218
  of follow-up patient calls, 314
  government regulations for, 308–309
  of injections, 162
  of laboratory test results, 232
  of maintenance issues, 139
  of medication administration, 32, 148
  of objective information, 112
  of patient education, 286, 288
  in quality control logs, 219
  for specimen collection, 222
  of subjective information, 111
  of vital signs, 109, 308
  of vitamin and supplement usage, 39
  of weight measurements, 126

Domestic violence, 348

Do-not-resuscitate (DNR) orders, 344, 345

Dorsalis pedis artery, 118

Dorsal recumbent position, 140

DOs (doctors of osteopathy), 4, 6, 279

Dosage calculations, 21–24, 126, 144–145

Double-booking, 297

DPOA (durable power of attorney), 105, 343, 344

Draping patients, 140–141, 164, 165, 266

Droplet precautions, 204

Drug Enforcement Administration (DEA), 161, 166, 167

Drug use. *See also* Medications; Substance use disorder
  patient education on, 287
  recreational, 113, 226
  testing for, 113, 226, 230, 255, 284
Durable medical equipment (DME), 197–198, 303
Durable power of attorney (DPOA), 105, 343, 344
Dyspnea, 120, 149, 194, 195, 263, 272

E

Ears. *See also* Hearing
  irrigation procedures, 164, 165
  medications for, 143, 149
Eating disorders, 46–47, 126, 127
Eating habits. *See* Diet and nutrition
Echocardiograms, 274
Economic abuse, 348
Ectopic pregnancy, 78
Eczema, 68
Education. *See* Patient education
Efferent neurons, 64
Ego integrity vs. despair, 97
EHRs. *See* Electronic health records
Elderly populations. *See* Older adults
Electrocardiograms (EKGs), 261–274
  abnormal rhythms on, 263–264
  adverse reactions to, 272
  artifacts within, 265, 267, 270–272
  cardiac cycle and, 60, 261, 262
  diagnosis with, 60, 134, 261
  lead placement for, 269–270
  patient preparation for, 266–267
  procedural steps for, 271–272
  supplies and equipment for, 267–268, 274
  transmitting results of, 273
  waveforms, intervals, and segments, 262
Electrodes, 194, 196, 264–272, 275

Electronic health records (EHRs)
  BMI calculation in, 127
  chart reviews, 303
  computerized provider order entry and, 171–172
  data entry and data fields, 315
  EKG results in, 273
  electronic medical records vs., 296
  growth charts in, 125
  laboratory test results in, 231
  medication orders and, 165–167
  patient-centered medical homes and, 278
  patient portals and, 9, 297, 312, 313, 317
  practice management systems and, 295–296
  referrals and, 305
  revenue cycle and, 310–312
  spirometry results in, 135
  storage of, 296
  updating information in, 170
Electronic medical records (EMRs)
  EKG results in, 273
  electronic health records vs., 296
  laboratory test results in, 231
  management of, 302–303
  medication information in, 111–112, 162
  updating information in, 170
Electronic prescribing, 165–167
Eligibility for health insurance, 299, 301, 303, 305, 310, 313
Email etiquette, 328
Emancipated minors, 343
Emergency action plans, 194–197
Emergency medical services (EMS), 184–185, 194, 300
Emergency Medical Treatment and Active Labor Act of 1986 (EMTALA), 338
Emergency medications, 194–196
Emergency situations, 110, 175, 184–188, 192, 194–197, 300
Emotional abuse, 348
Emotional disabilities, 101
Empathy, 101–102, 126, 320, 322–323, 329

EMRs. *See* Electronic medical records
Encounter forms (superbills), 302
Endemic diseases, 81
Endocardium, 59
Endocrine glands, 64
Endocrine system, 64, 67, 76–77, 87
Endocrinology and endocrinologists, 12, 134
End-of-life care
  advance directives for, 105, 343–345
  grief experiences during, 105–106
  hospice care as, 8, 102, 280, 288
  patient education during, 106
  terminal illnesses and, 8, 102, 105, 345
Endometriosis, 78
Endoplasmic reticulum, 50, 51
Endorsement, licensure by, 6
Endoscopy, 178, 208
Energy therapy, 14
Engineering controls, 205, 218
Enteral routes of administration, 28, 143
Environmental emergencies, 110
Environmental Protection Agency (EPA), 161
Environmental stressors, 99
Epicardium, 59
Epidemics, 81, 348
Epidermis layer of skin, 53, 54
Epididymis, 65
Epinephrine, 150, 188, 194
E-prescribing, 165–167
Epstein-Barr virus, 225
Erikson, Erik, 95–97
Erythema, 191
Erythrocytes. *See* Red blood cells
Esophagus, 47, 61
Essential nutrients, 33
Estradiol, 66
Estrogen, 65, 66, 124
Ethics and values, 350–351

Evacuated needle system, 244–245, 248
Evacuation plans, 110
Evisceration, 191
Examinations, 131–142
  accommodations during, 138
  for certification, 2, 6
  diagnostic measures and, 80
  draping during, 140–141
  eye, 31, 173, 283
  general, 131–133
  for licensure, 4–6
  mandated, 341
  mental state, 113
  pelvic, 124, 132
  positioning for, 140–142
  preparing for, 136–137
  privacy issues and, 136, 137
  rooms for, 131–133, 136, 138–139
  specialty, 134–135
  supplies and equipment for, 132, 133, 136
  telehealth and, 174
Excretion, 30, 36, 53, 54, 200, 224, 226
Exercise, 113, 123, 186, 287
Exocrine glands, 64
Expectorants, 16
Expiration dates, 31–32, 148, 159, 161, 163–164, 195, 227
Explanation of benefits, 305
Explicit bias, 352
Exposure control plans, 205, 218
Expressed consent, 324, 342
Eye contact, 102, 294, 321, 323, 327
Eyes. *See also* Vision
  examination of, 31, 173, 283
  irrigation procedures, 164
  medications for, 143, 148–149
  wash stations for, 215, 218

F

Facial expressions, 321, 323, 327
Fainting, 186, 242, 253, 263, 272, 275
Fallopian tubes, 65
Families
  in care coordination, 281
  communication with, 262, 281, 324
  in patient-centered medical homes, 278
  social worker assistance for, 280
  of terminally ill patients, 102
Family history reports, 112
Family practitioners, 12, 279
Farsightedness (hyperopia), 235
Fasting blood tests, 136, 222, 233, 242
Fats, 35, 37, 38, 62, 242, 287
Fat-soluble vitamins, 35, 36
Faxes, processing of, 314
FDA (Food and Drug Administration), 39, 161, 168, 226
Fecal occult blood tests (FOBTs), 226, 228, 283
Feedback, 294, 322
Fee-for-service (FFS) model, 10, 309, 311
Felonies, 346
Female reproductive organs, 65–66
Femoral artery, 118
Fever (pyrexia), 122
"Fight or flight" response, 64
Fingernails, 53
Fingersticks. *See Capillary punctures*
First aid, 175, 188, 213
First-degree burns, 192
First morning urine specimens, 227
Flagella, 50
Flat bones, 55

FOBTs (fecal occult blood tests), 226, 228, 283
Food and Drug Administration (FDA), 39, 161, 168, 226
Food intake. *See Diet and nutrition*
Forceps, 151, 177, 178, 181, 194
Foreign objects, removal of, 178
Formula method, 23
Fourth-degree burns, 192
Fowler's position, 141
Fractures, 187, 193
Frontal (coronal) plane, 52
Frostbite, 185
Fungi, 200, 222

G

Gallbladder, 61, 62
Gastroenterologists, 12
Gastroesophageal reflux disease (GERD), 73
Gastrointestinal system, 61–62, 73, 88
Gender identity and expression, 325
General examinations, 131–133
Generalized Anxiety Disorder 7-item questionnaire (GAD-7), 113
General practitioners (GPs), 12
Generativity vs. stagnation, 97
Generic medications, 146
Genetic Information Nondiscrimination Act of 2008 (GINA), 339
Genital herpes, 78
GERD (gastroesophageal reflux disease), 73
Gingko biloba, 41
Gloves
  biohazardous materials and, 216, 217
  disposable, 132, 209, 244
  for examinations, 132, 133
  for eye irrigation, 164

for infection control, 203, 204, 206–208
for injections, 151, 152, 157
nonsterile, 152, 157, 164, 189, 206–207
for phlebotomy, 244
removal of, 165, 206–207
for sanitization process, 211
sterile, 151, 175–177, 181, 189, 190, 208
for wound care, 189, 190

Glucometers, 224, 293

Glucosamine sulfate, 41

Glucose, 34–35, 136, 173–174, 222, 224–225, 232, 283, 287

Glucose tolerance test (GTT), 255

Glutaraldehyde, 211

Golden hour, 184

Golgi apparatus, 50, 51

Good Samaritan laws, 339

Gout, 69

GPs (general practitioners), 12

Graves' disease, 77

Greenstick fractures, 187

Grief, 99, 105–106, 288

Group A streptococcus testing, 224

Group ethics, 350

Growth charts, 125–126

Growth plate fractures, 187

GTT (glucose tolerance test), 255

Gynecology and gynecologists, 12, 135, 279

H

Hair follicles, 53, 54

Half-life of medications, 30

Hand hygiene
CDC recommendations for, 209
for examinations, 136
for eye and ear irrigation, 164, 165
for infection control, 204, 207–210, 212, 230, 292
patient education on, 292
surgical asepsis and, 175
for wound care, 181, 189

Hand sanitizers, 81, 209, 212, 292

hCG (human chorionic gonadotropin), 223

HCPCS (Healthcare Common Procedure Coding System), 304, 307, 309

Hct (hematocrit), 224, 232

Head circumference, 125

Heads of the European Radiological Protection Competent Authorities (HERCA), 339

Health care
ancillary services, 14
cardiac monitoring, 266, 274–275
complementary therapies, 14
coordination of. *See Care coordination*
delivery models and organization of, 7–8
disease states and. *See Diseases*
EKGs in. *See Electrocardiograms*
exams. *See Examinations*
general vs. specialty services, 12–13
holistic, 2, 4, 10, 12, 14, 277, 326
infection control in. *See Infection control*
injuries. *See Injuries*
inpatient, 7, 8, 278, 311
intake in. *See Intake process*
lab tests. *See Laboratory testing*
legal issues in. *See Legal and regulatory requirements*
for mental health. *See Mental health*
nutrition and. *See Diet and nutrition*
outpatient. *See Outpatient care*
payment models, 10–11, 277, 309, 311
pharmacology and. *See Medications*
preventive, 12, 279, 282–286, 298–299, 309, 311
provider and allied health roles, 4–6
safety in. *See Safety*
surgeries. *See Surgical procedures*
virtual. *See Telehealth*

Healthcare Common Procedure Coding System (HCPCS), 304, 307, 309

Health Information Technology for Economic and Clinical Health (HITECH) Act of 2009, 337

Health insurance
coinsurance and, 301, 306
copayments and, 299, 301, 306, 311, 312
deductibles and, 301, 306
eligibility verification, 299, 301, 303, 305, 310, 313
Medicaid, 170, 197
Medicare, 170, 197, 309
premiums for, 306
for telehealth visits, 172

Health Insurance Portability and Accountability Act of 1996 (HIPAA), 231, 290, 304, 327, 337, 340

Health maintenance organizations (HMOs), 11, 221

Health records. *See also Electronic health records*
audits of, 311
charting and, 303
of employees, 340
sections of, 111
sharing and exchange of, 308

Hearing. *See also Ears*
impairments in, 101, 325, 327
screening tests, 235–236

Heart, anatomy of, 59–60

Heart attack. *See Myocardial infarction*

Heart failure, 71

Heart rate. *See Pulse rate*

Heat exhaustion and heat stroke, 185

Height, 33, 125, 127, 274

APPENDIX: INDEX

Helicobacter pylori, 225
Hematocrit (Hct), 224, 232
Hematologic word roots, 87
Hematology and hematologists, 12, 222, 223
Hematopoiesis, 55
Hemoconcentration, 249
Hemoglobin (Hgb), 63, 224, 232
Hemoglobin A1C, 225, 232
Hemophilia, 71
Hemorrhage, 175, 188, 190
Hepatitis, 19, 203, 205, 218, 219, 284
Hepatologists, 12
Herbal supplements, 14, 20, 39–41
HERCA (Heads of the European Radiological Protection Competent Authorities), 339
Hernias, 78
Herpes, 78
Hgb (hemoglobin), 63, 224, 232
High blood pressure. See Hypertension
HIPAA (Health Insurance Portability and Accountability Act of 1996), 231, 290, 304, 327, 337, 340
HITECH (Health Information Technology for Economic and Clinical Health) Act of 2009, 337
HIV/AIDS, 113, 167, 170, 203, 205, 284, 341, 348
HMOs (health maintenance organizations), 11, 221
Holistic health care, 2, 4, 10, 12, 14, 277, 326
Holter monitoring, 134, 275
Home health care, 7, 102, 278, 288
Homeostasis, 53, 61, 64, 67, 109
Horizontal recumbent position. See Supine position
Hormones, 16, 47, 64, 155. See also specific hormones
Hospice care, 8, 102, 280, 288

Household measurements, 21–22
Human chorionic gonadotropin (hCG), 223
Hyperopia (farsightedness), 235
Hyperpnea, 120
Hypertension, 71, 115, 116, 174
Hyperthyroidism, 77
Hyperventilation, 120
Hypodermic syringes, 160
Hypoglycemia, 185
Hypoglycemics, 16
Hypotension, 117, 149
Hypothermia, 185
Hypothyroidism, 77
Hypovolemic shock, 185
Hypoxemia, 121

I

ICD-10 (International Classification of Diseases, 10th revision), 244, 303, 304, 307
ID (intradermal) injections, 28, 32, 143, 155, 157
Identification (defense mechanism), 103
Identification of patients, 30, 110, 147, 229, 243, 266, 301
Identity vs. role confusion stage, 96
Illnesses. See Diseases
IM (intramuscular) injections, 28, 29, 32, 143, 150, 155–158
Immune system, 57–58
Immunity, types of, 58
Immunizations. See Vaccinations
Immunoglobulins, 58
Impacted fractures, 187
Implicit bias, 352
Implied consent, 342
Incentive models, 311
Incisions, 175, 178–182, 189
Incontinence, 72

Indications for medications, 18–20, 150
Indigent programs, 306
Industry vs. inferiority stage, 96
Infection control, 203–219
  aseptic techniques for, 199, 207–208
  biohazardous materials and, 215–217
  for bloodborne pathogens, 203–205, 215
  disinfection and, 204, 207, 211–214
  gloves for, 203, 204, 206–207
  hand hygiene for, 204, 207–210, 212, 230, 292
  personal protective equipment for, 203–208, 213, 215–219
  post-exposure guidelines, 205, 218–219
  sanitization and, 211, 214
  standard precautions for, 203
  sterilization and, 211, 214–215
  transmission-based precautions for, 204
  universal precautions for, 203
Infectious diseases. See Communicable diseases
Inflammatory phase of wound healing, 191
Influenza, 200, 226
Informed consent, 136, 342–343, 346
Inguinal hernias, 78
Inhalation route of administration, 143, 168
Initiative vs. guilt stage, 96
Injections, 150–162
  documentation of, 162
  intradermal, 28, 32, 143, 155, 157
  intramuscular, 28, 29, 32, 143, 150, 155–158
  needles for, 28, 32, 132, 151–160
  of specialty medications, 168
  sterile technique for, 151–153
  storage of medications for, 161
  subcutaneous, 28, 32, 143, 154, 157
  syringes for, 132, 151–153, 156–160
  withdrawal techniques for, 159

Injuries. *See also* Wounds; *specific injuries*
  ancillary services for, 14
  burns, 34, 175, 184, 188, 192–193
  dislocations, 187, 193
  electrical, 188
  emergency care for, 184, 192
  fractures, 187, 193
  head, 170, 184, 188
  lower back, 141
  needlestick, 152, 157, 204, 219
  of pediatric patients, 110
  skeletal system as protection against, 54, 55
  skin as defense against, 54
  spinal, 185
  sprains, 69, 175, 186, 193
  strains, 175, 186, 193
  traumatic, 193
Inpatient care, 7, 8, 278, 311
Institute for Safe Medication Practices (ISMP), 27, 82
Insulin, 144, 154, 157, 160
Insulin shock, 188
Insulin syringes, 153, 157, 160
Insurance. *See* Health insurance
Intake process, 109–130. *See also Vital signs*
  anthropometric measurements and, 125–128
  chief complaints and, 111, 128, 193
  medication reconciliation and, 111
  menstrual status assessment and, 124
  pain assessment and, 124
  patient identification and, 110
  pediatric measurements and, 125–126
  personal and family history in, 112
  screenings and wellness assessments in, 113
Integumentary system, 53–54, 67–68, 87. *See also* Skin
Intellectual disabilities, 289
Intellectualization, 103
Intentional torts, 347
Interactions with medications, 19–20

International Classification of Diseases, 10th revision (ICD-10), 244, 303, 304, 307
Internists, 12, 279
Interpreters, 101, 325
Interrupted baselines, 265
Interstitial fluid, 57
Interviewing techniques, 322
Intestines, 61, 62
Intimacy vs. isolation stage, 97
Intimate partner violence, 284
Intradermal allergy testing, 236
Intradermal (ID) injections, 28, 32, 143, 155, 157
Intramuscular (IM) injections, 28, 29, 32, 143, 150, 155–158
Intravenous (IV) administration, 29, 143, 154
Introjection, 103
Inventory management, 315–316
Iodophors, 212
Irregular bones, 55
Irrigation, 164–165
Ishihara test, 235
ISMP (Institute for Safe Medication Practices), 27, 82

J

Jaeger eye charts, 235
The Joint Commission, 82, 110, 259
Justice, as ethical principle, 351

K

Kidney disease, 43–44
Kidney failure, 72
Kidneys, structure and function of, 60, 228
Kidney stones, 72
Kinesthetic communication, 321

Kinesthetic learning, 293, 294
Knee-chest position, 142
Korotkoff sounds, 114
Kübler-Ross, Elisabeth, 105–106

L

Labels
  for food products, 38
  for hazard notification, 205, 218
  for medications, 27, 31, 146–147, 159, 163
  for specimens, 222, 227, 254
Labia majora/minora, 66
Laboratory directories, 242, 243, 254, 255
Laboratory technicians, 5, 221
Laboratory testing, 221–234. *See also* Phlebotomy; Specimens
  as ancillary service, 14
  CLIA-waived, 221, 223, 226
  clinical, 221, 222
  errors in, 233–234
  point-of-care, 223–226
  quality control of, 227, 234
  requisition form for, 222–223, 227, 233, 243–244, 254
  results of, 231–234, 258–259, 313
Lacerations, 189, 193
Lancet devices, 252
Large intestine (colon), 61, 62
Larynx, 63
Lateral semi-prone recumbent position, 141
Laws. *See* Legal and regulatory requirements
Laxatives, 16, 47
Learning styles, 293, 294
Left lateral position, 141
Legal and regulatory requirements, 335–349. *See also* Consent; Privacy issues; *specific laws and regulations*
  chain of custody, 230–231, 255
  for controlled substances, 17, 166
  for disposal of medications, 161
  for documentation, 308–309

APPENDIX: INDEX

medical directives, 105, 343–345
for needlestick injuries, 204
Patient's Bill of Rights, 301, 335–336
for patients with disabilities, 100
for prescriptions, 165–166
reportable violations or incidents, 346–349
of Safety Data Sheets, 161

Letter formats, 328–329
Leukocytes. See White blood cells
Licensed practical nurses (LPNs), 5, 279
Licensure, 4, 6
Ligaments, 54, 186
Lipids. See Fats
Listening. See Active listening
Lithotomy position, 141
Liver, 61, 62
Living wills, 344
Long bones, 54, 55
Long-term care, 5, 280, 287, 288
Look-alike medications, 27
Low-cost medication programs, 287
LPNs (licensed practical nurses), 5, 279
Lumen of needles, 153, 245
Lungs, 63, 283
Lymphatic system, 57–58
Lymph nodes and nodules, 57, 58
Lysosomes, 50, 51

M

MACRA (Medicare Access and CHIP Reauthorization Act of 2015), 308
Magnetic resonance imaging (MRI), 80
Mail, processing of, 314
Male reproductive organs, 65
Malpractice, 342, 343, 346, 347
Mammography, 80, 283
Managed care models, 11
Mandated reporting laws, 348–349
Manipulative communication style, 321
Marijuana, 17
MARs (medication administration records), 30, 147, 162
MAs. See Medical assistants
Matrix, defined, 297
Maturation phase of wound healing, 191
Mayo stands, 176
MDs (medical doctors), 4, 6, 12, 279
Measurement systems, 21–22
Medicaid, 170, 197. See also Centers for Medicare & Medicaid Services
Medical asepsis, 199, 208
Medical assistants (MAs)
administrative. See Administrative assisting
anatomy principles for. See Anatomy and physiology
certification for, 2, 3, 6–7
communication by. See Communication
coordination of care. See Care coordination
education of patients. See Patient education
ethics and values, 350–351
in health care systems. See Health care
legal issues for. See Legal and regulatory requirements
licensing requirements for, 6
phlebotomy and. See Phlebotomy
professionalism of, 241, 319, 326–330, 332–333
roles and responsibilities, 2–3
scope of practice, 3
terminology for. See Medical terminology
Medical directives, 105, 343–345
Medical doctors (MDs), 4, 6, 12, 279
Medical emergencies, 175, 184–188, 192, 194–197
Medical ethics, 350
Medical laboratory technicians, 5, 221
Medical law. See Legal and regulatory requirements
Medical necessity, 197, 222, 302–308, 313
Medical receptionists, 5
Medical records. See also Electronic medical records
components of, 110, 169
for exam preparation, 136
legally ordered, 341
medications in, 31, 111–112, 147, 162
paper-based, 296, 302–303
privacy issues and, 296, 302, 340–341
sections of, 302
storage of, 296
symbols utilized in, 86
Medical terminology, 81–95
abbreviations, 82–85
achieving fluency in, 81
acronyms, 83–85
combining forms, 87, 90
directional, 95
in lay language, 93–94
positional, 94
prefixes, 86, 90–91
suffixes, 86, 90–92
symbols, 82, 86
word roots, 86–90
Medicare, 170, 197, 309. See also Centers for Medicare & Medicaid Services
Medicare Access and CHIP Reauthorization Act of 2015 (MACRA), 308
Medication administration records (MARs), 30, 147, 162
Medication orders, 146, 165–167
Medications. See also Routes of administration; specific names and types of medications
adverse reactions to, 12, 18–20, 111–112, 158
allergic reactions to, 18, 19, 22, 111–112, 149–150, 158
brand name, 146
classifications and indications, 15–16

controlled substances, 17–18, 161–163, 166–167
conversions and formulas, 24–25
disposal of, 31, 48, 161, 163
dosage calculations, 21–24, 126, 144–145
emergency, 194–196
e-prescribing of, 165–167
expiration dates of, 31–32, 148, 159, 161, 163–164, 195
forms of, 26, 146, 147, 168
generics, 146
half-life of, 30
indications and contraindications, 18–20, 150, 166
interactions involving, 19–20
labels for, 27, 31, 146–147, 159, 163
look-alike and sound-alike, 27
low-cost programs for, 287
measurement systems, 21–22
over-the-counter, 146, 149
patient education on, 148, 279, 287, 290
pharmacokinetics, 29–30
post-surgical, 183
during pregnancy, 29
reconciliation process for, 111, 286, 309
reconstitution of, 159
reference sources, 31, 32
refills of, 165, 167, 285, 290
rights of administration, 30–32, 147–148
side effects of, 18, 19
storage of, 161–163, 219
therapeutic effects of, 18, 19

Melanoma, 68
Melatonin, 41
Meningitis, 199
Menstruation, 65, 66, 124
Mental disabilities, 101
Mental health. *See also* Anxiety; *Depression*
common conditions affecting, 98
counseling services for, 173
psychosocial development and, 95–97
screenings for assessment of, 113

stressors impacting, 99–100
Metabolism, 20, 30, 36
Metric system, 21, 22
MI (myocardial infarction), 71, 184, 188, 195–196
Microbiology, 222, 223
Micro-collection devices, 251
Micro-organisms, 176, 189–191, 199–200, 207–208, 211, 229
Midsagittal plane, 52
Minerals, 14, 36–38, 54
Misdemeanors, 346
Mitochondria, 50
Mitral (bicuspid) valve, 59, 60
Mobile health units, 7
Monocytes, 58
Mononucleosis, 225
Monounsaturated fats, 35
Mouth (oral cavity), 61
MRI (magnetic resonance imaging), 80
Multicultural competence, 325–326, 352
Muscle, 57, 60, 64, 186
Muscle relaxants, 16
Muscular dystrophy, 70
Muscular system, 57, 70, 88
Myalgia, 70
Myocardial infarction (MI), 71, 184, 188, 195–196
Myocardium, 59
Myopathy, 70
Myopia (nearsightedness), 234
MyPlate, 33, 42

N

Nails, artificial, 209
Nasal swabs, 226
Naturally acquired immunity, 58
Nearsightedness (myopia), 234

Needles. *See also* Sharps containers
for acupuncture, 14
components of, 153, 245
for injections, 28, 32, 132, 151–160
injuries from, 152, 157, 204, 219
for phlebotomy, 244–245, 248, 251
Needle Safety and Prevention Act of 2000, 204
Negligence, 343, 347
Neonatologists, 13
Nephrologists, 13
Nervous system, 63–64, 67, 75, 117
Neurologic word roots, 87
Neurology and neurologists, 13, 134
Neurons, 63, 64
Nicotine. *See Tobacco use*
Nonessential nutrients, 33
Nonmaleficence, as ethical principle, 351
Nonparenteral routes of administration, 28, 143
Nonpathogens, 200
Nonverbal communication, 242, 319, 323–325, 327
Normal flora, 200
Nose, 63
No-shows, 313
No Surprise Act of 2021 (NSA), 339
Notice of Privacy Practices (NPP), 301
Nuclear medicine, 80
Nuclear pharmacies, 168
Nucleolus, 50
Nucleus and nuclear membrane, 50, 63
Nurse practitioners (NPs), 4, 146, 277, 279, 348
Nurses, 5, 279, 349
Nutrition. *See Diet and nutrition*
Nutritionists, 278, 280

O

Obesity, 35, 47, 125–127, 153, 174

Objective information, defined, 112

Oblique fractures, 187

Obstetrics and obstetricians, 13, 135

Obstructed airways, 184, 186

Occupational Safety and Health (OSH) Act of 1970, 338

Occupational Safety and Health Administration (OSHA)
on biohazardous materials, 215, 217
Bloodborne Pathogens Standard, 205, 215, 241
exposure control plans, 218
on reporting safety concerns, 318
on Safety Data Sheets, 213
specimen standards, 231
standard safeguards, 204

Occupational therapy/therapists, 5, 7, 14, 277, 280

Ocular medications, 143, 148–149

Oil (sebaceous) glands, 53, 54

Older adults. *See also* End-of-life care
abuse of, 348, 349
accommodations for, 138
burn treatment for, 192
communication with, 138, 323
day programs for, 287–289
depression among, 105
diet and nutrition for, 33
injections for, 155, 157
kidney disease in, 43
mental health screening for, 113
metabolism of, 30
phlebotomy and, 250
psychosocial crisis for, 97
safety considerations for, 110, 284

Oncologists, 13, 279

Open-ended questions, 111, 322

Open fractures, 187

Ophthalmic medications, 143, 148–149

Ophthalmologists, 13

Ophthalmoscopes, 132

Oral cavity (mouth), 61

Oral contraceptives, 20

Oral health services, 280, 283

Oral hypoglycemics, 16

Oral route of administration, 28, 29, 143, 168

Oral temperature, 122

Orthopedists, 13

Orthopnea, 120

Orthostatic hypotension, 117

OSH (Occupational Safety and Health) Act of 1970, 338

OSHA. *See* Occupational Safety and Health Administration

Osteoarthritis, 69

Osteoporosis, 69, 127, 283

OTC (over-the-counter) medications, 146, 149

Otic medications, 143, 149

Otolaryngologists, 13

Otoscopes, 132, 165

Outpatient care
accommodations in, 138–139
cardiac monitoring and, 266, 274–275
computer-based monitoring and, 273
coordination of, 282
EKGs in. *See* Electrocardiograms
exams. *See* Examinations
home health, 7, 102, 278, 288
hospice services through, 8
intake for. *See* Intake process
lab tests. *See* Laboratory testing
primary and specialty clinics for, 7
specialty testing, 234–238
surgeries. *See* Surgical procedures
virtual. *See* Telehealth

Ovaries, 65

Over-the-counter (OTC) medications, 146, 149

Overweight, 126, 127. *See also* Obesity

Oxygen therapy, 121

P

PACs (premature atrial contractions), 263, 264

Pain
abdominal, 47, 149, 183
analgesics for, 15, 17
assessment of, 124
burns and, 192
complementary therapies for, 14
cultural considerations, 326
detection of, 54, 64
muscular, 70, 186
sprains and, 186

Palpation, 115, 118

Pancreas, 61, 62

Pandemics, defined, 81. *See also* COVID-19 pandemic

Pap tests, 135, 283

Parasites, 200, 222

Parasympathetic nervous system, 64

Parenteral routes of administration, 28, 29, 143, 153–162

Par level of inventory, 316

Partial-thickness burns, 192

PAs (physician assistants), 4, 146, 277, 279, 348

Passive communication style, 321

Passive immunity, 58

Pathogens. *See also* Diseases; Infection control
bloodborne, 203–205, 215, 241
in chain of infection, 201, 208
immune system defense against, 57, 58
transmission of, 201, 208
types of, 200

Patient adherence, 233, 282, 286, 290–291

Patient-centered medical homes (PCMHs), 8, 277, 278, 280, 311

Patient dumping, 338

Patient education
on allergy testing, 236
on cardiac monitoring, 274, 275
on community resources, 287, 288

on diet and nutrition, 46, 280, 287
documentation of, 286, 288
on durable medical equipment, 197
during end-of-life care, 106
on hand hygiene, 292
on laboratory test results, 231
learning styles and, 293, 294
on medications, 148, 279, 287, 290
on oral health services, 280
on preventive care, 282, 286
on procedures, 137
telehealth and, 9, 173, 293
on wound healing, 183

Patient Health Questionnaires (PHQs), 113

Patient portals, 9, 297, 312, 313, 317

Patient Protection and Affordable Care Act of 2010, 278, 337

Patient Safety and Quality Improvement Act of 2005 (PSQIA), 339

Patient's Bill of Rights, 301, 335–336

Pay for Performance (P4P) model, 311

Payment models, 10–11, 277, 309, 311

PCMHs (patient-centered medical homes), 8, 277, 278, 280, 311

PCPs (primary care providers), 7, 8, 277–279, 282, 291, 304

PDR (Physicians' Desk Reference), 31, 32

Peak flow meters, 135, 238

Pediatricians, 13, 279

Pediatric patients
abuse of, 348, 349
anthropometric measurements for, 125–126
burn treatment for, 192
communication with, 139, 242, 325
consent issues for, 343
diet and nutrition for, 33
dosage calculations for, 21, 23–24, 144
hearing testing for, 236
injections for, 155–156
injuries of, 110
metabolism of, 30
pain assessment for, 124
phlebotomy and, 242, 251, 252
psychosocial crises for, 95–96
safety considerations for, 110, 125, 139
vision testing for, 234
vital sign ranges for, 116, 119, 120, 123

Pelvic cavity, 52

Pelvic examinations, 124, 132

Penis, 65

Pericardium, 59

Perineum, 66

Peripheral nerves, 63, 64

Peripheral nervous system (PNS), 64

Peristalsis, 61

Personal ethics, 350

Personal protective equipment (PPE). See also Gloves
for biohazardous materials, 215–217
for infection control, 203–208, 213, 215–219
for medication administration, 152
for specimen handling, 230
for venipuncture, 217, 244

Persons with disabilities, 100–101, 138, 139

Pertussis (whooping cough), 200

P4P (Pay for Performance) model, 311

PFT (pulmonary function test), 135, 237

Pharmacists, 5, 168, 277, 279

Pharmacokinetics, 29–30

Pharmacology. See Medications

Pharmacy technicians, 5

Pharynx, 61, 63

Phenols, 212

Phlebotomy, 241–259. See also Blood specimens; Venipuncture
capillary punctures, 224, 225, 251–253
patient preparation for, 242
postprocedure care, 253
skill requirements for, 241
verification of order details, 243–244

PHQs (Patient Health Questionnaires), 113

Physical abuse, 348

Physical avoidance, 103

Physical disabilities, 100–101, 138

Physical therapy/therapists, 5, 7, 14, 186, 277, 280

Physician assistants (PAs), 4, 146, 277, 279, 348

Physician Orders for Life-Sustaining Treatment (POLST), 345

Physicians
doctors of osteopathy, 4, 6, 279
general practitioners, 12
licensing requirements for, 4, 6
mandated reporting by, 349
medical doctors, 4, 6, 12, 279
primary care providers, 7, 8, 277–279, 282, 291, 304
specialists, 12–13, 279

Physicians' Desk Reference (PDR), 31, 32

Physiology. See Anatomy and physiology

Pinkeye (conjunctivitis), 200

Planes of body, 52

Plasma (blood), 246

Plasma membranes, 50

Platelets, 222, 246

PMSs (practice management systems), 295–296, 305, 310–312, 315

PNS (peripheral nervous system), 64

Point-of-care testing, 223–226

Point-of-service (POS) plans, 11

Poisoning, 184, 188

APPENDIX: INDEX

POLST (Physician Orders for Life-Sustaining Treatment), 345
Polyunsaturated fats, 35
Popliteal artery, 118
Positional terminology, 94
Positioning
    for electrocardiograms, 267
    for examinations, 140–142
    for eye irrigation, 164
    for phlebotomy, 242
Postanalytical errors, 234, 255
Posterior tibial artery, 118
Post-exposure guidelines, 205, 218–219
Post-traumatic stress disorder (PTSD), 98, 99
PPE. *See Personal protective equipment*
Practice management systems (PMSs), 295–296, 305, 310–312, 315
Preanalytical errors, 233, 255
Preauthorizations, 303–304, 313
Precertifications, 303–304
Preferred provider organizations (PPOs), 11
Prefixes, 86, 90–91
Pregnancy
    ectopic, 78
    medications during, 29
    nutrition during, 33, 34
    testing for, 124, 223, 227
    weight management during, 127
Prejudice. *See Biases; Stereotypes*
Premature atrial contractions (PACs), 263, 264
Premature ventricular contractions (PVCs), 264
Premeasured syringes, 160
Premiums, 306
Presbyopia, 235
Prescription drugs. *See Medications*
Preventive care, 12, 279, 282–286, 298–299, 309, 311
Primary care clinics, 7

Primary care providers (PCPs), 7, 8, 277–279, 282, 291, 304
PR intervals, 262
Prior authorizations, 198, 303–304
Privacy issues
    communication and, 322, 324, 327
    electrocardiograms and, 266, 272
    employee incidents and, 205, 219
    examinations and, 136, 137
    HIPAA, 231, 290, 304, 327, 337, 340
    medical records and, 296, 302, 340–341
    Notice of Privacy Practices, 301
    patient identification and, 110
    telephone calls and, 314, 327
    weight measurements and, 126
Probing questions, 322
Procedure codes, 307, 313. *See also CPT; HCPCS*
Professional ethics, 350–351
Professionalism, 241, 319, 326–330, 332–333
Progesterone, 65, 66, 124
Projection, 103
Proliferating phase of wound healing, 191
Prone position, 140
Proportion method, 22, 24
Prospective audits, 311
Prostate gland, 65
Proteins
    diabetes and, 42
    food sources of, 37
    kidneys and, 43, 228
    label requirements, 38
    types of, 34
PSQIA (Patient Safety and Quality Improvement Act of 2005), 339
Psychiatrists, 13, 280
Psychological abuse, 348
Psychologists, 280
Psychosocial care, 326
Psychosocial development (Erikson), 95–97

PTSD (post-traumatic stress disorder), 98, 99
Pulmonary circulation, 60
Pulmonary function test (PFT), 135, 237
Pulmonology, 135
Pulse oximeters, 121, 132, 135
Pulse rate
    anaphylactic shock and, 188
    bradycardia and, 93
    measurement of, 118, 147
    medications and changes in, 20
    orthostatic hypotension and, 117
    ranges by age, 119, 128
    tachycardia and, 93
Puncture wounds, 189
Purging behavior, 47
Purkinje fibers, 60, 262
PVCs (premature ventricular contractions), 264
P waves, 262–264, 272
Pyrexia (fever), 122

Q

QRS waves, 262–264, 272
QT intervals, 262
Quadrants of body, 52–53
Qualitative analysis, 226
Quality assurance (QA), 227, 233
Quality control (QC), 219, 227, 234
Quantitative analysis, 228
Quaternary ammonium, 212
Questioning techniques, 322

R

Radial pulse, 115, 118
Radiologists, 13
Radiology technicians, 5
Radiopharmaceuticals, 80, 168
Rales, 120, 121
Random urine specimens, 227
Rapid streptococcus testing, 224

Ratio and proportion method, 22
Rationalization, 103
RBCs (red blood cells), 222, 224, 246
RDNs (registered dietitian nutritionists), 280
Reaction formation, 103
Real-time adjudication (RTA), 296
Receptionists, 5
Reciprocity agreements, 6
Reconstitution, 159
Records. *See Health records; Medical records*
Rectal route of administration, 28, 143
Rectal temperature, 122, 141
Rectum, 62
Red blood cells (RBCs), 222, 224, 246
Red bone marrow, 55
Referrals
    care coordination and, 9, 12, 291
    in CPOE system, 171
    electronic, 305
    facilitation of, 304–305
    for hospice care, 102
    patient education on, 137, 290
    practice management systems and, 295
    screenings and, 234
    to support groups, 106
Refills of medications, 165, 167, 285, 290
Reflex hammers, 132
Regions of body, 52–53
Registered dietitian nutritionists (RDNs), 280
Registered nurses (RNs), 5, 279
Regression, 103
Regulatory requirements. *See Legal and regulatory requirements*
Renal calculi, 72
Renal failure, 72

Repetitive stress disorder (RSD), 70
Repression, 104
Reproductive systems, 65–66, 78–79, 89
Requisition forms, 222–223, 227, 233, 243–244, 254
RER (rough endoplasmic reticulum), 50, 51
Resheathing devices, 152
Respiratory rate, 119–121, 128, 188
Respiratory system, 63, 74, 87
Retrospective audits, 311
Revenue cycle
    billing in, 305–309, 312–313
    charge reconciliation in, 310–311
    codes and coding in, 244, 303, 304, 307–308, 313
    defined, 295
Rheumatoid arthritis, 69
Rhinitis, 74
Rhinovirus, 200
Rhonchi, 120, 121
Ribosomes, 50
Rights of medication administration, 30–32, 147–148
Risk management, 332
RNs (registered nurses), 5, 279
Root words, 86–90
Rough endoplasmic reticulum (RER), 50, 51
Routes of administration
    accuracy of, 31, 147
    allergic reactions and, 150
    enteral (nonparenteral), 28, 143
    formulations and, 26
    parenteral, 28, 29, 143, 153–162
    for specialty medications, 168
RSD (repetitive stress disorder), 70
RTA (real-time adjudication), 296
R waves, 271

S

SA (sinoatrial) node, 59, 60, 263
Safety. *See also Personal protective equipment*
    evaluations of, 318, 332
    of examination rooms, 132, 139
    of medication administration, 30–32, 111–112, 147–148, 151–152
    of older adults, 110, 284
    of pediatric patients, 110, 125, 139
    of vitamins and supplements, 40–41
Safety Data Sheets (SDSs), 161, 213, 215
Sagittal plane, 52
St. John's wort, 40
Sanitization, 211, 214
Sarcasm, 104
Saturated fats, 35
Schedules for controlled substances, 17–18
Scheduling appointments
    electronic vs. paper, 297
    for follow-ups, 193, 258, 290
    for hearing-impaired patients, 101
    methods for, 297
    practice management systems and, 295–296
    for referrals, 291
    for telehealth visits, 9, 293
Sciatica, 75
Scoliosis, 127
Scope of practice, 2, 3
Scratch testing, 236
Screenings
    anxiety, 113
    appointments and, 299, 300
    blood pressure, 283
    bone density, 283
    depression, 113, 284
    diabetes, 224, 283
    in incentive models, 311
    laboratory testing and, 224–228
    in preventive care, 283–286, 309
    referrals and, 234
    tobacco use, 113, 284
    vision and hearing, 234–235

APPENDIX: INDEX

Scrotum, 65
SDSs (Safety Data Sheets), 161, 213, 215
Sebaceous (oil) glands, 53, 54
Second-degree burns, 192
Security Rule (HIPAA), 340
Sedative-hypnotics, 16
Seizures, 15, 175, 188
Semi-Fowler's position, 141, 242, 267, 272
Seminal vesicles, 65
Seniors. See Older adults
SER (smooth endoplasmic reticulum), 50, 51
Serum samples, 246, 253, 254
Service animals, 101
Sesamoid bones, 55
Sexual abuse, 348
Sharps containers, 132–133, 152–153, 182, 216, 231, 244–245, 251–252
Shingles, 75
Shin splints, 70
Shock, 149–150, 185, 188
Short bones, 55
Shortness of breath. See Dyspnea
Side effects, 18, 19
Sign-language interpreters, 101
Simple carbohydrates, 35
Simple fractures, 187
Sims' position, 141
Sinoatrial (SA) node, 59, 60, 263
Sinus arrest, 263
Sinus bradycardia, 263
Sinus rhythms, 263
Sinus tachycardia, 263
Skeletal muscle, 57, 64
Skeletal relaxants, 16
Skeletal system, 54–56, 69, 88
Skin. See also Burns; Integumentary system
   biopsies and, 134
   cancer and, 68
   closure tapes for, 180, 181
   structure and function of, 53–54
Sliding scale of income, 306
Small intestine, 61, 62
Smoking. See Tobacco use
Smooth endoplasmic reticulum (SER), 50, 51
Smooth muscle, 57
Snellen eye charts, 234–235
Social workers, 280, 349
Socioeconomic stressors, 100
Somatic nervous system, 64
Somatic tremor, 265
Sound-alike medications, 27
Specialty care clinics, 7
Specialty examinations, 134–135
Specialty health care services, 12–13, 279
Specialty pharmacies, 167–168
Specialty testing, 234–238
Specimens. See also Laboratory testing
   blood. See Blood specimens
   chain of custody for, 230–231, 255
   collection of, 6, 222–228, 230–231
   disposal of, 231
   labels for, 222, 227, 254
   processing and handling, 229–230, 254–255
   stool, 226, 228
   transporting, 230, 257–258
   urine. See Urine specimens
Speech therapy/therapists, 7, 277, 280
Sphygmomanometers (blood pressure cuffs), 114–116, 132
Spinal cavity, 52
Spinal cord, 63, 64
Spiral fractures, 187
Spirometry, 135, 237
Spleen, 57, 58
Splinter forceps, 178
Sprains, 69, 175, 186, 193
Spun hematocrit, 224
SQ (subcutaneous) injections, 28, 32, 143, 154, 157
Stages of grief (Kübler-Ross), 105–106
Standard measurements, 21–22
Standard precautions, 203
Staples, surgical, 180–182
Stereotypes, 324, 330. See also Biases
Sterile technique, 151–153, 164, 175–177
Sterilization, 151, 176, 211, 214–215
Stethoscopes, 114, 115, 118, 132
ST intervals, 262
Stomach, 61, 62
Stool softeners, 16
Stool specimens, 226, 228
Strains, 175, 186, 193
Strep throat, 200
Streptococcus testing, 224
Stress testing, 272, 274
Strokes, 64, 75
Subcutaneous (SQ) injections, 28, 32, 143, 154, 157
Subcutaneous layer of skin, 53, 54
Subjective information, defined, 111
Sublimation, 104
Sublingual route of administration, 143
Subpoena duces tecum, 341
Substance use disorder, 47, 284, 288. See also Alcohol use; Drug use
Sudoriferous (sweat) glands, 53, 54
Suffixes, 86, 90–92
Sunburns, 192
Superbills (encounter forms), 302
Superficial burns, 192
Supine position, 140, 164, 242, 267
Supplements, 14, 20, 39–41

Suppression, 104
Surgical asepsis, 175–177, 208
Surgical procedures, 175–183
    diet following, 34, 183
    follow-up care for, 182–183
    incision/wound closure following, 180–182
    sterile field for, 175–177, 193
    suffixes related to, 92
    types of, 178–179
Sutures, 180–182
Sweat (sudoriferous) glands, 53, 54
Symbols, 82, 86
Sympathetic nervous system, 64
Syncope. *See Fainting*
Syringes, 132, 151–153, 156–160, 165, 245, 248
Systemic circulation, 60
Systolic pressure, 114–116, 119

T

Tachycardia, 93, 263, 264
Tachypnea, 120
Tapes for skin closure, 180, 181
TB (tuberculosis) tests, 155
T-cells, 57, 58
Teamwork, 324, 332
Telehealth
    advantages of, 298, 317
    barriers to access, 317
    communication and, 327
    conditions appropriate for, 173
    examinations through, 174
    insurance coverage for, 172
    patient education through, 9, 173, 293
    scheduling appointments for, 9, 293
    technical instruction for, 317
    telemedicine vs., 172
Telephone communication, 313, 314, 327

Temperature. *See also Body temperature*
    of blood samples, 254, 255, 257
    conversions for, 123
    of laboratory refrigerators, 227
    for medication storage, 161, 163, 219
    for sanitization, 211
    of saturated fats, 35
    for sterilization, 176, 214
    of urine specimens, 222
Templates, 314, 328
Temporal artery, 118
Temporal artery scanners, 122
Tendons, 54, 55, 57, 186
Terminal illnesses, 8, 102, 105, 345
Terminology. *See Medical terminology*
Testes, 65
Testicular torsion, 79
Testosterone, 65, 155
Therapeutic communication, 100, 294, 320, 326
Therapeutic effects, 18, 19
Therapeutic touch, 324
Thermometers, 122–123, 132, 163
Third-degree burns, 192
Third-party payers, 298, 299, 303–313, 328
Thoracic cavity, 52
Thready pulse, 118
Throat swabs, 224
Thymus, 57, 58
Title VII (Civil Rights Act of 1964), 338
Tobacco use
    blood pressure and, 115, 129
    body temperature readings and, 122
    patient education on, 287
    screening for, 113, 284
    spirometry and, 237
Toenails, 53
Tonsil swabs, 224
Topical route of administration, 28, 143

Torts, 342, 346–347
Touch, therapeutic, 324
Tourniquets, 190, 244, 249, 250
Tracers, in nuclear medicine, 80
Trachea (windpipe), 63
Transdermal route of administration, 143
Trans fats, 35
Transitional care, 282
Transportation, 230, 257–258, 280, 287
Transverse fractures, 187
Transverse plane, 52
Traumatic injuries, 193
Tricuspid valve, 59, 60
Trust vs. mistrust stage, 95
Tuberculin syringes, 160
Tuberculosis (TB) tests, 155
T waves, 262, 272
20/20 vision, 235
24-hour urine specimens, 228
Tympanic temperature, 122
Tympanometry, 235

U

Ultrasound, 80
Unconscious bias, 352
Underweight, 125, 127
Undoing (defense mechanism), 104
Unintentional torts, 347
United States Adopted Names (USAN) Council, 146
Universal precautions, 203
Unsaturated fats, 35
Ureters, 60
Urethra, 60
Urgent care, 14
Urinalysis, 222, 224
Urinary bladder, 60
Urinary incontinence, 72
Urinary system, 60, 72, 89

APPENDIX: INDEX

Urinary tract infections (UTIs), 72, 173
Urine specimens
  bacteria in, 230, 233
  collection of, 227–228
  disposal of, 231
  for drug tests, 226, 230
  errors involving, 233
  for pregnancy tests, 223
  processing and handling, 230
  temperature of, 222
Urologists, 13
USAN (United States Adopted Names) Council, 146
Uterus, 65, 66
Utilization reviews, 303
U waves, 262

V

Vaccinations
  active immunity through, 58
  allergic reactions to, 19
  CDC schedules for, 285
  for disease prevention, 81
  hepatitis B, 205, 218, 219
  injection of, 155, 160
  mobile health units and, 7
  storage of vaccines, 161
Vagina, 65
Vaginal route of administration, 28
Value-based model, 10, 309, 310
Values and ethics, 350–351
Varicella (chicken pox), 199
Vas deferens, 65
Veins and venules, 59, 60
Venipuncture
  order of draw for, 247
  patient preparation for, 242
  personal protective equipment for, 217, 244
  procedural steps for, 251
  site accessibility and preparation, 248–250
  standard precautions for, 203
  supplies and equipment for, 244–245
  verification of order details, 243

Venous bleeding, 190
Ventricles of heart, 59–60, 262, 264
Ventricular fibrillation, 264
Ventricular tachycardia, 264
Verbal abuse, 348
Verbal aggression, 104
Vials, 152, 159
Violence, 284, 348–349
Virtual health care. See Telehealth
Viruses, 199, 200, 211, 222, 225, 246
Vision. See also Eyes
  impairments in, 101, 323, 327
  screening tests, 234–235
Visual communication, 321
Visual learning, 293, 294
Vital signs. See also Blood pressure; Body temperature; Pulse rate
  documentation of, 109, 308
  factors affecting, 115, 121, 122, 129
  pulse oximetry, 121, 135
  respiratory rate, 119–121, 128, 188
  during stress testing, 274
Vitamins, 14, 35–40, 54
Voicemail, 314
Vowels, combining, 87, 90

W

Wandering baselines, 265, 272
Water
  body function and, 61
  diabetes and, 42
  excretion and loss of, 54
  food sources of, 37
  percentage in body, 34
Water-soluble vitamins, 36
Wave scheduling, 297
WBCs (white blood cells), 222, 246
Weight. See also Obesity
  conversions for, 23, 126, 145
  dosage calculations by, 21, 23–24, 126, 144–145
  gaining, 35, 46, 47

  loss of, 34, 35, 46
  management of, 127
  measurement of, 125–126
  nutrition considerations and, 33
  overweight, 126, 127
  underweight, 125, 127
Wellness assessments, 113
Wheelchairs, 100, 101, 139
Wheezing, 120, 121
White blood cells (WBCs), 222, 246
White-coat syndrome, 99, 113
WHO (World Health Organization), 81, 146
Whole blood samples, 246
Whooping cough (pertussis), 200
Willow bark, 41
Wills, 344
Windpipe (trachea), 63
Winged infusion set, 245
Wong-Baker faces rating scale, 124
Word roots, 86–90
Workplace controls, 205, 218
World Health Organization (WHO), 81, 146
Wounds
  abdominal, 184
  chest, 184
  classification of, 189
  closure of, 180–182
  dressing, 190
  gunshot, 341
  healing process, 183, 191
  hemorrhaging, 175, 190
Written communication, 314, 327–329

X

X-rays, 80

Y

Yellow bone marrow, 55